MINERAL
O

# MINERAL NUTRITION OF RICE

*Editor*

**Jeltsyn Rocha**

scitus academics

**Mineral Nutrition of Rice**

Edited by **Jeltsyn Rocha**

ISBN: 978-1-68117-710-6
Library of Congress Control Number: 2016958742


SCITUS Academics LLC,
616, Corporate Way, Suite 2, 4766,
Valley Cottage, NY 10989

www.scitusacademics.com



**Notice**



Printed in United States of America on Acid Free Paper

# PREFACE

Rice is one of the oldest cultivated crops on earth and half of the world's population subsists wholly or partially on rice. Applying nutrients to the crop is essential in managing soil fertility so the plants grow and develop normally. A number of crop problems can be related to inefficient management of nutrients and nutrient imbalances in the field. Rice crops need to have the optimum nutritional balance. Macro-elements are needed by plants in large amounts. These are carbon, hydrogen, oxygen, nitrogen, phosphorus, potassium, calcium, magnesium, and sulfur. While microelements are only needed in lesser quantities, often in trace amounts. These are iron, manganese, copper, zinc, molybdenum, boron, and chlorine. In this text we review key issues determining nutrient management strategies in irrigated and rainfed lowland riceland and present examples of nutrient management strategies. If rice crops have more or less than the required amount of nutrients, the yield can be greatly affected.

*Mineral Nutrition of Rice* focuses attention on rice crop nutrient necessities, assessment of soil nutrient delivering capacity, and features of soil microorganisms in a long-term fertilization experiment based on nutrient balance concepts. Also, the relationships between the microbial biomass and chemical properties of the soil, such as available N, P and K contents are highlighted. The investigation aimed at analyzing the effects of fertility on soil microbial biomass and soil nutrient supplying capacity, and at considering implications for the long-term management of paddy soil fertility.

Soil nutrient deficiency and unbalanced fertilization to rice crop had negative effect on the diversity of the microbial community and total microbial biomass in the soil. The long-term fertilizer experiment also showed that balanced application of N, P and K promoted microbial biomass growth and improvement of community composition. Unbalanced fertilization reduced microbial N and increased C/N ratio of the microbial biomass.

# TABLE OF CONTENTS

1

# THE STABLE LEVEL OF *GLUTAMINE SYNTHETASE 2* PLAYS AN IMPORTANT ROLE IN RICE GROWTH AND IN CARBON-NITROGEN METABOLIC BALANCE

**Aili Bao [1], Zhuqing Zhao [1], Guangda Ding [1], Lei Shi [1,2], Fangsen Xu [1,2] and Hongmei Cai [1]**

[1]Microelement Research Center, Key Laboratory of Arable Land Conservation (Middle and Lower Reaches of Yangtze River), Ministry of Agriculture, Huazhong Agricultural University, Wuhan 430070, China

[2]National Key Laboratory of Crop Genetic Improvement, Huazhong Agricultural University, Wuhan 430070, China

## ABSTRACT

Glutamine synthetase 2 (GS2) is a key enzyme involved in the ammonium metabolism in plant leaves. In our previous study, we obtained *GS2*-cosuppressed plants, which displayed a normal growth phenotype at the seedling stage, while at the tillering stage they showed a chlorosis phenotype. In this study, to investigate the chlorosis mechanism, we systematically analyzed the plant growth, carbon-nitrogen metabolism and gene expressions between the *GS2*-cosuppressed rice and wild-type plants. The results revealed that the *GS2*-cosuppressed plants exhibited a poor plant growth phenotype and a poor nitrogen transport ability, which led to nitrogen accumulation and a decline in the carbon/nitrogen ratio in the stems. Interestingly, there was a higher concentration of soluble proteins and a lower concentration of carbohydrates in the *GS2*-cosuppressed plants at the seedling stage, while a contrasting result was displayed at the tillering stage. The analysis of the metabolic profile showed a significant increase of sugars and organic acids. Additionally, gene expression patterns were different in root and leaf of *GS2*-cosuppressed plants between the seedling and tillering stage. These results indicated the important role of a stable level of *GS2* transcription during normal rice development and the importance of the carbon-nitrogen metabolic balance in rice growth.

**Keywords:** carbon-nitrogen; chlorosis; gene expression; *GS2*; metabolic profile; rice

# 1. INTRODUCTION

Nitrogen (N) is one of the essential macronutrients required for plant growth. It is also a major limiting factor, which determines plant biomass and crop yield [1,2]. N is not only a constituent of key molecules, such as amino acids, nucleic acids, chlorophyll, ATP and several plant hormones, it is also the regulator in many biological processes, such as amino acid metabolism, carbon metabolism and protein synthesis [3,4]. Additionally, carbon (C) plays a crucial role in plants' routine growth and development. Various C compounds, including glucose, sucrose, organic acids and other carbohydrates, provide both the C skeletons and the energy for ammonium ($NH_4^+$) assimilation. N compounds are synthesized by incorporating $NH_4^+$into the C skeletons. Amino acids and proteins, in particular enzymes, are essential for almost all cellular activities, including the C and N metabolic reactions [5]. Therefore, both C and N nutrients are essential for cellular functions. Recently, it has been recognized that cellular C and N metabolism must be tightly coordinated. Maintaining a coordination of carbon-nitrogen metabolism and an appropriate balance of carbohydrates to nitrogen metabolites, which also is referred to as the "C/N balance", is important for plant growth, development and yield production [5,6,7,8,9,10].

Glutamine synthetase (GS; EC 6.3.1.2) is a key enzyme for the assimilation of $NH_4^+$, which is derived from nitrate ($NO_3^-$), nitrogen fixation or generated by other reactions that release ammonium within the plant, into glutamine (Gln) [11,12,13]. The GS/GOGAT (glutamate synthase) cycle can generate two molecules of glutamate

(Glu). One, as the substrate, is cycled back to the $NH_4^+$ assimilation by the GS enzyme; the other one is exported out of the GS/GOGAT cycle to synthesize other types of amino acids [14]. In higher plants, there are two GS isoforms, cytosolic GS1 and chloroplastic GS2 [15,16]. Generally, there is a multigene family that encodes the cytosolic GS1, while only a single gene encodes the chloroplastic GS2 [17,18,19,20,21,22,23]. There is one exception that *Medicago truncatula* has two *GS2* genes [24]. To date, only the *OsGS2* gene is identified in rice that encodes chloroplastic GS2, which is mainly expressed in leaf [25].

Several studies have justified the importance of the GS2 enzyme in the assimilation of ammonium, especially the major function in photorespiratory ammonium re-assimilation, because mutants lacking the*GS2* gene were able to grow normally under non-photorespiratory conditions. For example, high light intensity tolerance and photorespiration capacity were observed in *GS2*-overexpressed transgenic tobacco plants [26]. Similarly, increased salt tolerance and photorespiration capacity were also found in transgenic rice [27]. The amount of GS2 protein decreased by 35% in *GS2*-silencing oil seed rape plants, while no changes in plant growth were observed when compared to the wild-type plants [28]. *GS2* deficiency in *Lotus japonicas* has an important effect on the nodulation process in legumes [29]. Moreover, barley *GS2* mutants died when grown in normal air, because they were unable to re-assimilate photorespiratory ammonium [30,31,32]. A recent study indicated that *GS2* genes may be related to the grain protein content of durum wheat [23].

Plant growth and crop production requires abundant nitrogen, which is generally the most common limiting nutrient for the growth and yield of crops worldwide. Large amounts of nitrogen fertilizers are applied to meet the high nitrogen requirements of crop plants. However, the application of large quantities of fertilizers to increase crop yield is not economically sustainable and also leads to environmental pollution. Reports pointed out that less than half of the applied nitrogen fertilizers were absorbed and used by crop plants, and the left nitrogen was inevitably lost to the atmosphere and leached into the underground water system, leading to severe environmental pollution [33]. A recent analysis showed that high N fertilizer input was the main reason for soil acidification in China [34]. Rice (*Oryza sativa*) is the main staple food in the world. As rice has the smallest genome among the major cereals and amount of genetic resources, it becomes a model cereal for science research [35]. Because of the important function of the GS enzyme in plant N metabolism, particular attention has been devoted to studies on GS transformation in higher plants, which is expected to be a good molecular method to analyze gene functions and a good strategy to improve nitrogen use efficiency.

Based on these aspects, we constructed the *GS2*-overexpressed transformants using *CaMV*35S promoter and obtained the transgenic rice plants by the *Agrobacterium*-mediated transformation method to improve the nitrogen use efficiency [36]. Interesting results were observed in these transgenic plants. In the $T_0$generation, transcripts of the *GS2* gene were shown to accumulate at higher levels, and no differences in the visible growth phenotype were observed; whereas, in the $T_1$ generation, the transgenic plants exhibited a chlorosis phenotype (yellow leaves) accompanied by a significant decline in the level of *GS2* messenger RNA (mRNA) and total GS activity, decreased plant height, few tillers and decreased dry weight. In addition, the transgenic plants displayed better performance when grown in a normal nutrient solution complemented with exogenous glutamine (Gln) [36]. Based on these results, we renamed the transgenic plants *GS2*-cosuppressed rice. In the present study, to determine the possible reason for the chlorosis phenotype of the transgenic plants, we systematically analyzed the differences in the plant growth, carbon-nitrogen metabolism and gene expression profile between the *GS2*-cosuppressed rice (homozygous $T_2$ generation of transgenic Line 87 with a decrease of 28% in GS activity in leaves) and wild-type Zhonghua 11 at the seedling stage and tillering stage. Additionally, in order to test the different response of the transgenic plants to the inorganic and organic nitrogen supplied in the environment, we planted these plants hydroponically under different nitrogen forms (supplied with ammonium nitrate, glutamine and both nitrogen forms). The results indicated the important role of a stable level of transcription of *GS2* mRNA for the normal development of rice and the carbon-nitrogen metabolic balance. The unbalanced carbon-nitrogen metabolic status and the excessively high expression level of *GS2* mRNA in the root may be the reasons for the chlorosis phenotype in the *GS2*-cosuppressed plants.

# 2. RESULTS

## 2.1. Growth Phenotype of GS2-Cosuppressed Plants at the Seedling and Tillering Stages

In our previous study, the *GS2*-cosuppressed plants exhibited a normal growth phenotype with a higher*GS2* mRNA transcriptional level at the seedling stage, while the chlorosis phenotype and a lower *GS2*mRNA transcriptional level was observed at the tillering stage [36]. Additionally, the *GS2*-cosuppressed plants displayed better performance when grown in a normal nutrient solution complemented with exogenous Gln [36]. To describe these phenotypes in detail, we measured the root length, plant height and the root and shoot dry weight of *GS2*-cosuppressed plants (homozygous $T_2$ generation of transgenic Line 87 with a decrease of 28% in GS activity in leaves) and wild-type plants at the seedling stage and the tillering stage under N, G (Gln) and N + G conditions. Additionally, the leaf SPAD (Soil and Plant Analyzer Development) value and photosynthesis parameters were also examined in *GS2*-cosuppressed plants and wild-type plants at the tillering stage under N, G and N + G conditions.

At the seedling stage, there was no obvious difference in the root length and plant height between the*GS2*-cosuppressed plants and wild-type plants (Figure 1A). At the tillering stage, there were significant ($p < 0.01$) decreases in the root length and plant height in *GS2*-cosuppressed plants compared to the wild-type plants (20.8% and 15.4% decreases in root length in the *GS2*-cosuppressed plants grown under N and G conditions, respectively; 25.9% decreases in plant height in *GS2*-cosuppressed plants grown under N + G conditions; Figure 1A). In addition, the root length of both *GS2*-cosuppressed plants and the wild-type plants decreased significantly after Gln was supplied to the nutrient solution, especially at the seedling stage. There were 58.3%–65% decreases in root length growth under G and N + G conditions when compared to the N condition (Figure 1A). For the root and shoot dry weight analysis, there were significant ($p < 0.05$) reductions in *GS2*-cosuppressed plants at both the seedling and tillering stages when compared to the wild-type plants under these three different growth conditions, except the root and shoot dry weight under the G condition at the seedling stage (Figure 1B). Compared to the wild-type plants, there were 20.8%–23.2% reductions in the root dry weight, and 8.6%–12.2% reductions in the shoot dry weight of *GS2*-cosuppressed plants were observed at the seedling stage; meanwhile, 36.2%–59.8% reductions in the root dry weight and 49.1%–80.9% reductions in the shoot dry weight of *GS2*-cosuppressed plants were observed at the tillering stage (Figure 1B). These results showed the different growth phenotypes between the *GS2*-cosuppressed plants and the wild-type plants at the tillering stage, especially with regard to the root and shoot dry weight.

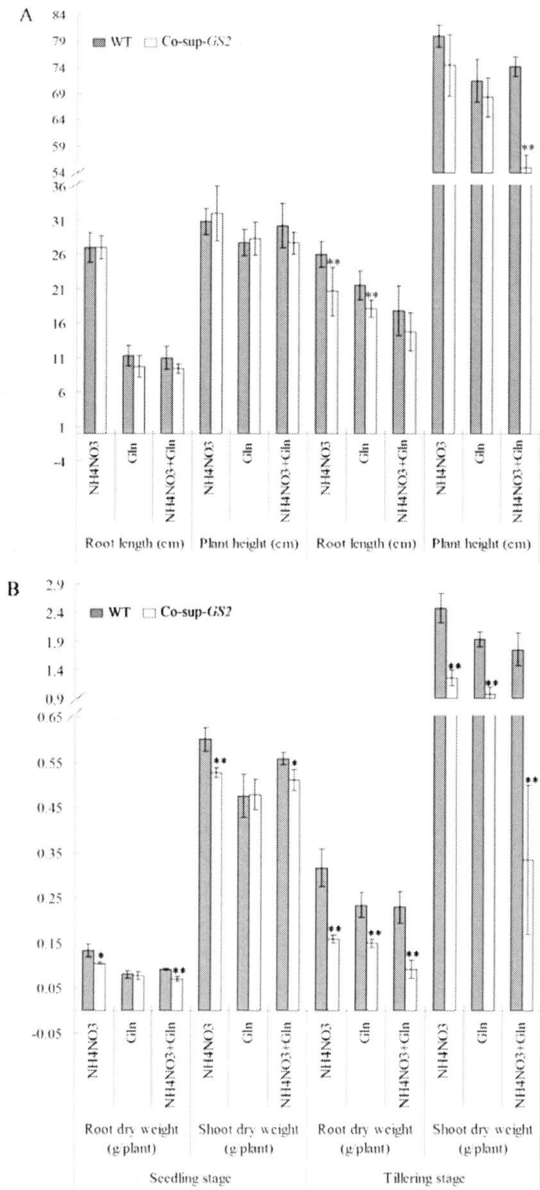


**Figure 1.** The root length and plant height (**A**), root dry weight and shoot dry weight (**B**) in the *GS2*-cosuppressed plants (Co-sup-*GS2*) and wild-type plants (WT) at the seedling stage and the tillering stage under N ($NH_4NO_3$), G (Gln) and N + G ($NH_4NO_3$ + Gln) conditions. Values are the mean ± SD of ten randomly-selected plants. *, ** Significant differences at the level of $p = 0.05$ and $p = 0.01$, respectively.

**Table 1.** The leaf SPAD value and photosynthetic parameters in the *GS2*-cosuppressed plants (Co-sup-*GS2*) and wild-type plants (WT) at the tillering stage under N ($NH_4NO_3$), G (Gln) and N + G ($NH_4NO_3$ + Gln) conditions.

| Treatment | SPAD at Tillering Stage | Photosynthesis Parameters at Tillering Stage | | | |
|---|---|---|---|---|---|
| | | Photosynthetic Rate (μmol $CO_2$ $m^{-2}\cdot s^{-2}$) | Stomatal Conductance (mmol $m^{-2}\cdot s^{-1}$) | Intercellular $CO_2$ Concentration (μL·$L^{-1}$) | Transpiration Rate (mmol $H_2O$ $m^{-2}\cdot S^{-1}$) |
| **$NH_4NO_3$** | | | | | |
| WT | 46.1 ± 2.9 | 28.24 ± 3.32 | 0.82 ± 0.06 | 287.75 ± 9.62 | 15.06 ± 1.10 |
| Co-sup-*GS2* | 38.3 ± 6.3 ** | 29.76 ± 3.24 | 1.01 ± 0.26 | 292.91 ± 8.36 | 15.99 ± 1.36 |
| **Gln** | | | | | |
| WT | 46.0 ± 2.2 | 33.24 ± 2.10 | 0.90 ± 0.12 | 278.39 ± 7.79 | 16.36 ± 1.56 |
| Co-sup-*GS2* | 41.1 ± 3.2 ** | 28.39 ± 1.54 ** | 0.71 ± 0.05 | 277.77 ± 1.32 | 12.99 ± 0.61 ** |
| **$NH_4NO_3$ + Gln** | | | | | |
| WT | 44.5 ± 2.4 | 30.83 ± 2.03 | 0.76 ± 0.10 | 274.75 ± 9.98 | 14.70 ± 1.61 |
| Co-sup-*GS2* | 42.3 ± 2.0 * | 29.53 ± 2.36 | 0.64 ± 0.02 | 268.03 ± 5.93 | 13.32 ± 0.74 |

Values are mean ± SD from ten randomly-selected plants. *, ** Significant differences at the level of $p = 0.05$ and $p = 0.01$, respectively.

The leaf SPAD value of the wild-type plants was stable under three different growth conditions, while the leaf SPAD value of the *GS2*-cosuppressed plants increased after the addition of Gln to the nutrient solution (Table 1). Additionally, the leaf SPAD value of the *GS2*-cosuppressed plants decreased significantly ($p < 0.05$) when compared to the wild-type plants, with 16.9%, 10.7% and 4.9% decreases for the N, G and N + G conditions, respectively (Table 1). However, there were no changes in the photosynthetic parameters (including photosynthetic rate, stomatal conductance, intercellular $CO_2$ concentration and transpiration rate) between the *GS2*-cosuppressed plants and the wild-type plants, except there were significant ($p < 0.01$) decreases in the photosynthetic rate (14.6% decrease) and transpiration rate (20.6% decrease) in the *GS2*-cosuppressed plants grown under the G condition when compared to the wild-type plants (Table 1).

## 2.2. Nitrogen Uptake by GS2-Cosuppressed Plants

As GS is the main enzyme that assimilates $NH_4^+$ into Gln, we analyzed the nitrogen uptake and transport ability of the *GS2*-cosuppressed plants at the tillering stage using $^{15}N$. The total carbon and nitrogen concentration and the carbon/nitrogen ratio were also determined in the roots, stems and leaves of *GS2*-cosuppressed plants and wild-type plants under N, G and N + G growth conditions at the tillering stage.

For the nitrogen uptake assay, the $NH_4NO_3$ in the nutrient solution was replaced by $^{15}NH_4{}^{15}NO_3$. After 1 h, 3 h, 8 h, 1 day and 3 days, the concentrations of total nitrogen and $^{15}N$ in the roots, stems and leaves were analyzed in the *GS2*-cosuppressed plants and wild-type plants. The results showed that there was no difference in the total nitrogen concentration in the root between the *GS2*-cosuppressed plants and the wild-type plants. The stem total nitrogen concentration of the *GS2*-cosuppressed plants was 16.5%–61.9% higher than that of the wild-type plants; while the leaf total nitrogen concentration was 5.5%–16.6% lower than that of the wild-type plants (Figure 2). Similarly, there was no difference in the $^{15}N$ concentration in the roots between the *GS2*-cosuppressed plants and the wild-type plants. The $^{15}N$ concentration in the stems of the*GS2*-cosuppressed plants was 11.4%–66.7% higher than that of the wild-type plants; while 3 d after the $NH_4NO_3$ in the nutrient solution was replaced with $^{15}NH_4{}^{15}NO_3$, the $^{15}N$ concentration in the leaves of the*GS2*-cosuppressed plants was 25.0% lower than in the wild-type plants (Figure 2). For the total carbon and nitrogen concentration analysis, significant ($p < 0.01$) increases in the total nitrogen concentration (26.0%, 32.7% and 18.1%) and significant ($p < 0.05$) decreases in the carbon/nitrogen ratio (20.2%, 24.0% and 17.9%) in the stem were observed in the *GS2*-cosuppressed plants grown under N, G and N + G conditions, respectively (Table 2). In addition, 3.8%, 5.3% and 9.9% decreases in the total nitrogen concentration were also observed in the *GS2*-cosuppressed plant leaves grown under the N, G and N + G conditions, respectively (Table 2). These results indicated a similar nitrogen uptake ability in roots between the *GS2*-cosuppressed plants and the wild-type plants, while a poor nitrogen transport ability from stems to leaves was observed, which led to nitrogen accumulation (especially the $NO_3^-$; data not shown here) and a decrease in the carbon/nitrogen ratio in the stems of the *GS2*-cosuppressed plants.

### 2.3. Soluble Proteins and Carbohydrates Determination in the GS2-Cosuppressed Plants

To evaluate the differences in the carbon and nitrogen metabolic status between the *GS2*-cosuppressed plants and the wild-type plants, we determined the concentrations of total soluble proteins and soluble carbohydrates in the roots, stems and leaves of *GS2*-

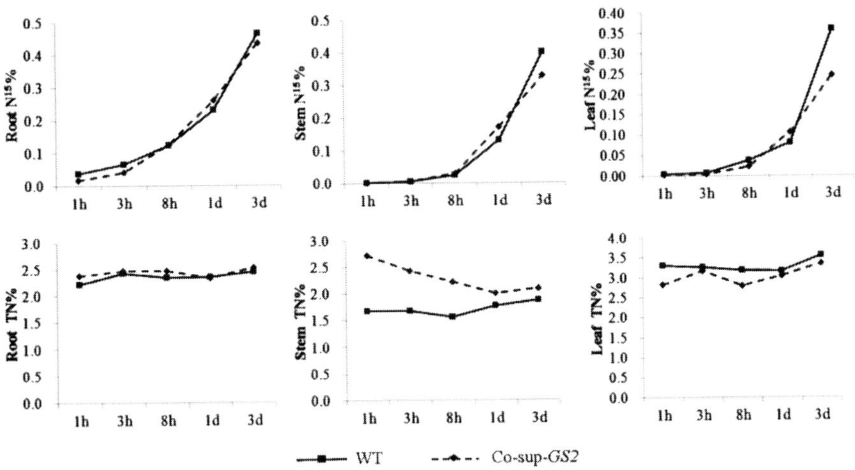


**Figure 2.** The $^{15}N$ ($^{15}N\%$) and total nitrogen content (TN%) in the roots, stems and uppermost leaves of the *GS2*-cosuppressed plants (Co-sup-*GS2*) and wild-type plants (WT) at 1 h, 3 h, 8 h, 1 day and 3 days after $NH_4NO_3$ in the nutrient solution was replaced with $^{15}NH_4{}^{15}NO_3$during the tillering stage. The values are the means from three biological replicated plant materials.

**Table 2.** The carbon content (C%), nitrogen content (N%) and carbon/nitrogen ratio (C/N) in the roots, stems and uppermost leaves of the *GS2*-cosuppressed plants (Co-sup-*GS2*) and wild-type plants (WT) at the tillering stage under N ($NH_4NO_3$), G (Gln) and N + G ($NH_4NO_3$ + Gln) conditions.

| Treatment | C% | | | N% | | | C/N | | |
|---|---|---|---|---|---|---|---|---|---|
| | Root | Stem | Leaf | Root | Stem | Leaf | Root | Stem | Leaf |
| **$NH_4NO_3$** | | | | | | | | | |
| WT | 38.64 ± 0.23 | 35.02 ± 0.52 | 38.81 ± 0.39 | 2.81 ± 0.13 | 2.50 ± 0.09 | 3.19 ± 0.05 | 13.75 ± 0.59 | 14.00 ± 0.41 | 12.16 ± 0.10 |
| Co-sup-*GS2* | 38.49 ± 0.49 | 35.11 ± 0.47 | 38.97 ± 0.80 | 3.16 ± 0.10 | 3.15 ± 0.15 ** | 3.07 ± 0.17 | 12.18 ± 0.53 | 11.17 ± 0.69 ** | 12.69 ± 0.41 |
| **Gln** | | | | | | | | | |
| WT | 41.18 ± 0.16 | 36.59 ± 0.30 | 39.78 ± 0.35 | 3.29 ± 0.20 | 2.84 ± 0.22 | 3.41 ± 0.10 | 12.53 ± 0.79 | 12.92 ± 0.86 | 11.68 ± 0.24 |
| Co-sup-*GS2* | 42.41 ± 0.30 | 37.00 ± 0.66 | 40.31 ± 0.73 | 3.21 ± 0.07 | 3.77 ± 0.07 ** | 3.23 ± 0.10 | 13.20 ± 0.40 | 9.82 ± 0.10 * | 12.48 ± 0.23 |
| **$NH_4NO_3$ + Gln** | | | | | | | | | |
| WT | 41.92 ± ND | 38.67 ± 0.36 | 42.64 ± 0.26 | 3.86 ± ND | 3.70 ± 0.07 | 4.16 ± 0.06 | 10.86 ± ND | 10.45 ± 0.17 | 10.25 ± 0.08 |
| Co-sup-*GS2* | ND | 37.54 ± 0.57 | 40.67 ± 1.14 | ND | 4.37 ± 0.13 ** | 3.75 ± 0.17 | ND | 8.58 ± 0.13 ** | 10.84 ± 0.19 |

Values are the mean ± SD from three biological replicated plant materials. *, ** Significant differences at the level of $p$ = 0.05 and $p$ = 0.01, respectively. ND no data

cosuppressed plants and wild-type plants under N, G and N + G growth conditions at the seedling and tillering stages. The results showed that there was a higher concentration of soluble proteins in the *GS2*-cosuppressed plants at the seedling stage, while there was a lower concentration of soluble proteins in the *GS2*-cosuppressed plants at the tillering stage compared to the wild-type plants (Figure

3). For example, at the seedling stage, compared to the wild-type plants, there was a 30.5% increase in the root soluble proteins in the *GS2*-cosuppressed plants under N + G conditions; there were 39.0% and 42.4% increases in soluble proteins in the stems under N and G conditions, respectively; and there was a 20.2% increase in the soluble proteins in the leaves under the N condition (Figure 3A). At the tillering stage, compared to the wild-type plants, there was a 39.8% decrease in the root soluble proteins of the *GS2*-cosuppressed plants under the G condition; there were 53.6% and 56.9% decreases in the soluble proteins in the stems under the N and G conditions, respectively; and there were 26.4%, 43.0% and 24.1% decreases in the soluble proteins in the leaves under the N, G and N + G conditions, respectively (Figure 3B).

In contrast, there was a lower concentration of soluble carbohydrates in the *GS2*-cosuppressed plants at the seedling stage, while there was a higher concentration of soluble carbohydrates in the *GS2*-cosuppressed plants at the tillering stage when compared to the wild-type plants (Figure 4). For example, at the seedling stage, compared to the wild-type plants, there were 30.0% and 46.7% decreases in the stem soluble carbohydrates of *GS2*-cosuppressed plants under the N and G conditions, respectively; and there were 25.7%, 31.8% and 23.2% decreases in soluble carbohydrates in the leaves under the N, G and N + G conditions, respectively; (Figure 4A). At the tillering stage, compared to the wild-type plants, there were 99.9% and 178.0% increases in the soluble carbohydrates in the stem, and there were 98.3% and 84.6% increases in the soluble carbohydrates in the leaves of *GS2*-cosuppressed plants under the N and G conditions, respectively (Figure 4B). These results suggested that the altered *GS2* expression level (higher*GS2* expression level at the seedling stage and lower *GS2* expression level at the tillering stage) affected the carbon and nitrogen metabolic status. There was an imbalance between the soluble protein and carbohydrate concentrations in the *GS2*-cosuppressed plants, especially in the stems and leaves.

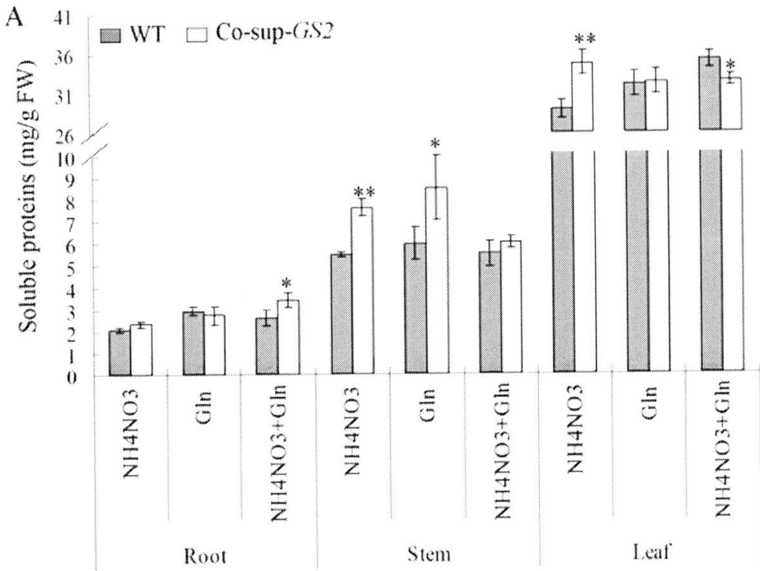


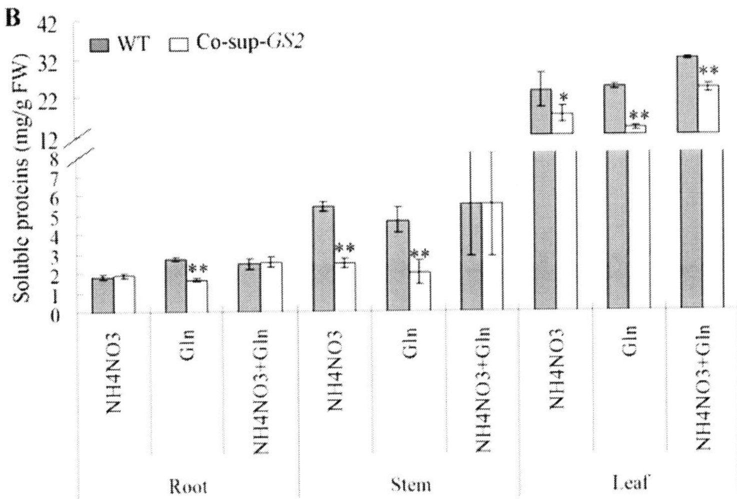


**Figure 3.** The concentration of soluble proteins in the roots, stems and uppermost leaves of *GS2*-cosuppressed plants (Co-sup-*GS2*) and wild-type plants (WT) at the seedling stage (**A**) and the tillering stage (**B**) under N ($NH_4NO_3$), G (Gln) and N + G ($NH_4NO_3$ + Gln) conditions. Values are the mean ± SD from three biological replicated plant materials. *, ** Significant differences at the level of $p = 0.05$ and $p = 0.01$, respectively.

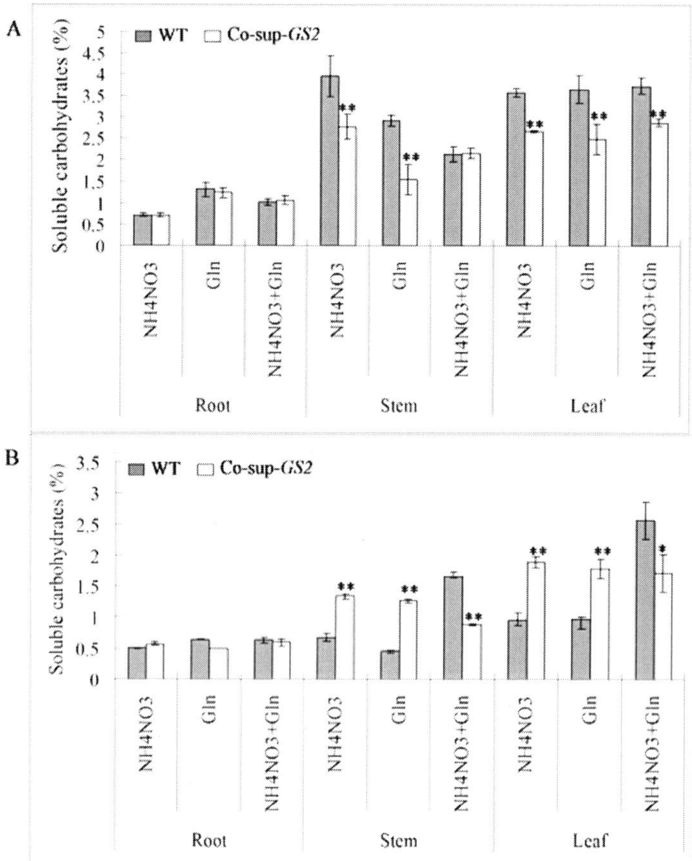


**Figure 4.** The concentration of soluble carbohydrates in the roots, stems and uppermost leaves of *GS2*-cosuppressed plants (Co-sup-*GS2*) and wild-type plants (WT) at the seedling stage (**A**) and the tillering stage (**B**) under N ($NH_4NO_3$), G (Gln) and N + G ($NH_4NO_3$ + Gln) conditions. Values are the mean ± SD from three biological replicated plant materials. *, ** Significant differences at the level of $p = 0.05$ and $p = 0.01$, respectively.

### 2.4. Metabolite Profiling Analysis in GS2-Cosuppressed Plants

To study the individual metabolites involved in the carbon and nitrogen metabolic pathway in detail, we analyzed the sugars, organic acids and free amino acids in the root and leaf tissues of *GS2*-cosuppressed plants and wild-type plants at the tillering stage under different N conditions. Figure 5 and Supplementary Figure S1 display the fold change corresponding to the ratio of *GS2*-cosuppressed plants/wild-type plants, calculated using the concentrations of these individual metabolites. Dramatic increases in the sugars, organic acids and free amino acids were observed in both the leaf and root tissues of the *GS2*-cosuppressed plants compared to the wild-type plants, especially for ascorbic acid (>37.7-fold), succinate (>312.4-fold) and methionine (>410.3-fold) in the leaf and xylitol (>46.3-fold), ascorbic acid (>14.2-fold), pyruvate (>808.1-fold) and ornithine (>19.9-fold) in the root (Figure 5; Supplementary Figure S1). Meanwhile, several metabolites had dramatically decreased concentrations, including glutaric acid (<0.10-fold) and glycine (<0.07-fold) in the leaf and glutamine (<0.04-fold), alanine (<0.004-fold) and leucine (<0.0006-fold) in the root (Figure 5;Supplementary Figure S1). However, the concentrations of total sugars, total organic acids and total free amino acids increased only slightly, a fold change ranging from 2.0–3.7 (data not shown here).

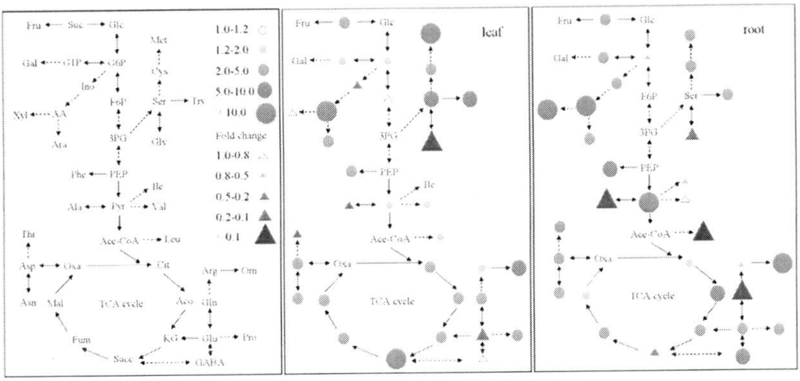


**Figure 5.** The fold change corresponds to the ratio of the concentration of individual metabolites involved in carbon and nitrogen metabolism in the *GS2*-cosuppressed plants relative to the wild-type plants for the uppermost leaves and roots at the tillering stage under N condition. Red dots indicate increased metabolites, and blue triangles indicate decreased metabolites. Glc, glucose; Suc, sucrose; Fru, fructose; F6P, frutose-6-P; G6P, glucose-6-P; G1P, glucose-1-P; Gal, galactose; Ino, inositol; AA, ascorbic acid; Ara, arabinose; Xyl, xylitol; 3PG, 3-P-glycerate; PEP, phosphoenolpyruvate; Pyr, pyruvate; Ace-CoA, acetyl-CoA; Cit, citrate; Aco, aconitase; KG, ketoglutarate; Succ, succinate; Fum, fumarate; Mal, malate; Oxa, oxaloacetate; Glu, glutamate; Gln, glutamine; Arg, arginine; Pro, proline; Orn, ornithine; GABA, aminobutyric; Asp, aspartate; Asn, asparagine; Ile, isoleucine; Met, methionine; Thr, threonine; Ala, alanine; Val, valine; Leu, leucine; Phe, phenylalanine; Try, tryptophan; Ser, serine; Gly, glycine; Cys, cysteine.

## 2.5. Gene Expression Analysis in GS2-Cosuppressed Plants

To determine the impact of the reduced *GS2* mRNA transcriptional level on the carbon-nitrogen metabolic genes' expression patterns, we analyzed the expression level of genes encoding NRT (nitrate transporter), NR (nitrate reductase), GS (glutamine synthetase), GOGAT (glutamate synthase), RUBISCO (ribulose-1,5-bisphosphate carboxylase/oxygenase) and PEPC (phosphoenolpyruvate carboxylase) by q-RT PCR. Figure 6A displays these genes in the carbon and nitrogen metabolic pathway in rice plants. Supplementary Table S1 lists the fold change corresponding to the ratio of the gene expression level in *GS2*-cosuppressed plants relative to wild-type plants in the roots and leaves at both the seedling and tillering stage under N, G and N + G conditions. The results showed that the expression levels of most genes were changed in the *GS2*-cosuppressed plants. Compared to the wild-type plants, the significantly ($p < 0.01$) higher *GS2* expression levels (35.06–537.49-fold) were observed in the roots of *GS2*-cosuppressed plants at both the seedling stage and the tillering stage under N, G and N + G conditions (Supplementary Table S1). However, significantly ($p < 0.05$) lower *GS2* expression levels (0.43–0.79-fold) were observed in the leaves of *GS2*-cosuppressed plants at both the seedling stage and the tillering stage under the N, G and N + G conditions, except a higher *GS2*expression level (2.35-fold) was observed in the leaves at the seedling stage under the N condition (Supplementary Table S1). Furthermore, different gene expression patterns were exhibited in the *GS2*-cosuppressed plants between the seedling stage and tillering stage. Additionally, opposite gene expression patterns were shown between the root and leaf tissues, particularly at the tillering stage. For example, the expression levels of the *NRT1;1*, *NRT1;2*, *NRT2*, *NR2*, *GS1;2*, *Fd-GOGAT1* and *NADH-GOGAT1* genes were significantly ($p < 0.05$) increased in the roots, while the expression levels of the *NR1*, *NR2*, *GS1;1*, *GS2*, *Fd-GOGAT2*, *NADH-GOGAT2*, *RUBISCO*, *PEPC1* and *PEPC2* genes were significantly ($p < 0.05$) decreased in the leaves under the N condition (Figure 6).

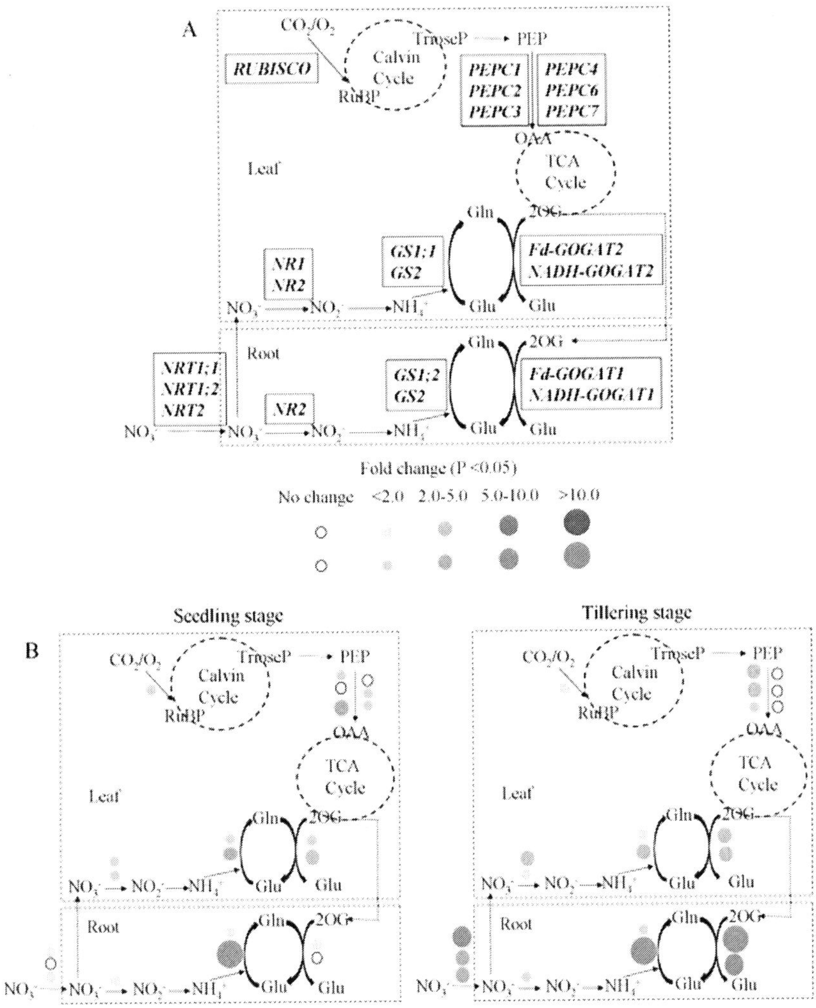
A
CO2/O2
Calvin Cycle
TriosePeP → PEP
RUBISCO
RuBP
PEPC1 PEPC2 PEPC3
PEPC4 PEPC6 PEPC7
OAA
TCA Cycle
Leaf
Gln
2OG
GS1;1 GS2
Fd-GOGAT2 NADH-GOGAT2
NR1 NR2
Glu
Root
NRT1;1 NRT1;2 NRT2
GS1;2 GS2
Fd-GOGAT1 NADH-GOGAT1
NR2
Fold change (P <0.05)
No change
<2.0
2.0-5.0
5.0-10.0
>10.0
B
Seedling stage
Tillering stage

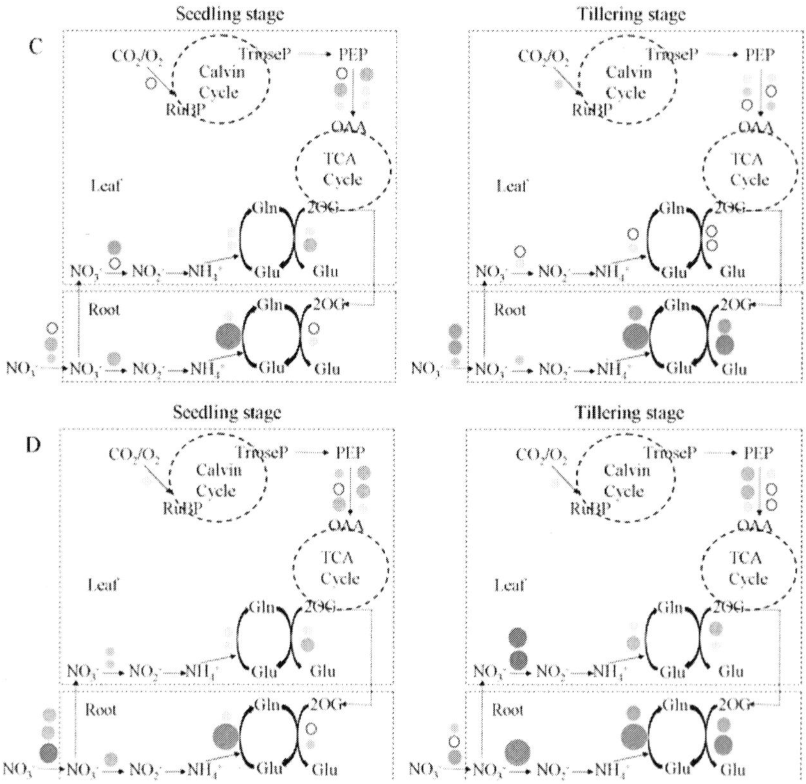


**Figure 6.** The fold change corresponds to the ratio of the gene expression level in the *GS2*-cosuppressed plants relative to the wild-type plants. (**A**) Diagrammatic representation of the key genes involved in the carbon and nitrogen metabolic pathway in rice plants. NRT, nitrate transporter; NR, nitrate reductase; GS, glutamine synthetase; GOGAT, glutamate synthase; RUBISCO, ribulose-1,5-bisphosphate carboxylase/oxygenase; PEPC, phosphoenolpyruvate carboxylase. Prominent changes in the gene expression level in the *GS2*-cosuppressed plants compared to wild-type plants at the seedling stage and tillering stage under N (**B**), G (**C**) and N + G (**D**) conditions. Red and blue dots indicate up- and down-regulated genes, respectively.

# 3. DISCUSSION

## 3.1. The Carbon-Nitrogen Metabolic Imbalance Is One of the Possible Reasons for the Chlorosis Phenotype in the GS2-Cosuppressed Plants

C and N are the essential elements for plant routine and fundamental growth and development. The optimal functioning and coordination of the C and N metabolism plays a very important role in plant growth and production [5,7,8,10]. Maintaining an appropriate balance or ratio of C and N nutrients is critical to sustain the optimal plant growth and development [5,8,10]. Because C and N resources change along with the environment, plants have developed a highly complex and sophisticated regulation system to adjust C and N uptake, transport and assimilation [10,37,38,39,40]. Schlüter *et al.* reported that the C, N and phosphorus balance played an important role in the stress adaptation of maize source leaf [41]. In the present study, our results showed an altered carbon and nitrogen metabolism in *GS2* transgenic plants. There were significant ($p < 0.05$) decreases of the carbon/nitrogen ratio in the stem tissue of *GS2*-cosuppressed plants. Furthermore, the opposite results between soluble protein and carbohydrate concentrations in the *GS2*-cosuppressed plants at both the seedling and the tillering stage indicated that the altered *GS2* expression level affected the carbon and nitrogen metabolic status. This type of carbon-nitrogen metabolic imbalance may be one of the reasons for the chlorosis phenotype of the *GS2*-cosuppressed plants. Early studies reported similar results that the C/N ratio, rather than the carbohydrate status alone, played the major role in the fresh weight, cotyledon size, chlorophyll and anthocyanin content in *Arabidopsis* [9]. Bao*et al.* reported that an imbalance of C-N metabolic status may cause the poor growth and yield in the *GS1;1*- and *GS1;2*-overexprssing transgenic rice [42]. Kusano *et al.* also reported that the rice *OsGS1;1* mutant showed an imbalance in tricarboxylic acid cycle metabolites, amino acids and sugars [43]. Additionally, variations in the leaf SPAD value, photosynthetic parameters, individual sugars, amino acids, organic acids and gene expression levels were observed in *GS2*-cosuppressed plants when compared to the wild-type plants in this study. Pérez-Delgado *et al.* also reported that the mutant plants lacking the plastidic isoform of Gln synthetase in *Lotus japonicas* accumulated high levels of several amino acids and organic acids, including intermediates of the Krebs cycle under photorespiratory active conditions [44].

### 3.2. The Incoordination between the Root and Leaf Tissues Is Another Possible Reason for the Chlorosis Phenotype in GS2-Cosuppressed Plants

In higher plants, a complex picture is emerging in which C/N signaling networks are subject to a “matrix effect” in which certain functions or interactions only occur under situations that are specific to a species, cell-type, developmental stage, metabolic status or environmental condition [8]. In addition to maintaining the carbon-nitrogen balance in the same organ and/or tissue, the tight coordination involves the sensing and signaling of the carbon/nitrogen balance between the source and sink tissues [5,8]. The $NO_3^-$ and/or $NH_4^+$are usually taken up by the root system and transported to the leaves for the inorganic nitrogen assimilation, while carbon metabolism primarily occurs in the leaves to provide both the carbon skeletons and energies for nitrogen assimilation [5,8]. Therefore, plants must develop a mechanism to sense the status of the nitrogen in the root system and the surrounding soil environment and coordinate with the sensory machinery in the leaves, where the photosynthetic output will be determined [5,8]. In this study, compared to the wild-type plants, the total nitrogen content of *GS2*-cosuppressed plants showed no significant difference in the root, while significantly increased in the stem and decreased in the leaf. This suggested that*GS2*-cosuppressed plants had similar capacities for nitrogen uptake from the environment and nitrogen export from the root to the stem, and they had poor nitrogen transport ability from the stem to the leaf, which led to dramatic nitrogen accumulation in the stem. Furthermore, the expression pattern of the *GS2*gene and other key genes involved in carbon and nitrogen metabolism was inconsistent between the root and leaf in the *GS2*-cosuppressed plants. These results showed an incoordination between the root and leaf tissues in *GS2*-cosuppressed plants. We hypothesized that this may be another reason for the chlorosis phenotype of the *GS2*-cosuppressed plants.

### 3.3. The Impact of Gln on Plant Growth and Carbon-Nitrogen Metabolism

Plants can capture nitrogen in a variety of different chemical forms, ranging from inorganic forms, such as $NO_3^-$ and $NH_4^+$, to as many as 20 different amino acids [45,46,47,48,49,50,51]. The uptake rates for amino acids are considerably lower compared to inorganic forms of nitrogen [45,47,48,51]. In general, it appears that plants can use most of the amino acids as a source of nitrogen, which depress plant growth relative to mineral sources of nitrogen [45,52]. Only a minority of amino acids can occasionally increase plant growth [50,52] or at least match plant growth on mineral forms of nitrogen [53]. In our study, we analyzed the growth phenotype, carbon-nitrogen metabolic status and gene expression profile of *GS2*-cosuppressed rice and wild-type plants under three different nitrogen conditions (N, G and N + G). Results showed that both the *GS2*-cosuppressed rice and wild-type plants could grow under Gln as the nitrogen source. However, Gln depressed the plant growth, particularly the root length and root dry weight. When compared to the N condition, the leaf SPAD value, total carbon or nitrogen content increased, while the leaf stomatal conductance, intercellular $CO_2$ concentration, transpiration rate and carbon/nitrogen ratio decreased under the G or N + G conditions. Additionally, Gln affected the gene expression patterns, particularly at the seedling stage. Similar results have been reported showing that, while plants generally have the capacity to take up many amino acids, these often negatively interfere with biomass production and even inhibit growth [54]. The model plant *Arabidopsis* has the capacity to acquire and utilize a number of amino acids for growth, including the amide glutamine (Gln) [48]. When grown with amino acids as the sole nitrogen source,*Arabidopsis thaliana* was only capable of achieving between 1% and 50% of its potential vegetative growth on an identical concentration of nitrate [48]. Results indicated that plants would be capable of growing when fed Gln, but Gln would contribute relatively little to plant growth compared to inorganic nitrogen sources of $NO_3^-$ and $NH_4^+$.

# 4. EXPERIMENTAL SECTION

## 4.1. Plant Materials and Growth Conditions

Seeds of the *GS2*-cosuppressed rice (the homozygous of $T_2$ generation of transgenic Line 87 with 28% decreased GS activity in leaves was used in this study) and wild-type Zhonghua 11 (*Oryza sativa* ssp.*japonica*) were germinated and sowed in sand. Seedlings with two leaves were then transplanted hydroponically in a normal nutrient solution using 1.44 mM·$NH_4NO_3$ as a nitrogen source (N), a nutrient solution without $NH_4NO_3$, but using 2.0 mM glutamine (Gln) as a nitrogen source (G), and a nutrient solution using both 1.44 mM·$NH_4NO_3$ and 2.0 mM·Gln as nitrogen sources (N + G). The composition of normal nutrient solution was described in detail by Yoshida *et al.* [55]. At the seedling stage (one week after transplanting) and the tillering stage (five weeks after transplanting), the roots, stems and leaves were harvested for the phenotype evaluation, the leaf SPAD value and photosynthesis capacity determination, the carbon-nitrogen metabolism and gene expression analysis. All of the plants were grown in the pot farm at Huazhong Agricultural University, Wuhan, China. The nutrient solution was refreshed every 3 days, and the pH value was kept at 5.5.

### 4.2. Nitrogen Uptake Assay

Seeds of the *GS2*-cosuppressed rice (transgenic Line 88 was used in this study) and wild-type Zhonghua 11 (*Oryza sativa* ssp. *japonica*) germinated and were sowed in sand in the pot farm at Huazhong Agricultural University. Seedlings with two leaves were transplanted into the normal nutrient solution described by Yoshida *et al.* [55]. Plants were transferred into a new nutrient solution, in which the $NH_4NO_3$ was replaced by $^{15}NH_4{}^{15}NO_3$, at the tillering stage (five weeks after transplanting). After 1 h, 3 h, 8 h, 1 day and 3 days, three biological replicated samples of roots, stems and uppermost leaves were harvested for the total N and $^{15}N$ concentration determination. A C/N analyzer (Elementar, Vario MAX CN, Germany) and an isotope mass spectrometer (ANCA-MS, Europa Scientific, Crewe, UK) were used to measure the concentrations of total C/N and $^{15}N$, respectively, as described in detail previously [42].

### 4.3. Determination of the Leaf SPAD Value and Photosynthetic Parameters

As described in detail previously [42], every ten randomly-selected plants of the *GS2*-cosuppressed rice and wild-type Zhonghua 11 grown under the N, G and N + G conditions at the tillering stage (five weeks after transplanting) were used for the leaf SPAD value and photosynthetic capacity determination. The SPAD value and the photosynthetic rate, transpiration rate, intercellular $CO_2$ concentration and stomatal conductance of upper, middle and bottom portion of the flag leaf in each plant were tested by a chlorophyll meter (SPAD-502) and a Li-6400XT portable photosynthesis system (Li-COR, Lincoln, NE, USA), respectively. The average mean was used in the further data analysis.

### 4.4. Determination of the Physiological Parameters

At the seedling stage (one week after transplanting) and the tillering stage (five weeks after transplanting), three biological replicated roots, stems and uppermost leaves of the *GS2*-cosuppressed rice and wild-type Zhonghua 11 grown under the N, G and N + G conditions were harvested for the concentrations of soluble proteins and carbohydrates analysis. All fresh samples were homogenized by grinding on ice with extraction buffer, which was described in detail previously [36,42]. After centrifuging (12,000× *g*, 20 min, 4 °C), the supernatant was used to analyze the concentration of soluble proteins by the Bradford method [56]. The pre-dried samples were boiled with boiling water to extract the soluble carbohydrates. Additionally, the concentration of soluble carbohydrates was measured colorimetrically by the anthrone method [57,58]. At the tillering stage (five weeks after transplanting), three biological replicated roots and uppermost leaves of*GS2*-cosuppressed rice and wild-type Zhonghua 11 grown under the N condition were harvested for the carbon-nitrogen metabolic profile analysis. Fifty milligrams of fresh sample were extracted with 1 mL extraction buffer (methanol/chloroform/water (3:1:1 *v*/*v*/*v*)) containing ten stable isotope compounds by a mixer mill at a frequency of 30 Hz for 3 min at 4 °C. The homogenates were then centrifuged at 15,000× *g* for 5 min at 4 °C. Four hundred microliters of supernatant were evaporated for further derivatization in a vacuum filled with 99.999% dry nitrogen. After evaporation, 20 μL methoxyamine hydrochloride were added to the sample for 30 h of derivatization at room temperature. Later, the sample was trimethylsilylated using 20 μL of MSTFA [*N*-Methyl-*N*-(trimethylsilyl)trifluoroacetamide] with 1% TMCS (Trimethylchlorosilane) at 37 °C with shaking for 1 h, and 20 μL *n*-heptane were added after silylation. The analysis of carbon and nitrogen metabolites by GC-TOF-MS and data analysis were performed as described by Kusano *et al.* [59,60] and Redestig *et al.* [61].

### 4.5. Gene Expression Analysis

At the seedling stage (one week after transplanting) and the tillering stage (five weeks after transplanting), three biological replicated roots and uppermost leaves of the *GS2*-cosuppressed rice and wild-type Zhonghua 11 grown under the N, G and N + G conditions were harvested for total RNA extraction (TRIzol reagent, Invitrogen, Darmstadt, Germany) and q-RT PCR analysis. The total RNA was treated by DNase I to remove the genomic DNA. The Superscript II reverse transcriptase (Invitrogen) was used to synthesize the first-strand cDNAs for q-RT PCR. The Primer Express Software (Foster City, CA, USA) and BLAST program in the database of the Institute for Genomic Research (TIGR, Available online:http://rice.plantbiology.msu.edu/) were used to design primers and check their specificity. Supplementary Table S2 lists the specific primers, both for tested genes and the rice *actin* gene (NM_197297). All of the experimental procedures were described in detail previously [36,42].

### 4.6. Statistical Analysis

The data were assessed with one-way ANOVA at $p < 0.05$ or $p < 0.01$ using SPSS 17.0 (SPSS Inc., Chicago, IL, USA).

## 5. CONCLUSIONS

In this study, we systematically analyzed the differences in the growth phenotype, carbon-nitrogen metabolic status and gene expression profile between *GS2*-cosuppressed rice and wild-type Zhonghua 11 at both the seedling stage and the tillering stage under three different nitrogen conditions (N, G and N + G). Results demonstrated the close relationships between the *GS2* mRNA levels and carbon-nitrogen metabolic status, as well as the plant growth phenotype. Figure 7 summarizes the differences between the seedling stage and the tillering stage in the *GS2* transgenic plants.

At the seedling stage, *GS2* was overexpressed under the control of the 35S promoter in the leaf tissue, which stimulated the expression levels of the *NR*, *GS* and *GOGAT* genes, resulting in an improvement in nitrogen reduction and assimilation for the increased production of amino acids and proteins. The content of carbohydrates decreased because of the large amount of carbon skeletons that were used to synthesize amino acids, and the expression levels of the *RUBISCO* and *PEPC* genes increased to produce more carbon skeletons. As fewer carbon skeletons could be transported into the root to participate in amino acid synthesis, the decreased *NRT*, *NR*, *GS* and *GOGAT* expression levels were displayed, which resulted in a decline in the nitrogen uptake, reduction and assimilation in the root. Additionally, *GS2* was excessively overexpressed (>35-fold) under the 35S promoter in the root, which could require a large amount of energy. This may be another factor causing the decreased nitrogen metabolic status in the roots of the *GS2*transgenic plants.

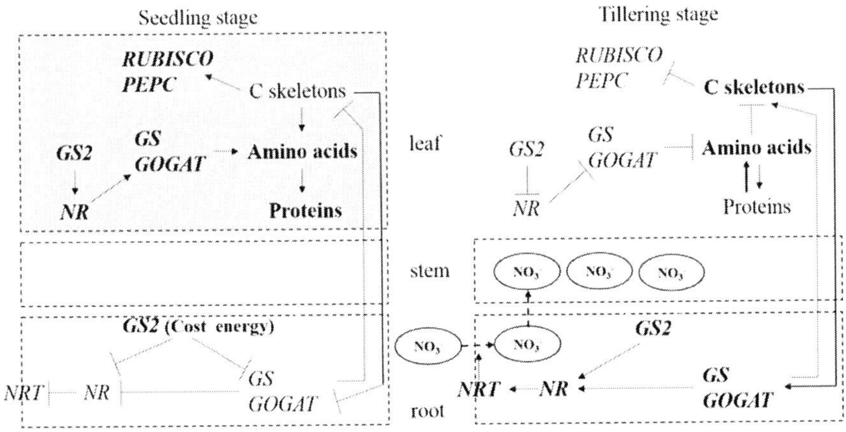


**Figure 7.** Summary of the differences between the seedling stage and the tillering stage in the *GS2* transgenic plant. The symbols ↑ and ⊤indicate induction and repression, respectively.

Although the *GS2* transgenic plants maintained a normal growth phenotype with green leaves at the seedling stage, the metabolic status was altered dramatically in both the root and leaf tissues because of the*GS2* overexpression. In this situation, plants must do something to maintain the metabolic status and complete the life cycle. From this point of view, the transgenic plants adjusted the *GS2* expression level in the leaves at the tillering stage. In the leaves, the *GS2* expression level decreased, which suppressed the *NR*,*GS* and *GOGAT* gene expression, resulted a decline in nitrogen reduction and assimilation, as well as decreased amino acid and protein production. However, the increased levels of free amino acids were observed in the metabolite profile analysis, which may have been caused by the protein degradation in the chlorotic leaves. In another case, the contents of the carbohydrates increased because few carbon skeletons were used to synthesize amino acids, and the expression levels of the *RUBISCO* and *PEPC* genes decreased to reduce the production of carbon skeletons. As more carbon skeletons were transported into the roots to participate in amino acids synthesis, increases in the *NRT*, *NR*, *GS* and *GOGAT* expression levels were observed, which resulted in an improvement in the uptake, reduction and assimilation of nitrogen in the roots. We concluded that the stable transcription level of *GS2* mRNA plays an important role in the normal development of rice and in the carbon-nitrogen metabolic balance. We hypothesized that the disrupted coordination of the carbon and nitrogen metabolic status and the excessively high expression level of *GS2*mRNA in the root were the possible reasons for the chlorosis phenotype in the *GS2*-cosuppressed plants.

## ACKNOWLEDGMENTS

This research was supported in part by grants from the National Natural Science Foundation of China (31000932), the Specialized Research Fund for the Doctoral Program of Higher Education, the Ministry of Education of China (20100146120017) and the Fundamental Research Funds for the Central Universities (2662013PY041). We thank Qifa Zhang and Xingming Lian for providing the plant materials.

## AUTHOR CONTRIBUTIONS

Fangsen Xu, Lei Shi and Hongmei Cai conceived of and designed the experiments; Aili Bao and Guangda Ding performed the experiments; Zhuqing Zhao and Hongmei Cai analyzed the data; Aili Bao and Guangda Ding contributed reagents; and Hongmei Cai wrote the manuscript. All authors read and approved the manuscript.

## CONFLICTS OF INTEREST

The authors declare no conflict of interest.

## REFERENCES

1. Lam, H.M.; Coschigano, K.T.; Oliveira, I.C.; Melo-Oliveira, R.; Coruzzi, G.M. The molecular-genetics of nitrogen assimilation into amino acids in higher plants. Annu. Rev. Plant Physiol. Plant Mol. Biol.1996, 47, 569–593.
2. Tabuchi, M.; Abiko, T.; Yamaya, T. Assimilation of ammonium ions and reutilization of nitrogen in rice (Oryza sativa L.). J. Exp. Bot. 2007, 58, 2319–2327.
3. Frink, C.R.; Waggoner, P.E.; Ausubel, J.H. Nitrogen fertilizer: Retrospect and prospect. Proc. Natl. Acad. Sci. USA 1999, 96, 1175–1180.
4. Crawford, N.M.; Forde, B.G. Molecular and developmental biology of inorganic nitrogen nutrition. InThe Arabidopsis Book;

Meyerowitz, E., Somerville, C., Eds.; American Society of Plant Biologists: Rockville, MD, USA, 2002.

5. Zheng, Z. Carbon and nitrogen nutrient balance signaling in plants. Plant Signal. Behav. 2009, 4, 584–591.

6. Krapp, A.; Ferrario-Méry, S.; Touraine, B. Nitrogen and signalling. In Advances in Photosynthesis; Foyer, C., Noctor, G., Eds.; Springer Netherlands: Dordrecht, The Netherlands, 2002; Volume 12, pp. 205–225.

7. Krapp, A.; Truong, H.N. Regulation of C/N interaction in model plant species. In The Efficiency of Nitrogen Utilization in Plants; Goyal, S., Tischner, R., Basra, A., Eds.; Enhancing Haworth Press: New York, NY, USA, 2005; pp. 127–173.

8. Coruzzi, G.M.; Zhou, L. Carbon and nitrogen sensing and signaling in plants: Emerging "matrix effects". Curr. Opin. Plant Biol. 2001, 4, 247–253.

9. Martin, T.; Oswald, O.; Graham, I.A. Arabidopsis seedling growth, storage lipid mobilization and photosynthetic gene expression are regulated by carbon: nitrogen availability. Plant Physiol. 2002, 128, 472–481.

10. Nunes-Nesi, A.; Fernie, A.R.; Stitt, M. Metabolic and signaling aspects underpinning the regulation of plant carbon nitrogen interactions. Mol. Plant 2010, 3, 973–996.

11. Miflin, B.J.; Lea, P.J. Ammonia assimilation. In The Biochemistry of Plants; Miflin, B.J., Ed.; Academic Press: New York, NY, USA, 1980; Volume 5, pp. 169–202.

12. Hirel, B.; Lea, P.J. Ammonium assimilation. In Plant Nitrogen; Lea, P.J., Morof Gaudry, J.F., Eds.; Springer-Verlag: Berlin, Germany, 2001; pp. 79–99.

13. Tobin, A.K.; Yamaya, T. Cellular compartmentation of ammonium assimilation in rice and barley. J. Exp. Bot. 2001, 53, 591–604.

14. Ireland, R.J.; Lea, P.J. The enzymes of glutamine, glutamate, asparagines and aspirate metabolism. InPlant Amino Acids: Biochemistry and Biotechnology; Singh, B.K., Ed.; Marcel Dekker: New York, NY, USA, 1999; pp. 49–109.

15. Mann, A.F.; Fenten, P.A.; Stewart, G.R. Identification of two forms of glutamine synthetase in barley (Hordeum vulgare L.). Biochem. Biophys. Res. Commun. 1979, 88, 515–521.

16. Hirel, B.; Gadal, P. Glutamine synthetase in rice: A comparative study of the enzymes from roots and leaves. Plant Physiol. 1980, 66, 619–623.

17. Hayakawa, T.; Kamachi, K.; Oikawa, M.; Ojima, K.; Yamaya, T. Response of glutamine synthetase and glutamate synthase isoforms to nitrogen sources in rice cell cultures. Plant Cell Physiol. 1990, 31, 1071–1077.

18. Kamachi, K.; Yamaya, T.; Maie, T.; Ojima, K. A role for glutamine synthetase in the remobilization of leaf nitrogen during natural senescence in rice leaves. Plant Physiol. 1991, 96, 411–417.

19. Zozaya-Garza, M.; Sengupta-Gopalan, C. Glutamine synthetase gene isolation from an alfalfa leaf cDNA library. Plant Physiol. 1999, 119, 1568.

20. Ishiyama, K.; Inoue, E.; Tabuchi, M.; Yamaya, T.; Takahashi, H. Biochemical background and compartmentalized functions of cytosolic glutamine synthetase for active ammonium assimilation in rice roots. Plant Cell Physiol. 2004, 45, 1640–1647.

21. Bernard, S.M.; Moller, A.L.; Dionisio, G.; Kichey, T.; Jahn, T.P.; Dubois, F.; Baudo, M.; Lopes, M.S.; Tercé-Laforgue, T.; Foyer, C.H.; et al. Gene expression, cellular localisation and function of glutamine synthetase isozymes in wheat (Triticum aestivum L.). Plant Mol. Biol. 2008, 67, 89–105.

22. Deng, Y.-W.; Zhang, Y.-D.; Chen, Y.; Wang, S.; Tang, D.-M.; Huang, D.-F. Isolation and characterization of a GS2 gene in melon (Cucumis melo L.) and its expression patterns under the fertilization of different forms of N. Mol. Biotechnol. 2010, 44, 51–60.

23. Gadaleta, A.; Nigro, D.; Giancaspro, A.; Blanco, A. The glutamine synthetase (GS2) gene is in relation to grain protein content of durum wheat. Funct. Integr. Genomics 2011, 11, 665–670.

24. Seabra, A.; Vieira, C.P.; Cullimore, J.V.; Garvalho, H.G. Medicago truncatula contains a second gene encoding a plastid located glutamine synthetase exclusively expressed in developing seeds. BMC Plant Biol. 2010, 10, 183. [PubMed]

25. Tabuchi, M.; Sugiyama, K.; Ishiyama, K.; Inoue, E.; Sato, T.; Takahashi, H.; Yamaya, T. Severe reduction in growth rate and grain filling of rice mutants lacking OsGS1;1, a cytosolic glutamine synthetase1;1. Plant J. 2005, 42, 641–651.

26. Oliveira, I.C.; Brears, T.; Knight, T.J.; Clark, A.; Coruzzi, G.M. Overexpression of cytosolic glutamine synthetase: Relation to nitrogen, light and photorespiration. Plant Physiol. 2002, 129, 1170–1180.

27. Hoshida, H.; Tanaka, Y.; Hibino, T.; Hayashi, Y.; Tanaka, A.; Takabe, T.; Takabe, T. Enhanced tolerance to salt stress in transgenic rice that overexpresses chloroplast glutamine synthetase. Plant Mol. Biol.2000, 43, 103–111.

28. Husted, S.; Mattsson, M.; Möllers, C.; Wallbraun, M.; Schjoerring, J.K. Photorespiratory NH4+production in leaves of wild-type and glutamine synthetase 2 antisense oilseed rape. Plant Physiol. 2002,130, 989–998.

29. García-Calderón, M.; Chiurazzi, M.; Espuny, M.R.; Márquez, A.J. Photorespiratory metabolism and nodule function: Behavior of Lotus japonicas mutants deficient in plastid glutamine synthetase. Mol. Plant. Microbe Interact. 2012, 25, 211–219.

30. Blackwell, R.D.; Murray, A.J.S.; Lea, P.J. Inhibition of photosynthesis in barley with decreased levels of chloroplastic glutamine synthetase activity. J. Exp. Bot. 1987, 38, 1799–1809.

31. Blackwell, R.D.; Murray, A.J.S.; Lea, P.J.; Joy, K.W. Photorespiratory amino donors, sucrose synthesis and the induction of CO2 fixation in barley deficient in glutamine synthetase and/or glutamate synthase. J. Exp. Bot. 1988, 39, 845–858.

32. Wallsgrove, R.M.; Turner, J.C.; Hall, N.P.; Kendall, A.C.; Bright, S.W.J. Barley mutants lacking chloroplast glutamine synthetase: Biochemical and genetic analysis. Plant Physiol. 1987, 83, 155–158.

33. Socolow, R. Nitrogen management and the future of food: Lessons from the management of energy and carbon. Proc. Natl. Acad. Sci. USA 1999, 96, 6001–6008.

34. Guo, J.H.; Liu, X.J.; Zhang, Y.; Shen, J.L.; Han, W.X.; Zhang, W.F.; Christie, P.; Goulding, K.W.T.; Vitousek, P.M.; Zhang, F.S. Significant acidification in major Chinese croplands. Science 2010, 327, 1008–1010.

35. Zhang, Q.F. Strategies for developing green super rice. Proc. Natl. Acad. Sci. USA 2007, 104, 16402–16409.

36. Cai, H.; Xiao, J.; Zhang, Q.; Lian, X. Co-suppressed glutamine synthetase 2 gene modifies nitrogen metabolism and plant growth in rice. Chin. Sci. Bull. 2010, 55, 823–833.

37. Gutiérrez, R.A.; Lejay, L.; Dean, A.; Chiaromonte, F.; Shasha, D.E.; Coruzzi, G.M. Qualitative network models and genome wide expression data define carbon/nitrogen-responsive molecular machines inArabidopsis. Genome Biol. 2007, 8.

38. Vidal, E.A.; Gutiérrez, R.A. A systems view of nitrogen nutrient and metabolite responses inArabidopsis. Curr. Opin. Plant Biol. 2008, 11, 521–529.

39. Pant, B.D.; Musialak-Lange, M.; Nuc, P.; May, P.; Buhtz, A.; Kehr, J.; Walther, D.; Scheible, W.R. Identification of nutrient responsive Arabidopsis and rapeseed microRNAs by comprehensive real-time PCR profiling and small RNA sequencing. Plant Physiol. 2009, 150, 1541–1555.

40. Vidal, E.A.; Araus, V.; Lu, C.; Parry, G.; Green, P.J.; Coruzzi, G.M.; Gutiérrez, R.A. Nitrate-responsive miR393/AFB3 regulatory module controls root system architecture in Arabidopsis thaliana. Proc. Natl. Acad. Sci. USA 2010, 107, 4477–4482.

41. Schlüter, U.; Colmsee, C.; Scholz, U.; Bräutigam, A.; Weber, A.P.; Zellerhoff, N.; Bucher, M.; Fahnenstich, H.; Sonnewald, U. Adaptation of maize source leaf metabolism to stress related disturbances in carbon, nitrogen and phosphorus balance. BMC Genomics 2013, 14.

42. Bao, A.; Zhao, Z.; Ding, G.; Shi, L.; Xu, F.; Cai, H. Accumulated expression level of cytosolic glutamine synthetase 1 gene (OsGS1;1 or OsGS1;2) alter plant development and the carbon-nitrogen metabolic status in rice. PLoS ONE 2014, 9, e95581.

43. Kusano, M.; Tabuchi, M.; Fukushima, A.; Funayama, K.; Diaz, C.; Kobayashi, M.; Hayashi, N.; Tsuchiya, Y.N.; Takahashi, H.; Kamata, A.; et al. Metabolomics data reveal a crucial role of cytosolic glutamine synthetase 1;1 in coordinating metabolic balance in rice. Plant J. 2011, 66, 456–466.

44. Pérez-Delgado, C.M.; García-Calderón, M.; Sánchez, D.H.; Udvardi, M.K.; Kopka, J.; Márquez, A.J.; Betti, M. Transcriptomic and metabolic changes associated with photorespiratory ammonium accumulation in the model legume Lotus japonicas. Plant Physiol. 2013, 162, 1834–1848.

45. Näsholm, T.; Kielland, K.; Ganeteg, U. Uptake of organic nitrogen by plants. New Phytol. 2009, 182, 31–48.

46. Kielland, K. Amino-acid-absorption by arctic plants-implications for plant nutrition and nitrogen cycling. Ecology 1994, 75, 2373–2383.

47. Lipson, D.; Näsholm, T. The unexpected versatility of plants: Organic nitrogen use and availability in terrestrial ecosystems. Oecologia 2001, 128, 305–316.

48. Forsum, O.; Svennerstam, H.; Ganeteg, U.; Nasholm, T. Capacities and constraints of amino acid utilization in Arabidopsis. New Phytol. 2008, 179, 1058–1069. [PubMed]

49. Marschner, H. Mineral Nutrition of Higher Plants, 2nd Ed. ed; Academic Press Limited: San Diego, CA, USA, 1997.

50. Cambui, C.A.; Svennerstam, H.; Gruffman, L.; Nordin, A.; Ganeteg, U.; Nasholm, T. Patterns of plant biomass partitioning depend on nitrogen source. PLoS ONE 2011, 6, e19211.

51. Thornton, B.; Robinson, D. Uptake and assimilation of nitrogen from solutions containing multiple sources. Plant Cell Environ. 2005, 28, 813–821.

52. Wang, H.-J.; Wu, L.-H.; Wang, M.-Y.; Zhu, Y.-H.; Tao, Q.-N.; Zhang, F.-S. Effects of amino acids replacing nitrate on growth, nitrate accumulation, and macroelement concentrations in pak-choi (Brassica chinensis L.). Pedosphere 2007, 17, 595–600.

53. Henry, H.A.L.; Jefferies, R.L. Free amino acid, ammonium and nitrate concentrations in soil solutions of a grazed coastal marsh in relation to plant growth. Plant Cell Environ. 2002, 25, 665–675.

54. Bollard, E.G. A comparative study of the ability of organic nitrogenous compounds to serve as sole nitrogen sources of nitrogen for the growth of plants. Plant Soil 1966, 25, 153–166.

55. Yoshida, S.; Forno, D.A.; Cook, J.H.; Gomez, K.A. Laboratory Manual for Physiological Studies of Rice, 3rd ed.; International Rice Research Institute: Manila, Philippine, 1976.

56. Bradford, M.M. A rapid and sensitive method for the quantitation of microgram quantities of protein utilizing the principle of protein binding. Anal. Biochem. 1976, 72, 248–254.

57. Morris, D.L. Quantitative determination of carbohydrates with Dreywood's anthrone reagent. Science1948, 107, 254–255.

58. Maness, N. Extraction and analysis of soluble carbohydrates. Methods Mol. Biol. 2010, 639, 341–370. [PubMed]

59. Kusano, M.; Fukushima, A.; Arita, M.; Jonsson, P.; Moritz, T.; Kobayashi, M.; Hayashi, N.; Tohge, T.; Saito, K. Unbiased characterization of genotype-dependent metabolic regulations by metabolomic approach in Arabidopsis thaliana. BMC Syst. Biol. 2007, 1.

60. Kusano, M.; Fukushima, A.; Kobayashi, M.; Hayashi, N.; Jonsson, P.; Moritz, T.; Ebana, K.; Saito, K. Application of a metabolomic method combining one-dimensional and two-dimensional gas chromatographytime-of-flight/mass spectrometry to metabolic phenotyping of natural variants in rice.J. Chromatogr. B Anal. Technol. Biomed. Life Sci. 2007, 855, 71–79.

61. Redestig, H.; Fukushima, A.; Stenlund, H.; Moritz, T.; Arita, M.; Saito, K.; Kusano, M. Compensation for systematic cross-contribution improves normalization of mass spectrometry based metabolomics data. Anal. Chem. 2009, 81, 7974–7980.

2

# RESPONSE OF NITROGEN-FIXING WATER FERN AZOLLA BIOFERTILIZATION TO RICE CROP

**K. Bhuvaneshwari • Pawan Kumar Singh**

Center for Advanced Study in Botany, Banaras Hindu University (B.H.U.), Varanasi 221005, India

## ABSTRACT

The water fern *Azolla* harbors nitrogen-fixing cyanobacterium *Anabaena azollae* as symbiont in its dorsal leaves and is known as potent $N_2$ fixer. Present investigation was carried out to study the influence of fresh *Azolla* when used as basal incorporation in soil and as dual cropped with rice variety Mahsoori separately and together with and without chemical nitrogen fertilizer in pots kept under net house conditions. Results showed that use of *Azolla* as basal or dual or basal plus dual influenced the rice crop positively where use of fern as basal plus dual was superior and served the nitrogen requirement of rice. There was marked increase in plant height, number of effective tillers, dry mass and nitrogen content of rice plants with the use of*Azolla* and N-fertilizers alone and other combinations. The use of *Azolla* also increased organic matter and potassium contents of the soil.

**Keywords:** Rice Water fern *Azolla* Crop response Soil enrichment

# INTRODUCTION

The use of biofertilizers and green manures is not only a need for sustainable agriculture but also an environment friendly and economically feasible scientific method. The integrated use of organic and inorganic fertilizers is desirable to sustain crop yields and maintenance of soil health (Meelu and Singh 1991; Prasanna et al. 2008). *Azolla* is a free-floating water fern and has agronomic importance due to its ability to fix nitrogen (Singh 1977). It forms a nitrogen-fixing symbiosis with the cyanobacterium *Anabaena azollae*, which is present in the leaf cavity of the fern (Watanabe 1982, spore 1992). *Azolla* is grown as a green manure before transplantation of rice or as an intercrop with the rice. Both the practices are reported to increase the growth and yield of rice (Singh 1989; Singh and Singh 1995).

In Asia, *Azolla* is the most commonly used green manure for rice crop, due to its high growth rate, nitrogen-fixing capacity and ability to scavenge nutrients from soil and water. The fern doubles its biomass in 2–5 days under ideal environmental conditions (Watanabe et al. 1989).*Azolla* can supply more than half of the required nitrogen to the rice crop and besides providing nitrogen it is beneficial in wetland rice fields for bringing number of changes which include preventing rise in pH, reducing water temperature, curbing $NH_3$ volatilization, suppressing weeds and mosquito proliferation (Pabby et al. 2004).

Therefore, the present study was undertaken to examine the feasibility of using *Azolla* as nutritional alternative for rice crop. Consequently, the main objective of this work was to study the influence of *Azolla* as green manure or dual crop on rice crop growth and development.

# MATERIALS AND METHODS

Pot incubation experiment was conducted between June and October 2012 under net house condition at the Institute of Agricultural Sciences, Banaras Hindu University (B.H.U.), Varanasi, India. Soil samples used in this experiment were collected from Khaira, a village near Varanasi, India. All the samples were brought to the laboratory, where sieving was done with 2-mm sieve. Part of the sieved soil was air dried and some chemical properties were determined (Table 1). Five kg of soil was weighed with a balance and kept into each, 48 pots having holes at the base. There were three pots per treatment and the control experiment was inclusive. Six seedlings of Mahsoori rice variety were transplanted in each pot. *Azolla* was used as green manure (basal) and dual (associated), at the rate of 0.012 kg pot$^{-1}$ (2 ton ha$^{-1}$) and in basal treatments it was incorporated in soil before transplanting. Equal shares of *A. pinnata* and *A. filiculoides* were mixed for achieving a more stable plant growth. A list of treatments along with the abbreviations used in the text and figure is given in Table 2.

**Table 1.** Initial soil properties at the start of the experiment

| Soil parameters | Value |
|---|---|
| Organic matter (OM), % | 3.12 |
| Phosphorus (P), ppm | 54.0 |
| Calcium (Ca), kg ha$^{-1}$ | 17.2 |
| Potassium (K), kg ha$^{-1}$ | 0.19 |
| Magnesium (Mg), kg/ha$^{-1}$ | 2.4 |
| pH | 6.6 |

Nitrogen applied to each treatment:

The following measurements were performed:

- Plant height (at 100 % heading).
- Number of fertile tillers per plant (at 100 % heading).
- Dry mass.
- Nitrogen, phosphorus (P) and potassium (K) content.
- Soil chemical analysis (organic matter, pH, P, K, Ca and Mg).

Sampling was performed 45 days after incorporating *Azolla.*

The pH of the soil was determined using pH meter with glass-column combination electrode in distilled water and 0.01 M $CaCl_2$ solution at a ratio of 1:2 soil solution. The organic matter was determined using Walkley and Black method (Jackson 1967). Total nitrogen was determined by Kjeldahl method (Jackson 1973). Exchangeable K, Ca and Mg were extracted using ammonium acetate, K was determined on flame photometer and Ca and Mg by EDTA titration.

Statistical analysis was performed by Tukey HSD test using the SPSS 16.0 (Statistical package for Social Sciences) software package.

**Table 2.** Details of treatments and abbreviations used in the text

| S. no | Treatments | Abbreviations | Treatment no |
|---|---|---|---|
| 1 | Without nitrogen (Control) | 0N | T1 |
| 2 | 30 kg $ha^{-1}$ nitrogen | 30N | T2 |
| 3 | 60 kg $ha^{-1}$ nitrogen | 60N | T3 |
| 4 | 90 kg $ha^{-1}$ nitrogen | 90N | T4 |
| 5 | 0N + Basal *Azolla* (BA) | 0N + BA | T5 |
| 6 | 30N + Basal *Azolla* (BA) | 30N + BA | T6 |
| 7 | 60N + Basal *Azolla* (BA) | 60N + BA | T7 |
| 8 | 90N + Basal *Azolla* (BA) | 90N + BA | T8 |
| 9 | 0N + BA + Dual *Azolla* (DA) | 0N + BA + DA | T9 |
| 10 | 30N + BA + Dual *Azolla* (DA) | 30N + BA + DA | T10 |
| 11 | 60N + BA + Dual *Azolla* (DA) | 60N + BA + DA | T11 |
| 12 | 90N + BA + Dual *Azolla* (DA) | 90N + BA + DA | T12 |
| 13 | 0N + Dual *Azolla* (DA) | 0N + DA | T13 |
| 14 | 30N + Dual *Azolla* (DA) | 0N + DA | T14 |
| 15 | 60N + Dual *Azolla* (DA) | 0N + DA | T15 |
| 16 | 90N + Dual *Azolla* (DA) | 0N + DA | T16 |

# RESULTS

Figure 1 shows the behavior of the rice plant height, influenced by *Azolla* incorporation and/or association as well as different nitrogen (N) rates. An increase for this character is seen in treatments where incorporated and/or associated *Azolla* was used. However, nitrogen dose and*Azolla* influence did not show significant differences, expect for the treatments in which 30 kg ha$^{-1}$ N doses with $T_6$ incorporated *Azolla* and 60 kg ha$^{-1}$ N doses with $T_{11}$ incorporated and associated *Azolla* were applied. Treatments from $T_7$ to $T_{12}$ and $T_{14}$ to $T_{16}$, in which incorporated and/or associated *Azolla* was used, presented the greatest plant height values, without showing significant differences among them. Treatment $T_9$ stood out, in which nitrogen was not applied and both ways of *Azolla* were performed. It was also observed that treatments where *Azolla* was used without nitrogen also showed better behavior with significant differences in relation to control, which presented a poor plant growth, just 67.25 cm high.

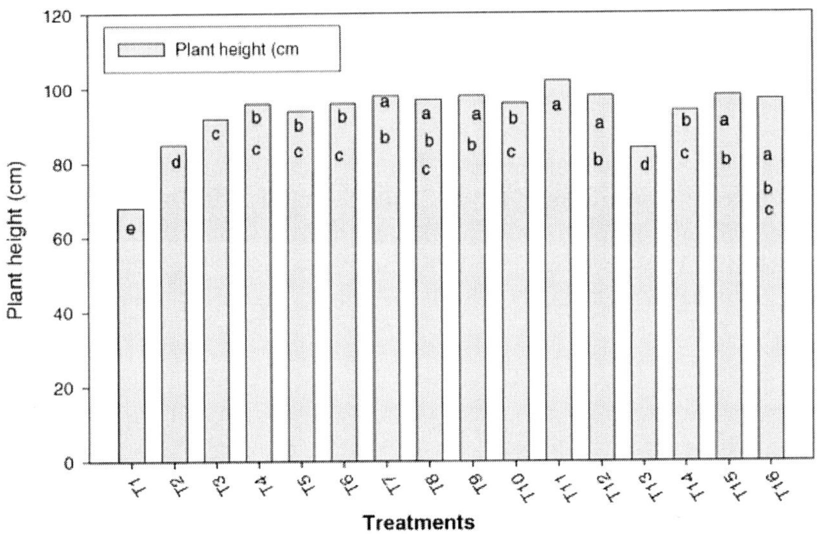


**Figure 1.** Influence of treatments on rice plant height

Figure 2 shows the number of effective tillers per plant. Nitrogen doses applied together with*Azolla* in this experiment influenced this variable as well. Treatments where *Azolla* was incorporated and/or associated ($T_8$, $T_{12}$, $T_{11}$, $T_{16}$, and $T_7$) stood out, for presenting the highest number of tillers per plant. (All the data are significant $p < 0.05$).

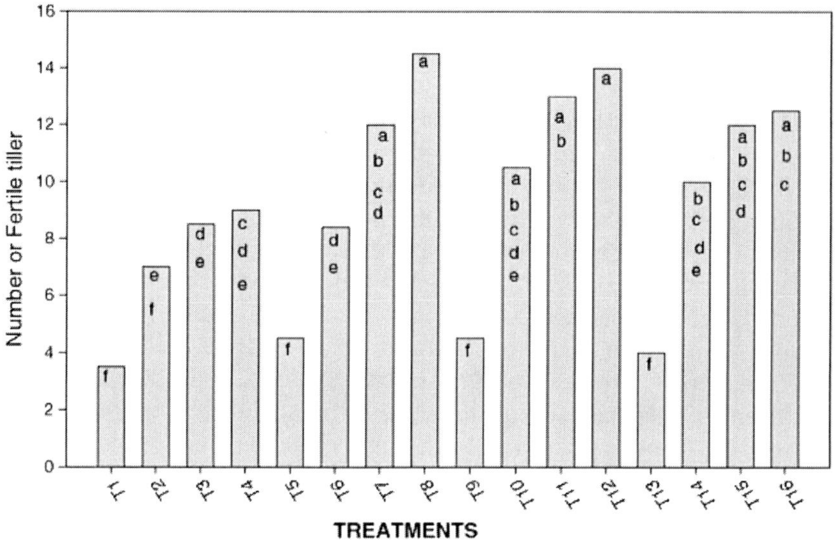


**Figure 2.** Influence of treatments on the number of fertile tillers *a, b, c, d, e, f, g, h, i* shows the significant differences on the basis of Tukey HSD

Figures 3 and 4 show nitrogen extracted by rice plants and plant dry mass at different variants, up to 100 % flowering. Like the number of tillers per plant and height, nitrogenous fertilization along with *Azolla* influenced nitrogen extracted by plants and dry mass production. Treatments $T_8$ and $T_{12}$ presented the highest nitrogen concentrations in plants. In both of them, incorporated *Azolla* and incorporated and associated *Azolla* at 90 kg ha$^{-1}$ N were used.

Figures 5 and 6 show the influence of associated and/or incorporated *Azolla* on phosphorus and potassium contents in rice plants, with different nitrogen doses, where both nutrients presented similar behavior to that of nitrogen, positively influenced by N fertilization and *Azolla*. In general, combining both ways of using *Azolla* surpassed the remaining treatments, followed by variants where *Azolla* was associated to rice crop, and where fern was incorporated.

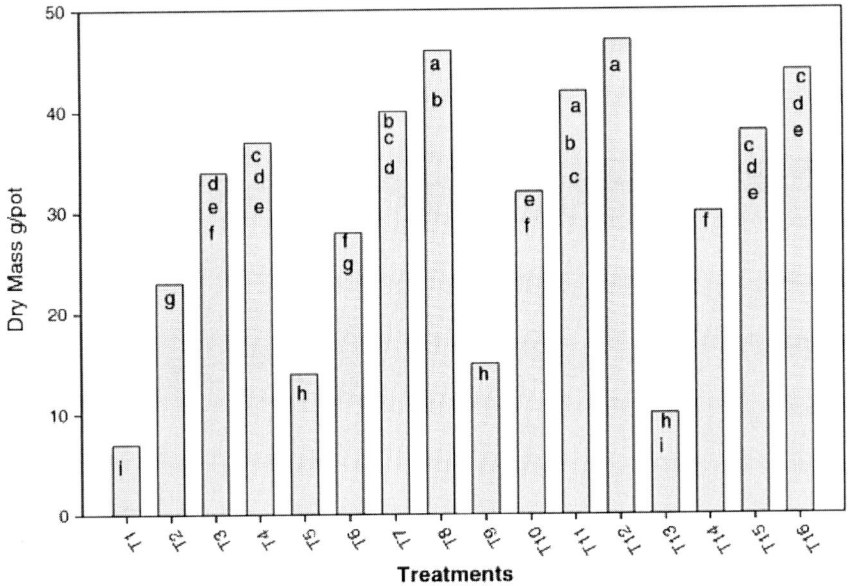


**Figure 3.** Influence of treatments on rice dry mass *a, b, c, d, e, f, g, h, i* shows the significant differences on the basis of Tukey HSD

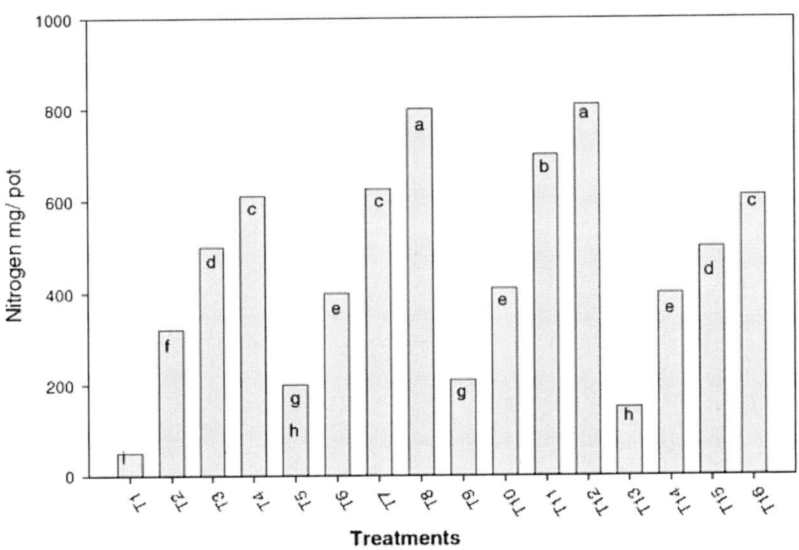


**Figure 4.** Influence of treatments on nitrogen content *a, b, c, d, e, f, g, h, i* shows the significant differences on the basis of Tukey HSD

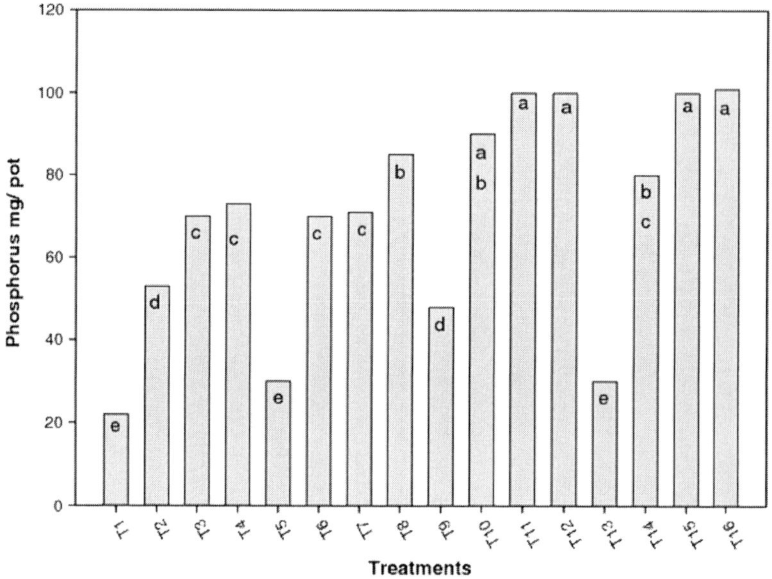


**Figure 5.** Influence of associated and incorporated Azolla on phosphorus contents in rice plants with different nitrogen doses *a, b, c, d, e, f, g, h, i* shows the significant differences on the basis of Tukey HSD

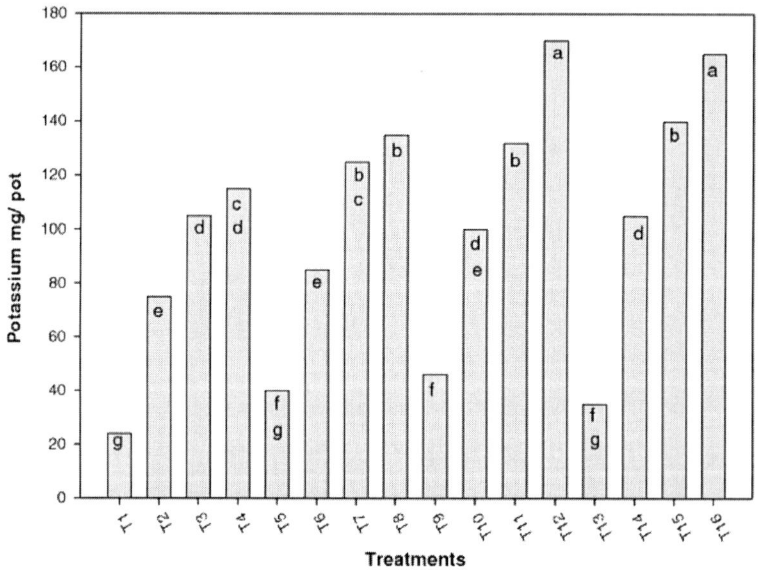


**Figure 6.** Influence of different treatments on potassium content in rice plants *a, b, c, d, e, f, g, h, i* shows the significant differences on the basis of Tukey HSD

When analyzing soil chemical features after incorporating *Azolla* (Table 3), it could be noticed that treatments did not influence pH, P, Ca and Mg. However, they did influence organic matter and potassium content. In this sense, the highest values were achieved by combining incorporated and associated *Azolla*, followed by treatments where *Azolla* was incorporated, leaving the third place of treatments in which the fern was associated to rice crop.

**Table 3.** Soil characteristic features after harvesting

| Treatments | pH | OM | P | K | Ca | Mg |
|---|---|---|---|---|---|---|
| T1 | 6.70c | 3.91ghi | 65.67abcd | 0.23e | 19.83 | 3.07 |
| T2 | 5.72bc | 3.89hi | 64.33abcd | 0.25cde | 19.67 | 3.67 |
| T3 | 6.72bc | 3.77i | 60.33cd | 0.24e | 20.33 | 3.67 |
| T4 | 6.72bc | 3.67i | 66.67ab | 0.25cde | 19.33 | 3.75 |
| T5 | 6.80ab | 4.47cde | 61.33bcd | 0.34ab | 19.50 | 3.00 |
| T6 | 6.71bc | 4.50cd | 60.00cd | 0.31ab | 19.58 | 3.00 |
| T7 | 6.78abc | 4.85ab | 61.00bcd | 0.29bcd | 19.67 | 3.04 |
| T8 | 6.76abc | 4.73bc | 66.67ab | 0.37a | 19.50 | 3.00 |
| T9 | 6.75abc | 4.70bc | 62.33bcd | 0.35ab | 20.08 | 3.00 |
| T10 | 6.80ab | 4.88ab | 68.67a | 0.31ab | 19.50 | 3.10 |
| T11 | 6.84a | 5.12a | 66.33abc | 0.3b | 19.50 | 3.10 |
| T12 | 6.77abc | 4.13fgh | 62.33bcd | 0.33ab | 19.58 | 3.12 |
| T13 | 6.82a | 4.16fgh | 64.33abcd | 0.24de | 19.33 | 3.04 |
| T14 | 6.80ab | 4.22def | 61.67bcd | 0.20e | 19.58 | 3.58 |
| T15 | 6.82a | 4.28def | 63.67abcd | 0.30bc | 19.25 | 3.54 |
| T16 | 6.77abc | 4.19efg | 69.66a | 0.31b | 19.67 | 3.33 |

a, b, c, d, e, f, g, h, i shows the significant differences on the basis of Tukey HSD

# DISCUSSION

An increase in plant height and number of tillers per plant was seen in the treatments where incorporated and/or associated *Azolla* was used. The highest value was achieved in treatment $T_{11}$, where 60 kg ha$^{-1}$ N was applied to rice plant (Figs. 1, 2). Treatment $T_9$ stood out, in which nitrogen was not applied and both ways of using *Azolla* were performed. This treatment seems to supply the nitrogen demands of rice plants. In, general terms, such behavior of rice height was caused by the influence of nitrogen content in the medium, which could be supplied through different ways and means, as reported earlier (Singh 1989; Baker 1999; Bhuvaneshwari2012; Bhuvaneshwari and Kumar 2013).

Like the number of tillers per plant and height, nitrogenous fertilization along with *Azolla*influenced nitrogen extracted by plants and dry mass production (Figs. 3, 4). Treatments combining both ways of using *Azolla* tended to produce more biomass than the remaining treatments with the same nitrogen dose. Therefore, combining incorporation and association of this fern not only serve to provide plants with significant amount of nitrogen, but also enables a better use of nitrogen added by mineral fertilization and thereby, a higher dry mass production. Similar results were recorded when *A. pinnata* was used by Manna and Singh (1990); Baker (2000); Bhuvaneshwari and Singh (2012).

For both above variables, it is highlighted the fact that nitrogen, phosphorus and potassium doses are inadequate for achieving good crop development, however, the influence of incorporated and/or associated *Azolla* allows a better use of nitrogen and better conditions for assimilating other nutrients, thus improving crop nutrition as reported by Samarajeewa (1999).

Treatment $T_8$ and $T_{12}$ presented the highest nitrogen concentration in the plants. In both of them, incorporated *Azolla* and 90 kg ha$^{-1}$ N were applied. The incorporation of this fern seems to maintain a higher soil nitrogen availability than its association, as observed by other workers (Singh 1989; Fageria et al. 1999; Baker 2000).

Regarding dry mass production and nitrogen content, in treatments where incorporated and associated *Azolla* were combined, value tended to be higher, compared to other treatments presenting the same nitrogen doses. This is caused by the influence of incorporated and associated *Azolla* on plant available nitrogen content in the soil, as a result of nitrogen release during fern decomposition, reduction in loss of nitrogen might have occured when applied as N fertilizer and that excreted into water by associated *Azolla* (de Macale et al. 2002).

Figures 5 and 6 show the influence of associated and incorporated *Azolla* on phosphorus and potassium contents in rice plants, combining both ways of using *Azolla* surpassed the remaining treatments, followed by the variants where *Azolla* was associated to rice crop, and where it was incorporated. This could be due to the influence of supplying these elements where fern is decomposed, as well as the effect on pH provoked by the associated *Azolla*, which increases the solubility of such elements. It was also reported that *Azolla* increased fertilizer efficiency, when applied in both ways (Pabby et al. 2004).

The soil chemical features are given in Table 3. Treatments did not influence pH, P, Ca and Mg. However, they did influence organic matter and potassium contents. Organic matter and potassium contents in the soil presented significant differences among treatments; the use of*Azolla* influenced both of them. The highest values were achieved by combining incorporated and associated *Azolla*, followed by treatments where *Azolla* was incorporated, third place was recorded given to the treatment in which fern was associated to rice crop. This is related to the contribution of *Azolla* after decomposition. Similar results were observed by other researchers (Singh 1979; Baker 1999).

The utilization of *Azolla* as a green manure benefits rice crop, obtaining the highest response when combining incorporation and association of this fern. It also favors nutrient absorption by rice and increases its yield, as well as organic matter content of the soil.

## ACKNOWLEDGMENTS

The first author is thankful to the department of science and Technology (DST), WOS-A, New Delhi, India for providing the funds. Thanks are also due to Head of Department of Botany and Prof. H. B. Singh, I.A.S. BHU, Varanasi for rendering laboratory and Net house facility.

## CONFLICT OF INTEREST

The authors declare that this research has no conflict of interest.

# REFERENCES


1. Baker ASS (1999) Nitrogen response of a Japonica and Indica variety under irrigated system. Report on experiments in rice research techniques course, vol 3. Tsukuba International center TBIC, Japan, pp 1–20
2. Baker R (2000) Experimental result in nitrogen response of rice. Disponible.http://www.3hawaii.edu/-jimi/publications.htm
3. Bhuvaneshwari K (2012) Beneficial effects of blue-green algae and *Azolla* in rice culture. Environ Conserv J 13(1 & 2):1–5
4. Bhuvaneshwari K, Kumar Ajay (2013) Agronomic potential of the association *Azolla-Anabaena*. Sci Res Report 3(1):78–82
5. Bhuvaneshwari K, Singh PK (2012) Organic rice production using organic manures and bio inoculants in alkaline soil. J Recent Adv Agric 1(4):128–134
6. de Macale MAR, Vlek PLG, San Valentine GD (2002) The role of *Azolla* cover in improving the nitrogen use efficiency of lowland rice. In: Proceedings of the conference sustaining food security and managing natural resource in Southeast Asia, Chiang Mai, Thailand
7. Fageria NK, Baliger VC (1999) Nitrogen management for low land rice production on dinceptisol. United States Department of Agriculture, Agricultural research Service, Tektran
8. Jackson ML (1967) Soil chemical analysis. Prentice Hall of India Pvt Ltd, New Delhi
9. Jackson ML (1973) Soil chemical analysis. Prentice Hall of India Pvt Ltd, New Delhi
10. Manna AB, Singh PK (1990) Growth and nitrogen fixation of *Azolla pinnata* and *Azolla caroliniana* as affected by urea in transplanted and direct seeded rice. Expl Agric 25:485–497
11. Meelu OP, Singh PK (1991) Integrated nutrient management through organic, bio and inorganic fertilization of crops. In: Meelu et al (eds) Micronutrients in soils and crops. Punjab Agricultural University, Ludhiana, pp 156–166
12. Pabby A, Prasanna R, Singh PK (2004) Biological significance of *Azolla* and its utilization in agriculture. Proc Indian Natl Sci Acad 70:299–333

13. Prasanna R, jaiswal P, Singh YV, Singh PK (2008) Influence of biofertilizers and organic amendments on nitrogenous activity and phototrophic biomass of soil under wheat. Aeta Agronomica Hungarica 56:149–159

14. Samarajeewa KBDP (1999) The effect of different timing of top dressing of nitrogen application and *Azolla* under low light intensity on the yield of rice (*Oryza sativa* L.) Report on experiments in rice research techniques course, vol 3. Tsukuba International Centre TBIC, Japan. International Co-operation Agency, Ibaraki, Japan, pp 71–79

15. Singh PK (1977) Multiplication and utilization of fern *Azolla* containing nitrogen fixing symbiont as green manure in rice cultivation. Riso 26:125–136

16. Singh PK (1979) Use of *Azolla* in rice production in India. Nitrogen and rice. International Rice Research Institute, Philippines, pp 407–418

17. Singh PK (1989) Use of *Azolla* in Asian agriculture. Appl Agric Res 4:149–161

18. Singh DP, Singh PK (1989) Growth and nitrogen fixation of *Azolla pinnata* and its effect on rice crop when incubated in different quantities after transplanting on rice. Thai J Agric Sci 22:25–35

19. Singh DP, Singh PK (1995) Response of *Azolla caroliniana* and rice to phosphorous enrichment of the *Azolla* inoculum and phosphorous fertilization during intercropping. Expt Agric 31:21–26

20. Spore (1992) *Azolla* a nitrogen source of rice farmers Bulletin of CTA no. 40 (CTA spore1992, 16P) Bimonthly bulletin of the technical center for agriculture and rural cooperation 40, p 5

21. Watanabe I (1982) *Azolla Anabaena* symbiosis—its physiology and use in tropical agriculture. In: Microbiology of tropical soil and plant productivity developments in plant and soil science, vol 5, pp 169–185

22. Watanabe I, Ventura W, Mascarina G, Eskew DL (1989) Fate of *Azolla* sp. and urea nitrogen applied to wetland rice (*Oryza sativa* L.). Biol Fertil Soils 8:102–110

# 3

# EFFECTS OF DIFFERENT FE SUPPLIES ON MINERAL PARTITIONING AND REMOBILIZATION DURING THE REPRODUCTIVE DEVELOPMENT OF RICE (ORYZA SATIVA L.)

**Raul Antonio Sperotto[1,2,3], Marta Wilton Vasconcelos[4], Michael Andrew Grusak[5] and Janette Palma Fett[1,2]**

[1]Centro de Biotecnologia, Universidade Federal do Rio Grande do Sul, 91501-970, Porto Alegre, RS, Brazil.

[2]Departamento de Botânica, Universidade Federal do Rio Grande do Sul, 91501-970, Porto Alegre, RS, Brazil.

[3]Centro de Ciências Biológicas e da Saúde, Centro Universitário UNIVATES, 95900-000, Lajeado, RS, Brazil.

[4]CBQF/Escola Superior de Biotecnologia, Universidade Católica Portuguesa, Rua Dr. António Bernardino de Almeida, 4200-072, Porto, Portugal.

[5] SDA/ARS Children's Nutrition Research Center, Department of Pediatrics, Baylor College of Medicine, 1100 Bates Street, Houston, TX 77030, USA.

# ABSTRACT

## Background

Minimal information exists on whole-plant dynamics of mineral flow through rice plants and on the source tissues responsible for mineral export to developing seeds. Understanding these phenomena in a model plant could help in the development of nutritionally enhanced crop cultivars. A whole-plant accumulation study, using harvests during reproductive development under different Fe supplies, was conducted to characterize mineral accumulation in roots, non-flag leaves, flag leaves, stems/sheaths, and panicles of Kitaake rice plants.

## Results

Low Fe supply promoted higher accumulation of Zn, Cu and Ni in roots, Mn, Ca, Mg and K in leaves and Zn in stems/sheaths and a smaller accumulation of Fe, Mn and Ca in roots and Zn and Ni in leaves. High Fe supply promoted higher accumulation of Fe in roots and Zn in leaves and a smaller accumulation of Fe in leaves and stems/sheaths and Zn, Cu and K in roots. Correlation analyzes indicated that fluctuations in Mn-Ca, Zn-Cu, Zn-Ni, Cu-Ni, Mo-S, Ca-Mg, Cu-Mn and Cu-Mg concentrations in response to different Fe supplies were positively correlated in at least four of the five organs analyzed.

## Conclusions

Mineral content loss analysis indicated that mineral remobilization from vegetative organs can occur in rice plants; however, for seeds to acquire minerals, vegetative remobilization is not absolutely required. Also, mineral remobilization from vegetative tissues in rice was greatly dependent of plant Fe nutrition. Remobilization was observed for several minerals from flag leaves and stems/sheaths, but the amounts were generally far below the total mineral accretion observed in panicles, suggesting that continued uptake and translocation of minerals from the roots during seed fill are probably more important than mineral remobilization.


**Keywords:** Biofortification Elemental analysis Ionomics Iron (Fe) Kitaake Mineral partitioning Reproductive development of rice

**Background**

Plants are the primary source of nutrients for human nutrition on a global basis. Staple seed crops, such as rice, supply the majority of daily dietary nutrients for billions of people. However, rice has a low density of mineral nutrients, and for those whose diets are high in staple foods, micronutrient malnutrition is widespread (Grusak and DellaPenna1999). Biofortification, which consists of the use of plant breeding and/or transgenic approaches to develop new cultivars with the potential to increase the nutrient concentration of edible portions of crop plants (White and Broadley2005), has emerged as one possible solution to alleviate malnutrition. Despite the increasing number of studies about the physiology and regulation of uptake of several minerals from the rhizosphere, the lack of knowledge about how minerals are moved into or out of vascular tissues, translocated to vegetative tissues and loaded into seeds is one of the barriers to seed biofortification (Colangelo and Guerinot2006).

Initial seed biofortification efforts for Fe and Zn in rice have focused on increasing the iron storage protein ferritin (Goto et al.1999; Vasconcelos et al.2003) or root ferric reductase activity (Vasconcelos et al.2004). The transgenic plants showed overaccumulation of minerals in leaves, but only a small increase in seeds. Grain Zn and Fe concentrations were increased in barley (*Hordeum vulgare*) expressing the Zn transporter *ZIP1* from *Arabidopsis thaliana* (Ramesh et al.2004), and were decreased in wheat (*Triticum aestivum*) expressing RNAi constructs that lowered *NAM* family gene expression (Uauy et al.2006). Vasconcelos et al. (2006) constitutively expressed the root ferric reductase *FRO2* from *A. thaliana* in soybean and observed that, in certain hydroponic growth conditions, the transgenic plants showed a threefold increase in leaf Fe concentration, but only a 10% increase in seed Fe. Similar results were found with the *brz* mutant of *Pisum sativum*, which overaccumulates Fe in leaves but has normal seed Fe concentrations (Grusak1994). Analysis of mineral overaccumulation mutants indicates that translocation of minerals to seeds is tightly regulated, and that simply increasing net mineral uptake into the plant will probably not result in seeds with higher mineral concentrations. Additional regulatory mechanisms or transport capabilities must be manipulated to improve remobilization and pass through of minerals from vegetative organs into seeds. Recently, over-expression of barley genes related to phytosiderophore synthesis resulted in enhanced Fe and Zn concentrations in rice unpolished and polished seeds (Masuda et al.2008; Masuda et al.2009). Enhanced expression of the three genes from the rice nicotianamine synthase family (*OsNAS* genes) also facilitated increases in Fe and Zn concentrations of rice grains (Lee et al.2009; Zheng et al.2010; Johnson et al.2011; Lee et al.2011). All of these results suggest that the most successful breeding or transgenic approaches will likely need to target multiple genes simultaneously (Waters and Grusak2008, Sperotto et al.2012).

It is accepted that minerals may be remobilized from vegetative sources (Hocking and Pate1977; Himelblau and Amasino2001), although a major portion of minerals in seeds are likely supplied through continuous uptake and translocation during reproductive growth to developing seeds. In wheat, Zn (Hocking1994) and Fe (Garnett and Graham2005) remobilization from leaves was observed. According to Jiang et al. (2007b), when $^{65}Zn$ is applied to rice leaves (either the flag leaf or the lowest senescent leaf), 45-50% is transported out of the treated leaf. From that Zn, more than 90% is translocated to other vegetative organs; little is partitioned to the panicle parts and even less to the grains. These results suggest that, in rice plants grown under sufficient or surplus Zn supply, most of the Zn accumulated in the grain originates from uptake by roots after flowering and not from Zn remobilization from leaves. In another study, Zn was applied to rice plants in various amounts and at various stages of plant development. Analysis of the total plant Zn and Zn content in individual organs at flowering and at maturity indicated that the presence of Zn in grains could be fully attributed to additional Zn uptake after flowering, except when application rates were very low (Jiang et al.2008). Under the latter conditions, roots, stems and sheaths contributed mostly to Zn allocation. None of the rice Zn-application treatments showed that the main portion of Zn loaded in grain was remobilized from leaves (Jiang et al.2008; Stomph et al.2009). Contrastingly, Wu et al. (2010) showed that large amounts of the Zn deposited in the rice grains at maturity had been retranslocated from other plant parts and not been transported directly after uptake to the grains in the grain-filling stage. Recently, Yoneyama et al. (2010) reported that Zn in the rice grains and partly in the husks may be actively supplied via the phloem after mobilization from the blades of the flag and upper leaves and also by xylem-to-phloem transfer in the nodes. Fe stored in the flag and upper leaves may be transported to the grains via the phloem. Fang et al. (2008) showed that foliar application of Zn and Se can influence the Zn, Se, and Fe content of rice grains; however, it was difficult to improve the Fe nutrition of rice grain by Fe spray, probably due to its limited mobility in the phloem. Waters and Grusak (2008) suggested that, in *Arabidopsis*, continuous uptake and translocation of minerals to source tissues during seed fill are as important, if not more important, than remobilization of previously stored minerals.

Uncovering the genetic architecture underlying mineral ion homeostasis in plants is a critical first step towards understanding the biochemical and physiological processes that regulate a plant's elemental composition. In this paper, we assess growth dynamics of the whole plant (panicles, non-flag leaves, flag leaves, stems/sheaths and roots) over the reproductive development of *Oryza sativa*. We also describe the concentrations and contents of ten mineral nutrients (Fe, Zn, Cu, Mn, Mo, Ni, Ca, Mg, K and S) in these organs over time. Additionally, we studied the net loss of mineral contents to investigate the potential of vegetative tissues as sources of stored minerals to be remobilized to panicles. To address the question of whether different Fe supplies could influence mineral partitioning and movement of minerals to panicles, we compared these parameters in plants treated with low, normal and high Fe concentrations.

## RESULTS

To test if different Fe supplies would influence mineral accumulation in rice organs, we cultivated Kitaake plants with 5, 20 or 200 μM of Fe(III)-HEDTA from the panicle exertion (PE) until the full maturity (FM) stage. Different Fe supplies caused slight growth changes in panicles collected at the grain filling (GF) stage, while no changes were seen at the full maturity stage (Figure1). High Fe concentration (200 μM) caused a decrease of about 50% in panicle dry weight compared to the control concentration (20 μM). However, no impact on dry weight was seen in other organs, possibly because the high Fe treatment used in this work did not lead to enough Fe accumulation to reach toxic levels (300 $\mu g\ g^{-1}$ DW – Sahrawat2004) in all aerial plant organs (Additional file1). A panicle weight reduction of about 22% (not statistically significant) was seen when plants were cultivated with limited Fe supply (5 μM), relative to 20 μM Fe controls. Therefore, the different Fe supplies used in this work during reproductive development did not result in different dry weight in most organs. Changes in mineral contents (Additional file2) were mainly dependent on changes in mineral concentrations.

Most of the changes in mineral concentrations resulting from different Fe supplies were found during full maturity stage. Panicle (along with flag leaf) was the organ with the least variation in mineral concentrations caused by different Fe supplies (Additional file1, Additional file3 and Additional file4). At GF stage, only Fe (Additional file1a), Ni (Additional file3k) and Mg (Additional file4f) concentrations

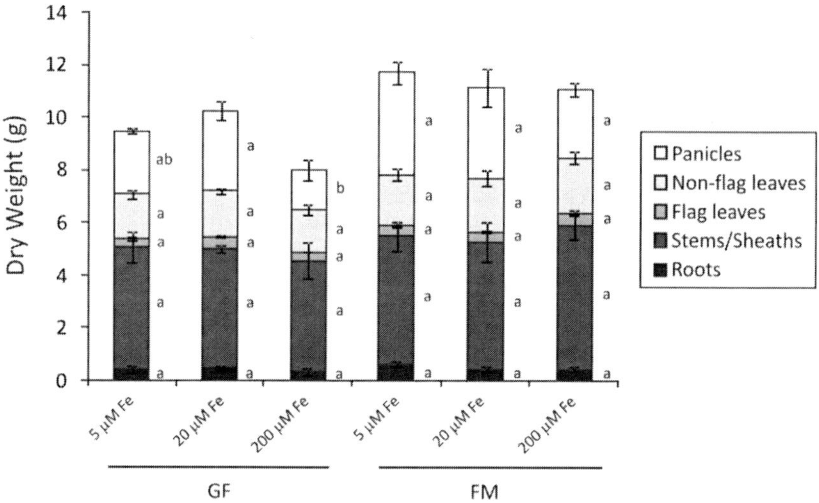


**Figure 1. Dry weight of rice organs.** Dry weight of panicles, non-flag leaves, flag leaves, stems/sheaths and roots collected during grain filling (GF) and full maturity (FM) stages of rice plants supplied with 5, 20 or 200 μM of Fe(III)-HEDTA from panicle exertion (PE) onwards. Values are the averages of at least three samples ± SE. Different letters indicate that the means (between different Fe supplies) are different by the Tukey HSD test ($P \leq 0.05$). Error bars may be too small to be visible in the figure.

showed differences due to the Fe supply. However, the decrease in panicle dry weight detected in plants cultivated with high Fe concentration during GF stage (< 50%; Figure1) resulted in decreased content in most of the minerals analyzed, except Fe, Mo and K (Additional file2). At FM stage, none of the minerals analyzed showed difference in the content between control (20 μM) and high Fe (200 μM) condition (Additional file2).

In non-flag leaves, no obvious mineral concentration dynamic could be detected. High Fe supply was responsible for higher Fe concentration (Additional file1b) and for lower Cu (Additional file1L), Mo (Additional file3g), Ca (Additional file4b) and S (Additional file4q) concentrations. Low Fe supply was responsible for higher Mn (Additional file3b) and Ni (Additional file3L) concentrations during GF and FM; Ca (Additional file4b) and Mg (Additional file4g) during FM and K (Additional file4L) during GF stage.

In flag leaves, most of the mineral concentrations (including Fe and Zn) were not affected by different Fe supplies. During GF stage, only Mo (Additional file3h), Mg (Additional file4h) and S (Additional file4r) concentrations were reduced by low and/or high Fe concentrations. During FM stage, along with Mo, Mg and S, the concentrations of Cu (Additional file1m), Mn (Additional file3c) and Ca (Additional file4c) also presented variations according to the Fe supply.

In stems/sheaths, most of the modifications in mineral concentrations found in plants collected at the GF stage were under high Fe supply. Only Fe (Additional file1d), Cu (Additional file1n) and Ni (Additional file3n) maintained similar concentrations independent of the Fe supply. During FM stage, Fe was the only mineral whose concentration increased at 200 μM Fe (Additional file1d). All the other minerals reached higher mineral concentrations at 5 μM Fe.

In roots, all the minerals analyzed, except K (Additional file4o) and S (Additional file4t), presented different concentrations when plants were cultivated with different Fe supplies. As expected, root Fe concentration was higher under 200 μM Fe (2.2X in GF and 4.2X in FM; Additional file1e). The opposite was found for Zn (Additional file1j), Cu (Additional file1o), Mo (Additional file3j) and Ni (Additional file3o), with higher concentrations under lower Fe supply. K (Additional file4o) and S (Additional file4t) concentrations were not affected by different Fe supplies.

Pearson's correlation analysis was performed in order to find relationships among the ten mineral concentrations in response to the different Fe supplies. As seen in Figure2, most of the correlations were found during full maturity (FM) stage, after a longer period under different Fe supplies. Negative correlations were found mainly in roots. During grain filling (GF) stage, the only pair of minerals positively correlated in every tested organ was Mn-Ca. These were also positively correlated during FM stage in all tested organs, along with Zn-Cu. Positive correlations at FM between the pairs Zn-Ni and Cu-Ni were found in four of the five tested organs, except in flag leaves. Similar dynamic was found for Mo-S and Ca-Mg, which were not correlated only in panicles. Cu-Mn and Cu-Mg were also positively correlated in four of the five tested organs, except in roots, showing a negative correlation in this organ (Figure2).

Differences in plant size were responsible for the high standard error in mineral contents (Additional file2). Therefore, partition quotient (PQ) values were calculated to allow comparison of the dynamics of partitioning of minerals between the reproductive development of rice plants cultivated with different Fe supplies (Figure3), since this approach is able to check if one mineral content is higher in one specific organ, regardless of differences in plant size. In general, non-flag leaves,

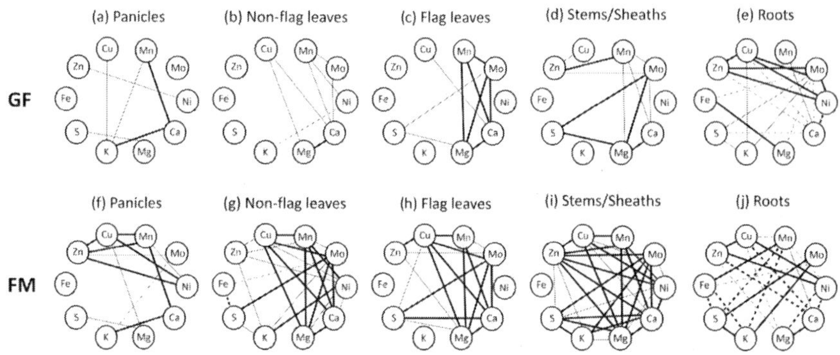


**Figure 2. Mineral correlation analyses.** Pearson's correlation analysis of ten mineral concentrations in panicles (**a** and **f**), non-flag leaves (**b** and **g**), flag leaves (**c** and **h**), stems/sheaths (**d** and **i**) and roots (**e** and **j**) of rice plants cultivated with 5, 20 and 200 µM of Fe(III)-HEDTA during grain filling (GF) and full maturity (FM) stages. Solid lines represent a significant positive correlation and dashed lines represent a significant negative correlation. Thinner lines indicate significance at the 0.05 level and thicker lines indicate significance at the 0.01 level.

flag leaves and roots were the organs which showed the higher mineral PQ variation according to Fe supply, whereas stems/sheaths was the organ with lower variation (Figure3). For Fe, PQ values above 100 were found only in roots (Figure3a), with higher values in plants cultivated with 200 µM Fe. In all the other organs, high Fe supply was responsible for the lowest Fe PQ value, especially during FM (Additional file5). Also, in this stage, control Fe supply (20 µM Fe) resulted in higher PQ values (Additional file5). For Zn, low Fe supply resulted in the lowest Zn PQ values in panicles, non-flag leaves and flag leaves, and high Fe supply resulted in the highest Zn PQ values (Figure3b). In stems/sheaths (during FM) and roots (during both stages), the opposite was found, with higher Zn PQ values under low Fe supply (Figure3b). Similar pattern was found for Cu (Figure3c) and Ni (Figure3f) PQ in roots. For Mn, no obvious pattern could be identified, except the higher PQ values in non-flag and flag leaves under Fe deprivation and in panicles and roots under Fe excess, both during FM (Figure3d). Mo (Figure3e) and S (Figure3j) were the minerals with the most stable PQ values. For Ca (Figure3g) and Mg (Figure3h) high PQ values were obtained in non-flag and flag leaves during FM stage under Fe starvation. Low Fe supply also resulted in extremely reduced Ca PQ values in roots (Figure3g), in relation to values seen in the other treatments.

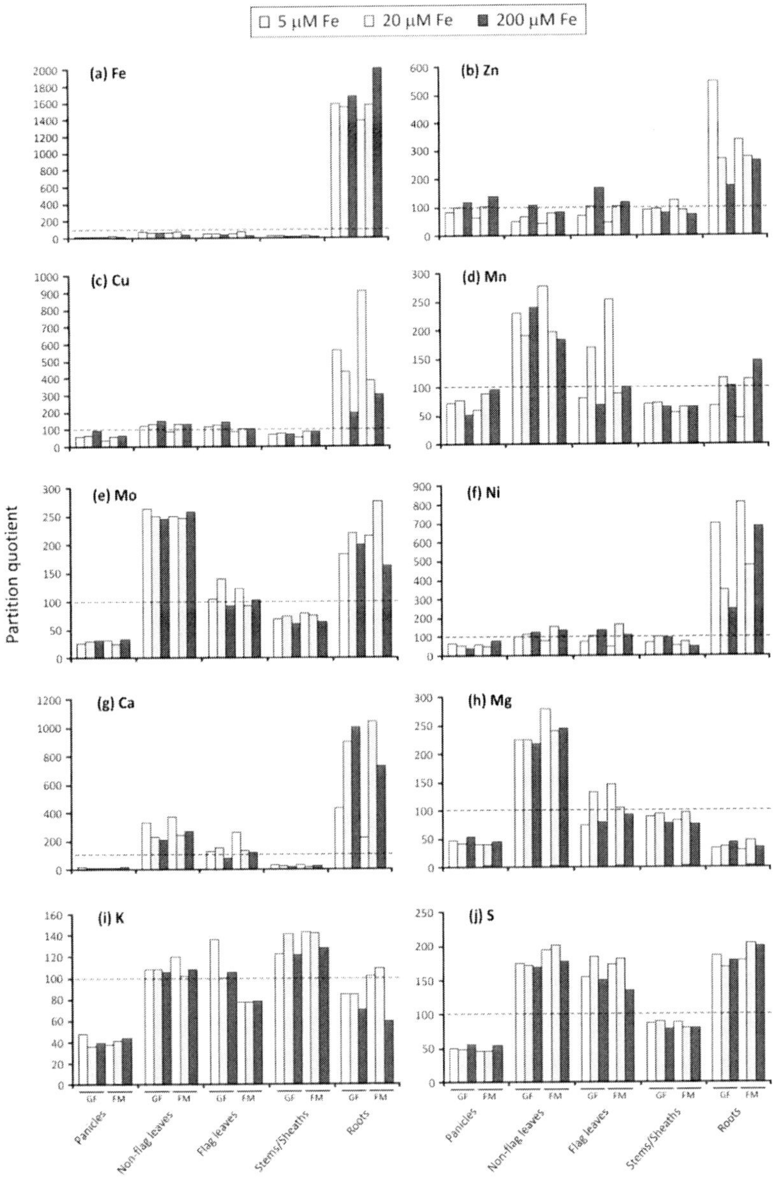


**Figure 3. Partition quotients (PQ) analyses.** Partition quotients of mineral elements in panicles, non-flag leaves, flag leaves, stems/sheaths and roots during grain filling (GF) and full maturity (FM) stages of rice plants supplied with 5, 20 or 200 µM of Fe(III)-HEDTA from panicle exertion onwards. Dashed horizontal line represents PQ of 100 (the percentage contribution of the organ to the plant's dry weight is the same as the percentage contribution to the plant's total content of the mineral being evaluated).

To investigate the potential of vegetative tissues as a source of stored minerals to be remobilized to panicles, we estimated the net loss of mineral content from non-flag leaves, flag leaves and stems/sheaths, by subtracting final mineral content from the prior time point which had the highest mineral content. As seen in Figure4, net loss of mineral content could be discerned under different Fe supplies. Under control Fe concentration (20 µM), all the minerals showed content loss from GF to FM stage (Figure4b), mostly from flag leaves but also from stems/sheaths. However, as the flag leaves' mineral content is much lower than the stems/sheaths' content, the maximum possible contribution to panicle mineral content, assuming that the total net loss of each mineral was translocated to panicles before the final collection point, is in general higher from stems/sheaths than from flag leaves. Different Fe supplies influenced the content loss of most of the minerals. Under limited Fe condition (5 µM), only Fe, Mn and Mg showed a net remobilization from stems/sheaths; and K from flag leaves. Under high Fe condition (200 µM), only K and S showed a net remobilization from flag leaves; and Ni from stems/sheaths. Surprisingly, no remobilization was found from non-flag leaves, except a minimum K remobilization under 20 µM Fe, which could have contributed at most only with 5% of total panicle K content (Figure4e). For most of the minerals analyzed, except Ni and Ca, the maximum possible contribution of remobilization from flag leaves and stems/sheaths to the final panicle's mineral content is less than 40%, being less than 20% for Fe, Zn, Cu, Mn and S. Ni and Ca remobilization from flag leaves and mostly from stems/sheaths could be responsible for more than 100% of the final panicle content (Figure4e), showing that remobilization does not necessarily correspond to mineral translocation to the panicles.

To determine whether different Fe supplies could result in different mineral export to developing seeds, we submitted rice plants to the same Fe conditions as the previous experiment (although 0 µM Fe was included in this analysis). In general, the dynamics of mineral concentrations of seeds (Additional file6) were similar to those of panicles; that is, higher Fe and lower Zn and Mo concentrations under 200 µM Fe. Fe, Cu, Mn, Mg and S showed the lowest and Zn, Mo and Ni showed the highest concentrations under Fe deprivation (Additional file6).

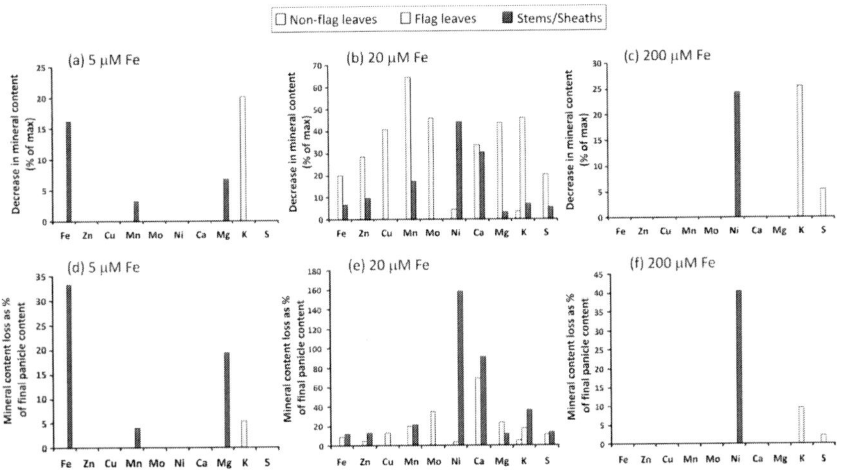


**Figure 4. Mineral remobilization analyses.** Percentage decrease in non-flag leaves, flag leaves and stems/sheaths mineral contents from grain filling to full maturity stages (**a**) and potential contribution of remobilized mineral to panicle mineral contents at the final time point (**b**).

# DISCUSSION

Plants are commonly faced with fluctuations in nutrient supply to the roots. To cope with these fluctuations, plants invoke a range of mechanisms, which include different uptake rates, changes in root morphology and physiology or storage and remobilization of mineral nutrients (Marschner1995). In this study, we characterized organ-specific changes in dry matter and mineral (Fe, Zn, Cu, Mn, Mo, Ni, Ca, Mg, K and S) content to monitor the net flow of minerals into and through the rice plant over the reproductive development and under different Fe supplies. Any increase in mineral content in one organ must have resulted from uptake and translocation from the soil, or from remobilization from one organ to another. By harvesting all the organs and tracking the mineral partitioning in these organs over time, remobilization can be estimated for each mineral. In this work we used the same remobilization definition used by Waters and Grusak (2008), which is defined as the net loss of stored or recycled mineral content from one organ over time, with the mineral loss representing movement into another organ.

Effects of low and high Fe supplies on mineral dynamics

As shown in Additional file2 and Figure3, low Fe supply (5 μM) allows higher accumulation of Zn, Cu and Ni in roots; Mn, Ca, Mg and K in leaves and Zn in stems/sheaths. On the other hand, low Fe supply allows a smaller accumulation of Fe, Mn and Ca in roots and Zn and Ni in leaves. Enhancement of Zn uptake under low Fe supply, either as a divalent cation or complexed to phytosiderophores (Zhang et al.1998), could explain its higher accumulation in roots. Several Fe transporters are able to transport also Zn and Mn (Korshunova et al.1999; Eckhardt et al.2001; Gross et al.2003; López-Millán et al.2004). Induction of Fe transporters under low Fe concentration could result in increased Zn uptake and translocation to stems/sheaths and increased Mn uptake and subsequent translocation to leaves, since Mn moves easily from root to shoot in the xylem-sap transpiration stream (Ramani and Kannan1987). Possibly, uptake of Mn and Cu may increase in rice plants under low Fe supply, because the presence of phytosiderophores in the rhizosphere may increase the availability of these ions both in the rhizosphere itself and in the apoplast (Zhang et al.1991). The complex Cu-phytosiderophore can be transported into root cells by Fe-phytosiderophore transporters, although with lower affinity (Briat et al.1995). Fertilizing a calcareous soil with an Fe-deficient solution increased Cu accumulation by roots and shoots in two wheat cultivars (Chaignon et al.2002). It has been suggested that Cu, Zn and Ni share a common uptake system (Kochian1991), which could explain the higher accumulation of Ni in roots under low Fe supply. In fact, Eckhardt et al. (2001) proposed that the Fe transporters IRT1 and IRT2 from tomato could also transport $Ni^{2+}$. Differently from our results, Silveira et al. (2007) detected increased Ca and K concentrations under Fe-deficiency in roots of rice, instead of in leaves. Possible explanations for such difference in Ca dynamic under low Fe supply are that we have used a different rice cultivar, a completely different technique for mineral detection (ICP-OES versus PIXE), different levels of Fe supply (5 μM Fe versus Fe deprivation) and we analyzed rice organs through the course of reproductive development instead of during vegetative development.

In rice, Fe toxicity seems to occur above 500 μg Fe $g^{-1}$ leaf dry weight (Audebert2006) and leads to a drastic reduction of root growth (Becker and Asch 2005). As shown in Figure1 and Additional file1, our plants cultivated with high Fe supply did not present reduction of root growth and did not reach toxic levels. However, the treatment resulted in decreased dry weight of panicles collected during grain filling (Figure1). In fact, depending on the site and the cultivars used, reported critical concentrations can range from 20 to 2,500 μg $g^{-1}$, indicating that factors other than Fe concentration influence the occurrence of Fe toxicity symptoms (Becker and Asch2005). In this way, the fluctuations in mineral accumulations found in the present work do not reflect the changes promoted by Fe toxicity. High Fe supply (200 μM) promoted a higher accumulation of Fe in roots and Zn in leaves. On the other hand, it promoted a smaller accumulation of Fe in leaves and stems/sheaths and Zn, Cu and K in roots (Additional file2, Figure3 and Additional file5). As expected, high Fe supply resulted in higher Fe accumulation in roots. However, root Fe measurements could be over-estimated. The oxidation ability of the rice root precipitates inactive Fe at the root apoplast and root-environment interface. The sampling technique used did not separate the existing oxidized Fe at the root surface. Thus, the root Fe content measured comprised the root Fe uptake and the oxidized Fe at the root surface. Most of this Fe seems to not be translocated to shoots, since smaller Fe PQ values were detected in leaves and stems/sheaths (Figure3), even with the increased Fe content in non-flag leaves (Additional file2). Under Fe-excess (500 mg $L^{-1}$), Silveira et al. (2007) reported that rice roots and also shoots accumulate higher Fe concentration. In that work, higher concentrations of Fe were detected in I409 plants, more susceptible to Fe toxicity. Shoot concentrations detected were up to 2.5X higher than in E108 plants (tolerant to Fe toxicity) after 10 days of treatment. The authors suggested, therefore, that E108 plants were more resistant to excess Fe due to the possible induction of avoidance mechanisms, allowing the plant to decrease Fe translocation to shoots. This avoidance mechanism was recently reviewed by Sperotto et al. (2010). In our work, Kitaake plants seem to use the avoidance mechanism, but additional studies are needed to confirm the hypothesis that Kitaake is an Fe-excess-tolerant rice cultivar.

In accordance with our results, Silveira et al. (2007) also detected higher Zn concentration in shoots of plants under Fe-excess. Also in accordance to our results, smaller K (Neue et al.1998; Ramirez et al.2002; Mehraban et al.2008) and Cu (Shao et al.2007; Silveira et al.2007) absorption rates under Fe-excess have already been reported in rice. It seems that, under Fe-excess, the relatively high ferrous iron concentration in the soil solution and uptake by the plant may result in K deficiency (Audebert2006). On the other hand, it appears that proper K supply may increase Fe exclusion from roots and reduce translocation of Fe to aerial plant organs, especially to upper leaves (Sahrawat2004).

Significant correlations were found among the ten mineral element concentrations in rice organs of plants facing different Fe supplies. In particular, Mn-Ca and Zn-Cu were positively correlated in all analyzed organs. Zn-Ni, Cu-Ni, Mo-S, Ca-Mg, Cu-Mn and Cu-Mg were positively correlated in four of the five organs (Figure2). Most of the available data about mineral correlation in plants were obtained in grains. As far as we know, this is the first work which tries to identify similar patterns of mineral fluctuations in different plant organs due to different Fe supplies. In this way, significant positive correlations between minerals suggest that different Fe supplies promote similar changes in their concentrations. Fe concentration was positively correlated with only two minerals (Mn and Mg) in roots (Figure2e and j). It is already known that Fe transporters can also transport Mn (Korshunova et al.1999; Eckhardt et al.2001; Gross et al.2003; López-Millán et al.2004) and high positive correlation between Fe and Mn was found in rice grains, along with Mn-Ca, Zn-Cu, Ca-Mg, and Cu-Mn (Jiang et al.2007a), in accordance with our findings. However, no Fe-Mn correlations were found in other rice organs. One possible explanation is that Mn moves easily from the root to the shoot in the xylem-sap transpirational stream (Ramani and Kannan1987), and the mobility of Fe is more regulated (Marschner 1995). The physiological significance of the correlation between Fe-Mg is unknown, but Jiang et al. (2007a) have already detected such relation in milled rice. These authors suggest that the high number of positive correlations in rice is probably due to the interaction between ions whose chemical properties are sufficiently similar, and such similarity allows the competition for site of absorption, transport and function in plant tissues. One example was shown by Kupper and Kupper (1998), which reported that the heavy metals (Hg, Cu, Cd, Ni, and Pb) might substitute Mg, the central atom of chlorophyll. This could help to explain the positive correlations we found between Cu and Mg in all the organs, except in roots (Figure2). Zeng et al. (2005) also found that Mn is positively associated with Ca in rice grains and Majumder et al. (1990) reported that uptake of Mn and Ca are positively correlated in rice cultivated in P-deficient soil, along with uptake of Ca and Mg.

Various molecules are known to bind minerals in rice organs and could explain some of the correlations detected, such as Ca-K in panicles, because both minerals bind to phytic acid in the aleurone layer of rice grain (Lin et al.2005). Similarly, many of the micronutrient correlations found in various organs could be attributed to nicotianamine or deoxymugineic acid, as these are known chelators of several metal cations in plant tissues (Curie et al.2009). However, further studies are needed to confirm the possibility of the same chelating molecules being involved in the mineral correlations detected.

Mineral remobilization versus continued supply from roots

The dynamics of mineral concentrations in seeds of plants cultivated with different Fe supplies showed that higher Fe supply results in higher Fe concentration in the seeds (Additional file6), implying that the uptake and transport systems were operating below capacity when plants were grown with lower Fe concentrations. As previously shown by Fang et al. (2008), it is difficult to improve the Fe nutrition of rice grain, even by Fe spray, possibly due to its limited mobility in the phloem. Probably, enhanced root uptake combined with leaf/stem/sheath efflux transport can be an effective way to increase the Fe concentration in rice grains.

Remobilization of reserves to supply rice seeds with minerals has been emphasized in previous studies (Jiang et al.2007b; Fang et al.2008; Jiang et al.2008; Wu et al.2010; Yoneyama et al.2010), but the contribution of stored minerals to total seed mineral content is unclear. According to Waters and Grusak (2008), it is expected that a minimal amount of each mineral is incorporated into structural or protein molecules and thus unavailable for mobilization, and that source tissues would have to accumulate minerals in excess of this minimal amount to allow mobilization to growing tissues such as seeds. This was the case for S in soybean leaves (Sunarpi and Anderson1996), where a soluble S pool was available for remobilization and an insoluble S pool could not be mobilized. The size of the soluble pool was dependent on S nutrition. In the present study, plants fertilized with a high Fe concentration (200 μM) showed only K and S remobilization from flag leaves and Ni from stems/sheaths (Figure4). In this case, vegetative tissues should have been able to store Fe quantities above the structural minimum, which would have provided excess Fe for remobilization. However, with the abundant Fe supply at the root level, continued uptake during seed fill may have reduced or precluded the need for remobilization to serve as a source of Fe for seeds. On the other hand, plants fertilized with low Fe concentration (5 μM) showed the highest net Fe remobilization (Figure4), probably due to reduced uptake during seed fill. Under limited Fe supply, stems/sheaths are the major Fe source for remobilization. A similar pattern was observed in other studies when Zn supply was very low. Under this condition, stems and sheaths contributed most to Zn allocation (Jiang et al.2008). All the minerals analyzed were subject to remobilization, mostly from flag leaves, but also from stems/sheaths (Figure4), when plants were fertilized with the control Fe concentration (20 μM). These results suggest that mineral remobilization from vegetative tissues can occur in rice plants; however, for seeds to acquire minerals this remobilization is not absolutely required. Remobilization results found for *Arabidopsis* plants byWaters and Grusak (2008) were not exactly consistent between experiments; differences were found in the minerals that were remobilized and the amounts remobilized. Crafts-Brandner (1992) also found inconsistent results in leaves of soybean, which remobilized P in one experiment, while in a second experiment no remobilization occurred, yet seeds of both experiments had comparable seed P concentrations. As shown by our results, mineral remobilization from vegetative tissues in rice is modified by plant Fe nutrition, because different Fe supplies alter the remobilization of several minerals. Also, a major proportion of mineral content in panicles probably comes from non-storage sources, that is, continued root uptake and translocation during the seed fill period. We did observe mineral remobilization mostly from flag leaves but also from stems/sheaths with 20 μM Fe, and at least a portion of these minerals was likely incorporated into panicles and seeds. In the unlikely event that 100% of the content of each mineral lost from vegetative tissues went to panicles, this could account for, at most, 20% of panicle Fe, Zn, Cu, Mn, Mg, K and S. However, at least for Zn, it is already known that most of the mineral transported out of the leaves (either the flag leaf or the lowest senescent leaf) is translocated to other vegetative organs instead of being partitioned to the panicles, and even less to the grains (Jiang et al.2007b). We can also discard the possibility of 100% Ni or Ca remobilization to panicles, since it would be responsible for more than 100% of the final panicle content (Figure4). However, if remobilized, a significant part of this Ni pool would be expected to be transported to the seeds, since it is already known that Ni rapidly re-translocates from leaves to young tissues in the phloem, particularly during reproductive growth. Indeed, up to 70% of Ni in the shoots was transported to the seeds of soybean (Tiffin 1971). In *Arabidopsis*, continuous uptake and translocation of minerals to source tissues during seed fill are as important, if not more important, than remobilization of previously stored minerals (Waters and Grusak 2008). As shown by our results, the flag leaf is the organ with highest percentage of mineral content loss. However, considering that flag leaves have extremely low mineral content, the maximum possible contribution to panicle mineral content would be from stems/sheaths, rather than from flag leaves.

## CONCLUSION

In summary, this study suggests that mineral accumulation throughout the reproductive development of rice organs can be affected by different Fe supplies. With respect to the translocation of minerals to panicles, remobilization from vegetative organs can occur in rice plants (and non-optimal Fe supplies can affect mineral remobilization), but apparently, for seeds to acquire minerals, vegetative remobilization is not absolutely required. In this way, continued uptake and translocation of minerals during seed fill are probably more important than remobilization of previously stored shoot minerals. Thus, in addition to targeting source tissues for increased mineral remobilization, researchers should also target root uptake and leaf/stem/sheath efflux transporters to increase mineral accumulation in the panicles and consequently in the rice seeds.

# METHODS

## Plant materials and growth conditions

Rice (*Oryza sativa* L.) seeds from the fast-growing cultivar Kitaake were germinated in Petri dishes with filter paper for 8 d before being transferred to hydroponic solution. Plants were grown in a controlled environment chamber with 16-h, 20°C day and 8-h, 15°C night at the USDA-ARS Children's Nutrition Research Center, Houston, TX. Relative humidity was maintained at 50% and photon flux density during the day was 350 µmol $m^{-2}$ $s^{-1}$, supplied by a mixture of incandescent bulbs and fluorescent lamps. The standard solution for hydroponically grown plants contained 1 mM $Ca(NO_3)_2$, 3 mM $KNO_3$, 0.5 mM $MgSO_4$, 0.75 mM $K_2SO_4$, 0.5 mM $KH_2PO_4$, 25 µM $CaCl_2$, 25 µM $MnSO_4$, 0.5 µM $ZnSO_4$, 0.5 µM $CuSO_4$, 0.5 µM $H_2MoO_4$, 0.1 µM $NiSO_4$, 0.1 mM $K_2SiO_3$, and 20 µM Fe(III)-HEDTA (N-hydroxyethyl-ethylenediaminetriacetic acid). All nutrients were buffered with 2 mM MES (2,4-morpholino-ethane sulfonic acid), pH 5.5 and growth solutions were replaced every 3 days. For treatments involving different Fe concentrations, Fe(III)-HEDTA concentration was adjusted to 5, 20 or 200 µM. Rice organs (panicles, non-flag leaves, flag leaves, stems/sheaths and roots) were collected at panicle exertion, grain filling and full maturity (R3, R5 and R9 stages, respectively, according to Counce et al.2000). De-husked unpolished seeds were analyzed at full maturity.

## Elemental analysis by ICP

All tissues were harvested and dried in a 60°C oven for 48 h. Dried tissues were predigested overnight in borosilicate glass tubes with 4 ml of redistilled 98.8% $HNO_3$. One milliliter of concentrated trace metal grade $HClO_4$ was added to the predigested tissues and heated at 100°C for 1 h, 150°C for 1 h, 180°C for 1 h and then at 210°C to dryness (1–2 h). Digestions were performed using a heating block (Model 1016, Tecator, Hoganas, Sweden) with an exhaust-collecting manifold. Digests were resuspended in 15 ml of redistilled 2% $HNO_3$. Concentrations of Fe, Zn, Cu, Mn, Mo, Ni, Ca, Mg, K and S were determined by inductively coupled plasma-optical emission spectroscopy (CIROS ICP Model

FCE12; Spectro, Kleve, Germany). Tomato leaves and rice flour standards (SRM 1573A and 1568A, respectively; National Institute of Standards and Technology, Gaithersburg, MD) were digested and analyzed along with the rice samples to ensure accuracy of the instrument calibration (Narayanan et al.2007). Mineral content was determined by multiplying each sample's concentration by dry weight. For estimation of net mineral content loss from non-flag leaves, flag leaves and stems/sheaths, the final mineral content of each organ was subtracted from the prior time point which had the highest mineral content. For minerals that had a decrease in content, the net loss was compared with final total panicle mineral content to determine the contribution of remobilized minerals to panicle mineral content.

### Partition quotient calculation

To evaluate the partitioning of minerals within a rice plant during its reproductive development and under different Fe supplies, changes in each tissue's content were normalized to changes in each tissue's weight, relative to the whole plant. The DW of each organ was calculated as a percentage of total plant weight at each time point (or at each Fe supply), and mineral content of each organ was calculated as a percentage of total plant mineral content at each time point (or at each Fe supply). Using these values, the normalized partitioning of each mineral within the plant was calculated by dividing each organ's percentage mineral content by its percentage DW, and multiplying by 100, which we refer to as the partition quotient (PQ), as described by Waters and Grusak (2008).

### Statistical analyses

When appropriate, data were subjected to analyses of variance (ANOVA) and means were compared by the Tukey HSD (Honestly Significant Differences) ($P \leq 0.05$). The Levene's test (for homogeneity of variance) was used prior to ANOVA. Data with unequal variances were subjected to Welch analysis and means were compared by the Dunnett-C test. Pearson's correlation analyses were carried out using two significance levels ($P \leq 0.05$ and 0.01). All the statistical analyzes were performed using the SPSS Base 19.0 for Windows (SPSS Inc., USA).

# DECLARATIONS

## Acknowledgements

This research was supported by HarvestPlus (Agreement number 6005–05), Conselho Nacional de Desenvolvimento Científico e Tecnológico (CNPq) and Coordenação de Aperfeiçoamento de Pessoal de Nível Superior (CAPES) to JPF, and by the USDA-ARS under Agreement number 58-6250-0-008 to MAG. The contents of this publication do not necessarily reflect the views or policies of the US Department of Agriculture, nor does mention of trade names, commercial products, or organizations imply endorsement by the US Government.

## Competing interests

The authors declare that they have no competing interests.

## Authors' contributions

MAG and JPF conceived and coordinated the study. RAS, MWV and MAG designed the experiments. RAS and MWV obtained the ICP data. RAS performed the statistical analyzes and drafted the manuscript. RAS, MAG and JPF prepared the final manuscript. All authors read and approved the final manuscript.

# REFERENCES

1. Audebert A: **Iron partitioning as a mechanism for iron toxicity tolerance in lowland rice.** In *Iron Toxicity in Rice-based Systems in West Africa, Africa Rice Center (WARDA)*. Edited by: Audebert A, Narteh LT, Kiepe P, Millar D, Beks B. Cotonou, Benin; 2006:34–46.
2. Becker M, Asch F: **Iron toxicity in rice-condition and management concepts.** *J Plant Nutr Soil Sci* 2005, **168:** 558–573.
3. Briat JF, Fobis-Loisy I, Grignon N, Lobréaux S, Pascal N, Savino G, Thoiron S, von Wirén N, Wuytswinkel O: **Cellular and molecular aspects of iron metabolism in plants.** *Biol Cell* 1995, **84:** 69–81.

4. Chaignon V, DiMalta D, Hinsinger P: **Fe-deficiency increases Cu acquisition by wheat cropped in a Cu-contaminated vineyard soil.** *New Phytol* 2002, **154:** 121–130.

5. Colangelo EP, Guerinot ML: **Put the metal to the petal: metal uptake and transport throughout plants.** *Curr Opin Plant Biol* 2006, **9:** 322–330.

6. Counce PA, Keisling TC, Mitchell AJ: **A uniform, objective and adaptative system for expressing rice development.** *Crop Sci* 2000, **40:** 436–443.

7. Crafts-Brandner SJ: **Significance of leaf phosphorus remobilization in yield production in soybean.***Crop Sci* 1992, **32:** 420–424.

8. Curie C, Cassin G, Couch D, Divol F, Higuchi K, Le Jean M, Misson J, Schikora A, Czemic P, Mari S: **Metal movement within the plant: contribution of nicotianamine and yellow stripe 1-like transporters.***Ann Bot* 2009, **103:** 1–11.

9. Eckhardt U, Mas Marques A, Buckhout TJ: **Two iron-regulated cation transporters from tomato complement metal uptake-deficient yeast mutants.** *Plant Mol Biol* 2001, **45:** 437–448.

10. Fang Y, Wang L, Xin Z, Zhao L, An X, Hu Q: **Effect of foliar application of Zinc, Selenium, and Iron fertilizers on nutrients concentration and yield of rice grain in China.** *J Agric Food Chem* 2008, **56:**2079–2084.

11. Garnett TP, Graham RD: **Distribution and remobilization of iron and copper in wheat.** *Ann Bot* 2005,**95:** 817–826.

12. Goto F, Yoshihara T, Shigemoto N, Toki S, Takaiwa F: **Iron fortification of rice seed by the soybean ferritin gene.** *Nat Biotechnol* 1999, **17:** 282–286.

13. Gross J, Stein RJ, Fett-Neto AG, Fett JP: **Iron homeostasis related genes in rice.** *Genet Mol Biol* 2003,**26:** 477–497.

14. Grusak MA: **Iron transport to developing ovules of Pisum sativum. 1. Seed import characteristics and phloem iron-loading capacity of source regions.** *Plant Physiol* 1994, **104:** 649–655.

15. Grusak MA, DellaPenna D: **Improving the nutrient composition of plants to enhance human nutrition and health.** *Annu Rev Plant Physiol Plant Mol Biol* 1999, **50:** 133–161.

16. Himelblau E, Amasino RM: **Nutrients mobilized from leaves of Arabidopsis thaliana during leaf senescence.** *J Plant Physiol* 2001, **158:** 1317–1323.

17. Hocking PJ, Pate JS: **Mobilization of minerals to developing seeds of legumes.** *Ann Bot* 1977, **41:**1259–1278.

18. Hocking PJ: **Dry-matter production, mineral nutrient concentrations, and nutrient distribution and redistribution in irrigated spring wheat.** *J Plant Nutr* 1994, **17:** 1289–1308.

19. Jiang SL, Wu JG, Feng Y, Yang XE, Shi CH: **Correlation analysis of mineral element contents and quality traits in milled rice (Oryza sativa L.).** *J Agric Food Chem* 2007, **55:** 9608–9613.

20. Jiang W, Struik PC, Lingna J, van Keulen H, Ming Z, Stomph TJ: **Uptake and distribution of root-applied or foliar-applied 65Zn after flowering in aerobic rice.** *Ann Appl Biol* 2007, **150:** 383–391.

21. Jiang W, Struik PC, van Keulen H, Zhao M, Jin LN, Stomph TJ: **Does increased Zn uptake enhance grain Zn mass concentration in rice?** *Ann Appl Biol* 2008, **153:** 135–147.

22. Johnson AAT, Kyriacou B, Callahan DL, Carruthers L, Stangoulis J, Lombi E, Tester M: **Constitutive overexpression of the OsNAS gene family reveals single-gene strategies for effective Iron- and Zinc-biofortification of rice endosperm.** *PLoS One* 2011, **6:** e24476.

23. Kochian LV: **Mechanisms of micronutrient uptake and translocation in plants. SSSA book series # 4.**In *Micronutrients in Agriculture*. 2nd edition. Edited by: Mortvedt JJ. Soil Science Society of America, Madison, WI; 1991:229–296.

24. Korshunova YO, Eide D, Clark WG, Guerinot ML, Pakrasi HB: **The IRT1 protein from Arabidopsis thaliana is a metal transporter with a broad substrate range.** *Plant Mol Biol* 1999, **40:** 37–44.

25. Kupper H, Kupper SM: **In situ detection of heavy metal substituted chlorophylls in water plants.***Photosynth Res* 1998, **58:** 123–133.

26. Lee S, Jeon US, Lee SJ, Kim YK, Persson DP, Husted S, Schjørring JK, Kakei Y, Masuda H, Nishizawa NK, An G: **Iron fortification of**

**rice seeds through activation of the nicotianamine synthase gene.** *Proc Nat Acad Sci USA* 2009, **106:** 22014–22019.

27. Lee S, Persson DP, Hansen TH, Husted S, Schjoerring JK, Kim YS, Kakei Y, Masuda H, Nishizawa NK, An G: **Bio-available zinc in rice seeds is increased by activation tagging of nicotianamine synthase.***Plant Biotechnol J* 2011, **9:** 865–873.

28. Lin L, Ockenden I, Lott JNA: **The concentrations and distribution of phytic acid-phosphorus and other mineral nutrients in wild-type and low phytic acid1–1 (lpa1–1) corn (Zea mays L.) grains and grain parts.** *Can J Bot* 2005, **83:** 131–141.

29. López-Millán A-F, Ellis DR, Grusak MA: **Identification and characterization of several new members of the ZIP family of metal transporters in Medicago truncatula.** *Plant Mol Biol* 2004, **54:** 583–596.

30. Majumder ND, Rakshit SC, Borthakur DN: **Genetic effect on uptake of selected nutrients in some rice (O. sativa L.) varieties in phosphorus deficient soils.** *Plant Soil* 1990, **123:** 117–120.

31. Marschner H: *Mineral Nutrition of Higher Plants.* 2nd edition. Academic, London; 1995.

32. Masuda H, Suzuki M, Morikawa KC, Kobayashi T, Nakanishi H, Takahashi M, Saigusa M, Mori S, Nishizawa NK: **Increase in iron and zinc concentrations in rice grains via the introduction of barley genes involved in phytosiderophore synthesis.** *Rice* 2008, **1:** 100–108.

33. Masuda H, Usuda K, Kobayashi T, Ishimaru Y, Kakei Y, Takahashi M, Higuchi K, Nakanishi H, Mori S, Nishizawa NK: **Overexpression of the barley nicotianamine synthase gene HvNAS1 increases iron and zinc concentrations in rice grains.** *Rice* 2009, **2:** 155–166.

34. Mehraban P, Zadeh AA, Sadeghipour HR: **Iron toxicity in rice (Oryza sativa L.) under different potassium nutrition.** *Asian J Plant Sci* 2008, **7:** 251–259.

35. Narayanan NN, Vasconcelos MW, Grusak MA: **Expression profiling of Oryza sativa metal homeostasis genes in different rice cultivars using a cDNA macroarray.** *Plant Physiol Biochem* 2007, **45:** 277–286.

36. Neue HU, Quijano C, Senadhira D, Setter T: **Strategies for dealing with micronutrient disorders and salinity in lowland rice systems.** *Field Crops Res* 1998, **56:** 139–155.

37. Ramani S, Kannan S: **Manganese absorption and transport in rice.** *Physiol Plant* 1987, **33:** 133–137.

38. Ramesh SA, Choimes S, Schachtman DP: **Over-expression of an Arabidopsis zinc transporter in Hordeum vulgare increases short-term zinc uptake after zinc deprivation and seed zinc content.***Plant Mol Biol* 2004, **54:** 373–385.

39. Ramirez L, Classen N, Ubiera A, Werner H, Movad AM: **Effect of phosphorus, potassium and zinc fertilizers on iron toxicity in wetland rice (Oryza sativa L.).** *Plant Soil* 2002, **239:** 197–206.

40. Sahrawat KL: **Iron toxicity in wetland rice and the role of other nutrients.** *J Plant Nutr* 2004, **27:** 1471–1504.

41. Shao G, Chen M, Wang W, Mou R, Zhang G: **Iron nutrition affects cadmium accumulation and toxicity in rice plants.** *Plant Growth Regul* 2007, **53:** 33–42

42. Silveira VC, Oliveira AP, Sperotto RA, Espindola LS, Amaral L, Dias JF, Cunha JB, Fett JP: **Influence of iron on mineral status of two rice (Oryza sativa L.) cultivars.** *Braz J Plant Physiol* 2007, **19:** 127–139.

43. Sperotto RA, Ricachenevsky FK, Stein RJ, Waldow VA, Fett JP: **Iron stress in plants: dealing with deprivation and overload.** *Plant Stress* 2010, **4:** 57–69.

44. Sperotto RA, Ricachenevsky FK, Waldow VA, Fett JP: **Iron biofortification in rice: It's a long way to the top.** *Plant Sci* 2012, **190:** 24–39.

45. Stomph TJ, Jiang W, Struik PC: **Zinc biofortification of cereals: rice differs from wheat and barley.***Trends Plant Sci* 2009, **14:** 123–124.

46. Sunarpi , Anderson JW: **Effect of sulfur nutrition on the redistribution of sulfur in vegetative soybean plants.** *Plant Physiol* 1996, **112:** 623–631.

47. Tiffin LO: **Translocation of nickel in xylem exudates of plants.** *Plant Physiol* 1971, **48:** 273–277.

48. Uauy C, Distelfeld A, Fahima T, Blechl A, Dubcovsky J: **A NAC gene regulating senescence improves grain protein, zinc, and iron content in wheat.** *Science* 2006, **314:** 1298–1301.

49. Vasconcelos M, Datta K, Oliva N, Khalekuzzaman M, Torrizo L, Krishnan S, Oliveira M, Goto F, Datta SK:**Enhanced iron and zinc accumulation in transgenic rice with the ferritin gene.** *Plant Sci* 2003, **164:**371–378.

50. Vasconcelos M, Musetti V, Li CM, Datta SK, Grusak MA: **Functional analysis of transgenic rice (Oryza sativa L.) transformed with an Arabidopsis thaliana ferric reductase (AtFRO2).** *Soil Sci Plant Nutr*2004, **50:** 1151–1157.

51. Vasconcelos M, Eckert H, Arahana V, Graef G, Grusak MA, Clemente T: **Molecular and phenotypic characterization of transgenic soybean expressing the Arabidopsis ferric chelate reductase gene FRO2.** *Planta* 2006, **224:** 1116–1128.

52. Waters BM, Grusak MA: **Whole-plant mineral partitioning throughout the life cycle in Arabidopsis thaliana ecotypes Columbia, Landsberg erecta, Cape Verde Islands, and the mutant line ysl1ysl3.***New Phytol* 2008, **177:** 389–405.

53. White PJ, Broadley MR: **Biofortifying crops with essential mineral elements.** *Trends Plant Sci* 2005,**10:** 586–593.

54. Wu CY, Lu LL, Yang XE, Feng Y, Wei YY, Hao HL, Stoffella PJ, He ZL: **Uptake, translocation, and remobilization of Zinc absorbed at different growth stages by rice genotypes of different Zn densities.** *J Agric Food Chem* 2010, **58:** 6767–6773.

55. Yoneyama T, Gosho T, Kato M, Goto S, Hayashi H: **Xylem and phloem transport of Cd, Zn and Fe into the grains of rice plants (Oryza sativa L.) grown in continuously flooded Cd-contaminated soil.** *Soil Sci Plant Nutr* 2010, **56:** 445–453.

56. Zeng YW, Shen SQ, Wang LX, Liu JF, Pu XY, Du J, Qiu M: **Correlation of plant morphological and grain quality traits with mineral element contents in Yunnan rice.** *Rice Sci* 2005, **12:** 101–106.

57. Zhang FS, Römheld V, Marschner H: **Diurnal rhythm of release of phytosiderophores and uptake rate of zinc in iron-deficient wheat.** *Soil Sci Plant Nutr* 1991, **37:** 671–678.

58. Zhang X, Zhang F, Mao D: **Effect of iron plaque outside roots on nutrient uptake by rice (Oryza sativa L.): Zinc uptake by Fe-deficient rice.** *Plant Soil* 1998, **202:** 33–39.

59. Zheng L, Cheng Z, Ai C, Jiang X, Bei X, Zheng Y, Glahn RP, Welch RM, Miller DD, Lei XG, Shou H:**Nicotianamine, a novel enhancer of rice iron bioavailability to humans.** *PLoS One* 2010, **5:** e10190.

4

# POLYMER-COATED UREA DELAYS GROWTH AND ACCUMULATION OF KEY NUTRIENTS IN AEROBIC RICE BUT DOES NOT AFFECT GRAIN MINERAL CONCENTRATIONS

**Terry J. Rose**

Southern Cross Plant Science, Southern Cross University, PO Box 157 Lismore, NSW 2480, Australia

## ABSTRACT

Enhanced efficiency nitrogen (N) fertilizers (EEFs) may improve crop recovery of fertilizer-N, but there is evidence that some EEFs cause a lag in crop growth compared to growth with standard urea. Biomass and mineral nutrient accumulation was investigated in rice fertilized with urea, urea-3,4-dimethylpyrazole phosphate (DMPP) and polymer-coated urea (PCU) to determine whether any delays in biomass production alter the accumulation patterns, and subsequent grain concentrations, of key mineral nutrients. Plant growth and mineral accumulation and partitioning to grains did not differ significantly between plants fertilized with urea or urea-DMPP. In contrast, biomass accumulation and the accumulation of phosphorus, potassium, calcium, magnesium, copper, zinc and manganese were delayed during the early growth phase of plants fertilized with PCU. However, plants in the PCU treatment ultimately compensated for this by increasing growth and nutrient uptake during the latter vegetative stages so that no differences in biomass or nutrient accumulation generally existed among N fertilizer treatments at anthesis. Delayed biomass accumulation in rice fertilized with PCU does not appear to reduce the total accumulation of mineral nutrients, nor to have any impact on grain mineral nutrition when biomass and grain yields are equal to those of rice grown with urea or urea-DMPP.

**Keywords:** controlled-release urea; nitrification inhibitor; nitrogen; phosphorus

# 1. INTRODUCTION

Global crop production relies heavily on the application of nitrogen (N) fertilizers to sustain high yields, and global demand for N fertilizers is predicted to increase further over the next decade [1]. Unfortunately, the N use efficiency of crop production is generally low, with crops rarely assimilating more than 50% of the fertilizer N applied [2]. While some of the fertilizer N is retained in the soil and may be available for uptake by subsequent crops, much of the N applied to crops and pastures is lost through leaching [3,4] or emitted as the gases $NH_3$ or $N_2O$ [5,6]. An unintended consequence of these losses is environmental damage, predominantly eutrophication of waterways due to N contamination, and increasing greenhouse gas emissions from agriculture as a result of $N_2O$ losses [2].

A number of agronomic management strategies have been suggested for enhancing N efficiency, including optimising N budgeting, N fertilizer placement, and timing [7,8] to better match soil N supply patterns with crop N demand. Another option is to use enhanced-efficiency fertilizers (EEF), which broadly comprise controlled-release N fertilizers and N fertilizers with urease or nitrification inhibitors [2]. A number of studies have investigated the impact of EEF *vs.* urea on crop yields, N use efficiency or nitrous oxide losses in dryland crops [9,10,11]. While N use efficiency was improved in some instances, the delayed N availability from controlled-release N fertilizers was also observed to delay biomass production, and ultimately reduce yield, compared to urea application in some seasons [10].

As yet, the impact of any delayed biomass accumulation pattern from EEFs on the accumulation of other mineral nutrients in crops, and the consequences for grain nutritional content, is not known. While delayed early nutrient accumulation can be compensated by increased uptake in later growth stages, moisture stress in later growing stages can limit nutrient uptake in a nutrient-specific manner [12]. Any impact on the concentrations of magnesium (Mg), calcium, (Ca), zinc (Zn) and copper (Cu) in grains are of particular importance because deficiencies of these nutrients in the diet are a major health concern [13]. The aim of the present study was to investigate whether any changes in growth patterns caused by EEF alter the accumulation of key nutrients in aerobically-cultivated rice (*Oryza sativa* L.) and whether these alterations impact on grain nutritional quality.

## 2. RESULTS

The accumulation of biomass, phosphorus (P), Mg, manganese (Mn) and Zn generally continued until maturity regardless of N fertilizer treatment, while peak accumulation of N, Ca and Cu generally occurred during early grain filling (108 days after sowing [DAS]) regardless of N fertilizer treatment (Figure 1). Peak accumulation of potassium (K) occurred earlier, at anthesis (93 DAS) in the urea and urea-3,4-dimethylpyrazole phosphate (DMPP) treatments, but at early grain filling (108 DAS) in the polymer-coated urea (PCU) treatment (Figure 1d).

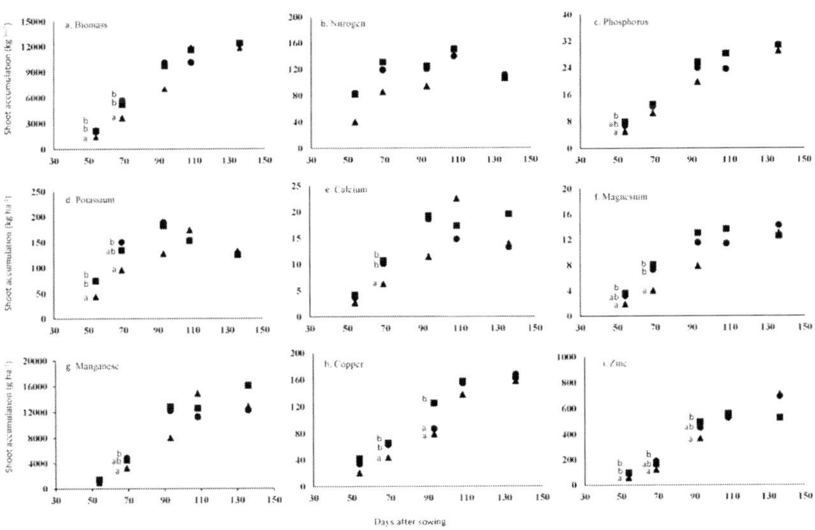


**Figure 1.** Accumulation of biomass (**a**), nitrogen (**b**), phosphorus (**c**), potassium (**d**), calcium (**e**), magnesium (**f**), manganese (**g**), copper (**h**) and zinc (**i**) throughout the growing season in shoots of rice fertilized with urea (circles), urea + urea-3,4-dimethylpyrazole phosphate

(DMPP) (squares) or polymer-coated urea (triangles). Treatments that do share a common letter within a given harvest (timepoint) are not significantly different at a $p \leq 0.05$. The absence of any letters at a given harvest (timepoint) indicates no significant differences among treatments.

Biomass data confirmed visual observations of delayed early growth in the PCU treatment, with significant reductions in biomass production at 54 DAS and 69 DAS in the PCU treatment compared to urea and urea-3,4-dimethylpyrazole phosphate (DMPP) treatments (Figure 1a). Despite these growth reductions, no significant reduction in early shoot N accumulation was observed in the PCU treatment at $p = 0.05$ (Figure 1b), although reductions were observed at $p < 0.1$ at 54 DAS. Notably, the urea-DMPP treatment did not result in increased shoot N accumulation compared to urea at any growth stage (Figure 1b).

The accumulation of macronutrients P, K, Ca and Mg was reduced in the PCU treatment compared to either or both of urea and urea-DMPP treatments at 54 DAS, 69 DAS or both harvest dates (Figure 1c–f). Similarly, the accumulation of the micronutrients Mn, Cu and Zn were delayed in the PCU treatment, with significantly lower shoot Mn (69 DAS), Cu (69 and 93 DAS) and Zn (54, 69 and 93 DAS) contents in the PCU treatment compared to urea-DMPP and urea treatments ($p < 0.05$; Figure 1g–i).

Grain yield and harvest index (proportion of crop biomass in grains at maturity) did not differ among treatments, with means of 5.07 $t \cdot ha^{-1}$ and 0.42 (Table 1). Similarly, N fertilizer treatment had no impact on grain nutrient concentrations and nutrient harvest indices (Table 1).

**Table 1.** Average rice nutrient harvest indices and grain nutrient concentrations in the field trial. Note: data are means from all three N treatments since there was no significant ($p = 0.05$) effect of N fertilizer type on grain yield, nutrient harvest indices or grain nutrient concentrations.

| | Grain Yield ($t \cdot ha^{-1}$) | Macronutrients ($mg \cdot g^{-1}$) | | | | | Micronutrients ($mg \cdot kg^{-1}$) | | |
|---|---|---|---|---|---|---|---|---|---|
| | | N | P | K | Ca | Mg | Cu | Mn | Zn |
| *Grain nutrient concentration* | 5.08 | 12.4 | 3.44 | 4.03 | 0.22 | 1.23 | 20.6 | 197 | 36.1 |
| *Nutrient harvest index* | 0.42 | 0.55 | 0.58 | 0.16 | 0.07 | 0.47 | 0.64 | 0.07 | 0.29 |

# 3. DISCUSSION

Controlled-release urea fertilizers have a sigmoidal N release pattern compared to the rapid mineralisation of urea N [14] and this resulted in the delayed biomass production in the CRU treatment compared to the urea and urea-DMPP treatments in the present study (Figure 1a). This delayed biomass production clearly demonstrates that, in the absence of other constraints, the availability of N heavily impacts on growth rates of upland rice, which has also been observed under varying N fertilizer regimes in flooded rice [15]. While urea-DMPP has been shown to reduce nitrification rates in controlled environments [16] and temperate environments [17], evidence in warmer subtropical environments is lacking. While nitrification rates were not measured in the present study, the fact that the urea-DMPP treatment had no impact on biomass production or N uptake compared to urea suggests that any effect of urea-DMPP on N dynamics is limited in subtropical conditions.

The macronutrient accumulation patterns throughout the season were typical of rice, with accumulation of biomass and P continuing until maturity while N and Ca accumulation peak during early grain filling [18]. The decline in the shoot K content between anthesis and maturity observed in the present study was also observed by Garcia *et al.* [18] and the same phenomenon occurs in wheat [19], although the reason for this net loss of K is not known. Nutrient concentrations in rice grains were also typical of the concentrations observed in field-grown rice [20].

The altered growth patterns in the PCU treatment affected the accumulation of key nutrients in shoots with significantly ($p < 0.05$) delayed uptake of all nutrients at one or more of the vegetative growth stages (tillering, jointing and anthesis). The exception was N (Figure 1), whose delayed accumulation was only significant at $p < 0.1$. This reflects the high variability in the N accumulation data, which is likely related to the uneven distribution of sugarcane (*Saccharum officinarum* L.) trash from the previous crop. Ultimately, however, there were no differences in nutrient accumulation among N fertilizer treatments at anthesis (93 DAS)-with the exception of Zn- and no differences in grain mineral concentrations at maturity (Table 1). In other words, nutrient uptake in all N treatments was finally congruent as the biomass production was also congruent. However, it is noteworthy that the 2014–2015 season was a wet season, with >500 mm precipitation falling from January-April. In seasons where topsoil drying is prevalent during mid-late summer (late tillering to anthesis, from around 60 DAS to 93 DAS in the present study) and

PCU-treated crops have higher biomass and nutrient accumulation rates, it is possible that the uptake of nutrients such as P and Zn, which are predominantly located in the 0–10 cm horizon (Table 2), may be restricted [21]. Moreover, by the same reasoning it is also possible that topsoil drying events earlier in the season may restrict the uptake of P and Zn in crops supplied with urea. In summary, there is no clear evidence that the delayed biomass accumulation observed in crops fertilised with PCU reduces the total accumulation of mineral nutrients in rice or has any impact on grain mineral nutrition when biomass and grain yields do not differ from crops fertilised with urea.

# 4. EXPERIMENTAL SECTION

A field trial was conducted near Woodburn, NSW, Australia, in the summer of 2014–2015, in a field previously under sugarcane. In the 5-month period following sugarcane harvest, the soil was rotary hoed twice, followed by offset discing, then rotary hoed twice more, and power harrowed immediately prior to planting rice. Soil samples were collected immediately prior to sowing and physiochemical properties are shown in Table 2.

Following the application of a pre-emergent herbicide (480 $g \cdot L^{-1}$ Clomazone at 600 $mL \cdot ha^{-1}$), rice (*cv.* Tachiminori) was sown on 7 December 2014 at 125 $kg \cdot seed \cdot ha^{-1}$ using a tined seeder at a row spacing of 150 mm. Plots 3 m × 8 m were established in triplicate 4 weeks after sowing to accommodate a completely randomized block trial investigating the impact of N fertilizer source on the accumulation of mineral nutrients in rice. The three N treatments were 80 $kg \cdot ha^{-1}$ N applied as urea, a commercial product with urea + 3,4-dimethylpyrazole phosphate (DMPP) at 1.84 kg DMPP active ingredient/t urea, and a commercial polymer-coated urea product (PCU). Fertilizer N rates above 80 $kg \cdot ha^{-1}$ in this region typically increase N uptake and grain yields but lead to severe crop lodging (unpublished data) and are not recommended.

Fertilizer-N was applied at around 35 DAS to avoid the accumulation of excess mineral N in the soil during early growth. The 5 months fallow period prior to rice planting in the rice-cane rotation in the Australian subtropics allows mineralization of organic N, and hence, around 100 $kg \cdot ha^{-1}$ mineral N was present in the soil to 900 mm depth assuming a bulk density of around 1 $g \cdot cm^{-3}$ (Table 2). Rainfall during the growing season recorded from the nearby Woodburn weather station was January–200 mm, February–217 mm, March–47 mm, and April–160 mm.

**Table 2.** Selected physiochemical properties of the 0–100 mm, 100–300 mm, 300–600 mm and 600–900 mm horizons at the Woodburn field site.

| | Soil Depth (mm) | | | |
|---|---|---|---|---|
| Property | 0–100 | 100–300 | 300–600 | 600–900 |
| Basic texture | clay loam | clay | clay | clay |
| Total carbon (%) | 2.3 | 2.1 | 1.1 | 2.1 |
| Total nitrogen (%) | 0.18 | 0.16 | 0.09 | 0.21 |
| KCl extractable ammonium (mg· $kg^{-1}$) | 9.9 | 11.3 | 12.5 | 12.2 |
| KCl extractable nitrate (mg· $kg^{-1}$) | 0.90 | 1.3 | 0.9 | 1.2 |
| pH (1:5 water) | 5.57 | 5.50 | 5.35 | 5.50 |
| EC (dS· $m^{-1}$) | 0.04 | 0.05 | 0.06 | 0.07 |
| Bray 1 phosphorus (mg· $kg^{-1}$) | 14.8 | 6.0 | 5.9 | 1.5 |
| Total acid extractable sulfur (mg· $kg^{-1}$) | 411 | 427 | 806 | 379 |
| Cation exchange capacity ($cmol^{+}$· $kg^{-1}$) | 27.3 | 27.3 | 25.0 | 26.3 |
| *Base cations (%)* | | | | |
| Calcium | 54.3 | 52.0 | 42.0 | 41.7 |
| Magnesium | 36.8 | 36.8 | 40.9 | 40.0 |
| Potassium | 2.3 | 1.8 | 1.5 | 1.2 |
| Sodium | 1.3 | 1.6 | 2.3 | 4.9 |
| Aluminium | 3.2 | 4.7 | 8.6 | 8.3 |
| *DPTA-extractable micronutrients* | | | | |
| Zinc (mg· $kg^{-1}$) | 2.5 | 1.3 | 1.3 | 0.9 |
| Manganese (mg· $kg^{-1}$) | 13 | 9 | 8 | 4 |
| Iron (mg· $kg^{-1}$) | 221 | 209 | 177 | 127 |
| Copper (mg· $kg^{-1}$) | 1.0 | 0.6 | 0.9 | not detectable |

Samples were measured at Environmental Analysis Laboratories (EAL), Southern Cross University, Lismore, Australia, using methods from Rayment and Lyons [22].

### 4.1. Measurements

Aboveground plant tissue was harvested at tillering (54 DAS), jointing (69 DAS), anthesis (93 DAS), mid grain filling (108 DAS) and maturity (136 DAS) by cutting two 1 m-lengths of row per plot at ground level. At maturity, samples were threshed by hand to separate grain and straw. All samples were dried in an air-forced oven at 60 °C for 5 days. Samples were analysed for nutrient concentration at Environmental Analysis Laboratories, Lismore, NSW, Australia. A 0.2 g subsample of finely ground tissue was digested with nitric acid in a MARS microwave oven (CEM Corp., USA) and concentrations of P, K, Mg, Ca, Zn, Mn, and Cu in the digest solutions were quantified using inductively coupled plasma optical emission spectroscopy (ICP-OES 4300D, Perkin Elmer, USA). Tissue N concentration was measured using a LECO TruMAC CNS analyser. The accumulation of sulphur (S) and iron (Fe) was not investigated because soils in the region are rich in these nutrients due to the presence of pyrite ($FeS_2$) in the subsoil [23], which results in excessive, rather than limiting, levels of S and Fe in crops grown.

### 4.2. Statistical Analyses

Nutrient accumulation, nutrient harvest index and grain nutrient concentration data were analysed using a two-way analysis of variance fitting N fertilizer treatment and block (replicate) in Genstat using a probability level of 0.05. Significance of differences between treatment mean values for each trait was tested using Duncan's multiple range test.

## 5. CONCLUSIONS

The use of PCU fertilizer caused a significant delay in early biomass production compared to both urea and urea-DMPP fertilizers, but ultimately this did lead to any reduction in the total accumulation of mineral nutrients at maturity or reductions in grain nutrient concentrations. However, it is possible that in seasons with a dry finish that limits nutrient uptake the delay in early growth observed in plants fertilized with PCU may have greater impacts on grain nutritional quality.

## CONFLICTS OF INTEREST

The author declares no conflict of interest.

## REFERENCES

1. Timilsena, Y.P.; Adhikari, R.; Casey, P.; Muster, T.; Gill, H.; Adhikari, B. Enhanced efficiency fertilizers: A review of formulation and nutrient release patterns. J. Sci. Food Agric. 2015, 95, 1131–1142.
2. Chen, D.; Suter, H.; Islam, A.; Edis, R.; Freney, J.R.; Walker, C.N. Prospects of improving efficiency of fertilizer nitrogen in Australian agriculture: A review of enhanced efficiency fertilizers. Soil Res. 2008,46, 289–301.
3. Burkitt, L.L. A review of nitrogen losses due to leaching and surface runoff under intensive pasture management in Australia. Soil Res. 2014, 52, 621–636.
4. Zhou, M.; Butterbach-Bahl, K. Assessment of nitrate leaching loss on a yield-scaled basis from maize and wheat cropping systems. Plant Soil 2014, 374, 977–991.

5. Macdonald, B.C.T.; Denmead, O.T.; White, I. Quantification of NOx and NH3 emissions from two sugarcane fields. Soil Res. 2014, 52, 833–840.

6. Schwenke, G.D.; Manning, W.; Haigh, B.M. Ammonia volatilisation from nitrogen fertilizers surface-applied to bare fallows, wheat crops and perennial-grass-based pastures on Vertosols. Soil Res. 2014,52, 805–821.

7. Nelson, K.A.; Motavalli, P.P.; Nathan, M. Nitrogen fertilizer sources and application timing affects wheat and inter-seeded red clover yields on claypan soils. Agronomy 2014, 4, 497–513.

8. Shenwu, L.; Wang, X.; Liu, G. A simple and reasonable calculation equation of balanced fertilization.Agronomy 2015, 5, 180–187.

9. Mahli, S.S.; Soon, Y.K.; Grant, C.A.; Lemke, R.; Lupwayi, N. Influence of controlled-release urea on seed yield and N concentration and N use efficiency of small grain crops grown on Dark Gray Luvisols. Can. J. Soil Sci. 2010, 90, 363–372.

10. Grant, C.A.; Wu, R.; Selles, F.; Harker, F.N.; Clayton, G.W.; Bittman, S.; Zebarth, B.J.; Lupwayi, N.Z. Crop yield and nitrogen concentration with controlled release urea and split applications of nitrogen as compared to non-coated urea applied at seeding. Field Crop Res. 2012, 127, 170–180.

11. Gao, X.; Asgedom, H.; Tenuta, M.; Flaten, D.N. Enhanced efficiency urea sources and placement effects on nitrous oxide emissions. Agron. J. 2015, 107, 265–277.

12. Rose, T.J.; Bloomfield, C.; Raymond, C.; King, G.J. Perturbation of nutrient source-sink relationships by post-anthesis stresses results in differential accumulation of key nutrients into wheat grain. J. Plant Nutr. Soil Sci. 2015, 178, 89–98.

13. White, P.J.; Broadley, M.R. Biofortification of crops with seven mineral elements often lacking in human diets–iron, zinc, copper, calcium, magnesium, selenium and iodine. New Phytol. 2009, 182, 49–84.

14. Chalk, P.M.; Craswell, E.T.; Polidoro, J.C.; Chen, D. Fate and efficiency of 15N-labelled slow- and controlled release fertilizers. Nutr. Cycl. Agroecosyst. 2015.

15. Dunn, B.W.; Dunn, T.S.; Beecher, H.G. Nitrogen timing and rate effects on growth and grain yield of delayed permanent-water rice in south-eastern Australia. Crop Pasture Sci. 2014, 65, 878–887.

16. Chen, D.; Suter, H.; Islam, A.; Edis, R. Influence of nitrification inhibitors on nitrification and nitrous oxide (N2O) emission from a clay loam soil fertilized with urea. Soil Biol. Biochem. 2010, 42, 660–664.

17. Weiske, A.; Benckiser, G.; Ottow, J.C.G. Effect of the new nitrification inhibitor DMPP in comparison to DCD on nitrous oxide (N2O) emissions and methane (CH4) oxidation during 3 years of repeated applications in field experiments. Nutr. Cycl. Agroecosyst. 2001, 60, 57–64.

18. Garcia, A.G.; Douradeo-Neto, D.; Basanta, M.D.V.; Ovejero, R.F.L.; Favarin, J.L. Logistic rice model for dry matter and nutrient uptake. Sci. Agric. 2003, 60, 481–488.

19. Rose, T.J.; Rengel, Z.; Bowden, J.; Ma, Q. Differential accumulation of phosphorus and potassium by canola cultivars compared to wheat. J. Soil Sci. Plant Nutr. 2007, 170, 404–411.

20. Dobermann, A.; Fairhurst, T.H. Nutrient Disorders and Nutrient Management; Potash and Phosphate Institute, Potash and Phosphate Institute of Canada and International Rice Research Institute: Singapore, 2000.

21. Ma, Q.; Rengel, Z.; Rose, T.J. The effectiveness of deep placement of fertilizers is determined by crop species and edaphic conditions in Mediterranean-type environments: A review. Aust. J. Soil Res. 2009,47, 19–32.

22. Rayment, G.E.; Lyons, D.J. Australian Laboratory Handbook of Soil and Water Chemical Methods; Inkata Press: Port Melbourne, Australia, 2011.

23. Huang, J.; Nhan, T.; Wong, V.N.L.; Johnston, S.G.; Lark, M.; Triantafilis, J. Digital soil mapping of a coastal acid sulfate soil landscape. Soil Res. 2014, 52, 327–339.

5

# WORLDWIDE GENETIC DIVERSITY FOR MINERAL ELEMENT CONCENTRATIONS IN RICE GRAIN

**Shannon R. Pinson** [*ab], **Lee Tarpley**[c], **Wengui Yan**[d], **Kathleen Yeater**[ef], **Brett Lahner**

[a] USDA–ARS Rice Research Unit, 1509 Aggie Drive, Beaumont, TX 77713

[b] present address, USDA–ARS Dale Bumpers National Rice Research Center, 2890 Highway 130 East, Stuttgart, AR 72160

[c] Texas A&M Univ. System, Texas A&M AgriLife Research, 1509 Aggie Dr., Beaumont, TX 77713

[d] USDA–ARS Dale Bumpers National Rice Research Center, 2890 Highway 130 East, Stuttgart, AR 72160

[e] USDA–ARS–SPA, 1001 Holleman Drive East, College Station, TX 77840

## ABSTRACT

With the aim of identifying rice (*Oryza* spp.) germplasm having enhanced grain nutritional value, the mineral nutrient and trace element concentrations (or ionome) of whole (unmilled) grains from a set of 1763 rice accessions of diverse geographic and genetic origin were evaluated. Seed for analysis of P, Mg, K, S, Ca, As, Cd, Co, Cu, Fe, Mn, Mo, Ni, Rb, Sr, and Zn concentrations by inductively coupled plasma mass spectrometry was produced over 2 yr in Beaumont, TX, under both flooded and unflooded watering regimes. The distributions of all element concentrations analyzed were skewed toward higher concentration. A significant portion of this ionomic variation has a genetic basis (broad sense heritabilities 0.14–0.75), indicating an ability to breed for improved grain concentration of all elements except possibly Ni. Variation in grain elemental concentrations was not strongly associated with plant height, heading time, or grain shape, suggesting these physiological factors are not of primary importance in controlling ionomic variation in rice grain. Accessions high in specific elements were sometimes found to have similar genetic or geographic origins, suggesting they share a heritable mechanism underlying their enhanced ionomes. For example, accessions with high Ca, Mg, or K were more common in the *indica* than in the *japonica*subgroup; low As was most common among temperate *japonica* accessions; and several lines high in Mo originated in Malaysia or adjacent Brunei.

---

With about half the world's human population dependent on rice (*Oryza* spp.) as a staple food, the grain provides the majority of dietary nutrients to billions of people. Unfortunately, rice grains are not dense in mineral nutrients, making nutrient deficiencies common among those dependent on rice as a dietary staple (Grusak and Della Penna, 1999). In addition to dietary supplementation and industrial food fortification, biofortification via the development of new crop cultivars with increased concentration of nutrients in their edible portions has been proposed as a possible solution to alleviate global malnutrition (e.g., Graham et al., 1999, 2001; Gregorio et al., 2000; White and Broadley, 2005; Bouis and Welch, 2010;Masuda et al., 2013; Rawat et al., 2013; Murgia et al., 2013). In fact, studies have documented improved health indicators from human consumption of crops biofortified for iron and β-carotene (Haas et al., 2005; van Jaarsveld et al., 2005; Low et al., 2007;Cercamondi et al., 2013). While most white (milled) rice in U.S. grocery stores is fortified by adding nutrients to the external surface of the milled rice grains (Flour Fortification Initiative, 2012), enhancement of the rice grain's nutritional value through genetic improvements could include both increasing concentrations of desirable elements (e.g., Fe, Zn, or Ca) and decreasing concentrations of undesirable elements (e.g., As or Cd) and could create new marketing strategies for nutritionally enhanced, value-added products. If the biofortification is accomplished through traditional breeding and selection, rather than through genetic engineering, then the nutritionally enhanced crops would not require special regulation or documentation and could thus be deployed more rapidly. Cultivars biofortified through traditional breeding methods would be able to acquire organic certification if grown under organic field conditions, and use of alleles conferring intermediate rather than extreme phenotypes found naturally functional among diverse rice accessions could be used to fine-tune grain element concentrations.

The most prevalent nutrient deficiencies worldwide are Fe and Zn, with estimates that more than 25% of the world's population are at risk of mild to severe deficiency in one or both elements and with each element attributable for the deaths of 0.8 million persons per year (World Health Organization [WHO], 2002, 2009; Maret and Sandstead, 2006). Because of significant interest in biofortifying grains for Fe and Zn, numerous studies have focused on the routes and mechanisms governing accumulation of Fe and Zn in crop grains (for reviews, see Stangoulis, 2010; Masuda et al., 2013). In that the seed serves as an energy and nutrient source for germinating seedlings, grain biofortification might also offer opportunity to enhance crop health. For example, reduced concentrations of P in seed have been associated with reduced germination and seedling vigor (Bolland and Baker, 1988;Robinson et al., 2012; White and Veneklaas, 2012), though the association may not be obligatory (Rose et al., 2013a). The first step toward breeding rice cultivars with an enhanced elemental composition (or ionome) is to understand the genetic diversity in germplasm collections available to breeders.

Rice is grown under a wide range of environmental conditions around the world. It is produced below sea level as well as in mountainside terraces as much as 1800 m above sea level, in tropical equatorial countries as well in the more temperate areas of Eastern and Western Europe. Although rice is most commonly produced under a shallow flood (8 to 20 cm water) in the United States, on a global view it is also commonly grown under upland (aerated rainfed) conditions and even under deep-water flood (more than 50 cm) in tropical areas that experience a monsoon season. Grassi et al. (2009) showed that a cultivar developed for upland production yielded more when grown flooded, indicating that an aerobic or unflooded production system limits rice yields even in the absence of water stress or drought. It has been shown that the concentrations of various elements in rice grain are so affected by the soil and other aspects of the environment under which a rice grain is produced that grain ionome profiles can be used to distinguish among rices produced in different countries and geographical regions of the world (Kelly et al., 2002; Gonzálvez et al., 2011; Li et al., 2012). This suggests that rice cultivars adapted to geographic regions where a particular element is especially lacking, or present in excess, may express genes for enhanced ability to mine those elements out of the soil and/or partition them to other organs once taken up by the plant's roots or compartmentalized in leaves. While Zn deficiency is widespread throughout the rice-growing regions of the world, deficiencies and toxicities of other elements (e.g., As, Ca, Fe, K, and Mo) are more specific to certain soil types or irrigation conditions. It is likely that landraces and cultivars adapted to these particular geographic regions may contain enhanced ability to absorb, exclude, or detoxify specific elements. One goal of the present study was to compare the grain ionome of 1763 diverse rice accessions to determine if rice accessions adapted to a particular region of the world or if those from a particular ancestral lineage were more likely to produce rice grains with reduced or elevated concentrations of one or more of the 16 elements (P, Mg, K, S, Ca, As, Cd, Co, Cu, Fe, Mn, Mo, Ni, Rb, Sr, Zn) we analyzed.

A second goal of the study was to evaluate correlations between the elements and plant traits, as these can implicate mechanisms of element uptake, transport, and grain accumulation. Because soil redox potential is known to significantly alter the availability of many soil mineral elements to plant uptake, seed from the diverse rice accessions was produced under both flooded and unflooded (flush irrigated) field conditions. While it is generally accepted that mineral elements may be remobilized from vegetative plant tissues to developing grains (Hocking and Pate, 1977; Himelblau and Amasino, 2001), recent study also indicates that major portions of mineral elements found in seeds have been supplied through root uptake and translocation during grain fill (Sperotto et al., 2012). It is difficult to know how to efficiently improve a process that is not already well understood. Thus, one barrier slowing the breeding and development of biofortified crops is a lack of understanding of the network of physicochemical and regulatory processes that are responsible for directing the element uptake by roots and subsequent translocation of the mineral elements into and out of vegetative tissues before they can be ultimately carried or loaded into developing grains. The third goal of this study, assuming sufficient differentiation existed, was to identify from among the 1763 widely diverse rice accessions those with extreme grain ionomes for use in further studies aimed at identifying genes, physiology, and biochemical factors underlying their differences in grain element concentrations.

## MATERIALS AND METHODS

### Genetic Materials

A total of 1763 highly diverse rice accessions (each a different genotype) collected from around the world (Supplemental Table S1) were compared for grain element concentrations. A majority (1748) are in the USDA Core Collection, which represents genetic diversity among ~20,000 accessions of rice germplasm originated from 116 countries (Yan et al., 2007, 2010). Among the five subgroup or ancestral lineages of rice (Garris et al., 2005; Zhao et al., 2011; Ren et al., 2013), this study included 578 accessions of the *indica* (IND) accessions, 412 temperate *japonica* (TEJ) accessions, 358 tropical *japonicas* (TRJ), 169*aus* (AUS), 63 *aromatic* (ARO) accessions, and 183 accessions considered admixtures (<60% of 72 simple sequence repeat markers from any one subgroup) among these subgroups (Agrama et al., 2010).

All *O. sativa* and *O. glaberrima* accessions in the USDA Rice Core Collection were planted, but those that did not produce sufficient quality and quantity of seed for grain analysis in the 2007 fields were eliminated from further study. To evaluate the suitability of identifying quantitative trait loci (QTLs) within preexistent mapping populations, 15 parents of widely studied biparental rice mapping populations were included in the study, 8 of which also represent modern (released after 1980) southern U.S. TRJ rice cultivars (Cybonnet, Cocodrie, Jefferson, Kaybonnet, Lemont, LaGrue, Saber, and Rosemont), and 7 of which were cultivars of international origin (Azucena [TEJ], Dragon Eyeball 100 [IND], Jasmine 85 [IND], Kasalath [IND], RT0034 [IND], TeQing [IND], and Zhe733 [IND]). With 'Gulfmont' and 'Cypress' included in the USDA Core Collection, a total of 10 modern southern U.S. rice cultivars were evaluated for their grain ionomes.

## Field-Plot Planting and Management

Seed samples for grain ionomic analyses were produced in small field plots in Beaumont, TX, using the same planting, field management, and harvest methods used in companion studies (Norton et al., 2012, 2014; Zhang et al., 2014). Because availability of many elements in soil is known to be greatly affected by soil redox potential, this rice grain study evaluated grains from the same set of diverse rice accessions grown over 2 yr under both flooded (anaerobic) and unflooded (aerobic, flush irrigated) irrigation schemes. All field plots were planted into soil classified as League clay (fine, smectitic, hypothermic Oxyaquic Dystrudert; Chen et al., 1989). Plots were fertilized 3 to 5 wk before planting with 33.6 kg/ha P and at the time of planting with 73 kg/ha N (as urea). Plots were drill-seeded approximately 2-cm deep into a dry seedbed using a Hege 80 Plot Seeder (Wintersteiger Inc., Salt Lake City, UT). Germination was initiated with the first flush irrigation, applied 1 d after planting. Additional flush irrigations were applied as needed to maintain soil moisture until seedlings of the shorter accessions were approximately

9-cm tall, at which time a 7- to 16-cm depth flood was applied and maintained on the flooded fields until the last plots per field were fully mature and hand-harvested. Unflooded fields received regular flush irrigations (once or twice a week) as necessary to prevent water stress while maintaining aerated soil conditions.

Use of small (13-cm) plot lengths, hereafter called hillplots, allowed each replication to be drill-seeded in a single day into a single paddy or irrigation area (Fig. 1A). Two replications of each Core accession were planted per water treatment (flooded versus unflooded) in both 2007 and 2008 at two different planting dates (replications) per year, with approximately 3 wk between planting dates. Because of storm damage, however, seed for grain analysis was obtained from a total of three flooded replications (both early and late plantings in 2007, early planting only in 2008) and three unflooded replications (early planting only in 2007, both early and late plantings in 2008). Experimental units consisted of a single hillplot per genotype (5 to 6 seeds per plot) per water treatment, with two planting replications per year. Hillplots were arranged in rows 25-cm apart, with each 240-cm field-row containing five individual hillplots, each separated by 47 cm. The relatively wide spacing between hillplots minimized plot-to-plot interactions from either shading or root-zone overlap. Field rows were arranged as five tiers of 100 rows each in a rectangular 28 × 20 $m^2$ field area surrounded by an irrigation levee, with a maximum distance of 34 m between plots in opposite corners of each replication. To evaluate variance due to field heterogeneity, 20 plots of check cultivars were planted in a 4 × 5 grid pattern throughout each treatment block (paddy). Each check-plot consisted of three to five hillplots (five planted, not all grew) per each of three check cultivars. Lemont was used to represent typical modern U.S. tropical *japonica* cultivars among the checks. TeQing, a cultivar from China, represented *indica* germplasm having taller plant height, later maturity, more numerous tillers (branches) per plant, and a larger root system than Lemont. The third check cultivar, Dragon Eyeball 100, is one of several rice cultivars valued by consumers in China for the high iron concentration of its unmilled, purple-bran kernels.

Lodging of the tall and/or weak-stemmed accessions was prevented by tying the main culms of each hillplot to a bamboo stake (Fig. 1B). The date of 50% heading was recorded for each hillplot. Days to heading (DHD) was calculated by subtracting the date of first irrigation after planting (0 to 1 d post planting) from the heading date recorded for each plot. Mature panicles were hand-harvested. Rough rice samples were dried to 12% moisture using an ambient-forced-air drier then stored at ambient temperature in sealed plastic boxes until subsampled for phenotypic analysis.

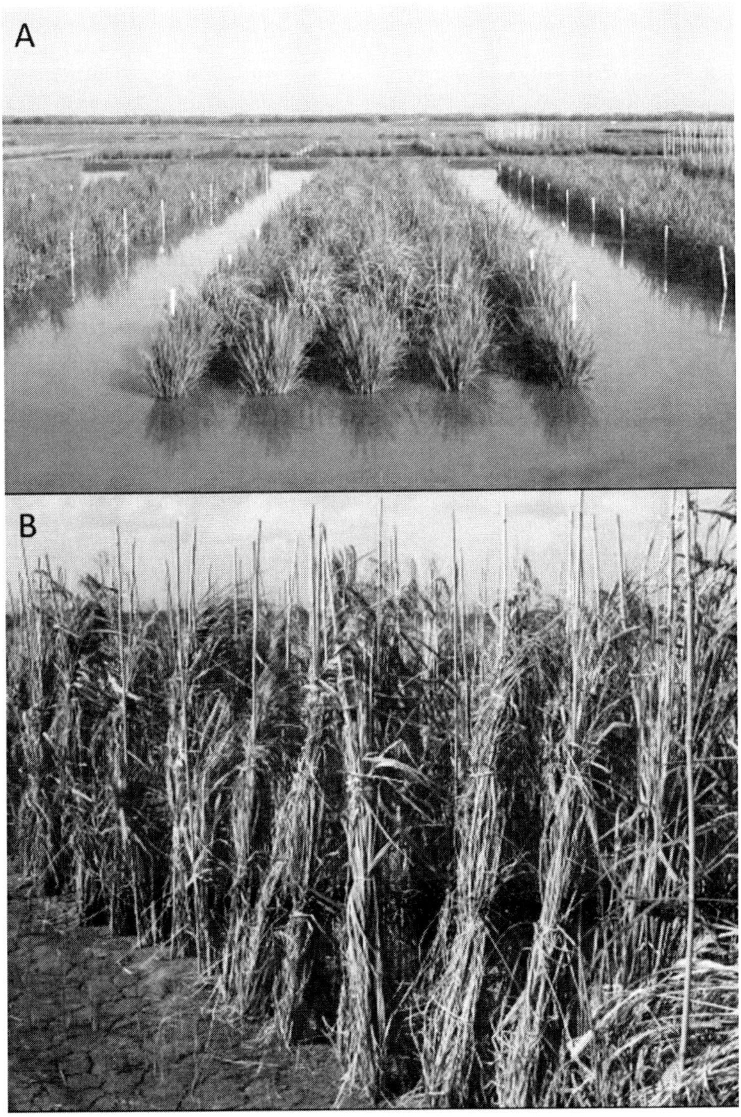


**Figure 1.** Field plots as observed (a) early and (b) late season, both flooded and unflooded (foreground and background in [a]). To minimize soil variance between plots and allow an entire replication to fit within a single irrigation paddy (field block), small hillplots were used, one per accession per field block. During midseason, plants of hillplots were tied to bamboo stakes to prevent lodging.

**Determination of Element Concentrations in Unmilled Rice Grain**

The concentrations of 16 elements were simultaneously determined in samples of brown (unmilled) rice grains using inductively coupled plasma mass spectrometry (ICP–MS). Unmilled rather than white (milled) kernels were evaluated to allow detection of variation in concentrations of elements that primarily accumulate in bran as well as those that accumulate primarily in endosperm and to prevent confounding the data with variance from potential milling differences (Hansen et al., 2012; Saenchai et al., 2012). The study of whole-grain brown rice makes this study consistent with, and more directly relevant to, biofortification research in other grain crops such as wheat (*Triticum aestivum* L.) (Salunke et al., 2012; Wu et al., 2013; Borrill et al., 2014), maize (*Zea mays* L.) (Baxter et al., 2012a), and pearl millet (*Pennisetum glaucum*) (Cercamondi et al., 2013) as well as prior studies in*Arabidopsis thaliana* (Vreugdenhil et al., 2004; Baxter et al., 2012b) and rice (e.g., Norton et al., 2012, 2014; Kuramata et al., 2013; Zhang et al., 2014). The convention in this report will be to report mineral concentrations as micrograms per gram grain dry weight (μg $g^{-1}$) and to present the five plant macronutrients first (P, Mg, K, S, Ca) in high to low order of their grain concentration, followed by the remaining 11 elements in alphabetical order (As, Cd, Co, Cu, Fe, Mn, Mo, Ni, Rb, Sr, Zn). The methods used to harvest and select seed for grain analysis are described in more detail by Zhang et al. (2014). Methods used to digest the kernels and then analyze them by ICP–MS are described elsewhere (Norton et al., 2012; Zhang et al., 2014). Briefly, 10 to 15 fully mature grains were hand-threshed from the tips of 3 panicles harvested per hillplot, then dehulled using a Satake TH035A sheller (Satake Engineering Co. Ltd.), on which the Zn-containing rubber lining the rollers (Stangoulis, 2010) was replaced with PU40 polyurethane plastic. From this, three complete (unbroken and unmilled) kernels were selected, (approximate weight 0.05 g) and digested with 1.0 mL concentrated $HNO_3$ in 16 × 100 mm Pyrex tubes at temperatures stepped from ambient to 110°C over a period of 12 h. Indium (EM Science) was added to the acid to a final concentration of 20 μg $L^{-1}$ as an internal standard. Samples were diluted to 10.0 mL and analyzed for their total elemental composition on a PerkinElmer Elan DRCe ICP–MS (PerkinElmer Corp.) using the following stable isotopes: P31, K39, Mg25, S34, Ca43, As75, Cd114, Co59, Cu65, Fe57, Mn55, Mo98, Ni60, Rb85, Sr88, and Zn66 and known natural isotopic abundances. To normalize data between machine runs to correct for drift, portions of the samples were combined and used as a matrix-matched standard, measured after every nine samples. Samples were normalized to the averaged signals of the best-measured elements and weights of seven samples per run (Lahner et al., 2003). All ICP–MS data on rice grain used in this study is publicly available at www.ionomicshub.org (accessed 9 Sept. 2014).

Preliminary Analyses of Effects Due to Water Management Treatment and Spatial Variance within Field Replications

The phenotypic variance observed for each element among the plots of repeated checks was examined further so that knowledge derived among the checks on magnitude of variance due to water treatment, planting time, and within-field spatial effects could be used to select statistical models most appropriate for evaluating the larger (1763 diverse accessions) data set. Using the Fit Model application of JMP version 9.0 (SAS Institute, 2010), the variance of each element response was first assessed on the basis of the partitions of sum of squares in models with Genotype, Water treatment, Year, Replication(within Year) (which also reflected differences in planting time), Tier(within Replication), Column(within Replication), and interaction terms. The water treatment (flooded vs. unflooded) effects were found to be so proportionally large for all 16 elements (>90.7%) that all other factors in the model had extremely minor effects in comparison. Therefore, flooded and unflooded data were kept separate in the following variance-partitioning analyses.

It was initially anticipated that a 3-wk difference in planting time between the two replications per year would result in a growing season so different that Replication(within Year) effects would be similar to Year effects. This hypothesis proved true with variance analyses indicating Replication effects in flooded and unflooded fields up to 30 times greater than Year effects. When variance was partitioned into Genotype, Replication, Tier(within Replication), Column(within Replication), and interaction effects, the terms reflecting within-field spatial variance (Tier, Column, and Tier × Column) were insignificant (at $\alpha = 0.05$) for the majority of elements. Even for those elements for which they were statistically significant (As, Co, Fe, Ni, and Rb flooded; Cd, Fe, Mn and Rb unflooded), they were relatively minor, with Genotype, Replication and Genotype × Replication together accounting for 90 to 97% of the variance attributed to all the model factors combined. In fact, Genotype was the single largest factor for most elements in both flooded and unflooded conditions. The few elements for which environmental factors (Replication and/or Genotype × Replication) were larger than Genotype effects were Ni and Sr flooded, and As, Ni, and Sr under unflooded conditions.

### Means and Comparisons among the 1763 Diverse Rice Accessions

In response to the large effects of water treatment seen among the check plots, and the small size and lack of useful trends observed for the within-field variance, comparisons made among the 1763 accessions were based on least squares means (LS means) calculated across the three replications per water treatment per accession using SAS (version 9.1, SAS Institute 2007). Partitioning of the variances per element into Subgroup, Geographic Region of Origin, and the interaction effects indicated significantly greater effects from Subgroup than Geographic Region of Origin, though both effects were statistically significant. Therefore, the results and discussion section focuses primarily on differences among ancestral subgroups rather than differences among accessions from different global regions, but all comparisons were made and considered during the data interpretations.

In addition to the grain element concentrations and DHD data collected from the 2007 and 2008 Texas hillplots, data on DHD, plant height (Ht, in cm), grain weight, and shape dimensions among the Core accessions from previous Arkansas flooded field evaluations of the USDA Core accessions (Yan et al., 2007) were analyzed. The following statistical analyses were performed using JMP version 9.0 (SAS Institute, 2010). Pearson correlations among the 16 elements, DHD, and grain dimensions included numerous pairwise comparisons, which can increase type I error. Therefore significance thresholds ($r \geq 0.310$ for both flooded and unflooded conditions) were determined using Bonferroni's adjustments (Abdi, 2007). Differences among various data subsets (e.g., water treatments, subgroups, or regions of origin) were tested for significance using ANOVA. The principal component analyses were performed using correlation matrices as input, thus all data were both standardized (Z-scale transformed) and mean-centered; unrotated results are provided.

## RESULTS AND DISCUSSION

### Trait Averages and Variances among 1763 Rice Accessions Grown Flooded and Unflooded

Data on the LS means, ranges, and variances of the grain element concentrations averaged over the 1763 accessions grown under both flooded and unflooded conditions are presented in Table 1. Soil chemistry and mineral element availability are known to differ between flooded (anaerobic, chemically reduced) and unflooded (oxidized) fields (De Datta, 1987; Daum et al., 2002; Zhang et al., 2004; Arao et al., 2009; Sahrawat, 2012). Some elements are more available for plant uptake when they are chemically reduced than when oxidized in aerobic soil, for example, Fe and As. The element with the largest observed change in grain concentration due to water treatment was As, with 30X higher concentrations in grains produced under flooded conditions than unflooded conditions. The elements next most sensitive to water treatment differences were Cd and Ni, which, in contrast to As, averaged 10X lower concentrations in grains grown under flooded rather than unflooded conditions. When making selections, breeders often seek to use growth conditions that maximize the phenotypic differences among genotypes. For most elements (all except Ni and As), a wider range in grain concentrations (max./min. ratios, Table 1) was observed under unflooded than under flooded conditions, initially suggesting that breeder selections for grain concentration of most elements might be more efficient in unflooded than flooded fields. Phenotypic variance is most useful when it is due to genetic rather than environmental effects. The proportion of total phenotypic variance explained by genotype is known as broad sense heritability (*H2*). As a point of reference, maturity (as measured by DHD) is generally considered a highly heritable trait in rice and had $H2 = 0.9$ under both flooded and unflooded conditions in this study. The heritabilities of the 16 elements ranged from 0.14 to 0.69 under flooded conditions (average 0.49) and from 0.23 to 0.75 under unflooded conditions (avg. 0.57) (Table 1). Fourteen of the 16 elements had $H2 > 0.5$ under one or both field conditions, indicating that grain element concentrations could be improved through breeder selections conducted on seed produced in one growing condition, if not both, for these 14 elements. Nickel had the lowest *H2* ($\leq 0.24$) under both flooded and unflooded conditions, followed by P ($H2 \approx 0.3$ under both conditions). Although genetic variability was statistically significant for both Ni and P, indicating the potential to make breeding improvement, with low relatively heritabilities, breeding progress would be expected to be slower than for elements with higher *H2*.

Partitioning of variance indicated that for all elements except As, Subgroup explained proportionally more variance (1.5 to 16 times more) than Geographic Region of Origin across both flooded and unflooded conditions (Supplemental Table S2). This is consistent with the fact that among the 1763 accessions in this study, accessions of multiple subgroups were collected from each of the 14 worldwide regions (Supplemental Fig. 1). In that the IND and AUS rice cultivars are more commonly grown in tropical regions with longer growing seasons than the regions where the more cold-tolerant TEJ accessions predominate, it was not unexpected to find that the TEJ subgroup has the lowest average DHD among the subgroups (Figs. 2 and 3). Because

**Table 1.** Summary of grain element concentrations (μg $g^{-1}$) from flooded and unflooded field studies of 1763 rice (*Oryza sativa* L.) accessions. Minimum (min.), maximum (max.), max./min. ratio, mean, standard deviation (SD), coefficient of variance (CV), and heritability (broad sense) based on least squares means calculated for 1763 accessions across three replications per water-irrigation treatment. Fl, flooded; Unfl, unflooded.

| | Fl | | | | | | | Unfl | | | | | | | |
|---|---|---|---|---|---|---|---|---|---|---|---|---|---|---|---|
| | Min. | Max. | Max./ Min. ratio | Mean | SD | CV | Herit-ability | Min. | Max. | Max./ Min. ratio | Mean | SD | CV | Herit-ability | Ratio of Fl/Unfl means |
| P | 2985 | 4734 | 1.6 | 3792 | 249 | 0.066 | 0.31 | 2198 | 4748 | 2.2 | 3455 | 283 | 0.082 | 0.29 | 1.1 |
| K | 2260 | 4541 | 2.0 | 2940 | 294 | 0.100 | 0.36 | 1565 | 4308 | 2.8 | 2738 | 295 | 0.108 | 0.61 | 1.1 |
| Mg | 1191 | 2006 | 1.7 | 1566 | 113 | 0.072 | 0.57 | 955 | 1916 | 2.0 | 1411 | 118 | 0.084 | 0.41 | 1.1 |
| S | 520 | 1757 | 3.4 | 1171 | 160 | 0.137 | 0.46 | 153 | 2912 | 19.1 | 1435 | 202 | 0.140 | 0.65 | 0.8 |
| Ca | 75.3 | 255.8 | 3.4 | 129.4 | 25.6 | 0.198 | 0.56 | 51.9 | 502.3 | 9.7 | 130.9 | 29.4 | 0.224 | 0.57 | 1.0 |
| As | 0.217 | 2.610 | 12.1 | 0.945 | 0.312 | 0.330 | 0.57 | 0.001 | 0.125 | 125.2 | 0.030 | 0.019 | 0.631 | 0.64 | 31.2 |
| Cd | 0.002 | 0.067 | 40.7 | 0.010 | 0.006 | 0.598 | 0.24 | 0.010 | 1.543 | 154.3 | 0.102 | 0.097 | 0.951 | 0.63 | 0.1 |
| Co | 0.010 | 0.241 | 23.8 | 0.052 | 0.022 | 0.425 | 0.57 | 0.004 | 0.240 | 62.5 | 0.037 | 0.020 | 0.555 | 0.67 | 1.4 |
| Cu | 1.756 | 5.397 | 3.1 | 3.340 | 0.565 | 0.169 | 0.46 | 3.300 | 11.354 | 3.4 | 6.444 | 1.100 | 0.171 | 0.75 | 0.5 |
| Fe | 1.55 | 16.56 | 10.7 | 11.45 | 1.40 | 0.122 | 0.47 | 0.09 | 25.89 | 287.6 | 12.04 | 3.18 | 0.264 | 0.73 | 1.0 |
| Mn | 14.35 | 46.51 | 3.2 | 24.72 | 4.15 | 0.168 | 0.58 | 15.37 | 76.00 | 4.9 | 35.94 | 7.70 | 0.214 | 0.55 | 0.7 |
| Mo | 0.063 | 2.059 | 32.4 | 0.429 | 0.118 | 0.274 | 0.69 | 0.084 | 2.006 | 24.0 | 0.388 | 0.105 | 0.271 | 0.53 | 1.1 |
| Ni | 0.298 | 6.036 | 20.3 | 1.573 | 0.495 | 0.315 | 0.14 | 4.073 | 37.628 | 9.3 | 10.963 | 2.359 | 0.215 | 0.23 | 0.1 |
| Rb | 3.93 | 24.48 | 6.2 | 10.78 | 2.53 | 0.235 | 0.64 | 0.30 | 35.81 | 120.9 | 11.77 | 4.10 | 0.348 | 0.73 | 0.9 |
| Sr | 0.303 | 1.425 | 4.7 | 0.555 | 0.134 | 0.241 | 0.68 | 0.140 | 2.035 | 14.5 | 0.417 | 0.121 | 0.290 | 0.64 | 1.3 |
| Zn | 15.72 | 65.01 | 4.1 | 24.29 | 3.55 | 0.146 | 0.50 | 19.34 | 63.13 | 3.3 | 29.99 | 4.07 | 0.136 | 0.47 | 0.8 |
| DHD | 52.5 | 129.5 | 2.5 | 90.4 | 14.3 | 0.159 | 0.91 | 54.5 | 118.6 | 2.2 | 93.7 | 13.5 | 0.144 | 0.87 | 1.0 |

of long-term cultural preferences and breeding selections, the TEJ subgroup also has the widest average grain width (GW), the shortest average grain length (GL), and thus the roundest (smallest GL/GW ratio) grain average among the subgroups (Fig. 4). Because of nonrandom differences among the subgroups, such as described here for grain shape and DHD, all further data analyses were conducted per individual subgroup as well as across all 1763 accessions.

Consistent with known changes in availability of elements in reduced (flooded) soil solution, average grain concentrations of As were higher, and Cd and Ni were lower in rice grains produced on flooded than on unflooded plants (Table 1). While other studies have reported reduced grain Fe under flooded conditions (Zhang et al., 2014), contrary to what one would expect on the basis of increased availability of Fe in soil solution, the mean grain Fe across the 1763 was not significantly different between the two water treatments. It has been suggested that altered grain accumulation of Fe and some other elements under flooded conditions may be due to the iron plaque (layer of oxidized Fe) that forms on the root surfaces of flooded rice plants and has been

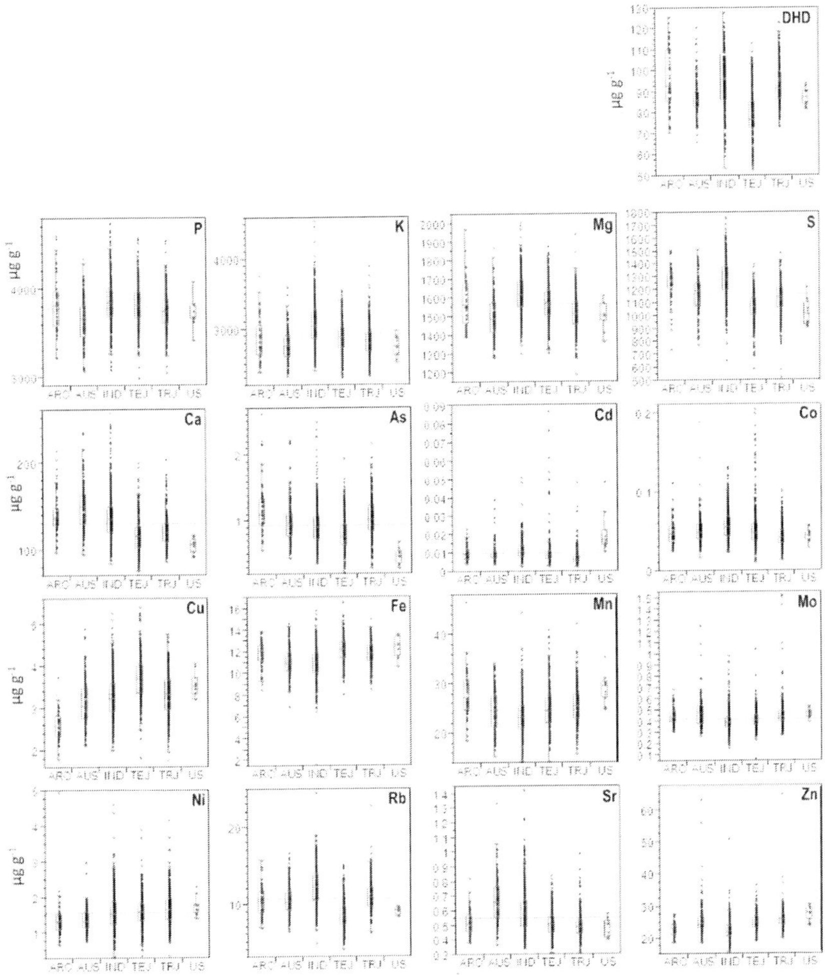


**Figure 2.** Mean data from 1763 diverse rice (*Oryza sativa* L.) accessions grown flooded and plotted per ancestral lineage or subgrouping. For comparison purposes, data from 10 modern southern U.S. rice cultivars are presented separately as well as included in the tropical *japonica* subgroup. The box represents data between the 25th and 75th percentiles, whiskers (error bars) indicate the 90th and 10th percentiles. Red lines inside the boxes represent the mean. The mean across all subgroups is indicated by the black line. ARO, *aromatic*; AUS, *aus*; IND, *indica*; TEJ temperate *japonica*; and TRJ, tropical *japonica*.

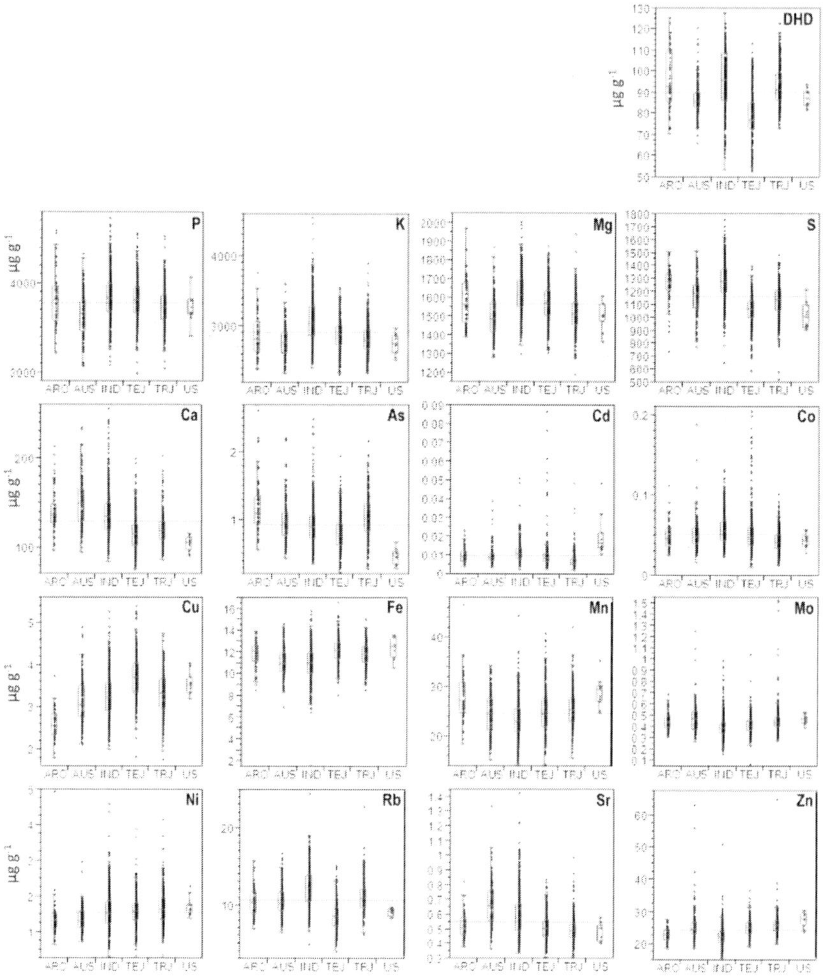


**Figure 3.** Mean data from 1763 diverse rice (*Oryza sativa* L.) accessions grown unflooded and plotted per ancestral lineage or subgrouping. For comparison purposes, data from 10 modern southern U.S. rice cultivars are presented separately as well as included in the tropical *japonica* subgroup. The box represents data between the 25th and 75th percentiles, whiskers (error bars) indicate the 90th and 10th percentiles. Red lines inside the boxes represent the mean. The mean across all subgroups is indicated by the black line. ARO, *aromatic*; AUS, *aus*; IND, *indica*; TEJ temperate *japonica*; and TRJ, tropical *japonica*.

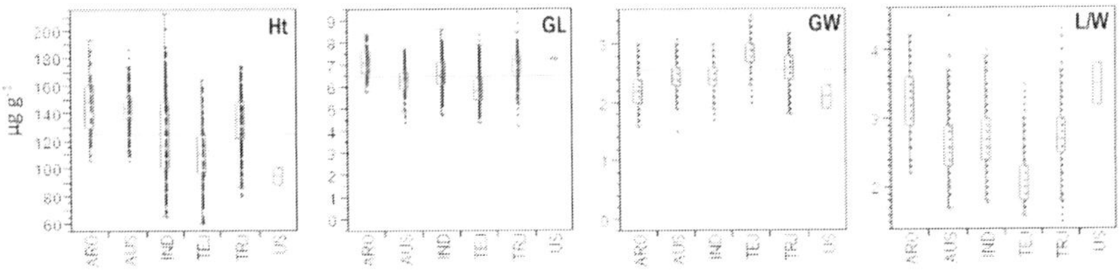


**Figure 4.** Trait means determined in other USDA Core Collection flooded field studies (Yan et al., 2007) plotted per ancestral lineage or subgrouping. For comparison purposes, data from 10 modern southern U.S. rice (*Oryza sativa* L.) cultivars are presented separately as well as included in the tropical *japonica* subgroup. The box represents data between the 25th and 75th percentiles, whiskers (error bars) indicate the 90th and 10th percentiles. Red lines inside the boxes represent the mean. The mean across all subgroups is indicated by the black line. ARO, *aromatic*; AUS, *aus*; IND, *indica*; TEJ temperate *japonica*; and TRJ, tropical *japonica*.

shown to increase the uptake or access of some elements (e.g., P, Zhang et al., 1999), but decrease plant uptake or access of others (e.g., Zn [Zhang et al., 1998; Wu et al., 2010], Se [Zhou et al., 2007], and As [Hu et al., 2005;Wu et al., 2012]). In addition to soil chemistry, changes in root morphology are also associated with soil aeration, with rice plants producing more surface-level roots under flooded conditions but deeper roots under unflooded growth conditions (Hoshikawa, 1989;Lafitte et al., 2001; Uga et al., 2012; Rose et al., 2013b). The surface-level roots are primarily in a soil zone that maintains some oxygen content, thus allowing access to mineral elements that are less soluble under the reduced conditions deeper in the flooded soil (De Datta, 1987, Rose et al., 2013b).

## Accessions with Elevated Grain Concentrations Were Identified for Each Element

The distributions of each of the 16 elements were positively skewed, with right-hand or positive tail longer than the left (negative) tail, and a population mean greater than (to the right of) both the median and the distribution peak (Figs. 2 and 3; Supplemental Table S1). The rarity of accessions in the extended upper tails (i.e., above the 90th percentiles, Figs. 2and 3) combined with the 2- to 200-fold range in grain concentration observed among the elements within this set of diverse rice accessions (Table 1) suggest that the rare accessions having exceptionally high grain-element concentrations may result from a mutation in one or a few genes of large effect. If the extreme phenotypes were due to a single mutation that was selected for (e.g., favored their adaptability to the soil chemistry characteristic of a particular region or location), then the accessions found extreme for a particular element would be expected to have similar ancestry (subgroup membership) and locations of origin. Indeed, five of the top 10 accessions in terms of mean grain Mo were TRJ accessions collected from either Malaysia or Brunei, adjacent island countries, suggesting they may share a heritable underlying mechanism that enhances grain Mo. These islands have acidic soils, and low pH decreases the bioavailability of Mo (Raun et al., 1998), suggesting that there might be a deficiency of available Mo in the soils of this geographic region. The wide range in heading dates (91 to 116 DHD) among these five high-Mo accessions supports the Pearson correlation data in indicating that heading time is not a determinant of grain Mo. Likewise, wide variations for plant height and grain shape were also noted among these high-Mo accessions from Malaysia and Brunei.

Of the 10 accessions with highest grain Cd under flooded conditions, all were members of the TEJ subgroup, four of which originated from Eastern Europe, and three of which were collected in Hungary. In contrast, a majority of accessions high for grain Cd under unflooded conditions were from the AUS subgroup. None of the accessions contained more than the codex alimentarius limit of 0.4 $\mu g\ g^{-1}$ Cd when grown flooded, but several accessions of the AUS, IND, and TEJ subgroups exceeded this concentration when grown unflooded. The distributions for grain Cd for all five subgroups were strongly positively skewed under both flooded and unflooded conditions, with a majority of the accessions being desirably low in grain Cd concentration. Interestingly, 5 of the 10 topmost accessions in terms of grain Co were also TEJ from Eastern Europe, though none of the accessions from Eastern Europe were high for both Cd and Co.

Like Cd, genes and mechanisms that reduce accumulation of As in grains are desired. The grain As concentrations in every one of the 1763 accessions was low ($<0.13\ \mu g\ g^{-1}$, Fig. 3) when grown unflooded, but higher (0.2 to 2.6 $\mu g\ g^{-1}$, Fig. 2) when grown flooded, focusing concerns about high grain As in rice plants exposed to reduced soil conditions. Among the 10 accessions with highest grain As grown flooded, four of the five subgroups (all except TEJ) are represented, with accessions originating from five different geographic regions (Fig. 6; Supplemental Table S1). In contrast, low grain As showed significant association with ancestral lineage with 7 of the 10 accessions selected for lowest grain As under flooded conditions being TEJ or admixtures with TEJ, and three being TRJ. In contrast, low grain As was uncommon among the IND and

AUS subgroups, with two IND but no AUS among the 20 accessions lowest for grain As. In a smaller set (~300) of diverse rice accessions grown in Bangladesh, China, and two U.S. sites (Texas and Arkansas), it was noted that the TEJ subgroup had the lowest average grain As (Norton et al., 2012). Interestingly, 2 of the 20 accessions lowest for grain As in the present study were modern U.S. rice cultivars (Gulfmont and Jefferson). In further agreement with Norton et al. (2012), the 10 modern U.S. cultivars observed herein were relatively low for grain As overall (Fig. 2).

## Correlations between Elements

The Pearson correlations ($r$) determined between traits among the 1763 accessions were calculated separately for flooded and unflooded data (Table 2). The correlations between flooded and unflooded LS means per element are shown in the boxes. Some interesting patterns can be seen among the correlations between the various elements. For example, Rb and K are chemical analogs and known to share plant uptake mechanisms, thus the fact that Rb and K are significantly and positively correlated under both flooded ($r = 0.45$) and unflooded ($r = 0.35$) conditions is as expected. The elements Ca and Sr are also chemical analogs and were very highly correlated under flooded conditions ($r = 0.80$) but were not correlated ($r = 0.29$) under unflooded conditions. Some of the other correlations observed were less readily explained, such as the positive correlations observed between Rb–As, Mn–Ca, and Cu–Ni and the negative correlations for Cu–Ca, Cu–As, P–Fe, and Rb–Fe under flooded conditions; and the positive correlation between As–Fe and the negative correlations between P–Fe, K–Fe, Cd–Fe, and Rb–As under flooded conditions. The strongest, most consistent element-to-element correlations were observed among the three essential macronutrients P, K, and Mg. These elements are not considered chemical analogs and are not known to share uptake mechanisms. When the data were analyzed separately by ancestral subgroups (data not shown), these elements remained highly correlated across all subgroups, indicating a widespread association among these elements in terms of grain accumulation. Strong positive associations between P, K, and Mg were also reported within two biparental rice mapping populations (Zhang et al., 2014). Significant P–K and P–Mg associations have also been reported in maize kernels (Baxter et al., 2012a) and seed of *A. thaliana* (Vreugdenhil et al., 2004; Baxter et al., 2012b). Among the 1763 accessions, individual exceptions to the strong positive correlations generally seen between grain P, K, and Mg could be found, such as Core accessions 310241 and 311625, which had high grain P but low grain K, and Core 311012 which had high grain K, but low concentrations of P and K.

**Table 2.** Correlations between traits in the flooded (upper right matrix) and unflooded (lower left matrix) studies. Correlations between traits (grain element concentrations [μg $g^{-1}$], grain shape, plant height, and days to heading) for the 1763 diverse rice accessions calculated from LS mean data across three field replications per water–irrigation treatment. The correlations for each trait presently observed under both flooded and unflooded conditions are underlined. Bold text indicates significance at α = 0.05. Bonferroni adjustments were used to account for the multiple comparisons made. DHD, days from planting to heading.

| | Macronutrients | | | | | Micronutrients | | | | | | | | | | | | Data from previous study† | | | |
|---|---|---|---|---|---|---|---|---|---|---|---|---|---|---|---|---|---|---|---|---|---|
| | P | K | Mg | S | Ca | As | Cd | Co | Cu | Fe | Mn | Mo | Ni | Rb | Sr | Zn | DHD | Height | Grain length | Grain width | L/W ratio |
| P | **0.37** | **0.66** | **0.72** | −0.02 | −0.02 | 0.14 | 0.01 | 0.04 | −0.09 | **−0.33** | −0.05 | −0.15 | −0.12 | 0.21 | −0.09 | −0.06 | 0.15 | 0.02 | −0.04 | 0.03 | −0.05 |
| K | **0.59** | **0.54** | **0.56** | 0.05 | 0.28 | 0.19 | −0.01 | 0.02 | −0.19 | −0.28 | 0.11 | −0.16 | −0.15 | **0.45** | 0.15 | −0.23 | **0.33** | 0.03 | −0.09 | −0.08 | −0.01 |
| Mg | **0.76** | 0.42 | **0.54** | −0.01 | 0.11 | 0.16 | 0.04 | 0.03 | −0.06 | −0.23 | 0.06 | −0.26 | −0.11 | 0.22 | 0.10 | −0.25 | 0.22 | −0.08 | −0.15 | −0.07 | −0.04 |
| S | −0.13 | −0.19 | −0.04 | 0.29 | 0.06 | 0.01 | 0.08 | 0.10 | −0.16 | −0.21 | −0.22 | −0.12 | −0.00 | 0.27 | 0.02 | −0.19 | **0.33** | 0.07 | 0.258 | −0.24 | 0.29 |
| Ca | 0.00 | 0.09 | 0.04 | −0.12 | **0.31** | 0.26 | −0.00 | 0.00 | **−0.39** | −0.17 | **0.37** | −0.12 | −0.16 | 0.26 | **0.80** | −0.19 | 0.23 | 0.27 | **−0.13** | −0.24 | 0.07 |
| As | −0.20 | −0.20 | −0.10 | 0.07 | −0.01 | −0.09 | −0.28 | −0.11 | **−0.44** | −0.15 | 0.04 | 0.09 | −0.22 | **0.38** | 0.107 | −0.03 | **0.37** | **0.37** | 0.09 | −0.08 | 0.10 |
| Cd | 0.14 | 0.14 | 0.15 | 0.06 | 0.07 | −0.14 | **0.49** | 0.06 | 0.21 | −0.07 | 0.03 | 0.02 | 0.25 | −0.02 | 0.07 | −0.10 | −0.16 | −0.19 | −0.08 | −0.07 | −0.01 |
| Co | 0.02 | −0.01 | −0.09 | 0.01 | −0.04 | 0.05 | 0.01 | 0.17 | −0.03 | 0.02 | −0.13 | −0.12 | 0.04 | −0.11 | 0.13 | 0.09 | −0.18 | −0.03 | −0.03 | 0.07 | −0.08 |
| Cu | −0.19 | −0.26 | −0.01 | 0.27 | −0.09 | 0.21 | −0.01 | −0.00 | **0.55** | 0.09 | −0.06 | −0.17 | **0.37** | −0.25 | −0.23 | 0.10 | **−0.39** | **−0.44** | −0.15 | 0.27 | −0.26 |
| Fe | **−0.37** | **−0.37** | −0.28 | 0.05 | −0.12 | 0.31 | −0.31 | 0.04 | **0.35** | **0.39** | 0.08 | −0.09 | 0.14 | **−0.38** | 0.01 | −0.03 | **−0.44** | −0.14 | −0.13 | 0.14 | −0.15 |
| Mn | 0.07 | 0.14 | 0.04 | −0.11 | 0.13 | 0.19 | −0.04 | 0.19 | −0.01 | −0.03 | **0.47** | 0.00 | −0.02 | −0.02 | 0.28 | −0.03 | 0.04 | −0.04 | −0.04 | −0.06 | 0.04 |
| Mo | −0.07 | −0.10 | −0.21 | −0.04 | −0.04 | −0.17 | 0.01 | −0.05 | −0.16 | −0.20 | −0.06 | **0.74** | −0.07 | 0.01 | −0.14 | 0.06 | 0.02 | 0.08 | 0.11 | −0.04 | 0.09 |
| Ni | 0.15 | 0.02 | 0.17 | 0.11 | 0.04 | −0.02 | 0.09 | 0.13 | 0.16 | 0.01 | −0.06 | −0.05 | 0.21 | −0.04 | −0.03 | 0.03 | −0.31 | −0.11 | 0.04 | 0.14 | −0.07 |
| Rb | 0.22 | **0.35** | 0.19 | 0.04 | 0.09 | **−0.31** | 0.22 | 0.07 | −0.21 | **−0.50** | −0.10 | 0.11 | 0.23 | **0.62** | 0.06 | −0.18 | **0.54** | 0.30 | 0.19 | −0.22 | 0.23 |
| Sr | −0.09 | 0.08 | 0.02 | 0.04 | 0.29 | 0.05 | 0.21 | −0.08 | 0.10 | −0.10 | 0.24 | −0.07 | 0.12 | 0.11 | **0.44** | −0.25 | −0.05 | 0.13 | **−0.20** | −0.16 | −0.03 |
| Zn | 0.03 | −0.16 | −0.03 | −0.07 | 0.02 | −0.01 | −0.10 | 0.10 | 0.14 | 0.08 | −0.02 | −0.04 | 0.07 | −0.14 | −0.03 | **0.32** | −0.07 | 0.10 | 0.10 | 0.16 | −0.04 |
| DHD | **0.33** | **0.40** | 0.24 | −0.09 | 0.01 | **−0.48** | 0.17 | 0.02 | **−0.39** | **−0.50** | −0.16 | 0.17 | 0.04 | **0.52** | −0.10 | −0.07 | **0.85** | 0.24 | 0.25 | −0.37 | **0.38** |
| **Height†** | 0.08 | 0.04 | −0.11 | −0.10 | 0.14 | −0.09 | 0.02 | 0.12 | **−0.36** | −0.31 | −0.04 | 0.13 | 0.09 | 0.30 | 0.04 | 0.05 | 0.25 | – | 0.15 | −0.06 | 0.11 |
| **Grain length†** | 0.08 | 0.01 | −0.08 | 0.15 | −0.11 | −0.16 | −0.01 | 0.07 | −0.20 | −0.15 | −0.12 | 0.18 | 0.04 | 0.14 | −0.19 | −0.01 | 0.27 | – | – | −0.27 | 0.79 |
| **Grain width†** | −0.15 | −0.09 | −0.17 | −0.06 | −0.06 | 0.24 | −0.20 | 0.08 | 0.20 | **0.36** | 0.03 | −0.10 | 0.01 | −0.26 | −0.04 | 0.11 | **−0.33** | – | – | – | −0.81 |
| **Grain L/W ratio†** | 0.13 | 0.06 | 0.05 | 0.12 | −0.03 | −0.23 | 0.11 | −0.02 | −0.24 | −0.30 | −0.07 | 0.16 | 0.00 | 0.22 | −0.10 | −0.07 | **0.36** | – | – | – | – |

† Plant height and grain shape dimensions (weight, length, width, L/W ratio) were as observed by Yan et al. (2007).

## Principal Components within Water Treatments and Subgroups

Principal component analysis (PCA) reinforced the importance of intercorrelation between P, K, and Mg in terms of grain concentration in that the first principal component (PC1) comprised P, K, and Mg along with Rb, Cu, Fe, and As regardless of flooding treatment (Fig. 5). Interestingly, the loading of each element onto the PC1 was consistent with the DHD correlations (Table 2), with P, K, Mg, and Rb loading positively and Cu and Fe loading negatively onto PC1 under both flooded and unflooded conditions, and As loading positively onto PC1 under flooded conditions, but negatively onto the unflooded PC1. The PC2 elements determined across all 1763 accessions under both flooded and unflooded conditions were Ca, Sr, and Mn. The PC1 explained approximately 20% of the variance among accessions under both flooded and unflooded conditions; PC2 explained an additional 11 to 13%. Together, the PC1 and PC2 explained approximately 30% of variance, and divided the accessions according to their ancestral

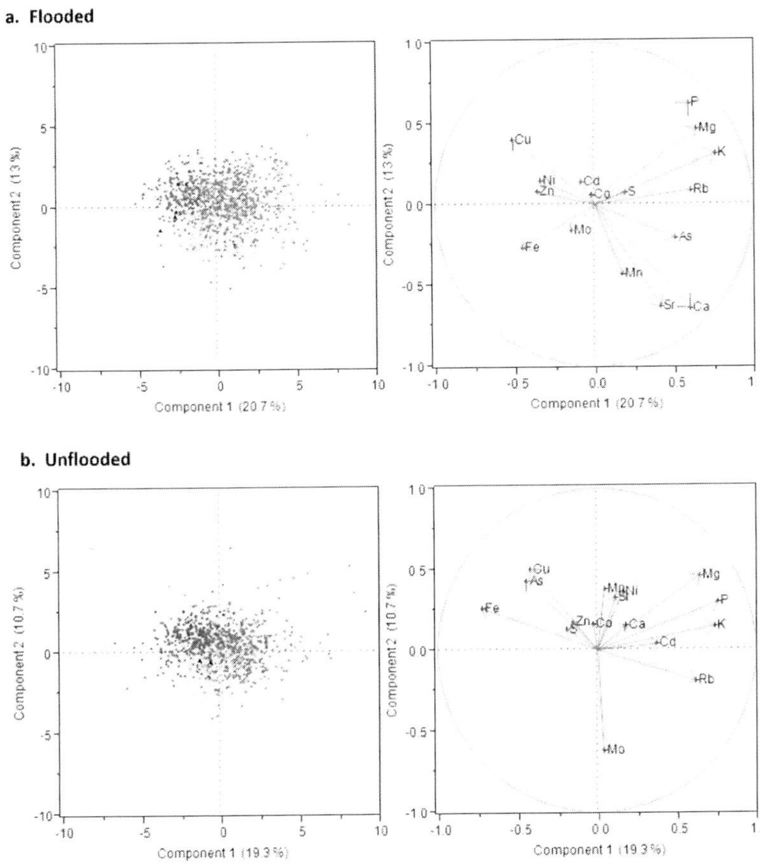


**Figure 5.** Principal components 1 and 2 (PC1 and PC2) determined from the entire set of 1763 diverse rice (*Oryza sativa* L.) accessions were similar under both (a) flooded and (b) unflooded conditions with the first two components (together explaining approximately 30% of the variance) and identifying ancestral subgroupings among the diverse rice accessions. Red dots indicate *indica* subgroup (IND) accessions, green = *aus*subgroup (AUS), light blue = tropical *japonica* subgroup (TRJ), purple = temperate*japonica* subgroup (TEJ), and dark blue triangles = modern U.S. TRJ accessions. The relatively low percentage of *aromatic* subgroup (ARO) accessions (gray) masks their presence in the figure. When data were analyzed per subgroup (Supplemental Fig. S2), the same elements were found important within each subgroup with P, K, Mg, and Rb consistently together in one of the main two components; Ca, Sr, Cu, Mn, and Mo in the second component; and As and Cu loading in nearly equal proportions between PC1 and PC2, with As reversing sign (positive versus negative loading) in the flooded versus unflooded data.

subgroups (Fig. 5). The subgroup identifications plus the preponderance of DHD-correlated elements loading on PC1 again raised the question of whether the observed correlations might be driven by nonrandom distribution of grain ionomics alleles among the subgroups. However, when the PCAs were conducted within each individual subgroup (Supplemental Fig. S2), what was most noteworthy was the consistency of the element groupings identified as the first and second principal components within and across the ancestral subgroups, and regardless of the field watering treatment.

### Correlations between Grain Element Concentrations and Grain Shape

Because it is known that some elements are more concentrated in the outer bran surface layers than in the starchy endosperm (Bryant et al., 2005; Liang et al., 2008; Lombi et al., 2009; Hansen et al., 2012), and that the surface to volume ratio is minimized with a round compared to long narrow grain shape, it was anticipated that grain shape might be a significant determinant of the grain ionome. To evaluate relationships between grain element concentrations and grain shape, this study included data on GL, GW, and roundness (GL/GW ratio) collected on the USDA Core Collection in prior studies (Yan et al., 2007). As mentioned earlier, the TEJ subgroup is, on average, shorter and rounder in grain shape than the other subgroups (Fig. 4), and being adapted to geographic regions with colder and shorter growing season, the TEJ also have shorter average DHD than the other rice subgroups (Fig. 2 and 3). This causes a relatively strong positive correlation between DHD and GW and GL/GW when data is analyzed across the 1763 diverse accessions (Table 2), but this association is not due to genetic linkage or physiological cause-and-effect relationship between low DHD and rounder grain shape but, rather, to breeding selections that favored nonrandom distribution of these traits among the ancestral subgroups. In contrast to the correlation seen between DHD and grain shape in Table 2, none of the elements were associated with GL, GW, or GL/GW under flooded conditions, and only Fe was weakly associated with GW under unflooded conditions. The associations between the grain elements and grain shape remained low or insignificant when the data were analyzed by individual subgroups or regions of origin (data not shown). Grain shape was not found to be as significant a determinant of grain ionomes as originally hypothesized, meaning that genes and mechanisms with stronger impact than bran:endosperm ratio alone exist among the rice accessions. The fact that grain shape did not prove to be a major determinant of grain ionomics means that differences in grain shape are not expected to confound future studies designed to identify genetic and molecular mechanisms controlling grain ionomics genes.

## Correlations between Elements and Days to Heading

Plants with a longer vegetative phase (later heading date) have a longer window of opportunity to mine mineral elements out of the soil, potentially building reserves in leaf tissues that can be later translocated to grains. It would follow, then, that extending the vegetative phase might be one method for increasing grain concentration of elements considered mobile within plants. Alternatively, later grain fill periods generally occur under cooler air and root zone temperatures, impacting transpiration rates which in turn affect root uptake rates, and rates of translocation of elements within plants (Quintana et al., 1999;Xiloyannis et al., 2001; Tani and Barrington, 2005). Additionally, soil chemistry and bioavailability of soil elements continue to change over time as the duration of flooding is extended (Somenahally et al., 2011b). With the PCA identifying six of the seven DHD-correlated elements as of primary importance, further evaluation of the associations between the grain element traits and DHD is warranted.

If an association between DHD and grain concentration of an element is due to duration-enhanced uptake and leaf storage of that element, then one might expect the element to increase with DHD over both flooded and unflooded field conditions, and for that element to be considered mobile as opposed to fixed or chemically bound within leaf and stem tissues. The elements P, K, Mg, Mo, S, and Ni are considered remobilized from leaves to newer leaves and/or grain (Raun et al., 1998) and were in abundant supply in the fertilized Texas field plots. As a chemical analog of K, Rb is also considered a remobilized element. The scatter plots of DHD by K and P (Fig. 6) are fairly representative of those for Rb and Mg, respectively. Both K and Rb were significantly correlated with DHD under both flooded and unflooded conditions, while P was significantly correlated with DHD under unflooded conditions. Like the P–DHD flooded correlation ($r = 0.15$), correlations with Mg (both $r = 0.2$) were positive but below the $\alpha = 0.05$ significance threshold. The graphs show a general upward trend, whether or not the correlations were above or below the threshold for statistical significance, as predicted if the increased grain concentrations were due to enhanced uptake of these elements by the plants over a longer vegetative phase followed by remobilization during grain fill. In contrast, Fe (Table 2, Fig. 6) and Cu (Table 2) are negatively associated with DHD under both flooded and unflooded conditions, which would be consistent with these elements being poorly remobilized within plants, making the Fe and Cu stored in vegetative tissues unavailable to the developing grain (Raun et al., 1998).

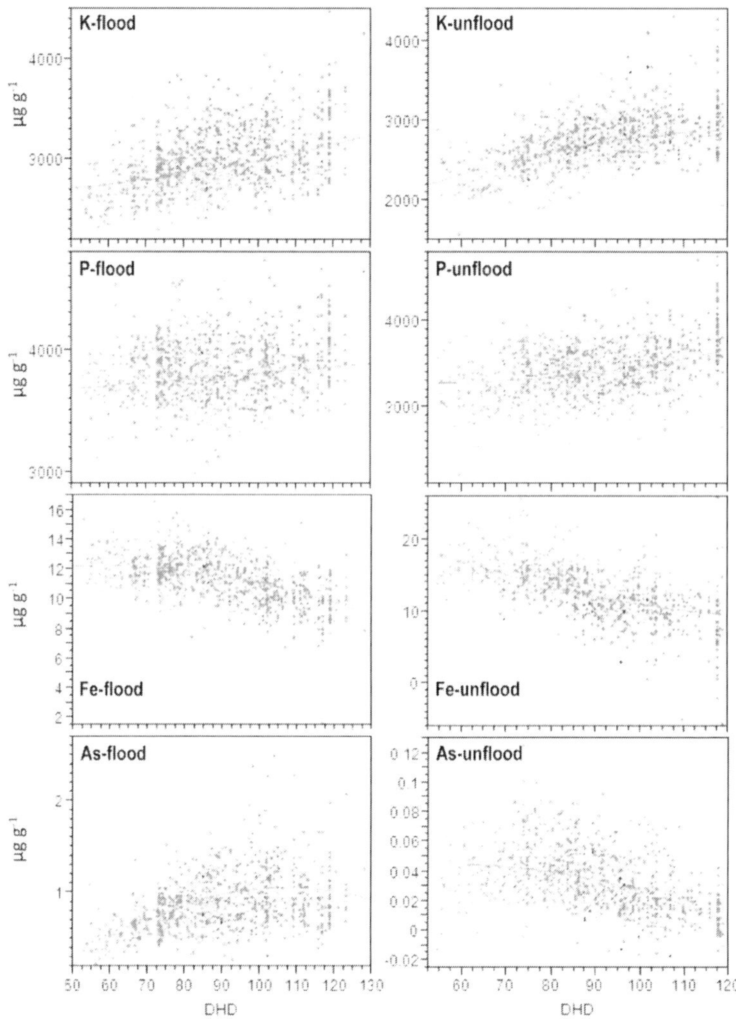


**Figure 6.** Scatter plots and quadratic means for K, P, Fe, and As, four elements whose grain concentrations were significantly associated with days from planting to heading (DHD) under flooded and/or unflooded field conditions across all 1763 accessions and within four of the five subgroups. Red dots indicate *indica* subgroup (IND) accessions, green =*aus* subgroup (AUS), light blue = tropical *japonica* subgroup (TRJ), purple = temperate *japonica* subgroup (TEJ), gray = *aromatic* subgroup (ARO), and dark blue triangles = modern U.S. TRJ accessions.

Arsenic is unique among the elements for having reversed association with DHD between the flooded (positive correlation) and unflooded (negative correlation) fields (Table 2, Fig. 6). Several reviews of current knowledge on the different forms of As in the rhizosphere under flooded and unflooded conditions and differences in their bioavailablity based on how they are taken up by plant roots and subsequently transported throughout or sequestered within specific cells or plant tissues have been published (Zhao et al., 2009, 2012; Carey et al., 2010, 2011; Tuli et al., 2010; Moore et al., 2011, 2013; Kuramata et al., 2013). With low grain As being more common among the TEJ, which are also noted for earlier heading, than among the IND and AUS, which are noted for longer vegetative stages in general, it came as no surprise that the average DHD among the 10 accessions with lowest grain As was less than the average DHD among the accessions with highest grain As (74 ±19 and 103 ±14, respectively). What is new and of particular interest here is the near-linear relationship between maximum observed grain As and DHD that results in a scatter plot with a narrower range in grain As among early-heading (mostly TEJ) accessions than among the later heading (mostly IND) accessions (Fig. 6). This lends support to reports that As availability in soil solution increases as the length of flooding period increases owing to an increase in the population of Fe-reducing microbes over time, which in turn results in increased release of reduced As into the soil solution under prolonged flooding (Somenahally et al., 2011a,2011b). Changes in As availability in soil solution during the growing season would also be consistent with As being the sole element for which ANOVA indicated less variance due to Subgroup than to Geographic Region since region of origin or collection site would be even more directly related to length of growing season and maturity differences than Subgroup.

Straighthead is a physiological disease in rice that is induced with application of As-based herbicide to the resistance screening nursery. It is interesting to note, therefore, that most rice accessions found to be resistant to straighthead disease are also early maturing, with none having greater than 92 DHD (Yan et al., 2004; Agrama and Yan, 2010; Pan et al., 2012).

The wide range in grain As observed among the accessions with a mid to late DHD (87 to 120 DHD, Fig. 6) increases the confidence in identifying lines as "As accumulators" (significantly above the grain As mean per DHD) versus "As excluders" compared with selections made among the lower grain As TEJ accessions with DHD from 50 to 65 d.

The linear association observed for maximum observed grain As concentration when plotted against DHD indicates two things. First, that one method for reducing grain As might be to produce early-maturing rice cultivars, within limits since early flowering has also been associated with reduced rice yield (Wu et al., 1998; Samonte et al., 2006). Second, that if one wants to identify and study differences in the uptake, transport, and/or sequestration mechanisms that ultimately affect grain As concentrations, one should not merely study late high-As lines compared with early low-As lines but should also compare "As accumulators" and "As excluders" of similar DHD to be more certain of comparing accessions with similar exposure to available soil As.

## Significance to Understanding and Knowledge in Plant Physiology

Deficiencies of micronutrients such as iron and zinc frequently limit plant growth and crop yields. If the mechanisms of uptake, distribution, and regulation of micronutrients were clearly understood, it might be feasible to breed plants better able to grow in soils now considered marginal and to increase crop biomass on soils now in cultivation. Furthermore, as most people rely on plants as their dietary source of micronutrients, plants that serve as better sources of essential nutrients would improve human health. The patterns of the grain ionome as displayed in the diverse accessions can suggest possible control mechanisms of element concentrations in the plant and identify appropriate genetic material to use in studies delimiting the mechanisms.

The correlations noted between grain elemental concentrations along with other accumulation patterns are of interest because they suggest the possibility of shared mechanisms or genes for root uptake and/or transport or partitioning between rice tissues or into rice grains, as noted previously for the chemical analogs Rb and K. As another example, the correlation between Ca and Mn under flooded conditions may partially reflect not only a shared intracellular transporter (as hypothesized by Fox and Guerinot, 1998), but also movement into the grain only at the early stages of seed formation when the seeds are still supplied by xylem (Oparka and Gates, 1981). In contrast, Mg, P, and K do not share uptake mechanisms, are not tightly chemically coupled with respect to soil solution levels in flooded vs. unflooded soil conditions (De Datta 1987), and were not found correlated in terms of their concentrations in plant vegetative tissues (Baxter et al., 2008; Baxter, 2009), yet they were found highly correlated in grains of this widely diverse set of rice germplasm, whether grown flooded or unflooded, as well as in seeds of *A. thaliana* (Baxter et al., 2008; Vreugdenhil et al., 2004) and maize (Baxter et al., 2012a). In rice, as in many cereal grains, most of the seed P is found in the form of a mixed K–Mg salt of phytic acid in the aleurone layer and germ (Bryant et al., 2005), so one possible explanation of the positive P–Mg–K intercorrelations might be that their levels are all driven by phytate levels in the grain. Vreugdenhil et al. (2004) found colocalization of QTLs for K, Ca, and P with a high phytate locus in *A. thaliana*suggesting that phytate levels were affecting P–K associations. However, in both the present and a prior study (Bryant et al., 2005) a phytateless mutant of rice did not display altered total grain P concentration compared with the parental line, suggesting that something other than, or in addition to, phytate levels in the bran is controlling total grain accumulation of P. Interestingly, Zhang et al. (2014) identified eight QTLs for grain K in a biparental mapping study, four of which were also associated with grain concentration of P, and two of which were correlated with concentrations of K, P, and Mg.

Further study with selected accessions may be able to clarify the factors underlying the strong correlations seen among P, K, and Mg in rice and other seeds. Among the 1763 accessions, rare exceptions to the strong P–K–Mg correlations could be found, such as in Core 311012, which was high in P and K but extremely low in Mg under both flooded and unflooded conditions, and Core 311625, which was high in P and Mg but low in grain K, regardless of flooded or unflooded field conditions. However, no accession had negative correlations between P and both Mg and K. For Core 310241, the P–K correlation was negative, with its grains being concentrated for P and low in K (more so under flooded conditions than unflooded), but with above-average grain Mg, the P–Mg correlation remained positive.

In addition to developing high-yielding, early-maturing lines to limit grain As concentrations as discussed above, another strategy suggested for reducing grain As would be to develop cultivars better suited to unflooded production (Marin et al., 1993; Williams et al., 2007; Xu et al., 2008). Because the flooding of rice fields affects more than just the rice plant, numerous plant traits are required for high yield potential under unflooded conditions. For example, in addition to increased tolerance to water stress, a high-yielding cultivar adapted to aerated production would need to compete well with weeds, be resistant to blast disease and stem borer insects, and, depending on the growth climate, would require increased tolerance to either heat or cold stress during pollination and grain fill. Furthermore, because Cd increases in availability under unflooded conditions, causing an increase in grain Cd in unflooded as compared with flooded rice, it may become necessary to add reduced Cd accumulation to the list of desired traits (Uraguchi and Fujiwara, 2012).

Observations of Particular Relevance to Efforts to Enhance Grain Ionomics of U.S. Rice

Modern U.S. rice cultivars are already, on average, comparatively high in grain Zn under flooded conditions (standard in the U.S.), though there were accessions found among the AUS and IND subgroups with twice this concentration. The U.S. rice cultivars were also notably low in K, S, Ca, Sr, and As, while higher than average for Cu and Cd. It must be remembered, however, that none of the accessions contained grain Cd high enough to be of dietary concern unless they were grown unflooded. The U.S. rices were less exceptional for any of the elements under unflooded conditions. Cross-progeny derived from parents in different ancestral subgroups can suffer from hybrid sterility because of genetic incompatibility; fortunately, other TRJ accessions were found high in K, S, Ca, and Sr that could be incorporated into U.S. breeding programs to raise the grain concentrations of these elements. With the U.S. cultivars already low for grain As among worldwide rices, research to identify novel As-excluding mechanisms would be required to further reduce grain As under the lengthy flood period and highly reduced soil conditions used in the present study. Since grain As varied most widely under moderate to late DHD, it may prove most fruitful to identify novel As-exclusion mechanisms in studies comparing accessions within these DHD groups.

## CONCLUSIONS

Though environmental variance was large for some elements (flooded: As, Cd, Co, Ni, Rb; unflooded: Cd, Mn, Ni, Rb), there was significant genetic variance for grain concentration of all 16 elements observed, suggesting that breeders could select for enhanced grain concentration of all 16 elements. The *H2* for the elements ranged from 0.14 to 0.75; the particularly low *H2* determined for grain Ni under both flooded and unflooded conditions indicate that breeding to alter grain Ni would be particularly confounded and slowed by environmental variance. For each element, germplasm accessions with extreme grain phenotypes were identified to support further genetic and physiological investigations. Shape was not as significant a determinant of grain ionome as originally hypothesized, but an extended vegetative phase (late maturity) was associated with concentrations of several grain elements. Highly similar sets of elements were identified by PCA as being of primary importance in explaining the variance across as well as within subgroups, and in flooded and unflooded conditions.

**Seed Availability**

Small quantities of seed of any of the 1763 accessions reported here may be obtained from the USDA–ARS Genetic Stocks-Oryza (GSOR) Collection at the USDA–ARS DBNRRC in Stuttgart, AR, where they are identified by the GSOR numbers provided in Supplementary Table 1. Instructions for requesting seed as well as the element concentration LS means provided here in Supplementary Table 1 can be found at http://ars.usda.gov/spa/dbnrrc/gsor(accessed 9 Sept. 2014). We ask that appropriate recognition be given when one or multiple of the accessions and grain ionomics data presented here contribute to future research.

# ACKNOWLEDGMENTS

This research was supported in part by the U.S. National Science Foundation, Plant Genome Research Program (grant #IOS 0701119) awarded to D.E.S, M.L.G., and S.R.M.P. We acknowledge the technical assistance of Faye Seaberg, Erin Franks, Richard Chase, Jerri Daniels, Yao Zhou, and Tiffanee Simar, without whom the planting, maintenance, and harvesting of such a large number of field plots would not have been possible.

# REFERENCES

1. ↵H. Abdi 2007. The Bonferroni and Šidák corrections for multiple comparisons. In: Salkind, N.J. , editor, Encyclopedia of measurement and statistics. Sage Publications, Thousand Oaks, CA. www.utdallas.edu/~herve/Abdi-Bonferroni2007-pretty.pdf (accessed 9 Sept. 2014). p. 103–107.
2. ↵Agrama, H.A., and W. Yan. 2010. Genetic diversity and relatedness of rice cultivars resistant to straighthead disorder. Plant Breed. 129:304–312.
3. ↵Agrama, H.A., W. Yan, M. Jia, R.G. Fjellstrom, and A.M. McClung. 2010. Genetic structure associated with diversity and geographic distribution in the USDA rice world collection. Nat. Sci. 2:247–291.

4. ↵Arao, T., A. Kawasaki, K. Baba, S. More, and S. Matsumoto. 2009. Effects of water management on cadmium and arsenic accumulation and dimethylarsinic acid concentrations in Japanese rice. Environ. Sci. Technol. 43:9361–9367.

5. ↵Baxter, I.R., O. Vitek, B. Lahner, B. Muthukumar, M. Borghi, J. Morrissey, M.L. Guerinot, and D.E. Salt. 2008. The leaf ionome as multivariable system to detect a plant's physiological status. Proc. Natl. Acad. Sci. USA 105:12081–12086.

6. ↵I.R. Baxter 2009. Ionomics: Studying the social network of mineral nutrients. Curr. Opin. Plant Biol. 12:381–386.

7. ↵Baxter, I.R., J.L. Gustin, A.M. Settles, and O.A. Hoekenga. 2012a. Ionomic characterization of maize kernels in the intermated B73 × Mo17 population. Crop Sci. 53:208–220.

8. ↵Baxter, I.R., C. Hermans, B. Lahner, E. Yakubova, and M. Tikhonova. 2012b. Biodiversity of mineral nutrient and trace element accumulation in Arabidopsis thaliana. PLoS ONE 7:E35121..

9. ↵Bolland, M.D.A., and M.J. Baker. 1988. High phosphorus concentrations in seed of wheat and annual medic are related to higher rates of dry matter production of seedlings and plants. Aust. J. Exp. Agric. 28:765–770.

10. ↵Borrill, P., J.M. Connorton, J. Balk, A.J. Miller, D. Sanders, and C. Uauy. 2014. Biofortification of wheat grain with iron and zinc: Integrating novel genomic resources and knowledge from model crops. Front. Plant Sci. 21:53..

11. ↵Bouis, H.E., and R.M. Welch. 2010. Biofortification—A sustainable agricultural strategy for reducing micronutrient malnutrition in the global south. Crop Sci. 50:S–20–S–32.

12. Bryant, R.J., J.A. Dot'sch, K.L. Peterson, J.N. Rutger, and V. Raboy. 2005. Phosphorus and mineral concentrations in whole grain and milled low phytic acid (lpa)1-1 rice. Cereal Chem. 82:517–522. d

13. ↵Carey, A.M., K.G. Scheckel, E. Lombi, M. Newville, Y. Choi, G.J. Norton, J.M. Charnock, J. Feldmann, A.H. Price, and A.A. Meharg. 2010. Grain unloading of arsenic species in rice. Plant Physiol. 152:309–319.

14. ↵Carey, A.M., G.J. Norton, C. Deacon, K.G. Scheckel, E. Lombi, T. Punshon, M.L. Guerinot, A. Lanzirotti, M. Newville, Y. Choi, A.H. Price, and A.A. Meharg. 2011. Phloem transport of arsenic

species from flag leaf to grain during grain filling. New Phytol. 192:87–98.

15. ↵Cercamondi, C., I. Egli, E. Mitchikpe, F. Tossou, C. Zeder, J. Hounhouigan, and R. Hurrell. 2013. Total iron absorption by young women from iron-biofortified pearl millet composite meals is double that from regular millet meals but less than that from post-harvest iron-fortifiedmillet meals. J. Nutr. 143:1376–1382.

16. ↵Chen, C.C., F.T. Turner, and J.B. Dixon. 1989. Ammonium fixation by high-charge smectite in selected Texas Gulf Coast soils. Soil Sci. Soc. Am. J. 53:1035–1040.

17. ↵Daum, D., K. Bogdan, M.K. Schenk, and D. Merkel. 2002. Influence of the field water management on accumulation of arsenic and cadmium in paddy rice. Dev. Plant Soil Sci. 92:290–291.

18. ↵S.K. De Datta 1987. Principles and practices of rice production. Robert Krieger Publishing Co., Malabar, FL.

19. ↵Flour Fortification Initiative. 2012. Answers to frequently asked questions about rice fortification. www.ffinetwork.org/about/faq/faq_rice_industry.html (accessed 13 Dec. 2012).

20. ↵Fox, T.C., and M.L. Guerinot. 1998. Molecular biology of cation transport in plants. Annu. Rev. Plant Physiol. Plant Mol. Biol. 49:669–696.

21. ↵Garris, A., T. Tai, J. Coburn, S. Kresovich, and S. McCouch. 2005. Genetic structure and diversity in Oryza sativa L. Genetics 169:1631–1638.

22. ↵Gonzálvez, A., S. Amrenta, and M. de la Guardia. 2011. Geographical traceability of "Arros de Valencia" rice grain based on mineral element composition. Food Chem. 126:1254–1260.

23. ↵Graham, R.D., D. Senadhira, S.E. Beebe, C. Iglesias, and I. Ortiz-Monasterio. 1999. Breeding for micronutrient density in edible portions of staple food crops: Conventional approaches. Field Crops Res. 60:57–80.

24. ↵Graham, R.D., R.M. Welch, and H.E. Bouis. 2001. Addressing micronutrient malnutrition through enhancing the nutritional quality of staple foods: Principles, perspectives and knowledge gaps. Adv. Agron. 70:77–142.

25. ↵Grassi, C., B.A.M. Bouman, A.R. Castañeda, M. Manzelli, and V. Vecchio. 2009. Aerobic rice: Crop performance and water use efficiency. J. Ag. Environ. Int. Dev. 103:259–270.

26. ↵Gregorio, G.B., D. Senadhira, H. Htut, and R.D. Graham. 2000. Breeding for trace mineral density in rice. Food Nutr. Bull. 21:382–386.

27. ↵Grusak, M.A., and D. DellaPenna. 1999. Improving the nutrient composition of plants to enhance human nutrition and health. Annu. Rev. Plant Physiol. Plant Mol. Biol. 50:133–161.

28. ↵Haas, J.D., J.L. Beard, L. Murray-Kolb, A. del Mundo, A. Feli, and G. Gregorio. 2005. Iron-biofortified rice increases body iron in Filipino women. J. Nutr. 135:2823–2830.

29. ↵Hansen, T.H., E. Lombi, M. Fitzgerald, K.H. Laursen, J. Frydenvang, S. Husted, D. Boualaphanh, A. Resurreccion, D.L. Howard, M.D. de Jonge, D. Paterson, and J.K. Schjoerring. 2012. Losses of essential mineral nutrients by polishing of rice differ among genotypes due to contrasting grain hardness and mineral distribution. J. Cereal Sci. 56:307–315.

30. ↵Himelblau, E., and R.M. Amasino. 2001. Nutrients mobilized from leaves of Arabidopsis thaliana during leaf senescence. J. Plant Physiol. 158:1317–1323.

31. ↵Hocking, P.J., and J.S. Pate. 1977. Mobilization of minerals to developing seeds of legumes. Ann. Bot. (Lond.) 41:1259–1278.

32. ↵K Hoshikawa. 1989. The growing rice plant: An anatomical monograph. Pub: Nobunkyo, Tokyo, Japan.

33. ↵Hu, Y., J.-H. Li, Y.-G. Zhu, Y.-Z. Huang, H.-Q. Hu, and P. Christie. 2005. Sequestration of As by iron plaque on the roots of three rice (Oryza sativa L.) cultivars in a low-P soil with or without P fertilizer. Environ. Geochem. Health 27:169–176.

34. ↵Kelly, S., M. Baxter, S. Chapman, C. Rhodes, J. Dennis, and P. Brereton. 2002. The application of isotopic and elemental analysis to determine the geographical origin of premium long grain rice. Eur. Food Res. Technol. 214:72–78.

35. ↵Kuramata, M., T. Abe, A. Kawasaki, K. Ebana, T. Shibaya, M. Yano, and S. Ishikawa. 2013. Genetic diversity of arsenic accumulation in rice and QTL analysis of methylated arsenic in rice grains. Rice 6:3..

36. ↵Lafitte, H.R., M.C. Champous, G. McLaren, and J.C. O'Toole. 2001. Rice root morphological traits are related to isozyme group and adaptation. Field Crops Res. 71:57–70.

37. ↵Lahner, B., J. Gong, M. Mahmoudian, E.L. Smith, K.B. Abid, E.E. Rogers, M.L. Guerinot, J.F. Harper, J.M. Ward, L. McIntyre, J.I. Schroeder, and D.E. Salt. 2003. Genomic scale profiling of nutrient and trace elements in Arabidopsis thaliana. Nat. Biotechnol. 21:1215–1221.

38. ↵Li, G., L. Nunes, Y. Wang, P.N. Williams, M. Zheng, Q. Zhang, and Y. Zhu. 2012. Profiling the ionome of rice and its use in discriminating geographical origins at the regional scale, China. J. Environ. Sci. (China) 25:144–154.

39. ↵Liang, J., Z. Li, K. Tsuji, K. Nakano, M.J.R. Nout, and R.J. Hamer. 2008. Milling characteristics and distribution of phytic acid and zinc in long-, medium- and short-grain rice. J. Cereal Sci. 48:83–91.

40. ↵Lombi, E., K.G. Scheckel, J. Pallon, A.M. Carey, Y.G. Zhu, and A.A. Meharg. 2009. Speciation and distribution of arsenic and localization of nutrients in rice grains. New Phytol. 184:193–201.

41. ↵Low, J.W., M. Arimond, N. Osman, B. Cunguara, F. Zano, and D. Tschirley. 2007. A food-based approach introducing orange-fleshed sweet potatoes increased vitamin A intake and serum retinol concentrations in young children in rural Mozambique. J. Nutr. 137:1320–1327.

42. ↵Maret, W., and H.H. Sandstead. 2006. Zinc requirements and the risks and benefits of zinc supplementation. J. Trace Elem. Med. Biol. 20:3–18.

43. ↵Marin, A.R., P.H. Masscheleyn, and W.H. Patrick. 1993. Soil redox-pH stability of arsenic species and its influence on arsenic uptake by rice. Plant Soil 152:245–253.

44. ↵Masuda, H., M.S. Aung, and N.K. Nishizawa. 2013. Iron biofortification of rice using different transgenic approaches. Rice J. 6:40..

45. ↵Moore, K.L., M. Schröder, Z. Wu, B.G.H. Martin, C.R. Hawes, S.P. McGrath, M.J. Hawkesford, J.F. Ma, F.-J. Zhao, and C.R.M. Grovenor. 2011. High-resolution secondary ion mass spectrometry reveals the contrasting subcellular distribution of arsenic and silicon in rice roots. Plant Physiol. 156:913–924.

46. ↵Moore, K.L., Y. Chen, A.M.L. van de Meen, L. Hughes, W. Liu, T. Geraki, F. Mosselmans, S.P. McGrath, C.R.M. Grovenor, and F.J. Zhao. 2013. Combined nanoSIMS and synchrotron X-ray fluorescence reveal distinct cellular and subcellular distribution patterns of trace elements in rice tissues. New Phytol. 201:104–115.

47. ↵Murgia, I., L. De Gara, and M.A. Grusak. 2013. Biofortification: How can we exploit plant science to reduce micronutrient deficiencies? Front. Plant Sci. 4:429..

48. ↵Norton, G.J., S.R.M. Pinson, J. Alexander, S. Mckay, H. Hansen, G. Duan, M.R. Islam, S. Islam, J.L. Stroud, F.-J. Zhao, S.P. McGrath, Y. Zhu, B. Lahner, E. Yakubova, M.L. Guerinot, L. Tarpley, G.C. Eizenga, D.E. Salt, A.A. Meharg, and A.H. Price. 2012. Variation in grain arsenic assessed in a diverse panel of rice grown in multiple sites. New Phytol. 193:650–664.

49. ↵Norton, G.J., A. Douglas, B. Lahner, E. Yakubova, M.L. Guerinot, S.R.M. Pinson, L. Tarpley, G.C. Eizenga, S.P. McGrath, F.-J. Zhao, M.R. Islam, S. Islam, G. Duan, Y. Zhu, D.E. Salt, A.A. Meharg, and A.H. Price. 2014. Genome wide association mapping of grain arsenic, copper, molybdenum and zinc in rice (Oryza sativa L.) grown at four international field sites. PLoS ONE 9(2):e89685..

50. ↵Oparka, K.J., and P. Gates. 1981. Transport of assimilates in the developing caryopsis of rice (Oryza sativa L.). Planta 152:388–396.

51. ↵Pan, X., Q. Zhang, W. Yan, M. Jia, A. Jackson, X. Li, L. Jia, B. Huang, P. Xu, F. Correa, and S. Li. 2012. Development of genetic markers linked to straighthead resistance through fine mapping in rice (Oryza sativa L.). PLoS ONE 7(12): E52540..

52. ↵Quintana, J.M., H.C. Harrison, J.P. Palta, J. Nienhuis, and K. Kmiecik. 1999. Xylem flow rate differences are associated with genetic variation in snap bean pod calcium concentration. J. Am. Soc. Hortic. Sci. 124:488–491.

53. ↵Raun, W.R., G.V. Johnson, and R.L. Westerman. 1998. Soil-plant nutrient cycling and environmental quality. Dep. Plant and Soil Sciences. Oklahoma State Univ., Stillwater, OK.

54. ↵Rawat, N., K. Neelam, V.K. Tiwari, and H.S. Dhaliwal. 2013. Biofortification of cereals to overcome hidden hunger. Plant Breed. 132:437–445.

55. ↵Ren, J., Y. Yu, F. Gao, L. Zeng, X. Lu, X. Wu, W. Yan, and G. Ren. 2013. Application of resistance gene analog markers to analyses of genetic structure and diversity in rice. Genome 56:1–11.

56. ↵Robinson, W.D., I. Carson, S. Ying, K. Ellis, and W.C. Plaxton. 2012. Eliminating the purple acid phosphatase AtPAP26 in Arabidopsis thaliana delays leaf senescence and impairs phosphorus remobilization. New Phytol. 196:1024–1029.

57. ↵Rose, T.J., L. Liu, and M. Wissuwa. 2013a. Improving phosphorus efficiency in cereal crops: Is breeding for reduced grain phosphorus concentration part of the solution? Front. Plant Sci. 4:444..

58. ↵Rose, T.J., S.M. Impa, M.T. Rose, J. Pariasca-Tanaka, A. Mori, S. Heuer, S.E. Johnson-Beebout, and M. Wissuwa. 2013b. Enhancing phosphorus and zinc acquisition efficiency in rice: A critical review of root traits and their potential utility in rice breeding. Ann. Bot. (Lond.) 112:331–345.

59. ↵Saenchai, C., C. Prom-u-tai, S. Jamjod, B. Dell, and B. Rerkasem. 2012. Genotypic variation in milling depression of iron and zinc concentration in rice grain. Plant Soil 361:271–278.

60. ↵K.L Sahrawat. 2012. Soil fertility in flooded and non-flooded irrigated rice systems. Arch. Agron. Soil Sci. 58:423–436.

61. ↵Salunke, R., N. Rawat, V.K. Tiwari, K. Neelam, G.S. Randhawa, H.S. Dhaliwal, and P. Roy. 2012. Determination of bioavailable-zinc from biofortified wheat using a coupled in vitro digestion/Caco-2 reporter-gene based assay. J. Food Compost. Anal. 25:149–159.

62. ↵Samonte, S.O.P.B., L.T. Wilson, and R.E. Tabien. 2006. Maximum node production rate and main culm node number contributions to yield and yield-related traits in rice. Field Crops Res. 96:313–319.

63. ↵SAS Institute. 2007. SAS 9.1.3 help and documentation. SAS Institute, Inc., Cary, NC.

64. ↵SAS Institute. 2010. JMP 9.0 basic analysis and graphing. SAS Institute, Inc., Cary, NC.

65. ↵Somenahally, A.C., E.B. Hollister, R.H. Loeppert, W. Yan, and T. Gentry. 2011a. Microbial communities in rice rhizosphere

altered by intermittent and continuous flooding in fields with long-term arsenic application. Soil Bio. Biochem. 43:1220–1228.

66. ↵Somenahally, A.C., E.B. Hollister, W. Yan, T. Gentry, and R.H. Loeppert. 2011b. Water management impacts on arsenic speciation and iron-reducing bacteria in contrasting rice-rhizosphere compartments. Environ. Sci. Technol. 45:8328–8335.

67. ↵Sperotto, R.A., M.W. Vasconcelos, M.A. Grusak, and J.P. Fett. 2012. Effects of different Fe supplies on mineral partitioning and remobilization during the reproductive development of rice (Oryza sativa L.). Rice 5:27..

68. ↵J. Stangoulis 2010. Technical aspects of zinc and iron analysis in biofortification of the staple food crops, wheat and rice. 19th World Congress of Soil Science, Soil Solutions for a Changing World. 1–6 Aug. 2010, Brisbane, Australia. Published on DVD. www.dfid.gov.uk/r4d/PDF/Outputs/Misc_Crop/Stangoulis-2499.pdf (accessed 31 May 2013).

69. ↵Tani, F.H., and S. Barrington. 2005. Zinc and copper uptake by plants under two transpiration rates. Part I. Wheat (Triticum aestivum L.). Environ. Pollut. 138:538–547.

70. ↵Tuli, R., D. Chakrabarty, P.K. Trivedi, and R.D. Tripathi. 2010. Recent advances in arsenic accumulation and metabolism in rice. Mol. Breed. 26:307–323.

71. ↵Uga, Y., E. Hanzawa, S. Nagai, K. Sasaki, M. Yano, and T. Sato. 2012. Identification of qSOR1, a major rice QTL involved in soil-surface rooting in paddy fields. Theor. Appl. Genet. 124:75–86.

72. ↵Uraguchi, S., and T. Fujiwara. 2012. Cadmium transport and tolerance in rice: Perspectives for reducing grain cadmium accumulation. Rice 5:5..

73. ↵van Jaarsveld, P.J., M. Faber, S.A. Tanumihardjo, P. Nestel, C.J. Lombard, and A.J.S. Benadé. 2005. β-Carotene-rich orange-fleshed sweetpotato improves the vitamin A status of primary school children assessed by the modified-relative-dose-response test. Am. J. Clin. Nutr. 81:1080–1087.

74. ↵Vreugdenhil, D., M.G.M. Aarts, M. Koornneef, H. Nelissen, and W.H.O. Ernst. 2004. Natural variation and QTL analysis for cationic mineral content in seeds of Arabidopsis thaliana. Plant Cell Environ. 27:828–839.

75. ↵White, P.J., and M.R. Broadley. 2005. Biofortifying crops with essential mineral elements. Trends Plant Sci. 10:586–593.

76. ↵White, P.J., and E.J. Veneklaas. 2012. Nature and nurture: The importance of seed phosphorus content. Plant Soil 357:1–8.

77. ↵Williams, P.N., A. Villada, C. Deacon, A. Raab, J. Figuerola, A.J. Green, J. Feldmann, and A.A. Meharg. 2007. Greatly enhanced arsenic shoot assimilation in rice leads to elevated grain levels compared to wheat and barley. Environ. Sci. Technol. 41:6854–6859.

78. ↵World Health Organization (WHO). 2002. Report reducing risks, promoting healthy life. WHO, Geneva, Switzerland.

79. ↵World Health Organization (WHO). 2009. Micronutrient deficiencies. Iron deficiency anaemia. http://www.who.int/nutrition/topics/ida/en/ (accessed 24 Dec. 2009).

80. ↵Wu, G., L.T. Wilson, and A.M. McClung. 1998. Contribution of rice tillers to dry matter accumulation and yield. Agron. J. 90:317–323.

81. ↵Wu, C.Y., L.L. Lu, X.E. Yang, Y. Feng, Y.Y. Wei, H.L. Hao, P.J. Stoffella, and Z.L. He. 2010. Uptake, translocation, and remobilization of zinc absorbed at different growth stages by rice genotypes of different Zn densities. J. Agric. Food Chem. 58:6767–6773.

82. ↵Wu, C., Z. Ye, H. Li, S. Wu, D. Deng, Y. Zhu, and M. Wong. 2012. Do radial oxygen loss and external aeration affect iron plaque formation and arsenic accumulation and speciation in rice? J. Exp. Bot. 63:2961–2970.

83. ↵Wu, B., F. Andersch, W. Weschke, H. Weber, and J.S. Beckera. 2013. Diverse accumulation and distribution of nutrient elements in developing wheat grain studied by laser ablation inductively coupled plasma mass spectrometry imaging. Metallomics 5:1276–1284.

84. ↵Xiloyannis, G., G. Celano, B. Montanaro, L. Dichio, and A.M. Sebastiani. 2001. Water relations, calcium and potassium concentration in fruits and leaves during annual growth in mature kiwifruit plants. Acta Hortic. 564:129–134.

85. ↵Xu, X.Y., S.P. McGrath, A.A. Meharg, and F.J. Zhao. 2008. Growing rice aerobically markedly decreases arsenic accumulation. Environ. Sci. Technol. 42:5574–5579.

86. ↵Yan, W., J. Rutger, H. Bockelman, and T. Tai. 2004. Germplasm accessions resistant to straighthead in the USDA rice core collection. In: Norman, R.J., Meullenet, J.-F., and Moldenhauer, K.A.K. , editors, B.R. Wells rice research studies 2003. Univ. of Arkansas, Agricultural Experiment Station, Research Series. 517: 97–102.

87. ↵Yan, W., J.N. Rutger, R.J. Bryant, H.E. Bockelman, R.G. Fjellstrom, M.H. Chen, T.H. Tai, and A.M. McClung. 2007. Development and evaluation of a core subset of the USDA Rice Germplasm Collection. Crop Sci. 47:869–876.

88. ↵Yan, W., H. Agrama, M. Jia, R. Fjellstrom, and A.M. McClung. 2010. Geographic description of genetic diversity and relationships in the USDA rice world collection. Crop Sci. 50:2406–2417.

89. ↵Zhang, M., S.R.M. Pinson, L. Tarpley, M.L. Guerinot, B. Lahner, E. Yakubova, and D.E. Salt. 2014. Mapping and validation of quantitative trait loci associated with concentration of 16 elements in unmilled rice grains. Theor. Appl. Genet.

90. ↵Zhang, Y., X. Lin, and W. Werner. 2004. Effects of aerobic conditions in the rhizosphere of rice on the dynamics and availability of phosphorus in flooded soil—A model experiment. J. Plant Nutr. Soil Sci. 167:66–71.

91. ↵Zhang, X., F. Zhang, and D. Mao. 1998. Effect of iron plaque outside roots on nutrient uptake by rice (Oryza sativa L.). Zinc uptake by Fe-deficient rice. Plant Soil 202:33–39.

92. ↵Zhang, X., F. Zhang, and D. Mao. 1999. Effect of iron plaque outside roots on nutrient uptake by rice (Oryza sativa L.). Phosphorus uptake. Plant Soil 209:187–192.

93. ↵Zhao, F.J., J.F. Ma, A.A. Meharg, and S.P. McGrath. 2009. Arsenic uptake and metabolism in plants. New Phytol. 181:777–794.

94. ↵Zhao, F.J., J.L. Stroud, M.A. Khan, and S.P. McGrath. 2012. Arsenic translocation in rice investigated using radioactive 73As tracer. Plant Soil 350:413–420.

95. ↵Zhao, K., C.-W. Tung, G.C. Eizenga, M.H. Wright, M.L. Ali, A.H. Price, G.J. Norton, M.R. Islam, A. Reynolds, J. Mezey, A.M. McClung, C.D. Bustamante, and S.R. McCouch. 2011. Genome-wide association mapping reveals a rich genetic architecture of complex traits in Oryza sativa. Nat. Commun. 2:467..

96. ↵Zhou, X.-B., W.-M. Shi, and L.-H. Zhang. 2007. Iron plaque outside roots affects selenite uptake by rice seedlings (Oryza sativa L.) grown in solution culture. Plant Soil 290:17–28.

6

# BIOFORTIFIED INDICA RICE ATTAINS IRON AND ZINC NUTRITION DIETARY TARGETS IN THE FIELD

**Kurniawan R.Trijatmiko[1,2], Conrado Dueñas[1], NikolaosTsakirpaloglou[1], LinaTorrizo[1], Felichi MaeArines[1]**

[1]Plant Breeding, Genetics, and Biotechnology Division, International Rice Research Institute, DAPO Box 7777, Metro Manila, Philippines.

[2] Centro Internacional de Agricultura Tropical, Cali, Colombia

## ABSTRACT

More than two billion people are micronutrient deficient. Polished grains of popular rice varieties have concentration of approximately 2 μg $g^{-1}$ iron (Fe) and 16 μg $g^{-1}$ zinc (Zn). The HarvestPlus breeding programs for biofortified rice target 13 μg $g^{-1}$ Fe and 28 μg $g^{-1}$ Zn to reach approximately 30% of the estimated average requirement (EAR). Reports on engineering Fe content in rice have shown an increase up to 18 μg $g^{-1}$ in glasshouse settings; in contrast, under field conditions, 4 μg $g^{-1}$ was the highest reported concentration. Here, we report on selected transgenic events, field evaluated in two countries, showing 15 μg $g^{-1}$ Fe and 45.7 μg $g^{-1}$ Zn in polished grain. Rigorous selection was applied to 1,689 IR64 transgenic events for insert cleanliness and, trait and agronomic performances. Event NASFer-274 containing rice nicotianamine synthase (*OsNAS2*) and soybean ferritin (*SferH-1*) genes showed a single locus insertion without a yield penalty or altered grain quality. Endosperm Fe and Zn enrichment was visualized by X-ray fluorescence imaging. The Caco-2 cell assay indicated that Fe is bioavailable. No harmful heavy metals were detected in the grain. The trait remained stable in different genotype backgrounds.

# INTRODUCTION

Micronutrient deficiencies or "hidden hunger" affect about 38% of pregnant women and 43% of preschool children worldwide and are most prevalent in developing countries[1]. More than 30% of the world's population is anemic[2]. Global studies estimate that approximately half of this is due to iron-deficiency anemia (IDA)[3]. IDA can affect productivity and cause serious health consequences, including impaired cognitive development in children, a weakened immune system, and increased risk of morbidity[4].

Zinc deficiency is a major cause of stunting among children[5]. About 165 million children with stunted growth run a risk of compromised cognitive development and physical capability[6,7]. Biofortification, the delivery of micronutrients via staple food crops, has been proposed to complement existing efforts for the alleviation of micronutrient deficiency[8].

Conventional breeding efforts for developing Fe-enriched polished rice face major challenges because of the limited variability in Fe concentration in polished grains among rice germplasm[9]. Engineering Fe- and Zn-biofortified rice has been extensively reviewed[10,11]. However, 15 years after the pioneering attempt[12] and numerous conventional breeding efforts[9], reaching the 30% EAR nutritional targets for iron and zinc concentrations in polished rice grains[8] still remains a major challenge[10]. This 30% EAR was calculated as 13 μg $g^{-1}$ Fe and 28 μg $g^{-1}$ Zn in polished grains taking into account of 90% micronutrient retention after processing and 10% bioavailability for Fe and 25% bioavailability for Zn[8]. These levels have been recommended by nutritionists to achieve potential biological impact in adult women and children.

The highest grain Fe concentration reported in glasshouse studies of genetically modified (GM) temperate japonica rice was a 4.2-fold increase[13], reaching 18 μg $g^{-1}$ from a baseline of 4.5 μg $g^{-1}$, while a maximum of a 6-fold increase was achieved[14] from a baseline of 1.2 μg $g^{-1}$ to 7 μg $g^{-1}$. An extensive study on the overexpression of three iron homeostasis genes[15] successfully obtained 8 μg $g^{-1}$ in the glasshouse; however, in confined field trials (CFT), the concentration declined to

4 μg $g^{-1}$, emphasizing the need for further improvement. Field trials are indispensable as recently reported16 to provide more realistic achievements closer to actual farming conditions. Maintaining the high-yield trait of the background popular genotype is crucial for farmer adoption. In addition, maintaining high yield could avoid selection of improved high-micronutrient lines due to concentration effect. As shown in wheat, grain Zn and grain yield concentration are often inversely correlated17. The high micronutrient grain concentration could be a bias when plant yield and milling degree are lower than in the comparative popular varieties.

Application of basic science achievements to the agricultural sector, particularly in the field of genetic engineering, is often underestimated. A large number of events need to be produced in order to apply rigorous selection18 to obtain transgenic events suitable for deregulation and farmer adoption. Our aim is to develop low-cost inbred biofortified (Fe-/Zn-dense) rice in popular indica varieties by translating the advances of fundamental science12,13,14,15 into a potential product. The product concept consists of achieving the Fe and Zn dietary target 14 μg $g^{-1}$ from the baseline of 2 μg $g^{-1}$ in the field, well-defined single-locus transgene integration, a good and stable agronomic performance under field settings. Limited number of thorough translational science studies has hindered GM crop development in the public sector.

We pursued the sink and source strategy by co-expressing *Sfer-H1* and *OsNAS2*genes in mega-variety IR64 and evaluated several combinations of promoters and transgenes. Ferritin is an iron storage protein capable of binding up to 4,500 Fe atoms per molecule19, and a major source of iron in vegetarian diets20. Ferritin in legumes has a long history of safe consumption; thus, it represents an attractive target protein for improving rice grain Fe concentration. Based on our earlier report21, we selected *SferH-1* gene instead of using *SferH-2* gene which encodes a more stable protein22.

In rice, iron is absorbed either directly or as a complex chelated by mugineic acid phytosiderophores23 such as 2′-deoxymugeneic acid (DMA). Biosynthesis of nicotianamine (NA), a precursor of DMA, is catalyzed by NA synthase24(NAS). Different NAS genes have been used to develop GM rice13,14,15. Three NAS genes (*OsNAS1*, *OsNAS2*, and *OsNAS3*) have been identified in rice24. We selected *OsNAS2* among the orthologues because its overexpression has been shown to be more effective for rice grain Fe enhancement13. For the selectable marker, we used *aph4* gene-encoding enzyme hygromycin B phosphotransferase25. Foods containing this protein have been approved for markets in nine countries including USA, Canada, Japan, Australia, South Korea, New Zealand, Taiwan, Mexico and Indonesia[26].

Here, we report on the development and characterization of potential candidate Fe- and Zn-dense transgenic events with a novel combination of promoter and gene orthologues for future release. This is the first report on achieving Fe and Zn biofortification nutrition targets in rice under field conditions. For broader impact, we introduced the genes to the widely grown IR64 indica cultivar, and bred the trait into other popular rice cultivars from South and Southeast Asia where Fe and Zn deficiencies are prevalent. Fe- and Zn-dense rice could eventually contribute to improve life quality in rural areas and a reduction in significant economic losses due to micronutrient deficiency[27].

# RESULTS

## Generation and selection of events

We generated global maps from updated data on micronutrient deficiency, rice consumption, and poverty distribution[2,7,28,29,30] to highlight the strong interconnection of micronutrient deficiency, poverty rate, and rice consumption (see Supplementary Fig. S1 online). An unequivocal overlap between all three of these issues is observed across the maps.

To select a product with the desirable trait of Fe- and Zn-dense rice and robust field performance, we generated and screened 1,689 independent IR64 transgenic events obtained through transformation of seven constructs containing Fe storage and/or chelator genes driven by various promoters (Fig. 1a, Supplementary Table S1 online). The flow of the entire screening process and validation strategy is presented in Fig. 1b.

We prioritized our selection based on the polished grain iron concentration. The highest number of plants showing intense staining when Perls' Prussian blue was used in $T_1$ grain sections was obtained from three constructs containing*OsNAS*2 under control of a 35S promoter and/or soybean ferritin under control of a glutelinA2 promoter[31] (Supplementary Table S1 online). The transformed plants derived from the construct containing *GluA2::SferH-1* in combination with *35S:OsNAS2* (Supplementary Table S1 online, coded as IRS495 or NASFer) gave the highest number of plants with intense staining, higher than the similar construct in which *SferH-1* is driven by glutelinB1 promoter (IRS493, Supplementary Table S1 online).

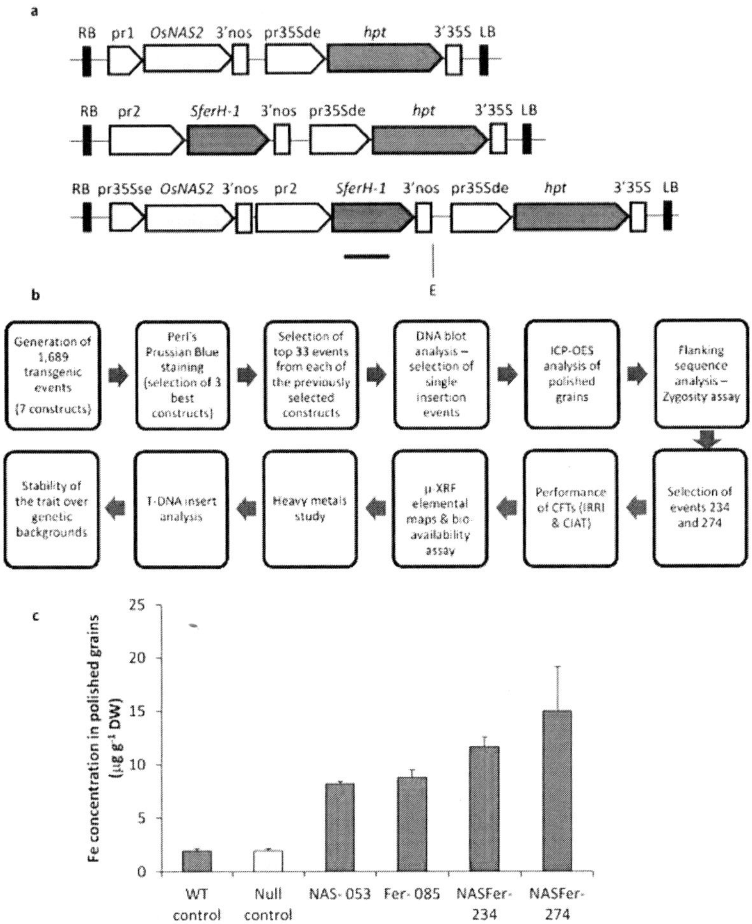


**Figure 1: Strategy for the development of biofortified high-iron rice and the Fe concentration achieved in $T_2$ polished seeds.**(a) Schematic diagram of the T-DNA constructs prepared for rice transformation for the purposes of our study. RB and LB represent the right and left borders of the T-DNA, respectively; pr1: represents the constitutive promoters pr35S with single enhancer (pr35Sse), maize ubiquitin promoter, or rice endosperm-specific promoter glutelinB1; pr2: represents the rice endosperm-specific promoters glutelinB1 or glutelinA2; pr35Sde represents the constitutive promoter pr35S with double enhancer; *OsNAS2*: *Oryza sativa* nicotianamine synthase 2; *SferH-1*:*Glycine max* ferritin subunit H-1; *hpt*: hygromycin phosphotransferase; 3′nos: 3′UTR of nopaline synthase; 3′35S: 3′UTR of 35S cauliflower mosaic virus gene. The horizontal line below *SferH-1* represents the deduced hybridization position of the digoxigenin-labeled cDNA probe; E: *Eco*RI. (**b**) Flow-chart displaying the steps that have been followed for the development of biofortified high-Fe/-Zn rice. (**c**) Fe concentration (µg $g^{-1}$ DW) of polished seeds harvested from $T_1$homozygous plants of representative NAS, Fer, and NASFer events, null segregant, and non-transformed rice under screenhouse conditions. Bars represent the means ± s.d. of three replicates.

We selected up to 33 events from each construct with the most intense Fe staining (Perls' Prussian blue) for copy number analysis (Supplementary Table S2 online). A majority of the transgenic events with intense staining contained multiple inserts, but events/lines with single-locus insertion were also identified (Supplementary Table S2 online). To accelerate the selection process, homozygous lines were selected in the segregating $T_1$ generation using a multiplexed PCR assay with three oligonucleotide primers (Supplementary Fig. S2 online) on selected events with high Fe concentration and have a single insert of the three selected constructs (Supplementary Table S2 online). The elemental analysis on homozygous $T_2$ polished seeds using inductively coupled plasma-optical emission spectrometry (ICP-OES) showed a significant 7.5-fold increase in Fe concentration, reaching 15 $\mu g\ g^{-1}$ from the 2 $\mu g\ g^{-1}$ baseline in the non-transformed IR64 control (Fig. 1c). This level of Fe concentration in polished grains was achieved in plants generated using the NASFer construct. Using the single-gene approach of *OsNAS2* or *SferH-1*, the maximum Fe concentration achieved in this study was 8.8 $\mu g\ g^{-1}$ (Supplementary Table S2online).

Quantitative RT-PCR confirmed enhanced expression of *OsNAS2* in roots and leaves of transgenic events (Fig. 2a,b). We also observed enhanced expression of *OsNAAT1* (Nicotianamine Aminotransferase 1) and *OsDMAS1*(Deoxymugineic Acid Synthase 1) genes in the transgenic events (Supplementary Fig. S3 online). The enhanced expressions of these three genes involved in deoxymugineic acid (DMA) biosynthesis lead to significant increase of NA and DMA concentrations in polished grains of transgenic events by up to thirty two- and thirty three-fold, respectively, compared to WT (Fig. 2c). Accumulation of ferritin in polished grains was detected by immunoblot assay (Fig. 2d).

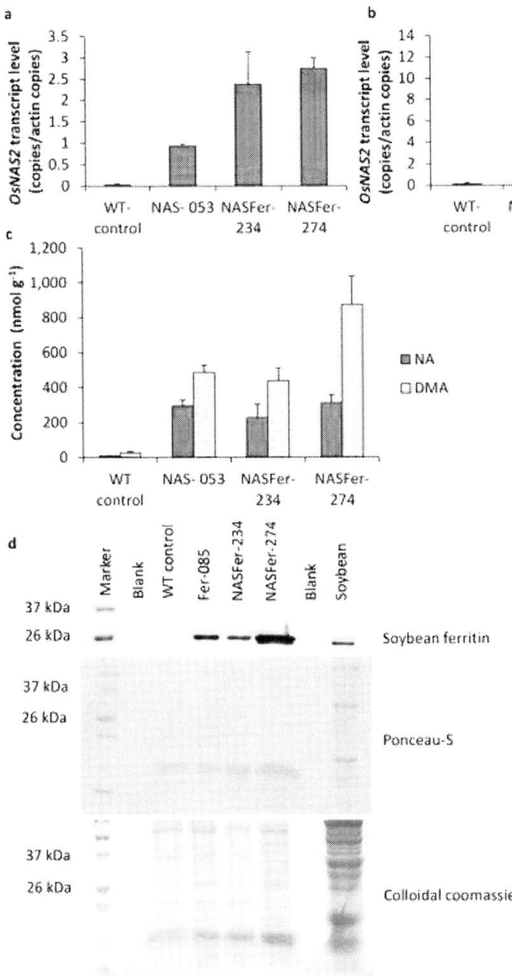


**Figure 2: Expression of transgenes in the representative events.** (**a**) Relative quantification of *OsNAS2* transcript levels of representative NAS and NASFer events and non-transformed rice in the roots of 8 days old seedlings. Bars represent the means ± s.d. of three biological replicates, each with three technical replicates of real-time RT-PCR. (**b**) Relative quantification of *OsNAS2*transcript levels of representative NAS and NASFer events and non-transformed rice in the leaves of 8 days old seedlings. Bars represent the means ± s.d. of three biological replicates, each with three technical replicates of real-time RT-PCR. (**c**) NA and DMA concentrations in $T_2$ homozygous polished seeds of representative NAS and NASFer events and non-transformed rice. Bars represent the means ± s.d. of three replicates. (**d**) Immunoblot analysis of soybean ferritin protein in $T_2$ polished seeds of representative Fer and NASFer events, non-transformed rice, and soybean. Ponceau-S staining of the membrane and colloidal coomassie staining of the gel served as loading controls.

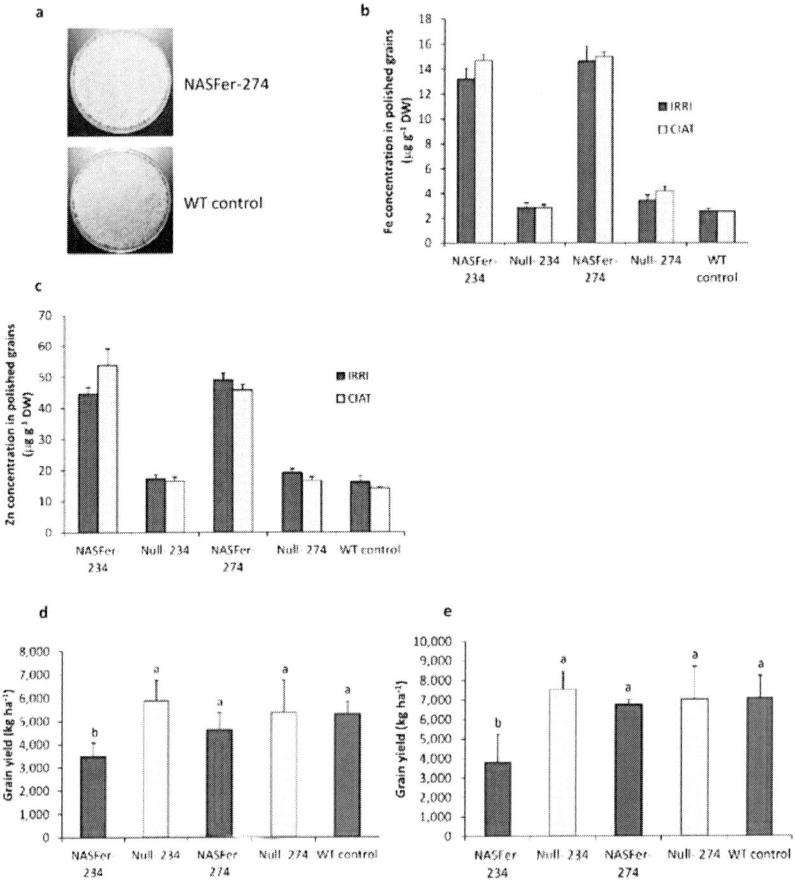


**Figure 3: Field trials for evaluation of target trait and agronomic characters of two lead events.** (**a**) Polished grains of lead event NASFer-274 and non-transformed rice. (**b**) Fe concentration (μg $g^{-1}$ DW) of $T_3$ polished seeds of lead events NASFer-234 and NASFer-274 under field conditions. Bars represent the means ± s.d. of three replicates. (**c**) Zn concentration (μg $g^{-1}$ DW) of $T_3$ polished seeds of lead events NASFer-234 and NASFer-274 under field conditions. Bars represent the means ± s.d. of three replicates. (**d**) Grain yield (kg $ha^{-1}$) of $T_3$ seeds of lead events NASFer-234 and NASFer-274 under field condition at IRRI. Bars represent the means ± s.d. of four replicates. Means labeled with different letters (**a,b**) differ significantly at the 5% level. (**e**) Grain yield (kg $ha^{-1}$) of $T_3$ seeds of lead events NASFer-234 and NASFer-274 under field condition at CIAT. Bars represent the means ± s.d. of four replicates. Means labeled with different letters (**a,b**) differ significantly at the 5% level.

## Field Trials in the Philippines and Colombia

Two high-Fe events with a single insert (NASFer-234 and NASFer-274) and no backbone integration beyond the T-DNA borders (Supplementary Table S2online) were evaluated in CFTs at IRRI-Philippines and CIAT-Colombia (Supplementary Fig. S4 online). Figure 3a shows that the rice samples were well milled after 2.5 minutes of milling by a Kett Mill laboratory milling machine. The absence of bran in our polished rice was confirmed by microscopy observation (Supplementary Fig. S5 online). We achieved the Fe target of 14.6–15.0 and 13.2–14.7 μg $g^{-1}$ (a 6-fold increase) for NASFer-274 and NASFer-234, respectively, in both locations (Fig. 3b). Additionally, these two transgenic events accumulated 2.7- to 3.8-fold more Zn when compared with the wild-type IR64 in both locations (Fig. 3c). This simultaneous increase in both Fe and Zn in single grains could have tremendous potential for alleviating both deficiencies.

Agronomic evaluation of the event NASFer-274 showed no yield penalty at both IRRI-Philippines and CIAT-Colombia (Fig. 3d,e), whereas the event NASFer-234 exhibited a lower yield in both locations when compared with IR64 and the null (negative segregant or azygous) (Fig. 3d,e). Grain quality testing on the most promising event (NASFer-274) did not reveal any difference in protein content, amylose content, gel consistency, seed size, and chalkiness (Supplementary Table S3 online).

## Elemental maps revealed significant increases of Fe and Zn localization in NASFer-274 endosperm

Synchrotron X-ray fluorescence microscopy (XFM) was used to map the localization of several metal cations transported by NA (Fe, Zn, Cu) as well as elements indicative of phytic acid and protein (P and S, respectively) in transversal sections of null and lead event NASFer-274 whole grain (Fig. 4a). The elemental maps corresponded well with the ICP-OES elemental results (Supplementary Table S4 online) and demonstrated that the grain of event NASFer-274 had higher localization of Fe in aleurone, sub-aleurone and outer endosperm layers relative to null grain. The Zn maps indicated less accumulation in the aleurone and much higher Zn localization in the sub-aleurone and outer endosperm layers of NASFer-274 grain. The localization pattern of P did not differ between NASFer-274 and null grain, indicating no difference in phytate distribution between the two grain types. The S elemental maps, by contrast, showed slightly higher endosperm localization in NASFer-274 grain and, in conjunction with the ICP-OES elemental results, suggest that protein may be slightly increased in NASFer-274 endosperm. The Cu elemental maps also indicated slightly higher Cu localization in NASFer-274 endosperm.

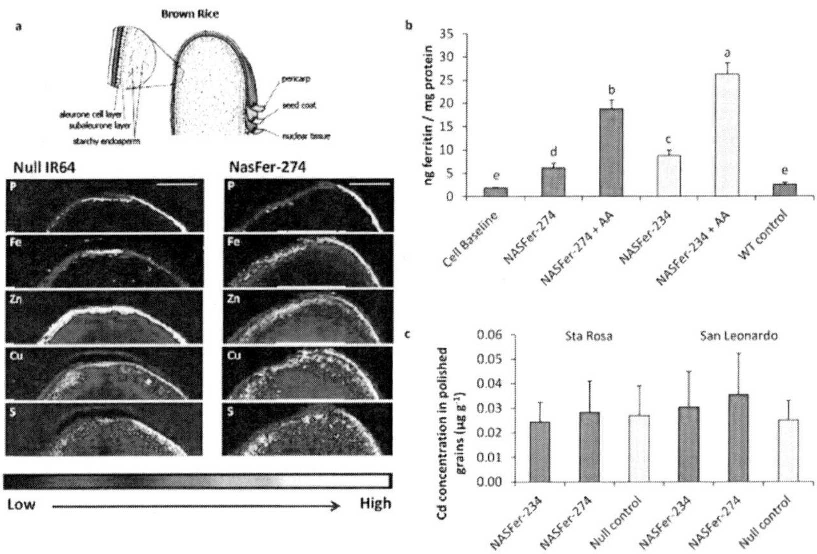


**Figure 4: Characterization of lead events.** (**a**) Grain elemental maps of brown grains of homozygous transgenic and null of NASFer-274. The color scale represents different elemental accumulations with black and white corresponding to the lowest and highest accumulations, respectively. The circled area in the diagram of brown rice (whole grain) indicates the grain layers presented in the XFM maps. (**b**) Fe bioavailability in grains of transgenic events NASFer-234 and NASFer-274 and a wild type (WT) in the absence/presence of ascorbic acid. Bars represent the means ± s.d. of three replicates. Means labeled with different letters (**a–e**) differ significantly at the 5% level. (**c**) Cd concentrations of polished seeds of transgenic events NASFer-234 and NASFer-274, nulls, and a wild type (WT) grown in high-Cd soils. Bars represent the means ± s.d. of three replicates.

## Enhanced Fe in the events is bioavailable

*In vitro* measurement of bioavailability in the new Fe-enhanced crops is important to predict level of Fe absorption in human. *In vitro* digestion/Caco-2 cell culture assays using $T_4$ polished grains showed an increase in Fe availability for both of our lead events; this increased bioavailability was more pronounced in the presence of ascorbic acid (Fig. 4b and Supplementary Table S5 online). Ascorbic acid was reported as the most efficient enhancer of the absorption of non-heme Fe32.

### Increased NA concentrations in the grain did not enhance grain heavy metal accumulation

Our data showed that cadmium (Cd), arsenic (As), and lead (Pb) concentrations in polished grains harvested from two CFTs were below detection limits by ICP-OES (Supplementary Table S4 online), indicating that increased NA concentrations in the grain did not enhance grain heavy metal accumulation. To further test the extent of possible Cd accumulation, high-Fe/-Zn rice lines were planted in pots containing Cd-contaminated soil from two different locations (0.104 and 0.246 μg $g^{-1}$ available Cd, respectively). A more sensitive ICP-MS (mass-spectrometry) analysis of harvested polished grains showed no significant difference between transgenic plants and controls, and all transgenic plants had Cd concentrations of <0.05 μg $g^{-1}$ (Fig. 4c).

### Characterization of integration sites of two lead events

DNA blot analysis using a single-cutter endonuclease within the T-DNA indicated single-copy insertions in our two lead events (Fig. 5a). Nevertheless, PCR-based assay analysis and sequencing indicated integration of two T-DNA copies oriented as an inverted repeat in both events (Fig. 5b,c, Supplementary Fig. S2 online, Supplementary Fig. S6 online, Supplementary Fig. S7 online). In agreement with previous studies33, the inverted T-DNA repeat of the two selected events did not trigger transgene silencing as shown by transcript expression and immunoblot analyses (Fig. 2a,b,d).

### Trait stability in different genotype backgrounds

The two selected events (274 and 234) were crossed with farmers' popular varieties from the Philippines (NSic Rc222), Indonesia (Ciherang), and Bangladesh (BR29). The ICP-OES Fe elemental measurement, carried out in the $F_2$ segregant grains, to gain an indication of trait stability in different genotypes showed concentrations ranging from 6 to 11 μg $g^{-1}$ for Fe (Fig. 6a) and from 33 to 45 μg $g^{-1}$ for Zn (Fig. 6b). This slight reduction, from 15 μg $g^{-1}$ in homozygous material to 11 μg $g^{-1}$, is expected since the $F_2$ bulk polished grains were segregated grains derived from heterozygous parents. In addition, the yield per plant of the crosses with event NASFer-274

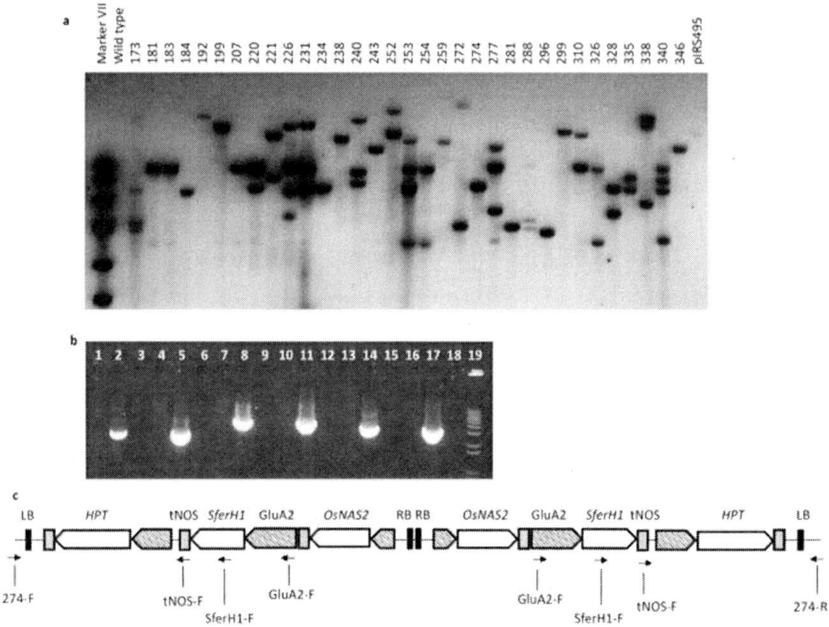


**Figure 5: Characterization of integration site of lead event.** (**a**) Genomic DNA blot hybridization from $T_0$ and non-transformed rice plants to determine the T-DNA insertion number of selected NASFer events. (**b**) PCR using non-transformed rice and lead event NASFer-274 with primer pairs tNOS-F and 274-upstream-flanking (lanes 1 and 2, expected product size: 2,877 bp), tNOS-F and 274-downstream-flanking (lanes 4 and 5, expected product size: 2,835 bp), GluA2-F and 274-upstream-flanking (lanes 7 and 8, expected product size: 4,664 bp), GluA2-F and 274-downstream-flanking (lanes 10 and 11, expected product size: 4,622 bp), SferH-1-RT-F and 274-upstream-flanking (lanes 13 and 14, expected product size: 3,517 bp), SferH-1-RT-F and 274-downstream-flanking (lanes 16 and 17, expected product size: 3,475 bp), blank (lanes 3, 6, 9, 12, 15, 18), and molecular weight markers (lane 19, 1 kb plus DNA ladder). (**c**) Schematic diagram of inverted T-DNA repeat configuration of lead event NASFer-274.

increased compared to the IR64 control, and was even higher in the event NASFer-234 (Fig. 6c) in this $F_1$population; therefore, the grain mineral concentration was most likely diluted because of the higher yield. Actual yield data should be obtained under field conditions on advanced backcross generations. We evaluated the Fe-polished seeds to obtain an indication of the trait stability. These data confirm the trend that this trait in general remains stable in different genotype backgrounds, even though there is some variation.

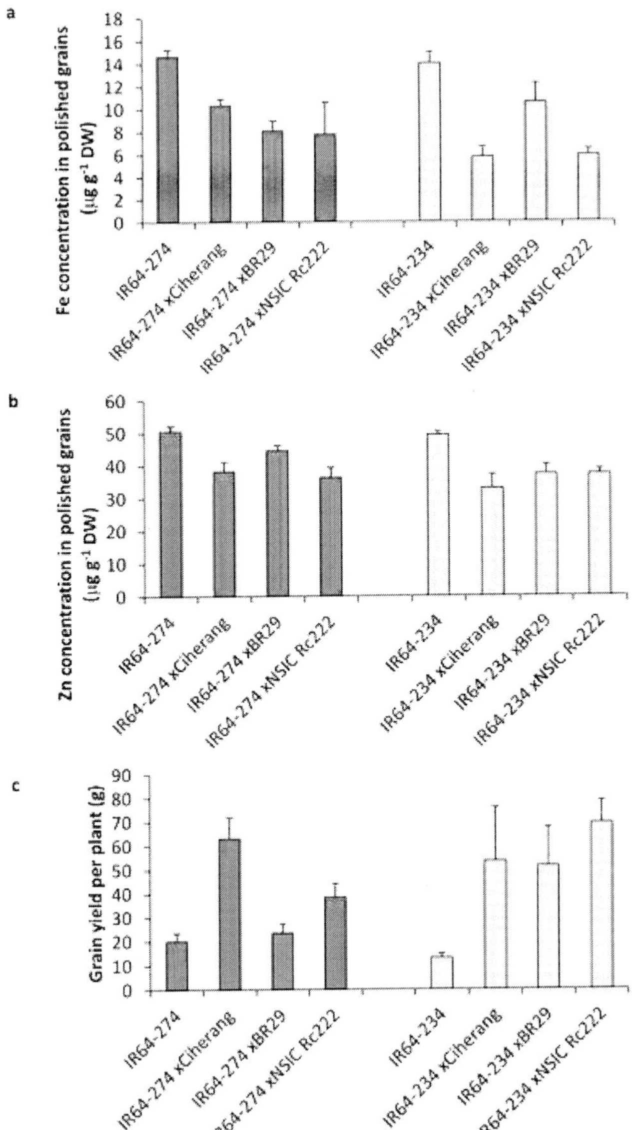


**Figure 6: Stability of Fe and Zn concentrations in different genetic backgrounds** (**a**) Fe concentration (μg $g^{-1}$ DW) of polished seeds harvested from $F_1$ plants derived from crossing between lead events and popular varieties. (**b**) Zn concentration (μg $g^{-1}$ DW) of polished seeds harvested from $F_1$ plants derived from crossing between lead events and popular varieties. (**c**) Grain yield of $F_1$plants derived from crossing between lead event and popular varieties. Bars represent the means ± s.d. of three replicates.

# DISCUSSION

More than three billion people consume rice as staple food, with an average consumption of 75.20 kg/capita/year28,29. Moreover, in countries with medium to high prevalence of Fe and Zn deficiencies2,7, polished rice consumption jumps up to 150 kg/capita/year. This shows the vast potential of biofortified rice to serve as a micronutrient-enriched product to alleviate the severe micronutrient deficiency in rural and urban populations with limited purchasing power and limited access to more diverse diets.

Our comprehensive studies focused on translating the state-of-the-art research on iron and zinc homeostasis genes10,11 needed to generate biofortified rice for potential release. We first over expressed NAS single transgene in indica rice, but the maximum Fe concentration in polished grain was only 8.2 μg $g^{-1}$ (Fig. 1c, Supplementary Table S2 online), lower than the concentration obtained previously in japonica rice13. This could be due to the difference in the varietal background, the favorable glasshouse versus screenhouse conditions, or plant yield dilution factor. Additionally, the baseline of grain Fe concentrations in the reported study13 was 4.5 μg $g^{-1}$, higher than the 2–3 μg $g^{-1}$ general baseline of popular indica varieties8. Recent evaluation across 1,763 rice germplasm accessions showed that grain Fe concentration is generally higher in the japonica subgroup34. We used indica rice since it is the popular varietal group in the target countries35.

Under field conditions, only two single-insert events from 1,689 generated events, reached the biofortification target to potentially fulfill the minimum of 30% of estimated average human requirement for Fe and Zn (Fig. 3b,c). This emphasizes the utmost importance of multiple construct evaluations and production of a large number of transgenic events to allow robust selection.

The two events with highest micronutrient concentrations in this study have different combination of promoters and gene orthologues than previously reported10,11. Here we selected the *SferH-1* gene, instead of using *SferH-2* gene which encodes a more stable protein22. Degradation of ferritin and the release of iron during cooking and gastric digestion are important for human absorption36and food safety. The *SferH-1* of the best performed events were driven by the GlutelinA2 (GluA2) promoter. GluA2 promoter directs strong expression as early as 7 DAF37 (Supplementary Fig. S8 online), whereas Globulin 1 (Glb1) promoter directs strong expression mainly at 17 DAF38. Translocation of Fe from leaves is highly dependent on the concurrent phloem loading of the other major assimilates such as sucrose39. Since the highest rate of sucrose unloading into developing grain occurs at 6–12 days after flowering40, likewise for Fe, accumulation of ferritin protein at early grain-filling would be beneficial to capture the Fe unloaded during this period. Furthermore, a recent study showed that, at 10 DAF, the central endosperm enters a programmed cell death stage and, by 16 DAF, the cells in the central region die41.

It is also important to note that our initial screening was performed in the screenhouse with paddy soil to minimize the glasshouse microclimate effects on the grain Fe and Zn. The genetic and environmental conditions play major roles for both Zn and Fe concentration in the grain. It was reported that concentration achieved in the glasshouse decreased when evaluated under field conditions15. In addition, grain Fe concentration was higher in unflooded conditions than in flooded conditions34. Field experiments are important because phenotyping under favorable conditions in tightly controlled pot experiment often do not represent conditions prevailing in the field, although it is useful for potential candidate gene assessment42,43.

Event NASFer-234 showed a yield penalty in the field trials, whereas no yield penalty was observed in NASFer-274 (Fig. 3d,e). One possible reason is endogenous gene disruption (knockout) since analysis of insertion sites showed that, in NASFer-234, T-DNA was integrated in the second exon of an endogenous gene on chromosome 6 (Supplementary Fig. S6 online). On the other hand, in NASFer-274, T-DNA was inserted in the 3′UTR of a gene on chromosome 3 (Supplementary Fig. S7 online), therefore it is not likely to disturb the function of the endogenous gene. Insertion after the stop codon in*Arabidopsis* rarely affects the expression of a disrupted genes44, which probably causes the absence of a yield penalty in event 274.

Further investigation of the insertion site showed that both events have two copies in one locus (Fig. 5b,c, Supplementary Fig. S2 online, Supplementary Fig. S6 online, Supplementary Fig. S7 online), indicating a gene dosage effect aside from position effect. This emphasizes the need for multiple transgene insertions to elevate iron up to the target concentration, which is in line with other efforts using multiple transgenes to reach a 6-fold Fe increase14,15. Having two copies of the same transgenes, encoding for two distinct proteins, instead of four different proteins represents an advantage, since the protein safety dossier studies required for biosafety deregulation would be fewer.

Since Zn-associated transporters can also co-transport Zn-mimic Cd45 we measured the concentration of Cd in the polished grains (Fig. 4c). Using ICP-OES, all transgenic plants grown in IRRI's CFTs had negligible Cd or other heavy metals. Concomitantly, in high-cadmium soil, there was no significant difference between NASFer-274 and -234 and their IR64 null (azygous) control counterparts, and the concentration is far below the Codex Alimentarius[46]threshold concentration of 0.4 μg $g^{-1}$. Similar to our findings, high-Zn japonica rice overexpressing *NAS* genes did not show an increase in grain Cd[11,47], suggesting that NA is highly specific in chelating zinc over cadmium[45]. However, further studies need to be performed to compare cultivation in flooded and upland conditions in order to give farming system recommendations to farmers in the future.

To effectively improve human nutritional status, it is essential for Fe and Zn in biofortified staple food to be bioavailable. Enhancement in Fe concentration in the biofortified crop may not be translated proportionally in similar increase of absorbed Fe, because of the possible simultaneous increase of Fe inhibitors or enhancers in the new product[48]. The *in vitro* screening employs a simulated gastric and intestinal digestion of food coupled with culture of human intestinal cells to indicate Fe biovailability in human intestine[48,49]. Here our result on Caco-2 cell assay revealed increased Fe bioavailability in both lead transgenic events (Fig. 4b), suggesting limited increase on Fe absorption inhibitors.

The values of grain Fe and Zn concentrations of the crossing material with other popular cultivars obtained in our study (Fig. 6a,b) indicated that the trait is potentially stable in multiple backgrounds. This is crucial for future breeding applications in different countries.

## CONCLUDING REMARKS

We have successfully accomplished the proof of concept on attaining Fe/Zn nutritional targets under flooded field conditions to fulfill 30% of EAR in the human diet in a well-characterized GM event of the widely consumed indica rice cultivar without a yield penalty. This achievement enables the future option to combine Fe, Zn and provitamin A traits in rice grain. The high-Fe and Zn rice could complement other current micronutrient intervention strategies such as supplementation and food fortification to alleviate nutritional deficiencies in rural regions and in urban poverty-stricken populations where these interventions are less effective.

# METHODS

## Online Methods

Generation of plant transformation vectors and transgenic rice

Construction of plant transformation vectors is described in the Supplementary Methods. Transformation of indica rice cv. IR64 was performed using an immature embryo as previously described50. Transgenic plants were grown in greenhouse conditions. The presence of a transgene in the transformants was confirmed by PCR as described in the Supplementary Methods.

## Selection of best constructs and events based on Fe staining

A semi-quantitative analysis of Fe concentration51 with brief modifications was performed on brown seeds for the mass screening of the generated transgenic events to select the best construct as described in the Supplementary Methods. Subsequently, selection of best events from the best constructs were performed using Perl's Prussian blue staining on polished seeds as described in the Supplementary Methods.

## Measurement of iron concentration in $T_1$ and $T_2$ grains

Polished grain samples (0.600–0.625 g) were digested in an ultrapure $HNO_3$–$HClO_4$ mixture in a microwave autoclave (Ultra Clave II, MLS GmbH, Leutkirch, Germany). Iron and zinc concentrations were determined using ICP-OES (Perkin Elmer ICP Optima 5300DV). The National Institute of Standards and Technology (NIST) rice flour standard 1568a and the Wageningen Evaluating Programs for Analytical Laboratories (WEPAL) IPE-135 were used as quality controls, and the samples were digested and analyzed using the same method as used for the rice samples.

## DNA blot analysis

Total DNA was prepared from leaves of $T_0$ plants as previously described53. EcoRI-digested DNA (10 μg) was separated by agarose gel electrophoresis, blotted to a nylon membrane, and hybridized with a SferH-1 (for IRS491 and IRS495) or hpt (for IRS433) probe labeled with digoxigenin (Roche Applied Science, Germany). Hybridization and detection were carried out as previously described54.

## T-DNA flanking sequence recovery

Genomic sequences flanking the T-DNA left border were amplified using inverse PCR or TAIL-PCR as described in the Supplementary Methods. Transgenic event-specific amplification products were excised from the agarose, purified using GeneClean Kit II (QBiogene), cloned into pGEM-T Easy (Promega), and sequenced. Identification of the insert position in the rice genome was performed using a BlastN algorithm55 at the National Center for Biotechnology Information (www.ncbi.nlm.nih.gov).

## Zygosity test of $T_1$ plants

Genomic DNA was isolated from leaves of $T_1$ plants as previously described53. A PCR-based assay using three oligonucleotides was performed as previously described18 to determine the zygosity of the $T_1$ plants.

Amplification and sequencing for confirmation of T-DNA inverted repeat configuration in event NASFer-274

A primer that is complementary to a genetic element within T-DNA insert was paired with either primer that is complementary to the upstream flanking sequence or primer that is complementary to the downstream flanking sequence to amplify genomic DNA of a homozygous $T_1$ NASFer-274 line with non-transformed IR64 as a negative control as described in the Supplementary Methods. Amplification products were excised from the agarose, purified using GeneClean Kit II (QBiogene), cloned into pGEM-T Easy (Promega), and sequenced.

## Relative quantification of transcript

Total RNA was isolated from leaves of wild-type and transgenic rice plants using Plant RNA Purification Reagent (Invitrogen, Carlsbad, California, USA) and purified using RNeasy Mini Kit (Qiagen, Valencia, California, USA). Real-time quantitative RT-PCR (qRT-PCR) was performed as described in the Supplementary Methods. The transcript level of the OsNAS2 transgene and endogenous OsNAAT1 and OsDMAS1 in transgenic and WT were normalized to the expression level of actin, using the relative standard curve method as previously described15.

### Immunoblot analysis

Grain protein was isolated as previously described21. Protein concentration was determined by the BCA method (Pierce, Rockford, IL). Protein samples were separated by SDS-PAGE, transferred to Invitrolon PVDF Filter Paper Sandwich membrane (Life Technologies, CA), and immunoblotted with a polyclonal anti-soybean ferritin56 at 1:2000 dilution. The anti-rabbit IgG-horseradish peroxidase (Bio-Rad) at 1:1000 dilution was used according to the manufacturer's instructions for secondary detection of the antibodies. The activity of horseradish peroxidase linked to the secondary antibody was detected with 4-chloro-1-naphthol colorimetric substrate (Bio-Rad).

### Determination of the NA concentration

$T_2$ seeds harvested from homozygous transgenic $T_1$ plants were analyzed for NA and DMA concentrations using the LC/ESI-TOF-MS method as previously described57.

### Synchrotron X-ray fluorescence microscopy (XFM)

The grain elemental maps of the homozygous transgenic and null of NASFer-274 were collected at the XFM beamline at the Australian Synchrotron as previously described13.

### Field evaluation

Confined field trials were conducted at IRRI-Philippines and CIAT-Colombia. The trials were planted in a randomized complete block design with four replications. Plot size was 4 rows x 15 hills (25 cm between rows and 20 cm between hills) with one plant per hill. Chemical properties of the soil at each CFT are presented in Supplementary Table S6 and S7 online. For IRRI CFT, NPKZn fertilizers were applied at a rate of 150-30-30-5 kg $ha^{-1}$. While P, K and Zn were applied in full before leveling, N was applied in three splits, once before leveling and twice as top dressing. For CIAT CFT, NPKZnFe fertilizers were applied at a rate of 400-130-220-26-104 kg $ha^{-1}$. While P, Zn and Fe were applied in full at the time of transplanting, N was applied in three splits, and K was applied in two splits. Six plants from each plot were randomly chosen for the evaluation of grain yield. The seeds of the six plants were then bulked and dehulled. The seeds were polished using a modified non-contaminating Kett Mill with a milling time of 2 min 30 sec as previously described13. Polished grain samples were sent to Waite Analytical Services, University of Adelaide, Australia, for metal quantification. Samples were digested using nitric/perchloric acid on a programmable digestion system in open glass tubes52. Iron, zinc, and other metal concentrations were determined using inductively coupled plasma-atomic emission spectrometry (SPECTRO CIROS Radial).

## High-Cd soil experiment

Seeds of selected high-Fe transgenic events (IR64-NASFer-274 and –234), as well as wild-type control seeds of IR64 and a bulk of nulls, were germinated in petri dishes. Young seedlings were transferred into soil for 14 days to establish normal plant growth. Later, five plants per event were transferred into pots containing high-Cd soil from two locations in the Philippines, Santa Rosa in the province of Laguna (Cd availability as determined by the Analytical Service Laboratory at IRRI was $0.1038 \pm 0.002881$ mg $kg^{-1}$) and San Leonardo in the province of Nueva Ecija (Cd availability was $0.246 \pm 0.005477$ mg $kg^{-1}$). Completely randomized designs with three replications were employed. The plants were grown in the glasshouse under flooded conditions. Mature seeds were harvested, polished, and submitted to Waite Analytical Services, University of Adelaide, for digestion using nitric/perchloric acid on a programmable digestion system in open glass tubes52, and cadmium concentration was determined using ICP-MS at Flinders University.

## Grain quality evaluation

Seed samples of non-transformed IR64, homozygous transgenic plants, and the null of NASFer-274 were evaluated for six seed quality traits, including physical traits, amylose content, protein content, and gel consistency in IRRI's Grain Quality and Nutrition Center Laboratory.

## *In vitro* iron bioavailability assessment

An *in vitro* digestion/Caco-2 cell culture model was used to assess Fe-bioavailability48,49. The rice samples were subjected to simulated gastric and intestinal digestion. Briefly, intestinal digestion is carried out in cylindrical inserts closed on the bottom by a semipermeable membrane and placed in wells containing Caco-2 cell monolayers bathed in culture medium. The upper chamber was formed by fitting the bottom of a Transwell insert ring (Corning) with a 15000 Da molecular weight cut-off (MWCO) membrane (Spectra/Por 2.1, Spectrum Medical, Gardena, CA). The dialysis membrane was held in place using a silicone ring (Web Seal, Rochester, NY). Iron uptake by the Caco-2 cell monolayers was assessed as previously described and by measuring ferritin concentrations in the cells48,49. The cells were maintained in Dulbecco's modified Eagle medium plus 1% antibiotic/antimycotic solution, 25 mmol/L HEPES, and 10% fetal bovine serum. Forty-eight hours prior to the experiment, the growth medium was removed from the culture wells, the cell layer was washed, and the growth medium was replaced with minimum essential medium (MEM) at pH 7.0. The MEM was supplemented with 10 mmol/L PIPES, 1% antibiotic/antimycotic solution, 4 mg/L hydrocortisone, 5 mg/L insulin, 5 μg/L selenium, 34 μg/L triiodothyronine, and 20 μg/L epidermal growth factor. This enriched MEM contained less than 80 μg Fe/L. All ingredients and supplements for cell culture media were obtained from GIBCO (Rockville, MD). The cells were used in the Fe uptake experiment at 13 days post-seeding. In these conditions, the amount of cell protein measured in each well was highly consistent between wells. On the experiment day, 1.5 mL of the digested sample was added to the inserts' upper chamber and incubated for 2 h. Then, the inserts were removed and 1 mL of MEM was added. Cell cultures were incubated for 22 h at 37 °C.

### Harvesting of Caco-2 cells for ferritin analysis

The protocols for ferritin and total protein content analyses were described previously48. Briefly, growth medium was removed from the culture well by aspiration and the cells were washed twice with a solution containing 140 mmol/L NaCl, 5 mmol/L KCl, and 10 mmol/L PIPES at pH 7.0. The cells were harvested by adding an aliquot of deionized water and placing them in a sonicator (Lab-Line Instruments, Melrose Park, IL). The ferritin and total protein concentrations were determined on an aliquot of the harvested cell suspension with a one-stage sandwich immunoradiometric assay (FER-IRON II Ferritin Assay, Ramco Laboratories, Houston, TX) and a colorimetric assay (Bio-Rad DC Protein Assay, Bio-Rad, Hercules, CA), respectively. Caco-2 cells synthesize ferritin in response to increases in intracellular Fe concentration. Therefore, we used the ratio of ferritin/total protein (expressed as ng ferritin/mg protein) as an index of cellular Fe uptake.

## ADDITIONAL INFORMATION

**How to cite this article**: Trijatmiko, K. R. *et al.* Biofortified indica rice attains iron and zinc nutrition dietary targets in the field. *Sci. Rep.* **6**, 19792;

# ACKNOWLEDGEMENTS

We thank M. Manzanilla, G. Borja, and P.B. Malabanan for technical assistance; F. Goto for providing the soybean ferritin polyclonal antibody; Lily Molina for ICP analysis at IRRI; Violeta Bartolome for statistical analysis; T. Kretzmar, A. Kohli and A. Macovei for reviewing the manuscript; and B. Hardy for editing the manuscript. This work was made possible through support provided by the grant from the HarvestPlus. Complementary funding from Global Rice Science Partnership (GRiSP) and the U.S. Agency for International Development (USAID-Development of Rice Biotechnology Products for Asia grant) is acknowledged. The contents of this manuscript are solely responsibility of the authors.

# REFERENCES

1. Iron deficiency anemia. WHO | Micronutr. Defic. at http://www.who.int/nutrition/topics/ida/en/[Date of access: 05/07/2015] (2014).
2. Stevens, G. a. et al. Global, regional, and national trends in haemoglobin concentration and prevalence of total and severe anaemia in children and pregnant and non-pregnant women for 1995–2011: a systematic analysis of population-representative data. Lancet Glob. Heal. 1, e16–e25 (2013).
3. Brotanek, J. M., Halterman, J. S., Auinger, P., Flores, G. & Weitzman, M. Iron deficiency, prolonged bottle-feeding, and racial/ethnic disparities in young children. Arch. Pediatr. Adolesc. Med. 159, 1038–1042 (2005).
4. Black, R. Micronutrient deficiency–an underlying cause of morbidity and mortality. Bull. World Health Organ. 81, 79 (2003).
5. Brown, K. H. et al. International Zinc Nutrition Consultative Group (IZiNCG) technical document #1. Assessment of the risk of zinc deficiency in populations and options for its control. Food Nutr. Bull. 25, S99–203 (2004).
6. Black, R. E. et al. Maternal and child undernutrition and overweight in low-income and middle-income countries. Lancet 382, 427–51 (2013).
7. Wessells, K. R. & Brown, K. H. Estimating the global prevalence of zinc deficiency: results based on zinc availability in national

food supplies and the prevalence of stunting. PLoS One 7, e50568 (2012).

8. Bouis, H. E., Hotz, C., McClafferty, B., Meenakshi, J. V. & Pfeiffer, W. H. Biofortification: a new tool to reduce micronutrient malnutrition. Food Nutr. Bull. 32, S31–40 (2011).

9. Graham, R., Senadhira, D., Beebe, S., Iglesias, C. & Monasterio, I. Breeding for micronutrient density in edible portions of staple food crops: Conventional approaches. F. Crop. Res. 60, 57–80 (1999).

10. Bashir, K., Takahashi, R., Nakanishi, H. & Nishizawa, N. K. The road to micronutrient biofortification of rice: progress and prospects. Front. Plant Sci. 4, 15 (2013).

11. Slamet-Loedin, I. H., Johnson-Beebout, S. E., Impa, S. & Tsakirpaloglou, N. Enriching rice with Zn and Fe while minimizing Cd risk. Front. Plant Sci. 6, 1–9 (2015).

12. Goto, F., Yoshihara, T., Shigemoto, N., Toki, S. & Takaiwa, F. Iron fortification of rice seed by the soybean ferritin gene. Nat. Biotechnol. 17, 282–6 (1999).

13. Johnson, A. A. T. et al. Constitutive overexpression of the OsNAS gene family reveals single-gene strategies for effective iron- and zinc-biofortification of rice endosperm. PLoS One 6, e24476 (2011).

14. Wirth, J. et al. Rice endosperm iron biofortification by targeted and synergistic action of nicotianamine synthase and ferritin. Plant Biotechnol. J. 7, 631–44 (2009).

15. Masuda, H. et al. Iron biofortification in rice by the introduction of multiple genes involved in iron nutrition. Sci. Rep. 2, 1–7 (2012).

16. Bruce, T. J. A. et al. The first crop plant genetically engineered to release an insect pheromone for defence. Sci. Rep. 5, 11183 (2015).

17. McDonald, G. K., Genc, Y. & Graham, R. D. A simple method to evaluate genetic variation in grain zinc concentration by correcting for differences in grain yield. Plant Soil 306, 49–55 (2008).

18. Heck, G. R. et al. Development and characterization of a CP4 EPSPS-based, glyphosate-tolerant corn event. Crop Sci. 45, 329–339 (2005).

19. Briat, J. F. & Lobreaux, S. Iron transport and storage in plants. Trends Plant Sci. 2, 187–193 (1997).

20. Lönnerdal, B. Soybean ferritin: implications for iron status of vegetarians. Am. J. Clin. Nutr. 89, 1680S–1685S (2009).

21. Oliva, N. et al. Large-scale production and evaluation of marker-free indica rice IR64 expressing phytoferritin genes. Mol. Breed. 33, 23–37 (2014).

22. Fu, X. et al. A novel EP-involved pathway for iron release from soya bean seed ferritin. Biochem. J. 427, 313–21 (2010).

23. Ishimaru, Y. et al. Rice plants take up iron as an Fe3+-phytosiderophore and as Fe2+. Plant J. 45, 335–46 (2006).

24. Inoue, H. et al. Three rice nicotianamine synthase genes, OsNAS1, OsNAS2, and OsNAS3 are expressed in cells involved in longdistance transport of iron and differentially regulated by iron. Plant J. 36, 366–81 (2003).

25. Kaster, K. R., Burgett, S. G., Rao, R. N. & Ingolia, T. D. Analysis of a bacterial hygromycin B resistance gene by transcriptional and translational fusions and by DNA sequencing. Nucleic Acids Res. 38, 6895–6911 (2010).

26. ISAAA GM Approval Database. Int. Serv. Acquis. Agri-biotech Appl. at http://www.isaaa.org/gmapprovaldatabase /default.asp [Date of access: 25/08/2015] (2015)

27. Khush, G. S., Lee, S., Cho, J., Il & Jeon, J. S. Biofortification of crops for reducing malnutrition. Plant Biotechnol. Rep. 6, 195–202 (2012).

28. FAOSTAT Food Supply Data Online Database. Food Agric. Organ. United Nations-Statistics Div. at http://faostat3.fao.org/home/E [Date of access: 27/08/2014] (2011).

29. USDA. United States Dep. Agric. at http://www. usda.gov/wps/portal/usda/usdahome?navid=DATA_STATISTIC S [Date of access: 27/08/2015] (2013).

30. World Bank Development Research Group. World Bank. at http://data.worldbank.org/[Date of access: 20/08/2014] (2015).

31. Paine, J. A. et al. Improving the nutritional value of Golden Rice through increased pro-vitamin A content. Nat. Biotechnol. 23, 482–7 (2005).

32. Teucher, Olivares & Cori. Enhancers of Iron Absorption: Ascorbic Acid and other Organic Acids. Int. J. Vitam. Nutr. Res. 74, 403–419 (2004).

33. Lechtenberg, B. et al. Neither inverted repeat T-DNA configurations nor arrangements of tandemly repeated transgenes are sufficient to trigger transgene silencing. Plant J. 34, 507–517 (2003).

34. Pinson, S. R. M. et al. Worldwide genetic diversity for mineral element concentrations in rice grain. Crop Sci. 55, 294–311 (2015).

35. Khush, G. S. Origin, dispersal, cultivation and variation of rice. Plant Mol. Biol. 35, 25–34 (1997).

36. Hoppler, M., Schönbächler, A., Meile, L., Hurrell, R. F. & Walczyk, T. Ferritin-iron is released during boiling and in vitro gastric digestion. J. Nutr. 138, 878–884 (2008).

37. Qu, L. Q., Xing, Y. P., Liu, W. X., Xu, X. P. & Song, Y. R. Expression pattern and activity of six glutelin gene promoters in transgenic rice. J. Exp. Bot. 59, 2417–24 (2008).

38. Qu, L. Q. & Takaiwa, F. Evaluation of tissue specificity and expression strength of rice seed component gene promoters in transgenic rice. Plant Biotechnol. J. 2, 113–25 (2004).

39. Grusak, M. A., Pearson, J. . & Marentes, E. The physiology of micronutrient homeostasis in field crops. F. Crop. Res. 60, 41–56 (1999).

40. Perez, C. M., Perdon, a. a., Resurreccion, a. P., Villareal, R. M. & Juliano, B. O. Enzymes of carbohydrate metabolism in the developing rice grain. Plant Physiol. 56, 579–583 (1975).

41. Kobayashi, H., Ikeda, T. M. & Nagata, K. Spatial and temporal progress of programmed cell death in the developing starchy endosperm of rice. Planta 237, 1393–1400 (2013).

42. Tuberosa, R. Phenotyping for drought tolerance of crops in the genomics era. Front. Physiol. 3, 1–26 (2012).

43. Gaudin, A. C. M., Henry, A., Sparks, A. H. & Slamet-Loedin, I. H. Taking transgenic rice drought screening to the field. J. Exp. Bot. 64, 109–17 (2013).

44. Wang, Y. H. How effective is T-DNA insertional mutagenesis? J. Biochem. Tech. 1, 11–20 (2008).

45. Olsen, L. I. & Palmgren, M. G. Many rivers to cross: the journey of zinc from soil to seed. Front. Plant Sci. 5, 30 (2014).

46. Codex Alimentarius, C. Codex Alimentarius Commision. Codex Stand. 193, 44 (2010).

# 7

# GENERATION AND FIELD TRIALS OF TRANSGENIC RICE TOLERANT TO IRON DEFICIENCY

**Takanori Kobayashi & Hiromi Nakanishi & Michiko Takahashi & Satoshi Mori & Naoko K. Nishizawa**

Graduate School of Agricultural and Life Sciences, The University of Tokyo

## ABSTRACT

Iron deficiency is a major cause of reduced crop yields worldwide, particularly in calcareous soils. Unlike barley, rice is highly susceptible to iron deficiency because of a low capacity to secrete mugineic acid family phytosiderophores (MAs), which are iron chelators secreted by graminaceous plants. We present an approach toward the generation along with field trials of transgenic rice lines exhibiting increased tolerance to iron deficiency. Cloning barley genes that encode biosynthetic enzymes for MAs enabled us to produce transgenic rice plants by introducing barley MAs biosynthesis-related genes. We tested three transgenic lines possessing barley genomic fragments responsible for MAs biosynthesis in a paddy field experiment on calcareous soil, which revealed tolerance of these lines to low iron availability. We also applied new approaches to generate iron-deficiency-tolerant rice lines, including the introduction of an engineered ferric-chelate reductase gene and manipulation of transcription factor genes regulating the iron deficiency response.

**Keywords:** Iron deficiency Field trial Mugineic acid family phytosiderophores Transgenic rice plants

## INTRODUCTION

Iron (Fe) is essential for most living organisms including plants. Although abundant in mineral soils, Fe is sparingly soluble under aerobic conditions at high soil pH, especially in calcareous soils, which account for about 30% of the world's cultivated soils. Fe deficiency is a widespread agricultural problem that reduces plant growth and crop yields [33, 36]. To take up and utilize Fe from the rhizosphere, higher plants have evolved two major strategies [34]: reduction (strategy I) and chelation (strategy II). The strategy I mechanism, utilized by nongraminaceous plants, includes induction of ferric-chelate reductase to reduce Fe at the root surface to the more soluble ferrous form and transport the ferrous ions generated across the root plasma membrane. In contrast, the strategy II mechanism, which is specific to graminaceous plants, is mediated by natural Fe chelators, the mugineic acid family phytosiderophores (MAs). Graminaceous plants synthesize and secrete MAs from their roots to solubilize Fe(III) in the rhizosphere [59], and the resulting Fe(III)–MAs complexes are taken up by roots through a specific transporter in the plasma membrane [5, 59].

In calcareous soils, the strategy II mechanism is more efficient than that of strategy I [33]. Tolerance to Fe deficiency is divergent among graminaceous plants and is thought to be dependent on the amount and kinds of MAs that they secrete. Rice, sorghum, and maize secrete only small amounts of 2'-deoxymugineic acid (DMA) among the MAs and thus are susceptible to low Fe availability. In contrast, barley secretes large amounts of MAs, including mugineic acid (MA), 3-epihydroxy-2'-deoxymugineic acid (epiHDMA), and 3-epihydroxymugineic acid (epiHMA), in addition to DMA, under Fe deficiency; therefore, it is more tolerant to Fe deficiency than other graminaceous plants [32, 37,52, 59].

We therefore hypothesized that introducing barley genes responsible for MAs biosynthesis into rice would lead to enhanced MAs production and tolerance in calcareous soils. We successfully produced various transgenic rice lines showing enhanced tolerance to low Fe availability by introducing barley MAs biosynthesis genes. Using selected lines, we carried out field trials on calcareous soil that revealed tolerance of these lines to low Fe availability. We also produced Fe-deficiency-tolerant rice lines using two other strategies: introduction of a reconstructed ferric-chelate reductase gene and manipulation of transcription factor genes controlling the expression of Fe-deficiency-induced genes. Future perspectives on generating further favorable and commonly acceptable transformants are described.

## Generation of Fe-deficiency-tolerant transgenic rice by introducing barley MAs biosynthesis genes

### Identification of genes responsible for MAs biosynthesis

The biosynthetic pathway of MAs (Fig. 1) has been identified through extensive biochemical and physiological studies [21, 30, 32, 37, 54]. Methionine is the precursor of MAs [37] and is adenosylated by *S*-adenosylmethionine (SAM) synthetase. Nicotianamine synthase (NAS) catalyzes the trimerization of SAM to nicotianamine (NA) [11]. All higher plants, including nongraminaceous plants, have the biosynthetic pathway to synthesize NA [29, 42], which serves as a common metal chelator involved in the internal transport of various micronutrients including Fe and zinc (Zn) [9, 62]. NA aminotransferase (NAAT) catalyzes the first step specific to graminaceous plants: transamination of NA to produce the 3''-oxo intermediate [20, 54]. DMA synthase (DMAS) subsequently reduces the 3''-oxo form to DMA [2]. All MAs share their biosynthetic pathway from methionine to DMA, which is then hydroxylated to form other MAs in some species, including barley.

Attempts to isolate the genes responsible for MAs biosynthesis have included "direct" approaches via enzyme purification and "indirect" approaches through screening the genes and proteins specifically induced in Fe-deficient roots. The former approach was applied to NAS and NAAT. *NAS* genes were first isolated from barley (*HvNAS1–7*) through the establishment of a NAS activity assay [11] and enzyme purification from Fe-deficient barley roots [13]. Two barley *NAAT* genes, *HvNAAT-A* and*HvNAAT-B*, were also cloned through the establishment of an enzyme activity assay [46] and enzyme purification [20, 60]. Expression of *HvNAS1*, *HvNAAT-A*, and *HvNAAT-B* is strongly induced by Fe deficiency and occurs almost exclusively in the roots [13, 60], suggesting direct involvement in MAs biosynthesis for the acquisition of Fe from the rhizosphere. Detection of NAS and NAAT enzyme activities in Fe-deficient roots of various graminaceous species revealed that NAS and NAAT activities are positively correlated with both the amounts of MAs secreted and Fe-deficiency tolerance [12, 19].

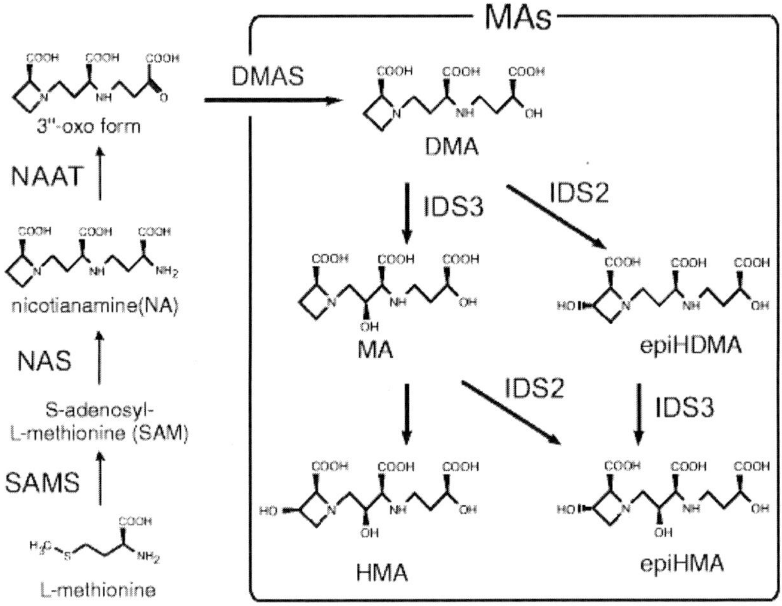


**Figure 1.** Biosynthesis pathway of mugineic acid family phytosiderophores (*MAs*). *SAMS*, *S*-adenosylmethionine synthetase; *NAS*, nicotianamine synthase; *NAAT*, nicotianamine aminotransferase; *DMAS*, deoxymugineic acid synthase; *IDS2*, iron-deficiency-specific clone no. 2; *IDS3*, iron-deficiency-specific clone no. 3; *DMA*, 2'-deoxymugineic acid; *MA*, mugineic acid; *HMA*, 3-hydroxymugineic acid; *epiHDMA*, 3-epihydroxy-2'-deoxymugineic acid; *epiHMA*, 3-epihydroxymugineic acid.

In the latter "indirect" approach, the differential hybridization method was applied with mRNA from Fe-deficient and Fe-sufficient barley roots. We cloned iron-deficiency-specific (*IDS*) genes specifically expressed in Fe-deficient barley roots [39, 49, 50]. Among these, *IDS2* and *IDS3* are homologous to 2-oxoglutarate-dependent dioxygenases, suggesting their possible involvement in the hydroxylation of MAs. By interspecies correlation between the expression of *IDS2–IDS3* and the capacity to secrete hydroxylated MAs, we deduced that IDS3 is the enzyme that hydroxylates the C-2' positions of DMA and epiHDMA, while IDS2 hydroxylates the C-3 positions of DMA and MA (Fig. 1; [40]). IDS3 was further confirmed to be the "MA synthase" by introducing the barley *IDS3* gene into rice [23]: transgenic rice plants secreted MAs in addition to DMA, while nontransformants secreted only DMA.

We also compared proteins of Fe-sufficient and Fe-deficient barley roots using two-dimensional polyacrylamide gel electrophoresis. Peptide sequencing of the induced proteins revealed that formate dehydrogenase (FDH) and adenine phosphoribosyltransferase (APRT), as well as the IDS3 protein, were induced in Fe-deficient roots [55]. The corresponding genes, *HvFDH* and *HvAPT*, were subsequently cloned [18, 55]. Both FDH and APRT are thought to function in scavenging the by-products (formate and adenine) that are released during the methionine cycle [36], thus supporting the production of MAs. Indeed, the methionine cycle works vigorously in roots to meet the increased demand for methionine in the synthesis of MAs [31]. We also applied a revised differential hybridization screening, identifying iron-deficiency-induced (*IDI*) genes from barley roots [70, 71, 72].*IDI1* and *IDI2* putatively encode enzymes catalyzing steps in the methionine cycle [26, 56].

Recent application of microarray techniques reconfirmed the induction of the abovementioned genes involved in MAs biosynthesis in Fe-deficient barley roots [41, 56]. The microarray approach also resulted in cloning of *DMAS* genes from rice (*OsDMAS1*), barley (*HvDMAS1*), wheat (*TaDMAS1*), and maize (*ZmDMAS1*). All of the corresponding encoding proteins were confirmed to possess the reductase activity to produce DMA [2].

## Introduction of barley genes responsible for MAs biosynthesis into rice

To produce transgenic rice plants with enhanced tolerance to Fe deficiency by increasing MAs production capacity, we introduced barley *HvNAS1*, *HvNAAT-A*, *HvNAAT-B*, and/or *IDS3* genes using either their genomic fragments or the *IDS3* gene promoter to confer inducibility to Fe deficiency. To introduce barley genomic fragments, we utilized the pBIGRZ1 vector [1], which was developed as a modified binary vector capable of transferring large-size DNA fragments into the rice genome. Rice cultivar Tsukinohikari was subjected to *Agrobacterium*-mediated transformation [10]. The transformants included those introduced with (a) a 13.5-kb genome fragment of the *HvNAS1* gene [14], designated "gNAS1"; (b) an 11-kb genome fragment of *HvNAAT* in which the *HvNAAT-A* and*HvNAAT-B* genes are tandemly located [61], designated "gNAAT"; (c) a 20-kb genome fragment of the *IDS3* gene [23], designated "gIDS3"; (d) a 7.6-kb genome fragment of *HvNAS1* plus an 11-kb genome fragment containing the *HvNAAT-A* and *HvNAAT-B* genes, designated "gNAS1-gNAAT"; (e) an *HvAPT* cDNA fragment fused downstream of the 2.2-kb *IDS3* promoter; (f) *HvNAS1*, *HvNAAT-A*, and *HvAPT* cDNA fragments each fused downstream of the 2.2-kb *IDS3* promoter; and (g) an *IDS3*cDNA fragment fused downstream of the cauliflower mosaic virus *35S* promoter [23]. Expression analysis revealed that the Fe-deficiency-induced expression was strongly conferred by genome fragments of the *HvNAS1*, *HvNAAT-A*, *HvNAAT-B*, or *IDS3* genes [14, 23, 61], confirming the potency of the barley promoter elements included in the genome fragments to drive Fe-deficiency-induced expression in rice plants. Although the barley promoters exhibit induction almost exclusively in Fe-deficient roots in native barley, they induced moderate expression in Fe-deficient leaves and prominent expression in Fe-deficient roots when introduced into rice.

To examine whether the transformants have enhanced tolerance to low Fe availability, the plants were cultured in pots filled with calcareous soils (pH 8.5–9.0; [61]) under controlled conditions in a greenhouse. Of the 36 gNAAT lines evaluated, ten showed remarkable tolerance to calcareous soils [61]. Nontransformants exhibited reduced growth and severe leaf chlorosis caused by Fe deficiency, whereas the gNAAT lines had greener and larger shoots. At harvest, the gNAAT lines possessed 4.2 and 4.1 times higher shoot dry weight and grain yield per pot than the nontransformants [61]. We also examined tolerance in calcareous soils for the other transformants. We found rice lines showing some tolerance to calcareous soils from all transgenes (a)–(g). In these lines, increased amounts or kinds of MAs secreted were thought to have contributed to enhanced Fe availability under Fe-limiting conditions.

## FIELD TRIALS OF FE-DEFICIENCY-TOLERANT RICE LINES

### Approval for using transgenics in field trials

For the field experiment, we first selected one line from each of (a) to (f) described above. Prior to culture in a quarantine field in Japan, we needed approval for Type 1 Use Regulations for living modified organisms from the Ministry of Agriculture, Forestry, and Fisheries in Japan. For that purpose, we performed evaluation tests on their priority in competition, possible production of harmful substances, and influence on biological diversity in relation to interspecific crossing. We performed the following tests on six lines of transgenic rice and the nontransformant: growth comparison in Andosol, stability of the transgene and expression beyond the first generation, determination of the interspecific crossing rate from transformants to nontransformants, evaluation of soil microorganism populations, evaluation of the residual effect of harmful compounds in postharvest soil, plowing-under effect of the dead transformants, carryover of *Agrobacterium*, tests on pollen shape, fertility, and dispersal distance, and tests on the germination rates of the seeds and tolerance to low temperature during early growth.

We confirmed stable inheritance of every transgene over at least three generations and found no harmful impacts on the environment in any of the abovementioned tests. Moreover, we detected no interspecific crossing from transformants to nontransformants. Based on these results, the transformants were approved for the quarantine field trials following the Type 1 Use Regulations.

## Field trials of the selected lines

A calcareous subsoil from Toyama Prefecture containing fossil shells (pH ~9.2; [38]) was used to establish a paddy field in the quarantine area of the Field Science Center of Tohoku University (Osaki, Miyagi, Japan; 38° 44' N; 140° 45' E). The paddy field in the first-year experiment was 7 m long, 14 m wide, and 0.5 m deep, with the external ridges completely covered with a vinyl sheet to avoid contamination from the surrounding Andosol at the site. The first-year experiment was conducted from April to October 2005, using the six transformant lines (a)–(f) and nontransformants (cv. Tsukinohikari). The following year, from April to October 2006, the second-year experiment was performed using the three most promising lines: gNAS1 (a), gIDS3 (c), and gNAS1–gNAAT (d). Experimental procedures of the second-year experiment were described by Suzuki et al. [57]. The paddy field in the second-year experiment was 6 m long and 4 m wide, and the experimental plots were arranged in a completely randomized design (Fig. 2b) including the three transgenic rice lines (gNAS1, gIDS3, and gNAS1–gNAAT) and nontransformants (NTs). Germinated seeds were grown for 45 days in a greenhouse, and seedlings were then transplanted (three per hill) into the calcareous paddy field.

Sixteen days after transplanting (DAT), chlorosis and growth retardation began to appear. By 42 DAT, the three transgenic rice lines were clearly superior to the NTs (Fig. 2a) both in leaf color and growth, although differences in performance were observed in individual plots. Using gIDS3 as an example, we saw no evident difference from NT on 16 DAT (Fig. 3a); chlorotic symptoms appeared in NTs but not in gIDS3 at 30 DAT (Fig. 3b). The clearest difference between gIDS3 and NTs was evident at 42 DAT (Fig. 3c). One week later (50 DAT), leaf chlorosis began to disappear, especially in NT plants close to the plot boundary adjacent to the transgenic gIDS3 rice plants (Fig. 3d), which suggests that NTs utilized MAs secreted by the transgenic rice.

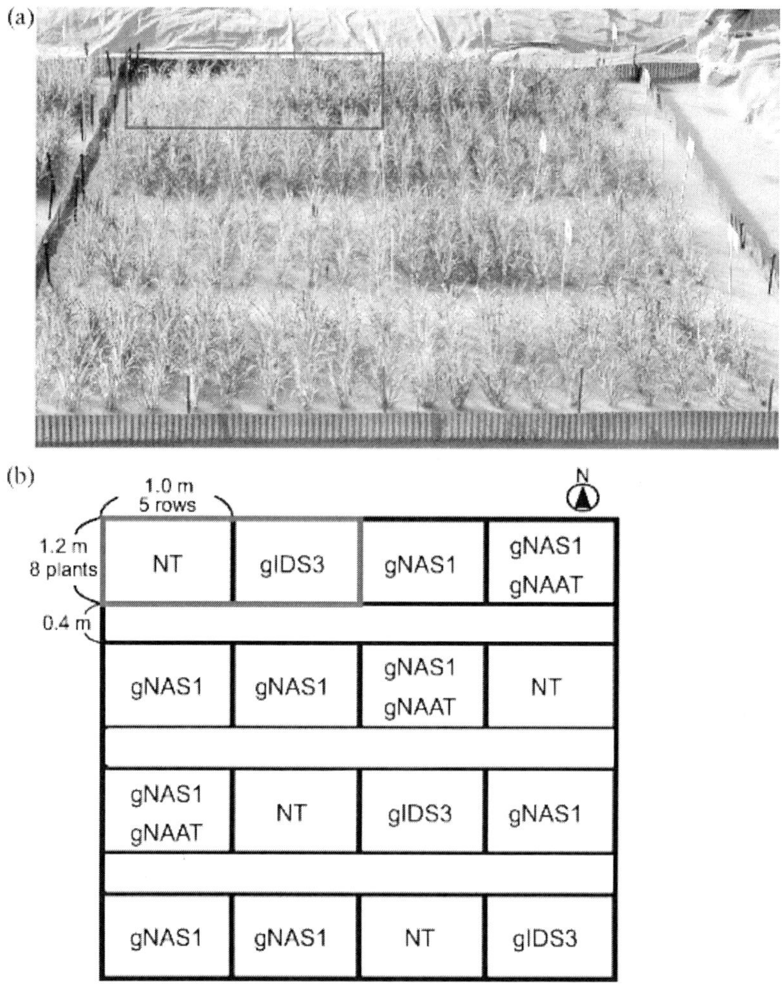


**Figure 2. a** Photograph (42 DAT) of the rice lines tested in a paddy field in the quarantine area of the Field Science Center of Tohoku University (Osaki, Miyagi, Japan) and **b** field layout. Each population contained five 1.2-m-long rows of rice with 20 cm between rows and 15 cm between hills. The *box* in the *upper left* indicates the two plots photographed on several occasions (Fig. 3). *NT*, nontransformant. Original figure: Suzuki et al. [57].

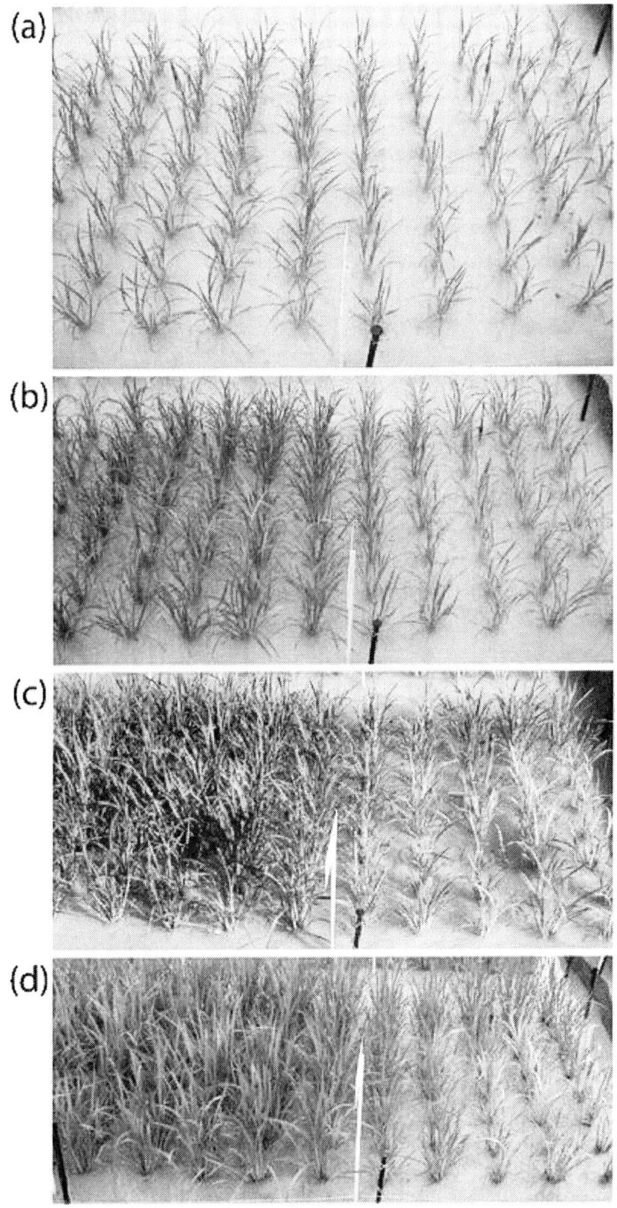


**Figure 3.** Visual comparison between gIDS3 (*left*) and NT (*right*) from 16 to 50 DAT, as illustrated in Fig. 2 but photographed from the opposite direction. **a** 16 DAT, **b** 30 DAT, **c** 42 DAT, and **d** 50 DAT. Original figure: Suzuki et al. [57].

From 16 to 42 DAT, plant height and the SPAD value (leaf color) of the three transformant lines were higher than those of NTs. In addition, the number of tillers per plant was higher in gIDS3 than in the other lines. By 42 DAT, however, all lines had about 15 tillers per plant. After 42 DAT, when soil Eh fell below 0 mV, all plant lines recovered their leaf color, and, consequently, the SPAD value of NT plants rose up to levels similar to that of transformants. The decrease in soil redox potential with time is thought to have resulted in the absorption of generated ferrous ion via the ferrous transporter OsIRT1 ("Introducing an engineered ferric-chelate reductase gene"; [16]).

At the time of grain harvest, the number of grains, 1,000-grain weights, and the grain yield of gNAS1 were higher than those of the NT and other lines. Plant height and the proportion of fully matured grains showed no significant difference among the lines. Timing of the decrease in soil redox potential might account for the relatively small differences in grain parameters between transformants and NTs, despite the clearly inferior performance of NTs during early growth. Indeed, in a prior experiment, NT seedlings grown in the same calcareous paddy field showed severe chlorosis, and many seedlings died in the early stages before the Eh fell below 0 mV [38]. Therefore, it is crucial for rice in calcareous paddy fields to survive the early stages of growth, when enhanced MAs production greatly supports Fe acquisition.

Interestingly, the concentrations of Fe and Zn in the rice grains of gIDS3 were significantly higher than those of NTs and the other lines, suggesting that MA synthesized by IDS3 contributed not only to improved Fe uptake from the soil but also to increased translocation to the grain. MAs have been suggested to be involved in long-distance transport of Fe and Zn inside rice plants [15, 58]. Since more hydroxylated MAs exhibit higher stability under mildly acidic conditions [67], MA synthesized by IDS3 would have been favorable for internal translocation of Fe and Zn.

In conclusion, our field trial of the transformants demonstrated that a transgenic approach to increase the tolerance of rice to low Fe availability is practical for improving agricultural productivity in calcareous paddy soils.

## Production of other transgenic rice plants tolerant to Fe deficiency

### Introducing an engineered ferric-chelate reductase gene

In strategy I plants, Fe uptake from the rhizosphere is mediated by ferrous ion transporters. Eide et al. [7] isolated the *Arabidopsis IRT1* gene, which is the dominant ferrous transporter in the Fe-uptake process [65]. Rice, in spite of being a strategy II plant, possesses homologs of the *Arabidopsis IRT1* gene, *OsIRT1* and *OsIRT2*, the ferrous transport capacity of which was demonstrated by functional complementation in yeast [3, 16]. *OsIRT1* expression is strongly induced in Fe-deficient roots, and *OsIRT2* is expressed similarly but at lower levels. Promoter β-glucuronidase (*GUS*) analysis indicated that *OsIRT1* is mainly expressed in the epidermis, exodermis, and inner layer of the cortex in Fe-deficient roots, as well as in companion cells of shoots. Moreover, an analysis using a positron-emitting tracer imaging system (PETIS) revealed that rice is able to take up both Fe(III)–DMA and $Fe^{2+}$. Thus, rice plants possess a system other than the MAs-based strategy II for Fe uptake [16]. In contrast to their ferrous-transporting ability, Fe-deficient rice roots do not induce ferric-chelate reductase activity [16], which is a hallmark of the strategy I response.

To take up ferrous ion directly using OsIRT1, without reducing ferric chelates, seems to be a consequence of adaptation of rice to waterlogged soils, in which the concentration of soluble ferrous iron increases with the decrease in soil redox potential [16, 57]. Because of the presence of OsIRT1, severe Fe deficiency is relatively rare in irrigated rice systems. Nevertheless, rice plants grown in calcareous soils exhibit Fe deficiency symptoms even under waterlogged conditions as noted previously because of their inability to induce ferric-chelate reductase and their low capacity to synthesize MAs. Therefore, we hypothesized that introducing ferric-chelate reductase into rice would enhance Fe deficiency tolerance, creating a complete strategy I system in addition to the rice endogenous strategy II.

For functional expression in plants, we modified and completely reconstructed the yeast ferric reductase gene, *FRE1*, to produce *refre1* (reconstructed *FRE1*; [47]). Since ferric-chelate reductase activity is inhibited by high pH, we then screened reductases with improved enzymatic activity at high pH [48]. Through screening of randomly mutagenized *refre1* derivatives, we obtained a variant designated *refre1/372*, whose encoding protein maintained strong reductase activity at pH 8–9. Transgenic tobacco plants with the introduced *refre1/372* under control of the *35S* promoter exhibited enhanced ferric-chelate reductase activity in roots and better growth when grown in calcareous soils [48].

Another concern in relation to the introduction of exogenous reductase genes into rice was the choice of an appropriate promoter. Vasconcelos et al. [64] introduced the *Arabidopsis* ferric-chelate reductase gene *FRO2* with its own promoter but observed no transgene mRNA expression. In *Arabidopsis*, expression of ferric-chelate reductase FRO2 and ferrous transporter IRT1 is similarly and coordinately regulated at transcriptional and posttranscriptional levels [4, 66]. Therefore, we chose the promoter of the rice ferrous transporter gene *OsIRT1* to drive the exogenous ferric-chelate reductase gene *refre1/372* [17].

Transgenic rice plants with the introduced *OsIRT1* promoter connected to *refre1/372*, successfully induced ferric-chelate reductase expression and activity in Fe-deficient roots, leading to higher Fe uptake than by vector controls, as revealed by a PETIS analysis. The transformants exhibited enhanced tolerance to low Fe availability in both hydroponic culture and calcareous soil (Fig. 4a). When grown in calcareous soil until harvest, the transformants had a 7.9 times higher grain yield than vector controls (Fig. 4b,c; [17]), demonstrating that creating a complete strategy I system in rice by enhancing ferric-chelate reductase activity is extremely effective in improving Fe deficiency tolerance.

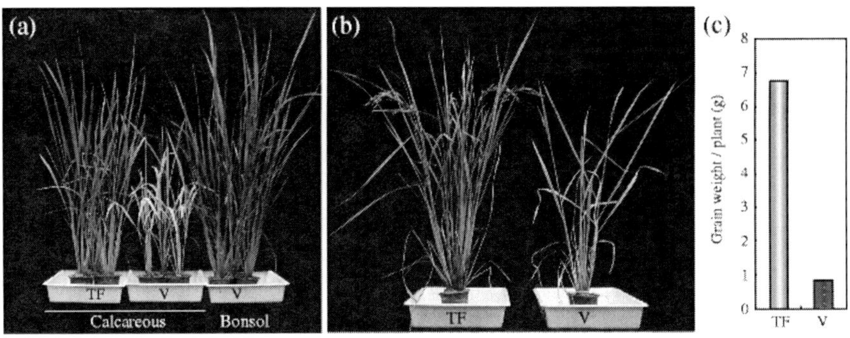


**Figure4.** Tolerance to Fe deficiency in transformants with the introduced *OsIRT1* promoter *refre1/372* grown in calcareous soil. **a** Transformants (*TF, left*) and vector controls (*V, center*) after 4 weeks of growth in a calcareous soil; vector controls (*V, right*) in bonsol (normal cultivated soil). **b** Transformant (*TF, left*) and vector control (*V, right*) after 17 weeks of growth in calcareous soil. **c** Grain yield after cultivation for 17 weeks in calcareous soil. Original figure: Ishimaru et al. [17].

## Manipulating transcription factors regulating the Fe deficiency response

The above studies have shown that introduction of only a single or a few genes is effective in conferring Fe deficiency tolerance if appropriate promoter(s) and gene(s) are utilized. However, further enhancement of Fe availability might be achieved by engineering multiple genes in a coordinated manner. The genetic enhancement of a wide range of related genes requires manipulation of basal regulatory systems, including transcription factors. Therefore, we also aimed to clarify the regulation mechanism controlling the Fe deficiency response in graminaceous plants.

Under low Fe availability, graminaceous plants induce various genes, many of which are involved in Fe acquisition and utilization [2, 26, 28, 36, 41]. Despite the number of Fe-deficiency-inducible genes isolated, little is known about the regulation of gene expression in response to Fe deficiency. Therefore, we applied a stepwise strategy to identify the molecular components regulating the expression of Fe-deficiency-responsive genes: establishment of a promoter assay system, identification of *cis*-acting elements, and identification of *trans*-acting factors that interact with the elements.

We introduced the promoter region of the barley *IDS2* gene connected to the *GUS* gene as a reporter into tobacco plants [73]. Transgenic tobacco plants induced GUS expression in Fe-deficient roots, basically reflecting the regulation pattern in native barley. Precise deletion and mutation analyses using numerous lines of transgenic tobacco identified the novel Fe-deficiency-responsive *cis*-acting elements, iron-deficiency-responsive element 1 and 2 (IDE1 and IDE2; [24]); these are the first identified elements related to micronutrient deficiencies in plants. IDE1 and IDE2 synergistically induce Fe-deficiency-responsive expression in tobacco roots. When introduced into rice, the pair IDE1 and IDE2 is able to induce Fe-deficiency-responsive expression both in roots and leaves [25]. Sequences similar to IDE1 or IDE2 were found in various Fe-deficiency-inducible promoters of barley, rice, tobacco, and *Arabidopsis* [6, 24, 26]. This suggests that gene regulation mechanisms involving IDEs are not only conserved among graminaceous (strategy II) plants but are also functional in nongraminaceous (strategy I) plant species.

Next, we searched for transcription factors that interact with IDEs. Very recently, we successfully identified two rice transcription factors, IDE-binding factor 1 (IDEF1) and IDEF2, which specifically bind to IDE1 and IDE2, respectively [27, 45]. IDEF1 and IDEF2 belong to uncharacterized branches of plant-specific transcription factor families ABI3/VP1 and NAC, respectively, and exhibit novel properties of sequence recognition. IDEF1 recognizes the CATGC sequence within IDE1, whereas IDEF2 predominantly recognizes CA[A/C]G[T/C][T/C/A][T/C/A] within IDE2 as the core binding site. Both *IDEF1* and *IDEF2* transcripts are constitutively expressed in rice roots and leaves.

In an attempt to improve Fe deficiency tolerance by modulating IDEF1 expression, we introduced*IDEF1* cDNA fused to either the constitutive *35S* promoter or the Fe-deficiency-inducible *IDS2*promoter. Transgenic rice seedlings with the introduced *35S* promoter *IDEF1* showed severe growth retardation during early growth, while those carrying the *IDS2* promoter *IDEF1* showed healthy growth. Notably, the *IDS2* promoter *IDEF1* transformants exhibited slower progression of leaf chlorosis in Fe-free hydroponic culture and also showed better growth when germinated on calcareous soil (Fig. 5; [27]).

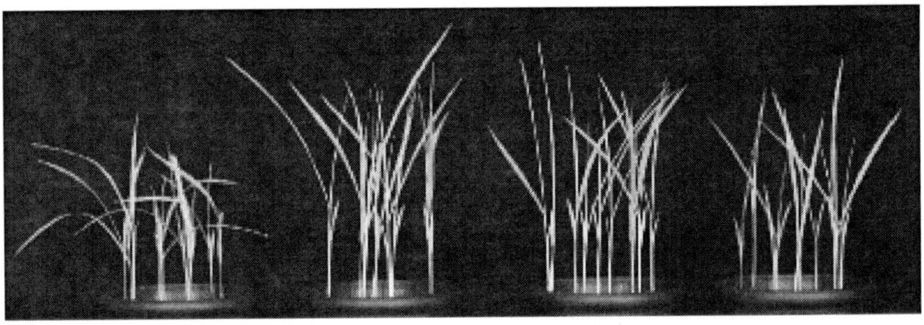


**Figure 5.** Tolerance to Fe deficiency in seedlings with the introduced *IDS2* promoter *IDEF1* germinated in a calcareous soil (*lines 9, 12,* and *13*) compared to nontransformants (*NT*) 17 days after sowing. Original figure: Kobayashi et al. [27].

To clarify the molecular mechanisms that regulate Fe acquisition, we also characterized Fe-deficiency-induced transcription factors. Microarray analyses revealed the upregulation of several transcription factor genes in barley and rice [41, 43], among which a bHLH transcription factor gene,*IRO2*, is of particular interest because of its pronounced transcriptional upregulation by Fe deficiency in shoots and roots of barley and rice [43]. The core sequence for OsIRO2 binding was determined to be CACGTGG [43].

We produced transgenic rice plants with enhanced or repressed OsIRO2 expression by introducing the *35S-OsIRO2* cassette or using the RNA interference technique [44]. In Fe-deficient hydroponic culture, OsIRO2-overexpressing lines showed enhanced MAs secretion and slightly better growth compared to nontransformants, whereas OsIRO2-repressed lines resulted in lower MAs secretion and hypersensitivity to Fe deficiency. Microarray and Northern blot analyses revealed that the expression level of OsIRO2 is positively related to various Fe-deficiency-induced genes in roots, including those responsible for MAs biosynthesis (*OsNAS1*, *OsNAS2*, *OsNAAT1*, *OsDMAS1*, and various genes involved in the methionine cycle) and Fe(III)–MAs uptake (*OsYSL15*). OsIRO2 also affects the expression of some Fe-deficiency-inducible transcription factor genes that possess OsIRO2-binding core sequences in their promoter regions [44]. Importantly, *OsIRO2* itself possesses multiple IDEF1-binding core sequences in its promoter region and is positively regulated by IDEF1 [27]. Based on these results, a sequential link in the Fe deficiency response involving IDEF1, IDEF2, OsIRO2, and its downstream Fe-deficiency-inducible transcription factors is proposed (Fig. 6; [27, 44,45]).

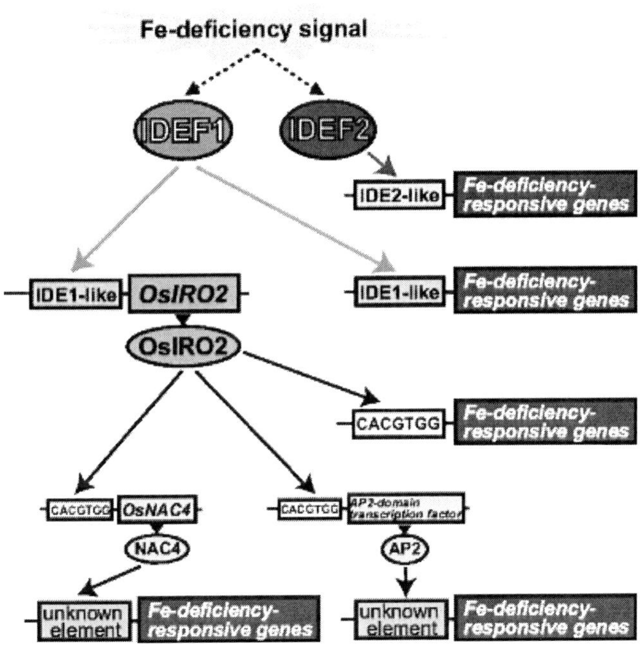


**Figure 6.** Proposed regulatory network for the induction of Fe-deficiency-responsive genes via IDEF1, IDEF2, and OsIRO2. Under Fe-deficient conditions, IDEF1 and IDEF2 transactivate the expression of Fe-deficiency-responsive genes by binding to the IDE1-like and IDE2-like elements, respectively [27, 45]. OsIRO2, which is induced by Fe deficiency and is positively regulated by IDEF1, binds to the CACGTGG element to activate another subset of Fe-deficiency-responsive genes, including two transcription factor genes: *OsNAC4* and the AP2 domain-containing gene. These transcription factors may then regulate Fe-deficiency-responsive genes lacking IDEs and CACGTGG in their promoter regions [44]. The induced expression of *IDEF1* in transgenic rice plants would effectively strengthen the overall regulatory pathway to confer tolerance to Fe deficiency.

In contrast to growth retardation observed in the *35S* promoter *IDEF1* transformants, the *35S*promoter *OsIRO2* transformants were healthy, not exhibiting any obvious defects. These differences in phenotypes of the transformants are thought to be related to the distinct nature of the two transcription factors.

## FUTURE PERSPECTIVES

We produced various lines of transgenic rice plants with enhanced tolerance to low Fe availability. Among these, tolerance of three selected lines (gNAS1, gIDS3, and gNAS1–gNAAT) in calcareous soil was demonstrated in field trials (Figs. 2, 3). Availability of Fe in rice fields is severely affected by soil type and redox potential, as well as numerous other environmental factors. An elaborate combination of previously adopted or new strategies will be needed to produce rice lines with even more tolerance to low Fe availability in problematic soils without loss of favorable agricultural traits. Manipulation of *DMAS* genes, which were recently cloned and thus have not been genetically modified, in the steps of MAs biosynthesis [2] would be of special interest. In addition, further clarification of the underlying mechanisms involved in Fe homeostasis is extremely important, including expressional regulation, secretion of MAs, and metal translocation inside the plants.

Understanding metal homeostasis also paves the way to fortifying rice grains with Fe and Zn. Previous efforts to enhance Fe in grains were performed by overexpressing ferritin, a common Fe storage protein in rice grain [8, 51, 63]. Our field trials revealed that the gIDS3 line is capable of accumulating more Fe in grains in both calcareous and Andosol paddy fields [35, 57]. Production and characterization of transgenic rice lines with introduced biosynthetic genes for MAs and ferritin genes in combination to enhance both Fe uptake and storage is in progress (Masuda et al. unpublished). Other advanced applications of our knowledge on Fe nutrition include the production of novel antihypertensive substrates. NA, the precursor of MAs, inhibits angiotensin-I-converting enzyme in humans and consequently reduces high blood pressure [22, 53]. We produced a yeast strain that highly accumulates NA by introducing the *Arabidopsis NAS* gene, *AtNAS2* [69]. Production and selection of rice lines with elevated levels of NA in grain by introducing the *HvNAS1* gene under the control of a seed-specific promoter of the rice glutelin gene is now under way [68].

Public acceptance of genetically modified organisms is still low. As a technical way to improve public acceptance, we modified the "marker-free vector" of the Cre/*loxP* DNA excision system [74] to construct a high-capacity binary vector for the transformation of rice, from which the sequence sandwiched between two *loxP* sites (including the selectable marker) can be removed by 17β-estradiol administration [68]. Many other approaches may aid public acceptance of transgenic plants, which have such high potential to increase food production, preserve the environment, and improve human health.

## REFERENCES

1. Akiyama K, Nakamura S, Suzuki T, Wisniewska I, Sasaki N, Kawasaki S. Development of a system of rice transformation with long genome inserts for their functional analysis for positional cloning. Plant Cell Physiol Supplement 1997;38:s94.
2. Bashir K, Inoue H, Nagasaka S, Takahashi M, Nakanishi H, Mori S, et al. Cloning and characterization of deoxymugineic acid synthase genes from graminaceous plants. J Biol Chem. 2006;43:32395–402.
3. Bughio N, Yamaguchi H, Nishizawa NK, Nakanishi H, Mori S. Cloning an iron-regulated metal transporter from rice. J Exp Bot 2002;53:1677–82.
4. Connolly EL, Campbell NH, Grotz N, Prichard CL, Guerinot ML. Overexpression of the FRO2 ferric chelate reductase confers tolerance to growth on low iron and uncovers posttranscriptional control. Plant Physiol. 2003;133:1102–10.
5. Curie C, Panavience Z, Loulergue C, Dellaporta SL, Briat JF, Walker EL. Maize yellow stripe1 encodes a membrane protein directly involved in Fe(III) uptake. Nature 2001;409:346–9.
6. Ducos E, Fraysse ÅS, Boutry M. NtPDR3, an iron-deficiency inducible ABC transporter in Nicotiana tabacum. FEBS Lett. 2005;579:6791–5.
7. Eide D, Broderius M, Fett J, Guerinot ML. A novel iron-regulated metal transporter from plants identified by functional expression in yeast. Proc Natl Acad Sci USA. 1996;93:5624–8.
8. Goto F, Yoshihara T, Shigemoto N, Toki S, Takaiwa F. Iron fortification of rice seed by the soybean ferritin gene. Nat Biotechnol 1999;17:282–6.
9. Hell R, Stephan UW. Iron uptake, trafficking and homeostasis in plants. Planta 2003;216:541–51.

10. Hiei Y, Ohta S, Komari T, Kumashiro T. Efficient transformation of rice (Oryza sativa L.) mediated byAgrobacterium and sequence analysis of the boundaries of the T-DNA. Plant J. 1994;6:271–82.

11. Higuchi K, Kanazawa K, Nishizawa NK, Chino M, Mori S. Purification and characterization of nicotianamine synthase from Fe deficient barley roots. Plant Soil. 1994;165:173–9.

12. Higuchi K, Kanazawa K, Nishizawa NK, Mori S. The role of nicotianamine synthase in response to Fe nutrition status in Gramineae. Plant Soil. 1996;178:171–7.

13. Higuchi K, Suzuki K, Nakanishi H, Yamaguchi H, Nishizawa NK, Mori S. Cloning of nicotianamine synthase genes, novel genes involved in the biosynthesis of phytosiderophores. Plant Physiol 1999;119:471–9.

14. Higuchi K, Watanabe S, Takahashi M, Kawasaki S, Nakanishi H, Nishizawa NK, et al. Nicotianamine synthase gene expression differs in barley and rice under Fe-deficient conditions. Plant J. 2001;25:159–67.

15. Inoue H, Takahashi M, Kobayashi T, Suzuki M, Nakanishi H, Mori S, et al. Identification and localisation of the rice nicotianamine aminotransferase gene OsNAAT1 expression suggests the site of phytosiderophore synthesis in rice. Plant Mol Biol. 2008;66:193–203.

16. Ishimaru Y, Suzuki M, Tsukamoto T, Suzuki K, Nakazono M, Kobayashi T, et al. Rice plants take up iron as an Fe3+ -phytosiderophore and as Fe2+. Plant J. 2006;45:335–46.

17. Ishimaru Y, Kim S, Tsukamoto T, Oki H, Kobayashi T, Watanabe S, et al. Mutational reconstructed ferric chelate reductase confers enhanced tolerance in rice to iron deficiency in calcareous soil. Proc Natl Acad Sci USA. 2007;104:7373–8.

18. Itai R, Suzuki K, Yamaguchi H, Nakanishi H, Nishizawa NK, Yoshimura E, et al. Induced activity of adenine phosphoribosyltransferase (APRT) in Fe-deficient barley roots: a possible role for phytosiderophore production. J Exp Bot. 2000;51:1179–88.

19. Kanazawa K, Higuchi K, Nishizawa NK, Fushiya S, Chino M, Mori S. Nicotianamine aminotransferase activities are correlated to the phytosiderophore secretions under Fe-deficient conditions in Gramineae. J Exp Bot. 1994;45:1903–6.

20. Kanazawa K, Higuchi K, Nishizawa NK, Fushiya S, Mori S. Detection of two distinct isozymes of nicotianamine aminotransferase in Fe-deficient barley roots. J Exp Bot. 1995;46:1241–4.

21. Kawai S, Takagi S, Sato Y. Mugineic acid-family phytosiderophores in root-secretions of barley, corn and sorghum varieties. J Plant Nutr. 1988;11:633–42.

22. Kinoshita E, Yamakoshi J, Kikuchi M. Purification and identification of an angiotensin I-converting enzyme inhibitor from soy sauce. Biosci Biotechnol Biochem. 1993;57:1107–10.

23. Kobayashi T, Nakanishi H, Takahashi M, Kawasaki S, Nishizawa NK, Mori S. In vivo evidence that Ids3 fromHordeum vulgare encodes a dioxygenase that converts 2'-deoxymugineic acid to mugineic acid in transgenic rice. Planta 2001;212:864–71.

24. Kobayashi T, Nakayama Y, Itai RN, Nakanishi H, Yoshihara T, Mori S, et al. Identification of novel cis-acting elements, IDE1 and IDE2, of the barley IDS2 gene promoter conferring iron-deficiency-inducible, root-specific expression in heterogeneous tobacco plants. Plant J. 2003;36:780–93.

25. Kobayashi T, Nakayama Y, Takahashi M, Inoue H, Nakanishi H, Yoshihara T, et al. Construction of artificial promoters highly responsive to iron deficiency. Soil Sci Plant Nutr. 2004;50:1167–75.

26. Kobayashi T, Suzuki M, Inoue H, Itai RN, Takahashi M, Nakanishi H, et al. Expression of iron-acquisition-related genes in iron-deficient rice is co-ordinately induced by partially conserved iron-deficiency-responsive elements. J Exp Bot. 2005;56:1305–16.

27. Kobayashi T, Ogo Y, Itai RN, Nakanishi H, Takahashi M, Mori S, et al. The novel transcription factor IDEF1 regulates the response to and tolerance of iron deficiency in plants. Proc Natl Acad Sci USA. 2007;104:19150–5.

28. Kobayashi T, Nishizawa NK. Regulation of iron and zinc uptake and translocation in rice. In: Hirano HY, Hirai A, Sano Y, Sasaki T, editors. Biotechnology in agriculture and forestry 62. Rice biology in the genomics era. Meppel: Springer; 2008. p. 321–35.

29. Ling HQ, Koch G, Bäumlein H, Ganal MW. Map-based cloning of chloronerva, a gene involved in iron uptake of higher plants encoding nicotianamine synthase. Proc Natl Acad Sci USA. 1999;96:7098–710.

30. Ma JF, Nomoto K. Two related biosynthetic pathways of mugineic acids in gramineous plants. Plant Physiol. 1993;102:373–8.

31. Ma JF, Shinada T, Matsuda C, Nomoto K. Biosynthesis of phytosiderophores, mugineic acids, associated with methionine cycling. J Biol Chem. 1995;270:16549–54.

32. Ma JF, Taketa S, Chang YC, Iwashita T, Matsumoto H, Takeda K, et al. Genes controlling hydroxylations of phytosiderophores are located on different chromosomes in barley (Hordeum vulgare L.). Planta 1999;207:590–6.

33. Marschner H. Mineral nutrition of higher plants, 2nd edn. London: Academic; 1995.Google Scholar

34. Marschner H, Römheld V, Kissel M. Different strategies in higher plants in mobilization and uptake of iron. J Plant Nutr. 1986;9:695–713.

35. Masuda H, Suzuki M, Morikawa KC, Kobayashi T, Nakanishi H, Takahashi M, et al. Increase in iron and zinc concentrations in rice grains via the introduction of barley genes involved in phytosiderophore synthesis. Rice 2008

36. Mori S. Iron acquisition by plants. Curr Opin Plant Biol. 1999;2:250–3.

37. Mori S, Nishizawa N. Methionine as a dominant precursor of phytosiderophores in Graminaceae plants. Plant Cell Physiol 1987;28:1081–92.Google Scholar

38. Morikawa CK, Saigusa M, Nakanishi H, Nishizawa NK, Hasegawa K, Mori S. Co-situs application of controlled-release fertilizers to alleviate iron chlorosis of paddy rice grown in calcareous soil. Soil Sci Plant Nutr. 2004;50:1013–21.

39. Nakanishi H, Okumura N, Umehara Y, Nishizawa NK, Chino M, Mori S. Expression of a gene specific for iron deficiency (Ids3) in the roots of Hordeum vulgare. Plant Cell Physiol 1993;34:401–10.

40. Nakanishi H, Yamaguchi H, Sasakuma T, Nishizawa NK, Mori S. Two dioxygenase genes, Ids3 and Ids2, from Hordeum vulgare are involved in the biosynthesis of mugineic acid family phytosiderophores. Plant Mol Biol. 2000;44:199–207.

41. Negishi T, Nakanishi H, Yazaki J, Kishimoto N, Fujii F, Shimbo K, et al. cDNA microarray analysis of gene expression during Fe-deficiency stress in barley suggests that polar transport of

vesicles is implicated in phytosiderophore secretion in Fe-deficient barley roots. Plant J. 2002;30:83–94.

42. Noma M, Noguchi M. Occurrence of nicotianamine in higher plants. Phytochemistry 1976;15:1701–2.

43. Ogo Y, Itai RN, Nakanishi H, Inoue H, Kobayashi T, Suzuki M, et al. Isolation and characterization of IRO2, a novel iron-regulated bHLH transcription factor in graminaceous plants. J Exp Bot. 2006;57:2867–78.

44. Ogo Y, Itai RN, Nakanishi H, Kobayashi T, Takahashi M, Mori S, et al. The rice bHLH protein OsIRO2 is an essential regulator of the genes involved in Fe uptake under Fe-deficient conditions. Plant J. 2007;51:366–77.

45. Ogo Y, Kobayashi T, Itai RN, Nakanishi H, Kakei Y, Takahashi M, et al. A novel NAC transcription factor IDEF2 that recognizes the iron deficiency-responsive element 2 regulates the genes involved in iron homeostasis in plants. J Biol Chem 2008;283:13407–17.

46. Ohata T, Kanazawa K, Mihashi S, Nishizawa NK, Fushiya S, Nozoe S, et al. Biosynthetic pathway of phytosiderophores in iron-deficient Graminaceous plants. Development of an assay system for the detection of nicotianamine aminotransferase activity. Soil Sci Plant Nutr. 1993;39:745–9.

47. Oki H, Yamaguchi H, Nakanishi H, Mori S. Introduction of the reconstructed yeast ferric reductase gene,refre1, into tobacco. Plant Soil 1999;215:211–20.

48. Oki H, Kim S, Nakanishi H, Takahashi M, Yamaguchi H, Mori S, et al. Directed evolution of yeast ferric reductase to produce plants with tolerance to iron deficiency in alkaline soils. Soil Sci Plant Nutr. 2004;50:1159–65.

49. Okumura N, Nishizawa NK, Umehara Y, Mori S. An iron deficiency-specific cDNA from barley roots having two homologous cysteine-rich MT domains. Plant Mol Biol 1991;17:531–3.

50. Okumura N, Nishizawa NK, Umehara Y, Ohata T, Nakanishi H, Yamaguchi H, et al. A dioxygenase gene (Ids2) expressed under iron deficiency conditions in the roots of Hordeum vulgare. Plant Mol Biol 1994;25:705–19.

51. Qu LQ, Yoshihara T, Ooyama A, Goto F, Takaiwa F. Iron accumulation does not parallel the high expression level of ferritin in transgenic rice seeds. Planta 2005;222:225–33.

52. Römheld V, Marschner H. Evidence for a specific uptake system for iron phytosiderophores in roots of grasses. Plant Physiol. 1986;80:175–80.

53. Shimizu E, Hayashi A, Takahashi R, Aoyagi Y, Murakami T, Kimoto K. Effects of angiotensin I-converting enzyme inhibitor from ashitaba (Angelica keiskei) on blood pressure of spontaneously hypertensive rats. J Nutr Sci Vitaminol. 1999;45:375–83.

54. Shojima S, Nishizawa NK, Fushiya S, Nozoe S, Irifune T, Mori S. Biosynthesis of phytosiderophores: in vitrobiosynthesis of 2'-deoxymugineic acid from L-methionine and nicotianamine. Plant Physiol. 1990;93:1497–503.

55. Suzuki K, Itai R, Suzuki K, Nakanishi H, Nishizawa NK, Yoshimura E, et al. Formate dehydrogenase, an enzyme of anaerobic metabolism, is induced by Fe-deficiency in barley roots. Plant Physiol. 1998;116:725–32.

56. Suzuki M, Takahashi M, Tsukamoto T, Watanabe S, Matsuhashi S, Yazaki J, et al. Biosynthesis and secretion of mugineic acid family phytosiderophores in zinc-deficient barley. Plant J. 2006;48:85–97.

57. Suzuki M, Morikawa KC, Nakanishi H, Takahashi M, Saigusa M, Mori S, et al. Transgenic rice lines that include barley genes have increased tolerance to low iron availability in a calcareous paddy soil. Soil Sci Plant Nutr. 2008;54:77–85.

58. Suzuki M, Tsukamoto T, Inoue H, Watanabe S, Matsuhashi S, Takahashi M, et al. Deoxymugineic acid increases Zn translocation in Zn-deficient rice plants. Plant Mol Biol 2008;66:609–17.

59. Takagi S. Naturally occurring iron-chelating compounds in oat- and rice-root washings. Soil Sci Plant Nutr. 1976;22:423–33.

60. Takahashi M, Yamaguchi H, Nakanishi H, Shioiri T, Nishizawa NK, Mori S. Cloning two genes for nicotianamine aminotransferase, a critical enzyme in iron acquisition (strategy II) in graminaceous plants. Plant Physiol. 1999;121:947–56.

61. Takahashi M, Nakanishi H, Kawasaki S, Nishizawa NK, Mori S. Enhanced tolerance of rice to low iron availability in alkaline

soils using barley nicotianamine aminotransferase genes. Nat Biotechnol. 2001;19:466–9.

62. Takahashi M, Terada Y, Nakai I, Nakanishi H, Yoshimura E, Mori S, et al. Role of nicotianamine in the intracellular delivery of metals and plant reproductive development. Plant Cell 2003;15:1263–80.

63. Vasconcelos M, Datta K, Oliva N, Khalekuzzaman M, Torrizo L, Krishnan S, et al. Enhanced iron and zinc accumulation in transgenic rice with the ferritin gene. Plant Sci. 2003;164:371–8.

64. Vasconcelos M, Musetti V, Li CM, Datta SK, Grusak MA. Functional analysis of transgenic rice (Oryza sativa L.) transformed with an Arabidopsis thaliana ferric reductase (AtFRO2). Soil Sci Plant Nutr. 2004;50:1151–7.

65. Vert G, Grotz N, Dedaldechamp F, Gaymard F, Guerinot ML, Briat JF, et al. IRT1, an Arabidopsistransporter essential for iron uptake from the soil and plant growth. Plant Cell 2002;14:1223–33.

66. Vert G, Briat JF, Curie C. Dual regulation of the Arabidopsis high-affinity root iron uptake system by local and long-distance signals. Plant Physiol 2003;132:796–804.

67. von Wirén N, Khodr H, Hider RC. Hydroxylated phytosiderophore species possess an enhanced chelate stability and affinity for iron(III). Plant Physiol. 2000;124:1149–57.

68. Wada Y, Ishimaru Y, Takahashi M, Nakanishi H, Mori S, Nishizawa NK. Engineering of hypotensive rice contain high amounts of nicotianamine for functional foods. In: Li CJ, et al., editors. Plant nutrition for food security, human health and environmental protection. Beijing: Tsinghua University Press; 2005. p. 424–5.

69. Wada Y, Kobayashi T, Takahashi M, Nakanishi H, Mori S, Nishizawa NK. Metabolic engineering ofSaccharomyces cerevisiae producing nicotianamine: potential for industrial biosynthesis of a novel antihypertensive substrate. Biosci Biotechnol Biochem. 2006;70:1408–15.

70. Yamaguchi H, Nakanishi H, Nishizawa NK, Mori S. Induction of the IDI1 gene in Fe-deficient barley roots: a gene encoding putative enzyme that catalyses the methionine salvage pathway for phytosiderophore production. Soil Sci Plant Nutr. 2000;46:1–9.

71. Yamaguchi H, Nakanishi H, Nishizawa NK, Mori S. Isolation and characterization of IDI2, a new Fe-deficiency induced cDNA from barley roots, which encodes a protein related to the a subunit of eukaryotic initiation factor 2B (eIF2B a). J Exp Bot. 2000;51:2001–7.

72. Yamaguchi H, Nishizawa NK, Nakanishi H, Mori S. IDI7, a new iron-regulated ABC transporter from barley roots, localizes to the tonoplast. J Exp Bot. 2002;53:727–235.

73. Yoshihara T, Kobayashi T, Goto F, Masuda T, Higuchi K, Nakanishi H, et al. Regulation of the iron-deficiency responsive gene, Ids2, of barley in tobacco. Plant Biotechnol. 2003;20:33–41.

74. Zuo J, Niu QW, Møller SG, Chua NH. Chemical-regulated, site-specific DNA excision in transgenic plants. Nat Biotechnol. 2001;19:157–61.

8

# OVEREXPRESSING OF *OSAMT1-3*, A HIGH AFFINITY AMMONIUM TRANSPORTER GENE, MODIFIES RICE GROWTH AND CARBON-NITROGEN METABOLIC STATUS

**Aili Bao, Zhijun Liang, Zhuqing Zhao and Hongmei Cai**

Key Laboratory of Arable Land Conservation (Middle and Lower Reaches of Yangtze River), Microelement Research Center, Ministry of Agriculture, Huazhong Agricultural University, Wuhan 430070, China

## ABSTRACT

*AMT1-3* encodes the high affinity $NH_4^+$ transporter in rice roots and is predominantly expressed under nitrogen starvation. In order to evaluate the effect of *AMT1-3* gene on rice growth, nitrogen absorption and metabolism, we generated *AMT1-3*-overexpressing plants and analyzed the growth phenotype, yield, carbon and nitrogen metabolic status, and gene expression profiles. Although*AMT1-3* mRNA accumulated in transgenic plants, these plants displayed significant decreases in growth when compared to the wild-type plants. The nitrogen uptake assay using a $^{15}N$ tracer revealed poor nitrogen uptake ability in *AMT1-3*-overexpressing plants. We found significant decreases in *AMT1-3*-overexpressing plant leaf carbon and nitrogen content accompanied with a higher leaf C/N ratio. Significant changes in soluble proteins and carbohydrates were also observed in *AMT1-3*-overexpressing plants. In addition, metabolite profile analysis demonstrated significant changes in individual sugars, organic acids and free amino acids. Gene expression analysis revealed distinct expression patterns of genes that participate in carbon and nitrogen metabolism. Additionally, the correlation between the metabolites and gene expression patterns was consistent in *AMT1-3*-overexpressing plants under both low and high nitrogen growth conditions. Therefore, we hypothesized that the carbon and nitrogen metabolic imbalance caused by *AMT1-3* overexpressing attributed to the poor growth and yield of transgenic plants.

**Keywords:** *AMT1-3*; carbon-nitrogen metabolism; $^{15}N$ tracer; overexpressing; rice

# 1. INTRODUCTION

Nitrogen (N) is one of the essential macronutrients required for plant growth and development and thus is often a major limiting factor for plant productivity and crop yield [1,2]. Nitrogen is not only a constituent of key cell molecules, such as amino acids, nucleic acids, chlorophyll, ATP and several plant hormones, but is also the pivotal regulator of numerous biological processes, including carbon metabolism, amino acid metabolism and protein synthesis [3,4]. Higher plants can absorb and use various forms of nitrogen components from the soil, most notably the inorganic ions ammonium ($NH_4^+$) and nitrate ($NO_3^-$). These ions are believed to be the principal nitrogen sources for plant growth in agricultural and most natural environments, as it is required in greater amounts than any other mineral nutrient [5]. Because ammonium assimilation requires less energy than nitrate, ammonium is the preferential nitrogen source for root uptake, particularly in nitrogen-deficient plants [6,7]. Carbon (C) is also essential for plants to keep their fundamental growth and development. Various carbohydrates, for example, glucose, sucrose and organic acids provide both the energy and the carbon skeletons for $NH_4^+$ assimilation to produce amino acids and proteins. The proteins, in particular enzymes, are essential for nearly all cellular activities. Several studies have emphasized the importance of the coordination of carbon and nitrogen metabolism [8,9,10,11,12]. The optimal functioning of the metabolic pathways for carbon and nitrogen assimilation in plants, and maintaining an appropriate balance or ratio of carbohydrates to nitrogen metabolites in the cell, which is referred to as the "carbon/nitrogen balance", are critical for determining plant growth, biomass accumulation and seed production [8,9,10,11,12].

Rice (*Oryza sativa*), a staple food for over half of the world's population, is one of the most important crops worldwide. $NH_4^+$ is the major available form of nitrogen that is used for growing rice plants in paddy fields and requires ammonium transporters (AMTs) in the root plasma membrane, which belong to the AMT/MEP/Rh (Ammonium Transporter/Methylamine Permease/Rhesus) protein superfamily with homologs in bacteria and fungi [13,14]. Several ammonia transporters, including bacterial AMT; plant AMT; and human RhAG, RhBG, and RhCG, have been suggested to support electroneutral $NH_3$ transport, $NH_3/H^+$symport, $NH_4^+$ transport, $NH_4^+/H^+$ antiport and $NH_4^+/H^+$ symport [15,16,17,18,19,20,21,22,23,24,25]. AMT/MEP proteins are integral membrane proteins that harbor 11 transmembrane helices and intracellular*C* terminals [26,27]. Biochemical studies have revealed that plant AMTs form trimers [16]. Recently, a different membrane protein type, aquaporins from the MIP (Major Intrinsic Proteins) superfamily, was also demonstrated to transport ammonia [28].

The cloning and expression analysis of *AMT* genes in several plant species have been reported to date.*Arabidopsis* harbors six AMT-type ammonium transporters, which are encoded by five genes (*AtAMT1-1*,*AtAMT1*-2, *AtAMT1-3*, *AtAMT1-5*, *AtAMT2-1*) expressed in the roots and one gene (*AtAMT1-4*) expressed in the pollen [29]. *AtAMT1-1* and *AtAMT1-3* are expressed in rhizodermal and cortical cells, where they confer high-capacity and high-affinity ammonium uptake [30,31]. In addition, reciprocal leaf and root expression of*AtAMT1-1* in response to nitrogen starvation has been reported by Engineer and Kranz [32]. *AtAMT1-2* is expressed in endodermal and cortical cells and most likely plays a major role in the uptake and retrieval of ammonium from the apoplast in the root with a lower-affinity [31]. However, *AtAMT2-1* is more highly expressed in shoots relative to roots, and no ammonium influx activity has been observed in the root [31,33,34]. *AtAMT1-5* is expressed in rhizodermal root cells and contributes 5%–10% to the overall ammonium uptake capacity [31]. *AtAMT1-4* is a pollen-specific high-affinity ammonium transporter in the plasma membrane [29]. Rice roots harbor four families of *AMT* genes: *OsAMT1*, *OsAMT2*, *OsAMT3* and*OsAMT4*. *OsAMT1* memb ers have been characterized as a high-affinity transport system (HAT), share a highly similar sequence to each other, while the other three families have been characterized as a low-affinity transport system (LAT) [13,35]. Sonoda *et al.* [35] demonstrated distinct expression patterns in the*OsAMT1* gene family. *OsAMT1-1* is constitutively expressed in the shoots but is stimulated by ammonium in the roots; *OsAMT1-2* expression is root-specific and ammonium-inducible, whereas *OsAMT1-3* is also expressed specifically in the roots but is repressed by nitrogen. *OsAMT2-1* encodes an ammonium transporter, which is more closely related to the yeast MEP transporter sequence and is constitutively expressed in the shoots and roots [36,37]. Several studies revealed a feedback regulation and a distinct nitrogen-dependent regulation for the rice *AMT* genes, which differs from that in tomato or *Arabidopsis*. Sonoda *et al.* identified cytosolic glutamine as a promising regulatory factor of the *OsAMT1* genes [35]. Additionally, *AMT* genes in several other plant species have been identified and characterized, including*Brassica napus* (*BnAMT1-2*) [38], *Lotus japonicas* (*LjAMT1-1*, *LjAMT2-1*) [39,40] and *Lycopersicon esculentum*(*LeAMT1-1*, *LeAMT1-2* and *LeAMT1-3*) [41,42,43].

Generally, the expression of the AMT1 isolated from different plant species are transcriptionally regulated. However, ectopically expressing of the *AtAMT1-1* gene under the control of a 35S promoter in transgenic tobacco plants revealed that the *AtAMT1-1* gene can also be post-transcriptionally regulated [44]. A post-translational regulation of ammonium transport activity has also been described for the AMT1 proteins in *Arabidopsis*. Loqué *et al.* reported that the cytosolic trans-activation domain in AMT was essential for ammonium uptake, a mutation in the cytosolic AMT1-1 *C* terminus attenuated the strict dependence on allosteric trans-activation [45,46]. The oligomerization of plant AMTs is critical for allosteric regulation of transport activity, in which the conserved cytosolic *C* terminus functions as a trans-activator [47]. AMT1-1 and AMT1-2 are allosterically regulated by *C*-terminal phosphorylation, which trans-inhibited the activation of AMT1 subunits in a trimeric complex [45,48,49]. AMT1-3 harbors a phosphomimic residue in its *C*terminus regulates both homo- and hetero-trimers in a dominant-negative fashion *in vivo* [47]. *C*-terminal phosphorylation of AMT1 is rapidly triggered by an external ammonium supply and decreases ammonium uptake by the roots and thereby quickly inactivating transport in a potentially toxic environment [49]. Additionally, Graff *et al.* [50] also reported that *N*-terminal cysteines affected the oligomer stability of the allosterically regulated ammonium transporter LeAMT1-1.

As we known, in agriculture, rice growth and yield requires abundant N. In order to meet the high production of rice, large amounts of synthetic N fertilizers are applied on arable land by farmers.

However, crop plants use less than half of the applied N fertilizers [51]. Zhang *et al.* [52] reported that the N use efficiency of midseason rice in China is less than 30%. The applications of large quantities of synthetic N fertilizers to increase crop yield are not economically sustainable and placed a heavy economic burden on farmers, and also result in environmental pollutions. Because of the high-affinity $NH_4^+$ uptake function of*AMT1-3* in rice, it is a good candidate gene for use in transformation strategies aimed at improving nitrogen use efficiency and rice yield. However, no study has been reported about the function of *AMT1-3* gene in rice growth and carbon-nitrogen metabolism to date. In order to evaluate the effect of *AMT1-3* gene on rice growth, nitrogen absorption and metabolism, we generated *AMT1-3*-overexpressing plants *via* the*Agrobacterium*-mediated transformation method using the *CaMV*35S promoter in this study, and analyzed the growth phenotype, yield, leaf SPAD (Soil and Plant Analyzer Development) value, photosynthesis, carbon and nitrogen metabolic status and gene expression profiles under four different N levels (0× N, 0.1× N, 1× N and 5× N) at both tillering and heading stages. Results revealed that the overexpressing of *AMT1-3*gene altered rice growth and development, yield, C/N ratio, soluble proteins and carbohydrates, carbon and nitrogen metabolites, gene expression patterns in transgenic plants when compared to the wild-type plants. Moreover, *AMT1-3* may act as a signal sensor to regulate plant growth in addition to its function in $NH_4^+$uptake in the root. Our results provided a new understanding of the function of *AMT1-3* genes in rice growth, yield, carbon and nitrogen metabolism, and a reference for the molecular breeding of the high nitrogen use efficiency rice cultivar using transgenic strategy.

# 2. RESULTS

## 2.1. Accumulated AMT1-3 mRNA Transcripts in $T_0$ Transgenic Plants

The complete mRNA sequence of *OsAMT1-3* (AF289479) was identified in the NCBI GenBank database using a key word search. The *OsAMT1-3* gene was amplified from the rice (Zhonghua 11, *Japonica*) genome and ligated into the pCAMBIA 1301S vector, which contained a *hygromycin resistance* gene driven by the*CaMV*35S promoter. The construct was then transformed into Zhonghua 11 using the *Agrobacterium*-mediated transformation method (Figure 1A). More than 50 independent $T_0$ transformants were generated, and 42 positive transformants were detected by PCR-directed analysis of the *hygromycin resistance* gene. Northern blot analysis of the transgene in these independent positive transgenic plants revealed that 21 (50%) transgenic plants harbored higher *OsAMT1-3* mRNA levels than the wild-type Zhonghua 11 (Figure 1B). Southern blot analysis showed 1–2 copies of transgene existed in the *OsAMT1-3*-overexpressing plants (Figures S1). To examine the effect of higher *OsAMT1-3* expression on plant growth, $T_1$ progeny of the 21*OsAMT1-3*-overexpressing plants and wild-type plants were grown hydroponically in normal and low nitrogen (0.1× N) nutrient solutions. Six-week-old plants were harvested to measure the plant height and fresh weight. Generally, transgenic lines exhibited a poorer growth than the wild-type plants under both normal and low nitrogen conditions. Figure 2 showed that the plant height and fresh weight of two transgenic lines (3–12, 3–39) were significantly ($p < 0.01$) decreased when compared with wild-type plants under both normal and low nitrogen conditions. To avoid confounding effects of the excessively higher*OsAMT1-3* gene expression on plant growth, we selected the $T_2$ generation of transgenic line 3–39 with single copy of transformed *AMT1-3*, which displayed higher *OsAMT1-3* levels than wild-type plants but were relatively lower among the 21 transgenic plants, for further analysis and was named *AMT1-3*-overexpressing plants.

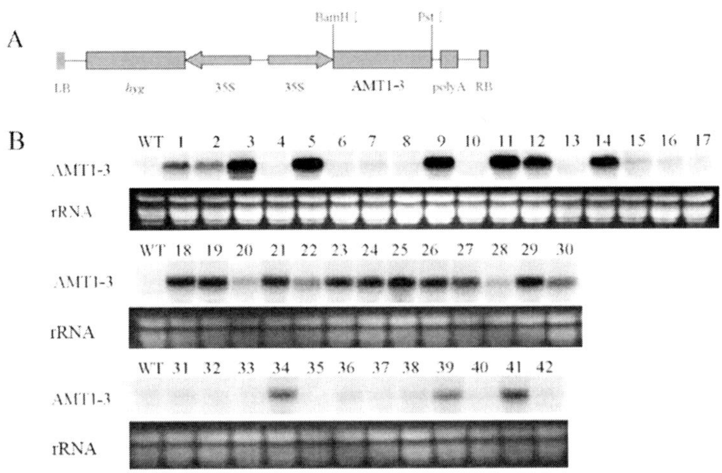


**Figure 1.** Generation of transgenic plants that overexpressing the*AMT1-3* gene. (**A**) The construct of the plasmid containing a derivative of the *CaMV* 35S promoter (35S), *AMT1-3* and the poly A terminator between the right (RB) and the left (LB) borders of the T-DNA. The*hygromycin resistance* gene (*hyg*) was located between the LB and the 35S promoter; (**B**) Northern blot analysis of the *AMT1-3* mRNA transcriptional levels in 42 positive transgenic plants of the $T_0$generation and the wild-type plants (WT).

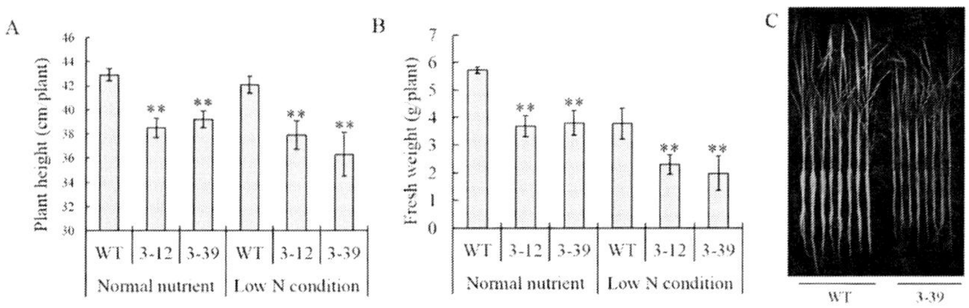


**Figure 2.** Phenotype analysis at the seedling stage. The growth phenotype (**A**), plant height (**B**) and plant fresh weight (**C**) of the *AMT1-3*-overexpressing plants (3–12, 3–39) and wild type plants (WT) at the seedling stage. Values are the mean ± s.d. of eight randomly selected plants. ** indicates the significant difference at the level of $p = 0.01$.

## 2.2. Effect of AMT1-3-Overexpressing on Growth Phenotype and Yield

As the *AMT1-3*-overexpressing plants displayed a poor growth phenotype at the seedling stage mentioned above, we analyzed the root length, plant height, root and shoot dry weight, leaf SPAD value and photosynthetic parameters of *AMT1-3*-overexpressing plants and wild-type plants at both tillering and heading stages grown hydroponically under four different nitrogen levels (0× N, 0.1× N, 1× N and 5× N) to test the poor growth phenotype at both vegetative and productive stages in more detail. The *AMT1-3*-overexpressing and wild-type plant yields at a mature growth stage in pots were also tested. The results revealed a significant ($p < 0.05$) decline in the root length and plant height and in the root and shoot dry weight in the *AMT1-3*-overexpressing plants compared to wild-type plants at both tillering and heading stages under the 0× N, 0.1× N, 1× N and 5× N conditions (Figure 3). At the tillering stage, a 17.7%–31.2%, 8%–15.8%, 60.7%–77.3% and 58%–79.1% decrease in the root length, plant height and the root and shoot dry weights of *AMT1-3*-overexpressing plants were observed, respectively (Figure 3A). At the heading stage, a 11.3%–21.6%, 6.9%–19.2%, 38.6%–55.2% and 42.3%–55.1% decrease in the root length, plant height and the root and shoot dry weights of *AMT1-3*-overexpressing plants were observed, respectively (Figure 3B). The leaf SPAD value and photosynthetic parameters did not significantly differ between the *AMT1-3*-overexpressing plants and wild-type plants, except for significant ($p < 0.05$) decreases in the photosynthetic rate and stomatal conductance in the leaves of *AMT1-3*-overexpressing plants compared with wild-type plants at the heading stage under the 1× N condition (Table 1). A yield analysis at the mature stage revealed decreases of 45.6%, 8.5%, 9.5% and 26.4% in *AMT1-3*-overexpressing plants compared with wild-type plants under the 0× N, 0.1× N, 1× N and 5× N conditions, respectively (Table 2). These results indicated that *AMT1-3*gene overexpressing could severely affect plant growth and development at both vegetative and productive stages under different nitrogen levels.

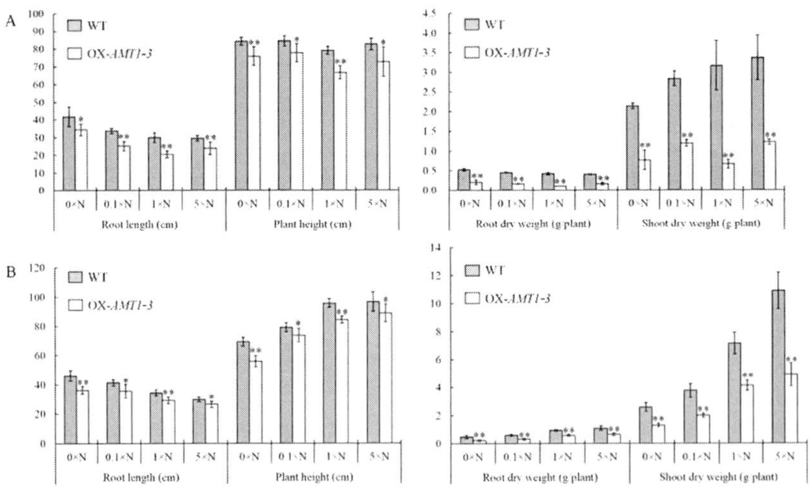


**Figure 3.** Phenotype analysis at the tillering and heading stages. The root length, plant height, root and shoot dry weight in the *AMT1-3*-overexpressing plants (we renamed 3–39 as OX-*AMT1-3*) and wild type plants (WT) at the tillering stage (**A**) and the heading stage (**B**) under 0× N, 0.1× N, 1× N and 5× N conditions. Values are the mean ± s.d. of ten randomly selected plants. *, ** indicate the significant differences at the level of $p = 0.05$ and $p = 0.01$, respectively.

### 2.3. Effect of AMT1-3-Overexpressing on Nitrogen Uptake and Accumulation

As *AMT1-3* is one of the high affinity ammonium transporter genes involved in $NH_4^+$ uptake in rice roots, we analyzed the $^{15}N$ and total N contents in roots, stems and leaves of *AMT1-3*-overexpressing plants and wild-type plants. We employed the $^{15}N$ tracer assay at the tillering stage to assess for differences in the nitrogen uptake ability in the root and in the nitrogen transport ability from the root to the

**Table 1.** The leaf SPAD value and photosynthetic parameters in the*AMT1-3*-overexpressing plants (OX-*AMT1-3*) and wild type plants (WT) at the tillering stage and the heading stage under 0× N, 0.1× N, 1× N, 5× N conditions.

| Treatment | SPAD | | Photosynthesis Parameters at Heading Stage | | | |
|---|---|---|---|---|---|---|
| | Tillering Stage | Heading Stage | Photosynthetic Rate (μmol $CO_2 \cdot m^{-2} \cdot s^{-2}$) | Stomatal Conductance (mmol$\cdot m^{-2} \cdot s^{-1}$) | Intercellular $CO_2$ Concentration ($\mu L \cdot L^{-1}$) | Transpiration Rate (mmol $H_2O \cdot m^{-2} \cdot S^{-1}$) |
| **0× N** | | | | | | |
| WT | 34.3 ± 2.4 | 32.7 ± 1.7 | 13.24 ± 1.47 | 0.28 ± 0.04 | 280.48 ± 1.12 | 7.54 ± 0.65 |
| OX-*AMT1-3* | 34.3 ± 2.5 | 33.0 ± 1.4 | 11.84 ± 2.34 | 0.25 ± 0.05 | 280.16 ± 8.55 | 6.71 ± 0.95 |
| **0.1× N** | | | | | | |
| WT | 40.7 ± 2.0 | 40.7 ± 2.2 | 10.58 ± 1.64 | 0.29 ± 0.02 | 297.52 ± 10.16 | 7.24 ± 0.25 |
| OX-*AMT1-3* | 42.3 ± 3.4 | 40.4 ± 1.2 | 12.88 ± 1.59 | 0.30 ± 0.05 | 287.51 ± 11.30 | 7.20 ± 0.71 |
| **1× N** | | | | | | |
| WT | 43.6 ± 2.0 | 47.1 ± 0.5 | 16.07 ± 1.78 | 0.41 ± 0.04 | 290.97 ± 8.26 | 7.49 ± 0.47 |
| OX-*AMT1-3* | 44.4 ± 1.3 | 46.5 ± 1.3 | 12.49 ± 1.76 * | 0.27 ± 0.09 ** | 278.65 ± 23.78 | 6.09 ± 1.47 |
| **5× N** | | | | | | |
| WT | 44.4 ± 1.5 | 48.4 ± 1.3 | 19.12 ± 3.45 | 0.53 ± 0.05 | 305.62 ± 15.74 | 7.85 ± 0.17 |
| OX-*AMT1-3* | 43.6 ± 4.0 | 47.4 ± 1.3 | 16.95 ± 2.39 | 0.48 ± 0.09 | 300.49 ± 14.01 | 7.86 ± 1.04 |

Values are mean ± s.d. from ten randomly selected plants. *, ** indicate the significant differences at the level of $p = 0.05$ and $p = 0.01$, respectively.

**Table 2.** The yield and its components in the *AMT1-3*-overexpressing plants (OX-*AMT1-3*) and wild type plants (WT) under 0× N, 0.1× N, 1× N, 5× N conditions.

| Treatment | Panicals/Plant | Filled Grains/Panicle | Seed Rate (%) | Thousand Grains Weight (g) | Yield (g/Plant) |
|---|---|---|---|---|---|
| **0× N** | | | | | |
| WT | 3.4 ± 0.3 | 19.1 ± 1.5 | 35.1 ± 1.5 | 24.46 ± 0.65 | 1.60 ± 0.11 |
| OX-*AMT1-3* | 2.5 ± 0.4 * | 15.6 ± 2.6 | 33.7 ± 1.2 | 22.89 ± 0.94 | 0.87 ± 0.05 ** |
| **0.1× N** | | | | | |
| WT | 4.0 ± 0.2 | 21.4 ± 3.5 | 36.4 ± 4.3 | 23.05 ± 0.74 | 2.00 ± 0.44 |
| OX-*AMT1-3* | 3.5 ± 0.2 | 21.9 ± 3.8 | 33.6 ± 4.8 | 23.68 ± 0.91 | 1.83 ± 0.23 |
| **1× N** | | | | | |
| WT | 11.5 ± 1.1 | 44.9 ± 4.9 | 66.9 ± 5.9 | 24.98 ± 0.21 | 12.78 ± 0.42 |
| OX-*AMT1-3* | 11.6 ± 0.6 | 39.5 ± 4.3 | 64.8 ± 6.1 | 25.35 ± 0.31 | 11.56 ± 0.87 |
| **5× N** | | | | | |
| WT | 14.6 ± 0.9 | 32.5 ± 2.3 | 65.9 ± 10.9 | 22.77 ± 0.75 | 10.80 ± 0.41 |
| OX-*AMT1-3* | 15.6 ± 0.7 | 23.3 ± 0.6 ** | 54.0 ± 4.4 | 21.87 ± 0.91 | 7.95 ± 0.26 ** |

Values are mean ± s.d. from ten randomly selected plants. *, ** indicate the significant differences at the level of $p = 0.05$ and $p = 0.01$, respectively.

stem and from the stem to the leaf between *AMT1-3*-overexpressing plants and wild-type plants. The results indicated that*AMT1-3*-overexpressing plants harbored lower $^{15}N$ contents in the roots, stems and leaves, especially three days after $NH_4Cl$ in the nutrient solution was refreshed by $^{15}NH_4Cl$ (Figure 4). Furthermore, we analyzed the total carbon and nitrogen contents in the roots, stems and leaves of *AMT1-3*-overexpressing plants and wild-type plants under the 0× N, 0.1× N, 1× N and 5× N conditions at this stage. Because we performed two independent assays, the plant materials differed from the materials used in the $^{15}N$ tracer assay. The results indicated significant ($p < 0.05$) decreases in the leaf carbon and nitrogen contents in *AMT1-3*-overexpressing plants compared with wild-type plants under the 0× N, 0.1× N, 1× N and 5× N conditions (Table 3). There were 4.6%, 9.9%, 5.9% and 5.8% decreases in the leaf carbon content, whereas decreases of 4.7%, 13.4%, 15.5% and 8.6% in the leaf nitrogen content under the 0× N, 0.1× N, 1× N and 5× N conditions were observed, respectively, which resulted in leaf carbon/nitrogen ratio increases of 11.7%, 11.6% and 9.4% under the 0.1× N, 1× N and 5× N conditions, respectively (Table 3). These results suggest that *AMT1-3*-overexpressing plants exhibited a poor nitrogen transport ability. The nitrogen transport from stems to leaves was especially attenuated, which caused a higher carbon/nitrogen ratio in the leaves.

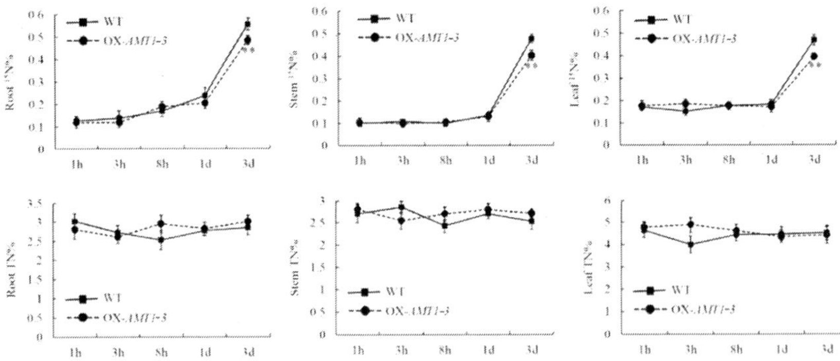


**Figure 4.** Nitrogen uptake analysis. The $^{15}N$ ($^{15}N$%) and total nitrogen content (TN%) in the roots, stems and leaves of the *AMT1-3*-overexpressing plants (we renamed 3–39 as OX-*AMT1-3*) and wild type plants (WT) at 1, 3, 8 h, 1 and 3 day after $NH_4Cl$ in the nutrient solution was replaced with $^{15}NH_4Cl$ during the tillering stage. Values are the mean ± s.d. of six randomly selected plants. ** indicates the significant difference at the level of $p = 0.01$.

## 2.4. Effect of AMT1-3-Overexpressing on Soluble Proteins and Carbohydrates Concentrations

As the nitrogen and carbon contents were changed by the overexpressing of *AMT1-3* mentioned above, we wanted to evaluate the differences of carbon and nitrogen metabolic status between *AMT1-3*-overexpressing plants and wild-type plants. Therefore, we assessed the concentrations of soluble proteins and carbohydrates in the roots, stems and leaves of *AMT1-3*-overexpressing plants and wild-type plants at both tillering and heading stages under the 0× N, 0.1× N, 1× N and 5× N conditions. Our

**Table 3.** The carbon content (C%), nitrogen content (N%) and carbon/nitrogen ratio (C/N) in the roots, stems and leaves of the *AMT1-3*-overexpressing plants (OX-*AMT1-3*) and wild type plants (WT) at the tillering stage under 0× N, 0.1× N, 1× N, 5× N conditions.

| Treatment | C% | | | N% | | | C/N | | |
|---|---|---|---|---|---|---|---|---|---|
| | Root | Stem | Leaf | Root | Stem | Leaf | Root | Stem | Leaf |
| **0× N** | | | | | | | | | |
| WT | 38.54 ± 0.60 | 38.26 ± 0.43 | 40.10 ± 0.20 | 1.76 ± 0.06 | 0.96 ± 0.04 | 2.14 ± 0.03 | 21.85 ± 0.77 | 39.79 ± 1.05 | 18.71 ± 0.25 |
| OX-*AMT1-3* | 36.36 ± ND | 36.07 ± 1.63 | 38.25 ± 0.39 ** | 1.62 ± ND | 1.02 ± 0.03 | 2.04 ± 0.09 | 22.39 ± ND | 35.26 ± 0.61 ** | 18.80 ± 0.67 |
| **0.1× N** | | | | | | | | | |
| WT | 38.47 ± 0.07 | 38.88 ± 0.10 | 40.52 ± 0.16 | 2.10 ± 0.14 | 1.40 ± 0.11 | 2.91 ± 0.18 | 18.34 ± 1.17 | 27.80 ± 2.20 | 13.94 ± 0.81 |
| OX-*AMT1-3* | 39.13 ± 0.76 | 37.53 ± 0.39 | 36.51 ± 0.35 ** | 2.13 ± ND | 1.39 ± 0.07 | 2.52 ± 0.15 * | 17.17 ± ND | 26.97 ± 1.59 | 15.57 ± 0.85 * |
| **1× N** | | | | | | | | | |
| WT | 37.48 ± 0.60 | 37.00 ± 0.36 | 41.46 ± 0.25 | 2.72 ± 0.004 | 2.44 ± 0.08 | 3.75 ± 0.08 | 13.77 ± 0.20 | 15.19 ± 0.49 | 11.05 ± 0.16 |
| OX-*AMT1-3* | ND | 36.21 ± 0.46 | 39.01 ± 0.13 ** | ND | 2.37 ± 0.21 | 3.17 ± 0.14 ** | ND | 15.36 ± 1.24 | 12.33 ± 0.59 * |
| **5× N** | | | | | | | | | |
| WT | 37.69 ± 0.61 | 36.96 ± 0.18 | 41.46 ± 0.25 | 2.85 ± 0.16 | 3.04 ± 0.08 | 3.98 ± 0.08 | 13.27 ± 1.00 | 12.15 ± 0.31 | 10.41 ± 0.15 |
| OX-*AMT1-3* | 37.21 ± ND | 36.08 ± 0.78 | 39.04 ± 0.72 ** | 2.56 ± ND | 2.96 ± 0.02 | 3.43 ± 0.23 * | 14.52 ± ND | 12.18 ± 0.21 | 11.39 ± 0.60 * |

Values are mean ± s.d. from three biological replications. *, ** indicate the significant differences at the level of $p < 0.05$ and $p < 0.01$, respectively. ND: no data.

results demonstrated that most of the soluble proteins were in the leaves, whereas most of the soluble carbohydrates resided in the stems. Interestingly, the soluble proteins increased with increasing nitrogen levels, whereas an opposite trend was observed for soluble carbohydrates, which decreased with increasing nitrogen levels at both the tillering and heading stages (Figure 5 and Figure 6). The soluble protein and carbohydrate concentrations in*AMT1-3*-overexpressing plants were noticeably distinct from those of wild-type plants (Figure 5 and Figure 6). Compared to wild type plants, there were 18.5%, 4.9%, 14.3% decreases and 22.3% increase of soluble proteins in *AMT1-3*-overexpressing plants at tillering stage under 0× N, 0.1× N, 1× N and 5× N conditions, respectively. While an opposite change pattern displayed at heading stage that there were 8.6%, 5.8%, 7.8% increases and 1.3% decrease of soluble proteins in *AMT1-3*-overexpressing plants under 0× N, 0.1× N, 1× N and 5× N conditions, respectively (data not show here). For soluble carbohydrates, 15.5%, 18.5%, 2.1% and 10.4% decreases displayed in *AMT1-3*-overexpressing plants at tillering stage, while 3.8% decrease, 19.0% increase, 10.6% decrease and 28.1% increase displayed in *AMT1-3*-overexpressing plants at heading stage under 0× N, 0.1× N, 1× N and 5× N conditions, respectively (data not show here). Additionally, there was a certain change in the concentrations of root, stem and leaf soluble proteins and carbohydrates in *AMT1-3*-overexpressing plants when compared to wild type plants (Figure 5 and Figure 6). For example, soluble proteins analysis at the tillering stage revealed significant ($p < 0.05$) increases in the root under the 0.1× N (30.6%) and 1× N (66.9%) conditions and in the leaf under the 5× N (40.4%) condition, as well as significant ($p < 0.05$) decreases in the stem under the 5× N (34.3%) condition and in the leaf under the 0× N (22.2%) and 1× N (19.5%) conditions. However, an analogous analysis at the heading stage revealed significant ($p < 0.05$) increases in the root under the 0× N (14.1%) and 5× N (29.8%) conditions and in the spikelet under the 1× N (10.5%) and 5× N (12.4%) conditions, as well as significant ($p < 0.05$) decreases in the stem under the 5× N (40.8%) condition (Figure 5). An analysis of soluble carbohydrates at the tillering stage demonstrated significant ($p < 0.05$) increases in the root under the 5× N (14.5%) condition and in the stem under the 1× N (25.9%) condition, as well as significant ($p < 0.05$) decreases in the stem under the 5× N (34.3%) condition and in the leaf under the 0× N (29.3%) and 1× N (34.0%) conditions. An analogous analysis at the heading stage indicated significant ($p < 0.05$) increases in the stem under the 0.1× N (22.6%) and 5× N (119.3%) conditions and in the leaf under the 0× N (14.1%) condition (Figure 6). These results suggest that the overexpressing of the *AMT1-3* gene altered carbon and nitrogen metabolic statuses in transgenic plants.

## 2.5. Effect of AMT1-3-Overexpressing on Carbon and Nitrogen Metabolites

To study the individual metabolites involved in the carbon and nitrogen metabolic pathways, we analyzed the sugars, organic acids and free amino acids in the roots and leaves of *AMT1-3*-overexpressing plants and wild-type plants at the tillering stage under the 0× N and 5× N conditions. Figure 7 and supplementary Figure S2 displays the fold change that corresponds to the ratio of *AMT1-3*-overexpressing plants/wild-type plants calculated by the concentration of these individual metabolites. For the total sugars, total organic acids and total free amino acids, the results indicated similar patterns between the roots and leaves, where the total sugars and total free amino acids decreased and the total organic acids increased in *AMT1-3*-overexpressing plants under the 0× N condition, and the total sugars and total organic acids decreased and the total free amino acids increased in *AMT1-3*-overexpressing plants under the 5× N condition (data not shown). The fold change of individual sugars, organic acids and free amino acids in *AMT1-3*-overexpressing plants compared with wild-type plants indicates that *AMT1-3* overexpressing yielded larger metabolite content variations in the roots than the leaves and under the 0× N condition than the 5× N condition. In*AMT1-3*-overexpressing plant leaves, when compared with wild-type plants, dramatic increases in xylitol (>21.9-fold) and succinate (>277.6-fold) and dramatic decreases in benzoic acid

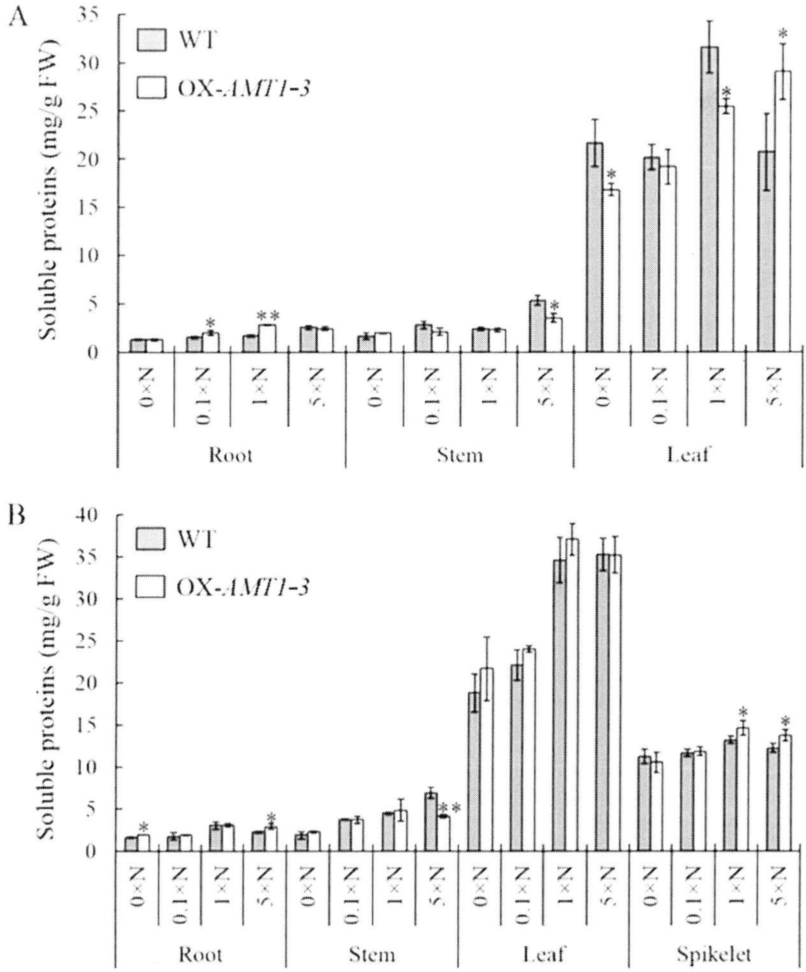


**Figure 5.** Soluble proteins analysis. The concentration of soluble proteins in the roots, stems and leaves of the *AMT1-3*-overexpressing plants (we renamed 3-39 as OX-*AMT1-3*) and wild type plants (WT) at the tillering stage (**A**) and the heading stage (**B**) under 0× N, 0.1× N, 1× N and 5× N conditions. Values are the mean ± s.d. from three biological replications. *, ** indicate the significant differences at the level of $p = 0.05$ and $p = 0.01$, respectively.

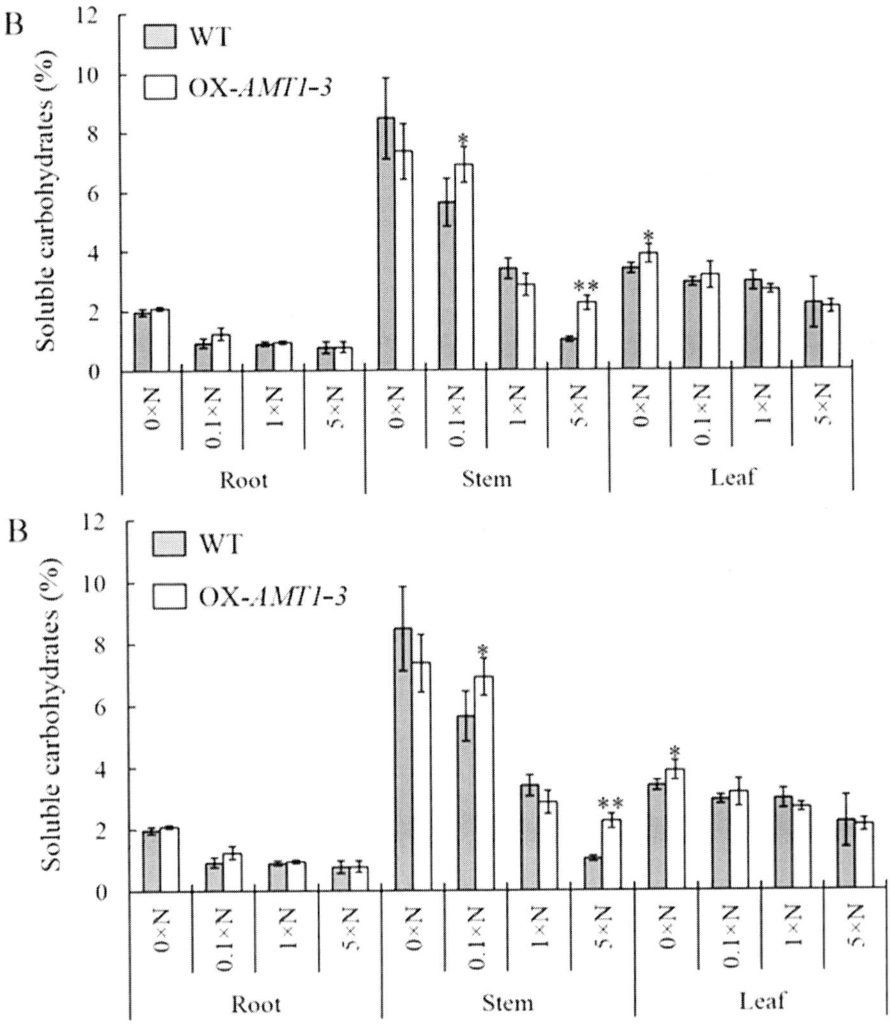


**Figure 6.** Soluble carbohydrates analysis. The concentration of soluble carbohydrates in the roots, stems and leaves of the *AMT1-3*-overexpressing plants (we renamed 3–39 as OX-*AMT1-3*) and wild type plants (WT) at the tillering stage (**A**) and the heading stage (**B**) under 0× N, 0.1× N, 1× N and 5× N conditions. Values are the mean ± s.d. from three biological replications. *, ** indicate the significant differences at the level of $p = 0.05$ and $p = 0.01$, respectively.

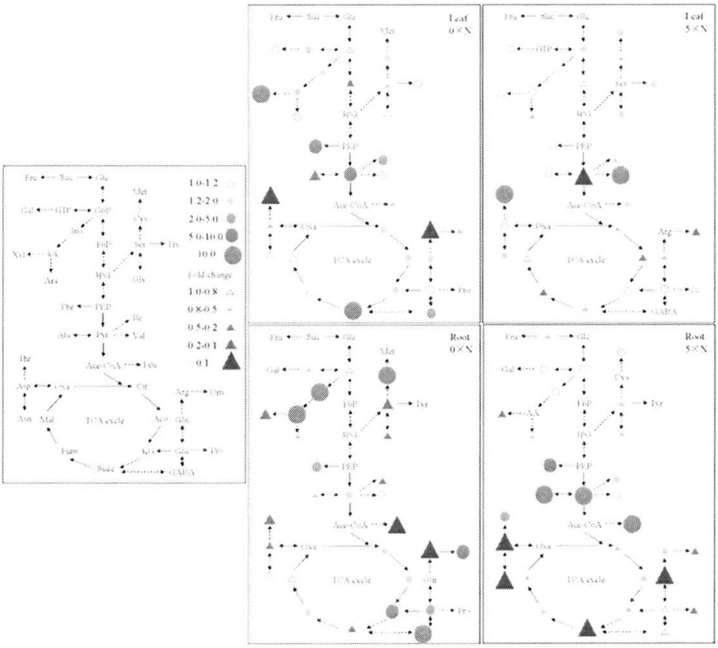

**Figure 7.** Metabolites analysis. Fold change corresponds to the ratio of the concentration of individual metabolites involved in carbon and nitrogen metabolism in the *AMT1-3*-overexpressing plants relative to the wild type plants for the leaves and roots at the tillering stage under 0× N and 5× N conditions. Glc, glucose; Suc, sucrose; Fru, Fructose; F6P, Frutose-6-P; G6P, Glucose-6-P; G1P, Glucose-1-P; Gal, galactose; Ino, Inositol; AA, Ascorbic acid; Ara, Arabinose; Xyl, Xylitol; 3PG, 3-P-glycerate; PEP, P-enolpyruvate; Pyr, Pyruvate; Ace-CoA, acetyl-CoA; Cit, Citrate; Aco, Aconitase; KG, Ketoglutarate; Succ, Succinate; Fum, Fumarate; Mal, Malate; Oxa, oxaloacetate; Glu, Glutamate; Gln, Glutamine; Arg, Arginine; Pro, Proline; Orn, Ornithine; GABA, Aminobutyric; Asp, Aspartate; Asn, Asparagine; Ile, Isoleucine; Met, Methionine; Thr, Threonine; Ala, Alanine; Val, Valine; Leu, Leucine; Phe, Phenylalanine; Try, Tryptophan; Ser, Serine; Gly, Glycine; Cys, Cysteine. Red dots indicate increased metabolites and blue triangles indicate decreased metabolites.

(<0.01-fold), arginine (<0.04-fold) and threonine (<0.03-fold) were observed under the 0×N condition. However, dramatic increases in threonine (>42.8-fold) and valine (>32.5-fold) and dramatic decrease in pyruvate (<0.07-fold) were observed under the 5× N condition (Figure 7 and Figure S2). In *AMT1-3*-overexpressing plant roots, when compared with wild-type plants, dramatic increases in inositol

(>21.2-fold), ascorbic acid (>96.5-fold), aminobutyric acid (>526.6-fold) and cysteine (>20.0-fold) and dramatic decreases in arginine (<0.07-fold) and leucine (<0.001-fold) were observed under the 0× N condition. However, dramatic increases in benzoic acid (>14.0-fold), pyruvate (>684.7-fold), alanine (>63.3-fold) and leucine (>21.0-fold) and dramatic decreases in succinate (<0.10-fold), glutamine (<0.06-fold), aspartate (<0.05-fold) and asparagine (<0.005-fold) were observed under the 5× N condition (Figure 7 and Figure S2).

## 2.6. Effect of AMT1-3-Overexpressing on Gene Expression Level

To analyze the impact of higher *AMT1-3* mRNA levels on the expression patterns of key genes involved in carbon and nitrogen metabolism, the expression levels of genes encoding NRT (nitrate transporter), NR (nitrate reductase), GS (glutamine synthetase), GOGAT (glutamate synthase), RUBISCO (ribulose-1,5-bisphosphate carboxylase/oxygenase) and PEPC (phosphoenolpyruvate carboxylase) were analyzed by q-RT PCR. Figure 8A displays these genes in the carbon and nitrogen metabolic pathways in rice plants.Supplementary Table S1 lists the fold changes that correspond to the ratio of *AMT1-3*-overexpressing plants/wild-type plants calculated by the relative gene expression level in roots and leaves at the tillering stage under the 0× N, 0.1× N, 1× N and 5× N conditions. The results demonstrated that although *AMT1-3* was constitutively overexpressing under the 35S promoter, these genes displayed distinct expression patterns under different nitrogen levels.

Under the 0× N condition, compared with wild-type plants, the roots of *AMT1-3*-overexpressing plants displayed significantly decreased *NTR1;1* and *Fd-GOGAT1* levels ($p < 0.01$) and significantly increased *NRT2*and *NADH-GOGAT1* levels ($p < 0.01$), whereas the leaves of *AMT1-3*-overexpressing plants displayed significantly decreased levels for most of the genes assayed (*NR1, NR2, GS1;1, GS2, Fd-GOGAT2, RUBISCO,PEPC1, PEPC2, PEPC3, PEPC7*) ($p < 0.05$), except one gene (*NADH-GOGAT2*), which significantly increased ($p < 0.01$) (Figure 8B, Supplementary Table S1). Under the 0.1× N condition, compared with wild-type plants, the roots of *AMT1-3*-overexpressing plants displayed significantly increased *NRT1;2* and *GS1;2* levels ($p < 0.01$) and significantly decreased *NRT2, NR2, Fd-GOGAT1* and *NADH-GOGAT1* levels ($p < 0.05$), which differed from the results obtained under the 0× N condition, where the leaves of *AMT1-3*-overexpressing plants displayed significant increases in most of the genes assayed (*NR2, GS2, NADH-GOGAT2, RUBISCO,PEPC1, PEPC2, PEPC4, PEPC7*)

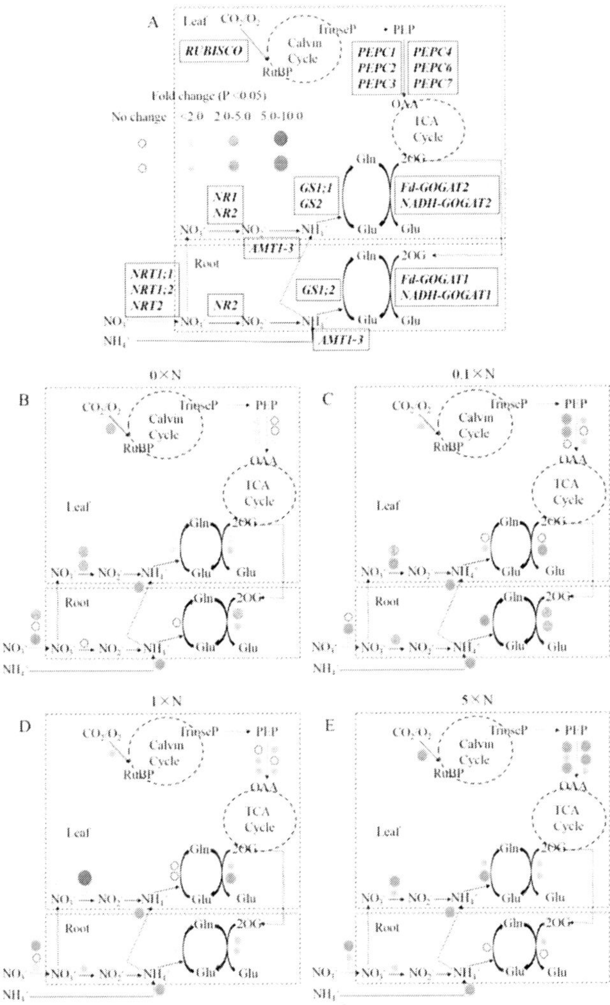


**Figure 8.** Gene expression analysis. Fold change corresponds to the ratio of the gene expression level in the *AMT1-3*-overexpressing plants relative to the wild type plants. (**A**) Diagrammatic representation of the key genes involved in the carbon and nitrogen metabolic pathway in rice plants. NRT, nitrate transporter; NR, nitrate reductase; GS, glutamine synthetase; GOGAT, glutamate synthase; RUBISCO, ribulose-1,5-bisphosphate carboxylase/oxygenase; PEPC, phosphoenolpyruvate carboxylase. Prominent changes in the gene expression level in the*AMT1-3*-overexpressing plants compared to wild type plants at the tillering stage under 0× N (**B**); 0.1× N (**C**); 1× N (**D**) and 5× N (**E**) conditions. Red and blue dots indicate up- and down-regulated genes, respectively.

($p < 0.05$), except one gene (*NR1*), which significantly decreased ($p < 0.01$) (Figure 8C, Supplementary Table S1). Under the 1× N condition, compared with wild-type plants, the roots of *AMT1-3*-overexpressing plants displayed significantly increased *NRT1;1*, *NR2*, *Fd-GOGAT1* and *NADH-GOGAT1* levels ($p < 0.05$) and significantly decreased *NRT2* and *GS1;2* levels ($p < 0.05$), whereas the leaves of*AMT1-3*-overexpressing plants displayed similar results to those obtained under the 0.1× N condition, where most of the genes significantly increased (*Fd-GOGAT2*, *NADH-GOGAT2*, *RUBISCO*, *PEPC2*, *PEPC3*, *PEPC4*,*PEPC7*) ($p < 0.05$) , except the *NR* genes (*NR1* and *NR2*), which significantly decreased ($p < 0.05$) (Figure 8D,Supplementary Table S1). Under the 5× N condition, the expression levels of the detected genes were significantly increased ($p < 0.05$) in the roots and leaves of *AMT1-3*-overexpressing plants compared with wild-type plants, except one gene (*NRT2*), which significantly decreased ($p < 0.05$) (Figure 8E, Table S1).

## 3. DISCUSSION

As *OsAMT1* members, including *OsAMT1-1*, *OsAMT1-2* and *OsAMT1-3*, have been characterized as high-affinity $NH_4^+$ transport genes in rice [13,35], we expected to obtain *OsAMT1*-overexpressing transgenic rice plants with higher ammonium uptake capacity, improved nitrogen use efficiency and a low nitrogen tolerance using the *Agrobacterium*-mediated transformation method. Although we generated *AMT1-2-*,*AMT1-3*-overexpressing plants, we failed to obtain *AMT1-1*-overexpressing plants. Unexpectedly, *AMT1-3*-overexpressing plants displayed poor growth, but no significant differences between *AMT1-2*-overexpressing plants and wild-type plants were observed. In order to understand why poor growth phenotype exhibited in *AMT1-3*-overexpressing transgenic rice plants and evaluate the effect of *AMT1-3*gene on the rice growth, nitrogen absorption and metabolism, we analyzed the growth phenotype, yield, carbon and nitrogen metabolic status and gene expression profiles of the *OsAMT1-3*-overexpressing rice and wild-type Zhonghua 11 under four different N levels (0× N, 0.1× N, 1× N and 5× N) at both tillering and heading stages in detail. Results showed that despite the higher *AMT1-3* mRNA levels in transgenic plants, the root length, plant height, root and shoot biomass and yield were significantly decreased in *AMT1-3*-overexpressing plants compared with wild-type plants (Figure 2 and Figure 3; Table 2). The contents of total carbon and nitrogen, soluble proteins and carbohydrates, individual metabolites (such as sugars, organic acids, amino acids), the expression patterns of key genes involved in carbon and nitrogen metabolic pathway changed significantly in *AMT1-3*-overexpressing plants (Figure 5, Figure 6, Figure 7 and Figure 8; Table 3). The discordant of carbon and nitrogen metabolic status in transgenic plants caused by the *OsAMT1-3*overexpressing may be the main reason for poor growth and yield in our investigation. Similar results were reported that overexpressing of *OsAMT1-1* gene caused decreased shoot and root biomass in transgenic lines during seedling and early vegetative stage, especially when grown under high ammonium nutrition [53,54]. However, completely different results were reported by Ranathunge *et al.* [55] that transgenic rice lines overexpressing the *OsAMT1-1* gene had higher plant growth rate and grain yield, especially under suboptimal $NH_4^+$ levels.

As we known, both carbon and nitrogen nutrients are essential for various cellular functions. Recently, cellular carbon and nitrogen metabolism was demonstrated to be tightly coordinated [8,9,10,11,56]. In addition to independent utilization, the coordination and optimal functioning of the metabolic pathways governing nitrogen and carbon assimilation in plants were demonstrated to be critical for plant growth and, ultimately, biomass accumulation and yield production [10,56]. Maintaining an appropriate balance or carbohydrate to nitrogen metabolite ratio in the cell, which is referred to as the "carbon/nitrogen balance", is extremely important for regulating plant growth, development and production yield [8,9,11]. In our study, we found 4.6%–9.9% and 4.7%–15.5% decreases in *AMT1-3*-overexpressing plant leaf C and N content, respectively, which resulted in a higher (9.4%–11.7% increases) leaf C/N ratio in *AMT1-3*-overexpressing plant leaves (Table 3). Additionally, distinct changes between the soluble protein and carbohydrate concentrations were observed in *AMT1-3*-overexpressing plants (Figure 5 and Figure 6). Therefore, combined with our results, we hypothesized that the carbon and nitrogen metabolic imbalance caused by*AMT1-3* overexpressing attributed to the poor growth and yield of transgenic plants.

To further study the impact of higher *AMT1-3* mRNA levels at both the physiological and molecular level, we analyzed the individual carbon and nitrogen metabolites and the gene expression levels in the roots and leaves of *AMT1-3*-overexpressing plants and wild-type plants. Consistent results of the metabolite concentrations and gene expression levels were showed in this study. Under the 0× N growth condition, given an almost complete lack of nitrogen (a residual amount of nitrogen may reside in water) in the nutrient solution, the nitrogen uptake, reduction and assimilation levels declined in leaves.

The expression level of *NRT1;1*, which encodes a low-affinity $NO_3^-$ transporter [57], was repressed, whereas *NRT2*, which encodes a high-affinity $NO_3^-$ transporter [58], was induced in the root. Although the *AMT1-3* gene was overexpressing under the 35S promoter, the $NH_4^+$ concentration in roots and leaves significantly decreased. Together with the lower $NO_3^-$ uptake and transport by NRTs in roots and leaves, the expression levels of the genes (*NR1*, *NR2*, *GS1;1*, *GS2*, *Fd-GOGAT1* and *Fd-GOGAT2*) involved in $NO_3^-$ reduction and $NH_4^+$assimilation were significantly decreased, which resulted in reduced total free amino acids and soluble proteins (Figure 5, Figure 7 and Figure 8). During $NH_4^+$ assimilation, numerous organic acids provided carbon skeletons to produce a variety of amino acids [59]; therefore, an accumulation of total organic acids may have been observed because of the decreased nitrogen assimilation status in leaves of *AMT1-3*-overexpressing plants (Figure 8). The expression levels of *RUBISCO*, *PEPC1*, *PEPC2*, *PEPC3* and *PEPC7* were decreased, which lead to a decline in total sugars and soluble carbohydrates in leaves of *AMT1-3*-overexpressing plants (Figure 6, Figure 7 and Figure 8). Under the 5× N growth condition, given the much higher nitrogen content in the nutrient solution, higher levels of nitrogen uptake, reduction and assimilation were observed in both roots and leaves of *AMT1-3*-overexpressing plants. The expression of low-affinity $NO_3^-$ transporter genes (*NRT1;1* and *NRT1;2*) [57] were induced, whereas the expression of the high-affinity $NO_3^-$ transporter gene *NRT2* [58] was repressed in the root, which resulted in more $NO_3^-$ absorption and higher expression of genes (*NR1*, *NR2*, *GS1;1*, *GS2*, *Fd-GOGAT1*, *Fd-GOGAT2* and *NADH-GOGAT2*) involved in $NO_3^-$ reduction and $NH_4^+$ assimilation. As a result, total free amino acids and soluble proteins accumulated in leaves of *AMT1-3*-overexpressing plants, which depleted total organic acids to provide carbon skeletons for amino acid production. This large consume of organic acids promoted the breakdown of sugars. Conversely, the expression levels of *RUBISCO*, *PEPC1*, *PEPC2*, *PEPC3*, *PEPC4*, *PEPC6* and *PEPC7*dramatically increased in leaves of *AMT1-3*-overexpressing plants to produce more carbohydrates (Figure 7).

Plants have evolved a complex profile of responses to cope with changes in soil nitrogen availability, which is mediated by a stringent control of expression and/or activity of proteins involved in nitrogen transport and assimilation [59]. Recent studies on nutrient effects in plants have focused on their potential roles as signaling molecules in addition to their roles as building blocks of organic matter or cofactors [60]. Nitrogen sensing appears to regulate a variety of physiological and developmental processes in plants [8,61]. For example, $NO_3^-$ is a positive signal required for the induction of $NO_3^-$ uptake and its reduction, and the metabolized products of $NO_3^-$, $NH_4^+$ and its assimilation products Glu and Gln are believed to exert negative effects on $NO_3^-$ uptake and reduction [35,62,63,64,65]. Bacterial and fungal AMTs have been demonstrated to act as transceptors with dual functions as ammonium transporters and receptors that mediate ammonium-triggered changes in morphology or the transcription of target genes [66]. Plant AMTs may also be transceptors. For example, AMT1-3 can regulate lateral root branching in response to localized ammonium supplies [67]. More recent reports have demonstrated that *OsAMT1-3* is expressed specifically in roots but repressed by nitrogen, which indicates that *OsAMT1-3* participates not only in ammonium uptake but also in ammonium sensing in rice [14,35]. In this study, we expected to enhance ammonium uptake capacity in roots and to improve nitrogen fertilizer use efficiency and yield formation by overexpressing the*AMT1-3* gene in rice. In contrast, our transgenic plants grew poorly and displayed a low yield production and an unbalanced carbon and nitrogen metabolic status (Figure 3; Table 2 and Table 3). We hypothesized that the *AMT1-3* transcriptional level may act as a signal sensor to regulate carbon and nitrogen metabolism in rice. *AMT1-3* is a high-affinity $NH_4^+$ transporter gene, its transcriptional level is mainly expressed in rice roots under low nitrogen in the environment and repressed with nitrogen supplementation [13,35] The high transcriptional level of *AMT1-3* in our transgenic rice may mimic a nitrogen starvation signal in the environment and thus retard plant growth and development to ensure the plant can complete its entire life cycle. Recently, Gaur *et al.* validated *OsAMT1-3* as a biomarker for detecting available nitrogen pools both inside cells and in the soils around the root [14]. Similar results were reported by Yuan *et al.* who attempted to increase the ammonium uptake capacity via ectopic expression of *AMTs*; however, this largely failed because their transport capacities are tightly regulated by ammonium [31]. In addition, excess ammonium intake deregulates cellular pH homeostasis and primary metabolism [68]. Therefore, plant roots repress ammonium uptake at elevated ammonium supplementation [49,64]. Furthermore, several published works have demonstrated that *C*-terminal phosphorylation can mediate intermonomeric trans-inhibition of ammonium transport in plant roots and that the allosteric regulation of transporter activities even extends to heteromeric AMT protein complexes in *Arabidopsis* [47,49]. Additionally, *N*-terminal cysteines were demonstrated to affect oligomer stability of the allosterically regulated ammonium transporter LeAMT1-1 [50]. Thence, the post-transcriptional and post-translational regulation of plant AMT cannot be ignored in further studies.

# 4. MATERIALS AND METHODS

## 4.1. Constructs and Transformation

"Ammonium transporter 1-3, rice" was used as the keywords to search the NCBI database (National Center for Biotechnology Information; Available online: http://www.ncbi.nlm.nih.gov) and the complete*OsAMT1-3* mRNA sequence (AF289479) was found. The full-length cDNA of *OsAMT1-3* gene was amplified by PCR from the rice (Zhonghua 11, *Japonica*) genome using the forward primer 5'-CATAGGACTCCTGTGTTGAGCGCGCGTCGA-3' and reverse primer 5'-CTGCCTGCAGGTACTACTAGCTCAGCTCCT-3', which contained the enzyme site of BamHI and PstI, respectively. Then the cDNA fragment was ligated into the pCAMBIA 1301S vector which driven by *CaMV*(Cauliflower Mosaic Virus) 35S promoter. All the procedures of DNA manipulation were according to the standard molecular techniques [69,70]. The chimeric gene was transformed into Zhonghua 11, a *japonica* rice cultivar, to obtain the *AMT1-3*-overexpressing transgenic plants by the *Agrobacterium tumefaciens*-mediated transformation method [71].

## 4.2. Plant Growth Conditions

Seeds of the wild type and *AMT1-3*-overexpressing rice germinated and were sowed in sand. The wild type and *AMT1-3*-overexpressing seedlings with four leaves were transferred into the experimental pots under the 0× N (fertilized with 0.15 g $P_2O_5$ and 0.2 g K per kg soil), 0.1× N (fertilized with 0.02 g·N, 0.15 g $P_2O_5$ and 0.2 g·K·per·kg soil), 1× N (fertilized with 0.2 g N, 0.15 g $P_2O_5$ and 0.2 g K per kg soil) and 5× N (fertilized with 1 g·N, 0.15 g·$P_2O_5$ and 0.2 g K·per kg·soil) conditions. The yield and its components were analyzed at the mature stage. In addition, the wild type and *AMT1-3*-overexpressing seedlings with four leaves were transplanted hydroponically under the 0× N (without $NH_4NO_3$), 0.1× N (with 1/10 $NH_4NO_3$), 1× N (normal nutrient solution described by Yoshida *et al.* [72]) and 5× N (with 5-fold $NH_4NO_3$) conditions. The culture solution was refreshed every 3 days. At the tillering stage and the heading stage, the roots, stems and leaves were harvested for the growth phenotype, leaf SPAD value and photosynthetic capacity analysis; for the carbon and nitrogen content, soluble proteins and carbohydrates concentrations determination; for the metabolic profiling and gene expression investigation.

### 4.3. Northern Blot, Southern Blot and Gene Expression Analysis

Leaf total RNA of the wild type and transgenic plants was extracted using TriZol reagent (Invitrogen, Karlsruhe, Germany), and 18 μg total RNA was used for Northern blotting to check whether the expression level of *OsAMT1-3* gene was accumulated in transgenic plants. Hybridizations were performed with a $^{32}$P-labeled probe, which is a partial specific fragment of *OsAMT1-3* gene. For Southern blot, genomic DNA was extracted from the leaves of transgenic plants by the CTAB method, and 4 μg of genomic DNA was digested by BamHI. The DNA was then transferred to a Hybond N+ nylon membrane (Amersham, Buchinghamshire, UK) for Southern blot analysis. Hybridizations were performed with a P32-labeled partial DNA fragment of the *hygromycin* gene. The results were detected by autoradiography. All the experimental procedures were according to the instructions described by Sambrook *et al.* [69] previously. For q-RT PCR assay, both roots and leaves of the wild type and *AMT1-3*-overexpressing plants were harvested from three biological replications under four different nitrogen conditions (0× N, 0.1× N, 1× N and 5× N) at the tillering stage. Total RNA was extracted using TriZol reagent (Invitrogen) and treated with DNaseI (Invitrogen) to avoid the genomic DNA contamination. The first-strand cDNAs were synthesized using Superscript III reverse transcriptase (Invitrogen). Table S2 listed the gene-specific and *actin* primers. Q-RT PCR assay was then performed in an ABI PRISM 7500 real-time PCR system (Applied Biosystems, Foster City, CA, USA).

### 4.4. Nitrogen Uptake Assay

Seeds of the wild type and *AMT1-3*-overexpressing rice germinated and were sowed in sand. At the 3-leaf stage, seedlings were transplanted hydroponically into the normal nutrient solution described by Yoshida *et al.* [72], except that 1.44 mM $NH_4NO_3$ was replaced by 2.88 mM $NH_4Cl$. At the tillering stage, the $NH_4Cl$ in the nutrient solution was replaced with $^{15}NH_4Cl$. Three biological replicated roots, stems and leaves were harvested at the time of 1, 3, 8 h, 1 and 3 days after $^{15}N$ replacement. Then the $^{15}N$ and total N content were analyzed by an isotope mass spectrometer (ANCA-MS, Europa Scientific, Crewe, UK) and by a C/N analyzer (Elementar,

Vario MAX CN, Germany), respectively. Additionally, the total carbon and nitrogen content in roots, stems and leaves of wild type and *AMT1-3*-overexpressing plants under four different nitrogen conditions (0× N, 0.1× N, 1× N and 5× N) at the tillering stage were also determined by the C/N analyzer.

## 4.5. Physiological Parameters Determination

At the tillering stage, a chlorophyll meter (SPAD-502) was used to determine the SPAD value in flag leaves of the wild type and *AMT1-3*-overexpressing plants; a Li-6400XT portable photosynthesis system (Li-COR, Lincoln, NE, USA) was used to determine the photosynthetic parameters in flag leaves of the wild type and*AMT1-3*-overexpressing plants. Ten randomly selected plants were determined. The results were the average value of the upper, middle and bottom portion of each flag leaf. For soluble proteins analysis, three biological replicated roots, stems and leaves of the wild type and *AMT1-3*-overexpressing plants under four different nitrogen conditions (0× N, 0.1× N, 1× N and 5× N) were harvested at both the tillering and heading stages. Fresh samples were ground and homogenized with the Trizma extraction buffer described by Melo *et al.* [73] on ice. After centrifuging (12,000× *g*, 20 min, 4 °C), the supernatant was used to measure the soluble protein concentration based on the protocols of Bradford [74] protein assay with the bovine serum albumin as a standard protein. For soluble carbohydrates analysis, three biological replicated roots, stems and leaves of the wild type and *AMT1-3*-overexpressing plants under four different nitrogen conditions (0× N, 0.1× N, 1× N and 5× N) were harvested at both the tillering and heading stages. All the samples were dried and ground to powder. The soluble carbohydrates were extracted with boiling water and centrifuged at 12,000× *g*for 10 min. The supernatant was used to measure the soluble carbohydrate concentration according to the anthrone procedure [75,76]. For individual carbon and nitrogen metabolites analysis, three biological replicated roots and leaves of the wild type and *AMT1-3*-overexpressing plants under 0× N and 5× N conditions were harvested at the tillering stage. The individual metabolites involved in carbon and nitrogen metabolism were determined using GC-TOF-MS method from 50 mg fresh samples. The sample extraction, the data pre-treatment and normalization, the alignments and the metabolite identification were performed as described by Kusano *et al.* [77,78] and Redestig *et al.* [79].

## 5. CONCLUSIONS

In this study, we obtained the *AMT1-3*-overexpressing transgenic rice plants and systematically analyzed the effect of *AMT1-3* overexpressing on the rice growth, carbon-nitrogen metabolic status and gene expression profile at both the tillering and heading stages under four different nitrogen conditions (0× N, 0.1× N, 1× N and 5× N). Our results indicated that the overexpressing of *AMT1-3* gene caused a poor growth and yield in transgenic plants. The unbalanced carbon-nitrogen metabolic status might be the main reason. However, how *AMT1-3* overexpressing could lead to the carbon-nitrogen imbalance is still on going.

## ACKNOWLEDGMENTS

This work was supported in part by grants from the National Natural Science Foundation of China (31000932); the Fundamental Research Funds for the Central Universities (2662013PY041) and the Specialized Research Fund for the Doctoral Program of Higher Education, the Ministry of Education of China (20100146120017). We thank Xingming Lian for providing the plant materials.

## AUTHOR CONTRIBUTIONS

Zhuqing Zhao and Hongmei Cai conceived and designed the experiments, Aili Bao and Zhijun Liang performed the experiments, Zhuqing Zhao and Hongmei Cai analyzed the data, Aili Bao and Zhijun Liang contributed reagents, Hongmei Cai wrote the manuscript. All authors read and approved the manuscript.

## CONFLICTS OF INTEREST

The authors declare no conflict of interest.

# REFERENCES


1. Lam, H.M.; Coschigano, K.T.; Oliveira, I.C.; Melo-Oliveira, R.; Coruzzi, G.M. The molecular-genetics of nitrogen assimilation into amino acids in higher plants. Ann. Rev. Plant Physiol. Mol. Biol. 1996, 47, 569–593.

2. Tabuchi, M.; Abiko, T.; Yamaya, T. Assimilation of ammonium ions and reutilization of nitrogen in rice (Oryza sativa L.). J. Exp. Bot. 2007, 58, 2319–2327.

3. Frink, C.R.; Waggoner, P.E.; Ausubel, J.H. Nitrogen fertilizer: Retrospect and prospect. Proc. Natl. Acad. Sci. USA 1999, 96, 1175–1180.

4. Crawford, N.M.; Forde, B.G. Molecular and developmental biology of inorganic nitrogen nutrition. InThe Arabidopsis Book; Meyerowitz, E., Somerville, C., Eds.; American Society of Plant Biologists: Rockville, MD, USA, 2002.

5. Howitt, S.M.; Udvardi, M.K. Structure, function and regulation of ammonium transporters in plants.Biochim. Biophys. Acta 2000, 1465, 152–170.

6. Bloom, A.J.; Sukrapanna, S.S.; Warner, R.L. Root respiration associated with ammonium and nitrate absorption and assimilation by barley. Plant Physiol. 1992, 99, 1294–1301.

7. Gazzarrini, S.; Lejay, L.; Gojon, A.; Ninnemann, O.; Frommer, W.B.; von Wirén, N. Three functional transporters for constitutive, diurnally regulated, and starvation-induced uptake of ammonium intoArabidopsis roots. Plant Cell 1999, 11, 937–948.

8. Coruzzi, G.M.; Zhou, L. Carbon and nitrogen sensing and signaling in plants: Emerging "matrix effects". Curr. Opin. Plant Biol. 2001, 4, 247–253.

9. Martin, T.; Oswald, O.; Graham, I.A. Arabidopsis seedling growth, storage lipid mobilization and photosynthetic gene expression are regulated by carbon: Nitrogen availability. Plant Physiol. 2002, 128, 472–481.

10. Krapp, A.; Truong, H.N. Regulation of C/N interaction in model plant species. In Enhancing the Efficiency of Nitrogen Utilization in Plants; Goyal, S., Tischner, R., Basra, A., Eds.; Haworth Press: New York, NY, USA, 2005; pp. 127–173.

11. Zheng, Z. Carbon and nitrogen nutrient balance signaling in plants. Plant Signal. Behav. 2009, 4, 584–591.

12. Nunes-Nesi, A.; Fernie, A.R.; Stitt, M. Metabolic and signaling aspects underpinning the regulation of plant carbon nitrogen interactions. Mol. Plant 2010, 3, 973–996.

13. Loqué, D.; von Wirén, N. Regulatory levels for the transport of ammonium in plant roots. J. Exp. Bot.2004, 55, 1293–1305.

14. Gaur, V.S.; Singh, U.S.; Gupta, A.K.; Kumar, A. Understanding the differential nitrogen sensing mechanism in rice genotypes through expression analysis of high and low affinity ammonium transporter genes. Mol. Biol. Rep. 2012, 39, 2233–2241.

15. Wang, M.Y.; Glass, A.; Shaff, J.E.; Kochian, L.V. Ammonium uptake by rice roots. Plant Physiol. 1994,104, 899–906.

16. Ludewig, U.; Wilken, S.; Wu, B.; Jost, W.; Obrdlik, P.; El Bakkoury, M.; Marini, A.-M.; André, B.; Hamacher, T.; Boles, E.; et al. Homo- and hetero-oligomerization of ammonium transporter-1 NH4+uniporters. J. Biol. Chem. 2003, 278, 45603–45610.

17. Bakouh, N.; Benjelloun, F.; Hulin, P.; Brouillard, F.; Edelman, A.; Chérif-Zahar, B.; Planelles, G. NH3 is involved in the NH4+ transport induced by the functional expression of the human RhC glycoprotein.J. Biol. Biochem. 2004, 279, 15975–15983.

18. Khademi, S.; O'Connell, J.; Remis, J.; Robles-Colmenares, Y.; Miercke, L.J.; Stroud, R.M. Mechanism of ammonia transport by Amt/MEP/Rh: Structure of AmtB. Science 2004, 305, 1587–1594.

19. Ripoche, P.; Bertrand, O.; Gane, P.; Birkenmeier, C.; Colin, Y.; Cartron, J.-P. Human Rhesusassociated glycoprotein mediates facilitated transport of NH3 into red blood cells. Proc. Nat. Acad. Sci. USA 2004,101, 17222–17227.

20. Zheng, L.; Kostrewa, D.; Bernèche, S.; Winkler, F.K.; Li, X.-D. The mechanism of ammonia transport based on the crystal structure of AmtB of Escherichia coli. Proc. Natl. Acad. Sci. USA 2004, 101, 17090–17095.

21. Benjelloun, F.; Bakouh, N.; Fritsch, J.; Hulin, P.; Lipecka, J.; Edelman, A.; Planelles, G.; Thomas, S.R.; Chérif-Zahar, B. Expression of the human erythroid Rh glycoprotein (RhAG) enhances both NH3 and NH4+ transport in HeLa cells. Pflüg. Arch. 2005, 450, 155–167.

22. Mak, D.-O.D.; Dang, B.; Weiner, I.D.; Foskett, J.K.; Westhoff, C.M. Characterization of ammonia transport by the kidney Rh glycoproteins RhBG and RhCG. Am. J. Physiol. 2006, 290, F297–F305.

23. Mayer, M.; Dynowski, M.; Ludewig, U. Ammonium ion transport by the AMT/Rh homologue LeAMT1;1. Biochem. J. 2006, 396, 431–437.

24. Fong, R.N.; Kim, K.S.; Yoshihara, C.; Inwood, W.B.; Kustu, S. The W148L substitution in the Escheria coli ammonium channel AmtB increase flux and indicates that the substrate is an ion. Proc. Natl. Acad. Sci. USA 2007, 104, 18706–18711.

25. Ortiz-Ramirez, C.; Mora, S.I.; Trejo, J.; Pantoja, O. PvAMT1;1, a highly selective ammonium transporter that functions as H+/NH4+ symporter. J. Biol. Chem. 2011, 286, 31113–31122.

26. Marini, A.M.; André, B. In vivo N-glycosylation of the mep2 high-affinity ammonium transporter ofSaccharomyces cerevisiae reveals an extracytosolic N-terminus. Mol. Microbiol. 2000, 38, 552–564.

27. Thomas, G.H.; Mullins, J.G.; Merrick, M. Membrane topology of the Mep/Amt family of ammonium transporters. Mol. Microbiol. 2000, 37, 331–344.

28. Litman, T.; Søgaard, R.; Zeuthen, T. Ammonia and urea permeability of mammalian aquaporins. InHandbook of Experimental Pharmacology; Springer: Berlin, Germany, 2008; pp. 327–358.

29. Yuan, L.; Graff, L.; Loqué, D.; Kojima, S.; Tsuchiya, Y.N.; Takahashi, H.; von Wirén, N. AtAMT1;4, a pollen-specific high-affinity ammonium transporter of the plasma membrane in Arabidopsis. Plant Cell Physiol. 2009, 50, 13–25.

30. Loqué, D.; Yuan, L.; Kojima, S.; Gojon, A.; Wirth, J.; Gazzarrini, S.; Ishiyama, K.; Takahashi, H.; von Wirén, N. Additive contribution of AMT1;1 and AMT1;3 to high-affinity ammonium uptake across the plasma membrane of nitrogen-deficient Arabidopsis roots. Plant J. 2006, 48, 522–534.

31. Yuan, L.; Loqué, D.; Kojima, S.; Rauch, S.; Ishiyama, K.; Inoue, E.; Takahashi, H.; von Wirén, N. The organization of high-affinity ammonium uptake in Arabidopsis roots depends on the spatial arrangement and biochemical properties of AMT1-type transporters. Plant Cell 2007, 19, 2636–2652.

32. Engineer, C.B.; Kranz, R.G. Reciprocal leaf and root expression of AtAmt1.1 and root architectural changes in response to nitrogen starvation. Plant Physiol. 2007, 143, 236–250.

33. Sohlenkamp, C.; Shelden, M.; Howitt, S.; Udvardi, M. Characterization of Arabidopsis AtAMT2, a novel ammonium transporter in plants. FEBS Lett. 2000, 467, 273–278.

34. Sohlenkamp, C.; Wood, C.C.; Roeb, G.W.; Udvardi, M.T. Characterization of Arabidopsis AtAMT2, a high-affinity ammonium transporter of the plasma membrane. Plant Physiol. 2002, 130, 1788–1796.

35. Sonoda, Y.; Ikeda, A.; Saiki, S.; von Wirén, N.; Yamaya, T.; Yamaguchi, J. Distinct expression and function of three ammonium transporter genes (OsAMT1;1–1;3) in rice. Plant Cell Physiol. 2003, 44, 726–734.

36. Marini, A.M.; Soussi-Boudekou, S.; Vissers, S.; André, B. A family of ammonium transporters inSaccharomyces cerevisiae. Mol. Cell. Biol. 1997, 17, 4282–4293.

37. Suenaga, A.; Moriya, K.; Sonoda, Y.; Ikeda, A.; von Wirén, N.; Hayakawa, T.; Yamaguchi, J.; Yamaya, T. Constitutive expression of a novel-type ammonium transporter OsAMT2 in rice plants. Plant Cell Physiol. 2003, 44, 206–211.

38. Pearson, C.J.; Finnegan, P.M.; Schjoerring, J.K. Regulation of the high-affinity ammonium transporter (BnAMT1;2) in the leaves of Brassica napus by nitrogen status. Plant Mol. Biol. 2002, 49, 483–490.

39. Salvemini, F.; Marini, A.M.; Riccio, A.; Patriarca, E.J.; Chiurazzi, M. Functional characterization of an ammonium transporter gene from Lotus japonicus. Gene 2001, 270, 237–243.

40. Simon-Rosin, U.; Wood, C.; Udvardi, M.K. Molecular and cellular characterization of LjAMT2;1, ammonium transporter from the model legume Lotus japonicus. Plant Mol. Biol. 2003, 51, 99–108.

41. Lauter, F.R.; Ninnemann, O.; Bucher, M.; Riesmeier, J.W.; Frommer, W.B. Preferential expression of an ammonium transporter and of two putative nitrate transporters in root hairs of tomato. Proc. Natl. Acad. Sci. USA 1996, 93, 8139–8144.

42. Von WireÂn, N.; Gazzarrini, S.; Gojon, A.; Frommer, W.B. The molecular physiology of ammonium uptake and retrieval. Curr. Opin. Plant Biol. 2000, 3, 254–261.

43. Becker, D.; Stahnke, R.; Fendrick, I.; Frommer, W.B.; Vanderleyden, J.; Kaiser, W.M.; Hedrich, R. Expression of the ammonium transporter gene LeAMT1;2 is induced in tomato roots upon association with N2 fixing bacteria. Planta 2002, 215, 424–429.

44. Yuan, L.; Loqué, D.; Ye, F.; Frommer, W.B.; von Wirén, N. Nitrogen-dependent posttranscriptional regulation of the ammonium transporter AtAMT1;1. Plant Physiol. 2007, 143, 732–744.

45. Loqué, D.; Lalonde, S.; Looger, L.L.; von Wirén, N.; Frommer, W.B. A cytosolic trans-activation domain essential for ammonium uptake. Nature 2007, 446, 195–198.

46. Loqué, D.; Mora, S.I.; Andrade, S.L.A.; Pantoja, O.; Frommer, W.B. Pore mutations in ammonium transporter AMT1 with increased electrogenic ammonium transport activity. J. Biol. Chem. 2009, 284, 24988–24995.

47. Yuan, L.; Gu, R.; Xuan, Y.; Smith-Valle, E.; Loqué, D.; Frommer, W.B.; von Wirén, N. Allosteric regulation of transport activity by heterotrimerization of Arabidopsis ammonium transporter complexes in vivo. Plant Cell 2013, 25, 974–984.

48. Neuhäuser, B.; Dynowski, M.; Mayer, M.; Ludewig, U. Regulation of NH4+ transport by essential cross talk between AMT monomers through the carboxyl tails. Plant Physiol. 2007, 143, 1651–1659.

49. Lanquar, V.; Loqué, D.; Hörmann, F.; Yuan, L.; Bohner, A.; Engelsberger, W.R.; Lalonde, S.; Schulze, W.X.; vonWirén, N.; Frommer, W.B. Feedback inhibition of ammonium uptake by a phosphodependent allosteric mechanism in Arabidopsis. Plant Cell 2009, 21, 3610–3622.

50. Graff, L.; Obrdlik, P.; Yuan, L.; Loqué, D.; Frommer, W.B.; von Wirén, N. N-terminal cysteines affect oligomer stability of the allosterically regulated ammonium transporter LeAMT1;1. J. Exp. Bot. 2011,62, 1361–1373.

51. Socolow, R. Nitrogen management and the future of food: Lessons from the management of energy and carbon. Proc. Natl. Acad. Sci. USA 1999, 96, 6001–6008.

52. Zhang, F.; Cui, Z.; Fan, M.; Zhang, W.; Chen, X.; Jiang, R. Integrated soil–crop system management: Reducing environmental risk while increasing crop pro-ductivity and

improving nutrient use efficiency in China. J. Environ. Qual. 2011, 40, 1051–1057.

53. Hoque, M.S.; Masle, J.; Udvardi, M.K.; Ryan, P.R.; Upadhyaya, N.M. Over-expression of the riceOsAMT1-1 gene increases ammonium uptake and content, but impairs growth and development of plants under high ammonium nutrition. Funct. Plant Biol. 2006, 33, 153–163.

54. Kumar, A.; Kaiser, B.N.; Siddiqi, M.Y.; Glass, A.D.M. Functional characterization of OsAMT 1.1overexpression lines of rice, Oryza sativa. Funct. Plant Biol. 2006, 33, 339–346.

55. Ranathunge, K.; EI-Kereamy, A.; Gidda, S.; Bi, Y.-M. OsAMT1;1 transgenic rice plants with enhanced NH4+ permeability show superior growth and higher yield under optimal and suboptimal NH4+conditions. J. Exp. Bot. 2014, 65, 965–979.

56. Krapp, A.; Ferrario-Méry, S.; Touraine, B. Nitrogen and signaling. In Advances in Photosynthesis; Foyer, C., Noctor, G., Eds.; Kluwer Academic Publishers: Dordrecht, The Netherlands, 2002.

57. Lin, C.M.; Koh, S.; Stacey, G.; Yu, S.-M.; Lin, T.-Y.; Tsay, Y.F. Cloning and functional characterization of a constitutively expressed nitrate transporter gene, OsNRT1, from rice. Plant. Physiol. 2000, 122, 379–388.

58. Araki, R.; Hasegawa, H. Expression of rice (Oryza sativa L.) genes involved in high-affinity nitrate transport during the period of nitrate induction. Breed. Sci. 2006, 56, 295–302.

59. Lea, P.J.; Morot-Gaudry, J.F. Plant Nitrogen; Springer-Verlag: New York, NY, USA, 2001.

60. Coruzzi, G.; Bush, D.R. Nitrogen and carbon nutrient and metabolite signaling in plants. Plant Physiol.2001, 125, 61–64.

61. Foyer, C.H.; Parry, M.; Noctor, G. Markers and signals associated with nitrogen assimilation in higher plants. J. Exp. Bot. 2003, 54, 585–593.

62. Scheible, W.R.; GonzaÂles-Fontes, A.; Lauerer, M.; MuÈller-RoÈber, B.; Caboche, M.; Stitt, M. Nitrate acts as a signal to induce organic acid metabolism and repress starch metabolism in tobacco. Plant Cell1997, 9, 783–798.

63. Dzuibany, C.; Haupt, S.; Fock, H.; Biehler, K.; Migge, A.; Becker, T. Regulation of nitrate reductase transcript level by glutamine accumulating in the leaves of a ferredoxin-dependent glutamate

synthase-deficient gluS mutant of Arabidopsis thaliana, and by glutamine provided via the roots. Planta1998, 20, 515–522.

64. Rawat, S.R.; Silim, S.N.; Kronzucker, H.J.; Siddiqi, M.Y.; Glass, A.D.M. AtAMT1gene expression and NH4+ uptake in roots of Arabidopsis thaliana: Evidence for regulation by root glutamine levels. Plant J.1999, 19, 143–152.

65. Ferrario-MeÂry, S.; Masclaux, C.; Suzuki, A.; Valadier, M.H.; Hirel, B.; Foyer, C.H. Glutamine and a-ketoglutarate are metabolite signals involved in nitrate reductase gene transcription in untransformed and transformed tobacco plants deficient in ferredoxin-glutamine-a-ketoglutarate aminotransferase. Planta2001, 213, 265–271.

66. Tremblay, P.L.; Hallenbeck, P.C. Of blood, brains and bacteria, the Amt/Rh transporter family: Emerging role of Amt as a unique microbial sensor. Mol. Microbiol. 2009, 71, 12–22.

67. Lima, J.E.; Kojima, S.; Takahashi, H.; von Wirén, N. Ammonium triggers lateral root branching inArabidopsis in an AMMONIUM TRANSPORTER1;3—Dependent manner. Plant Cell 2010, 22, 3621–3633.

68. Hachiya, T.; Watanabe, C.K.; Fujimoto, M.; Ishikawa, T.; Takahara, K.; Kawai-Yamada, M.; Uchimiya, H.; Uesono, Y.; Terashima, I.; Noguchi, K. Nitrate addition alleviates ammonium toxicity without lessening ammonium accumulation, organic acid depletion and inorganic cation depletion inArabidopsis thaliana shoots. Plant Cell Physiol. 2012, 53, 577–591.

69. Sambrook, J.; Fritsch, E.F.; Maniatis, T. Molecular Cloning: A Laboratory Manual, 2nd ed.; Cold Spring Harbor Laboratory Press: Cold Spring Harbor, NY, USA, 1989.

70. Maniatis, T.A.; Fritsch, E.F.; Sambrook, J. Molecular Cloning: A Laboratory Manual; Cold Spring Harbor Laboratory Press: Cold Spring Harbor, NY, USA, 1992.

71. Hiei, Y.; Ohta, S.; Komari, T.; Kumashiro, T. Efficient transformation of rice (Oryza sativa L.) mediated by Agrobacterium and sequence analysis of the boundaries of the T-DNA. Plant J. 1994, 6, 271–282.

72. Yoshida, S.; Forno, D.A.; Cook, J.H.; Gomez, K.A. Laboratory Manual for Physiological Studies of Rice, 3rd eds; International Rice Research Institute: Manila, Philippine, 1976.

73. Melo, P.M.; Lima, L.M.; Santos, I.M.; Carvalho, H.G.; Cullimore, J.V. Expression of the plastid-located glutamine synthetase of Medicago truncatula: Accumulation of the precursor in root nodules reveals anin vivo control at the level of protein import into plastids. Plant Physiol. 2003, 132, 390–399.

74. Bradford, M.M. A rapid and sensitive method for the quantitation of microgram quantities of protein utilizing the principle of protein binding. Anal. Biochem. 1976, 72, 248–254.

75. Morris, D.L. Quantitative determination of carbohydrates with Dreywood's anthrone reagent. Science1948, 107, 254–255.

76. Maness, N. Extraction and analysis of soluble carbohydrates. Methods Mol. Biol. 2010, 639, 341–370.

77. Kusano, M.; Fukushima, A.; Arita, M.; Jonsson, P.; Moritz, T.; Kobayashi, M.; Hayashi, N.; Tohge, T.; Saito, K. Unbiased characterization of genotype-dependent metabolic regulations by metabolomic approach in Arabidopsis thaliana. BMC Syst. Biol. 2007, 1, 53.

78. Kusano, M.; Fukushima, A.; Kobayashi, M.; Hayashi, N.; Jonsson, P.; Moritz, T.; Ebana, K.; Saito, K. Application of a metabolomic method combining one-dimensional and two-dimensional gas chromatographytime-of-flight/mass spectrometry to metabolic phenotyping of natural variants in rice.J. Chromatogr. B Anal. Technol. Biomed. Life Sci. 2007, 855, 71–79.

79. Redestig, H.; Fukushima, A.; Stenlund, H.; Moritz, T.; Arita, M.; Saito, K.; Kusano, M. Compensation for systematic cross-contribution improves normalization of mass spectrometry based metabolomics data. Anal. Chem. 2009, 81, 7974–7980.

9

# ROUTE AND REGULATION OF ZINC, CADMIUM, AND IRON TRANSPORT IN RICE PLANTS (*ORYZA SATIVA* L.) DURING VEGETATIVE GROWTH AND GRAIN FILLING: METAL TRANSPORTERS, METAL SPECIATION, GRAIN CD REDUCTION AND ZN AND FE BIOFORTIFICATION

**Tadakatsu Yoneyama [1,*], Satoru Ishikawa [2] and Shu Fujimaki [3]**

[1]Department of Applied Biological Chemistry, The University of Tokyo, Tokyo 113-8657, Japan

[2]Soil Environment Division, National Institute for Agro-Environmental Sciences, Tsukuba, Ibaraki 305-8604, Japan

[3]Quantum, Beam Science Center, Japan Atomic Energy Agency, Takasaki, Gunma 370-1292, Japan

## ABSTRACT

Zinc (Zn) and iron (Fe) are essential but are sometimes deficient in humans, while cadmium (Cd) is toxic if it accumulates in the liver and kidneys at high levels. All three are contained in the grains of rice, a staple cereal. Zn and Fe concentrations in rice grains harvested under different levels of soil/hydroponic metals are known to change only within a small range, while Cd concentrations show greater changes. To clarify the mechanisms underlying such different metal contents, we synthesized information on the routes of metal transport and accumulation in rice plants by examining metal speciation, metal transporters, and the xylem-to-phloem transport system. At grain-filling, Zn and Cd ascending in xylem sap are transferred to the phloem by the xylem-to-phloem transport system operating at stem nodes. Grain Fe is largely derived from the leaves by remobilization. Zn and Fe concentrations in phloem-sap and grains are regulated within a small range, while Cd concentrations vary depending on xylem supply. Transgenic techniques to increase concentrations of the metal chelators (nicotianamine, 2′-deoxymugineic acid) are useful in increasing grain Zn and Fe concentrations. The elimination of OsNRAMP5 Cd-uptake transporter and the enhancement of root cell vacuolar Cd sequestration reduce uptake and root-to-shoot transport, respectively, resulting in a reduction of grain Cd accumulation.


**Keywords:** cadmium; iron; metals in grains; metal speciation; metal transporter; rice (*Oryza sativa* L.); xylem-to-phloem transport; zinc

## 1. INTRODUCTION

Zinc (Zn) and iron (Fe) are required by plants in response to demands for plant growth, which is underlined by cellular metabolisms [1,2], while cadmium (Cd) is not essential for plants and is toxic at high levels. Likewise, Zn and Fe are essential in the human metabolism and their deficiency may lead to various diseases, while Cd is toxic and at high doses may even cause severe diseases like *Itai-Itai* disease (Table 1).

**Table 1.** Demands and toxicity of Zn, Cd, and Fe for plants and impacts of their dietary deficiency or excess on humans.

| Metal | Demands/Toxicity for Plants | Deficiency Diseases/Excess Toxicity for Humans |
|---|---|---|
| Zn | Demand: Cofactor of over 300 enzymes including DNA- and RNA-polymerases; Excess toxicity: Unregulated binding of Zn to S-, N- and O-containing molecules | Deficiency: Stunting, diarrhea, pneumonia; Excess toxicity: Interference of Fe and Cu uptake in the intestines |
| Cd | Toxicity: Binding to protein SH-residues, exchanges with divalent cations such as $Zn^{2+}$ and $Ca^{2+}$, and excessive production of reactive oxygen species | Excess toxicity: *Itai-itai* disease (spinal and leg bone pain) caused by Cd accumulation in the liver and kidneys resulting in tubular renal dysfunction, osteoporosis, cancer, and cardiovascular diseases |
| Fe | Demand: Proteins involved in redox and electron transport, Leaf pigment formation; Toxicity: Free Fe can generate toxic levels of oxygen and hydroxyl free radicals through the Fenton reaction | Deficiency: Anemia, impaired mental development; Iron overload: Excessive accumulation of Fe in the liver, heart, and pancreas, Hemosiderosis; Hemochromatosis |

Literature sources: Palmgren *et al.* [3], White and Broadley [4], and Clemens *et al.* [5].

Zinc and Fe in the grains of cereals such as rice are essential elements for humans. However, humans' intake of Zn and Fe is generally not sufficient [3,6,7]. In contrast, Cd, which is sometimes contained at high levels in the rice grains grown in Cd-contaminated soils, is toxic for humans [8]. Therefore, it is necessary to enrich rice grains with Zn and Fe and to decrease their Cd content [9].

Fukushima *et al.* [8] reported that, in the district where "*Itai-Itai* disease" was endemic, soil Cd levels ranged from 0.4 to 8 $mg \cdot kg^{-1}$ (dry soil) and those of brown rice were correlated, varying between 0.2 to 2 $mg \cdot kg^{-1}$ (dry weight), while in the case of Zn levels, although soil Zn levels varied greatly from 50 to 1200 $mg \cdot kg^{-1}$, those of brown rice had a much smaller range from 20 to 30 $mg \cdot kg^{-1}$. (Names of rice plant parts are shown in Figure 1).

Recent field studies in Thailand by Simmons *et al.* [10] on Cd, Zn, and Fe accumulation in rice grains (unpolished rice) under Cd/Zn contaminated soils, containing 2.9–284 $mg \cdot kg^{-1}$ Cd, 254–8036 $mg \cdot kg^{-1}$ Zn, and 0.5–25 $mg \cdot kg^{-1}$ Fe, indicated that the harvested grains contained variable concentrations of Cd ranging from 0.02 to 5.0 $mg \cdot kg^{-1}$, but relatively constant concentrations of Zn (from 15 to 25 $mg \cdot kg^{-1}$) and Fe (from 7.5 to 12.7 $mg \cdot kg^{-1}$), although the concentrations of all three metals varied greatly in the stems and leaves. Thus, Zn and Fe levels in rice grains are little affected by the availability of Zn and Fe in the soil, while grain Cd levels vary greatly.

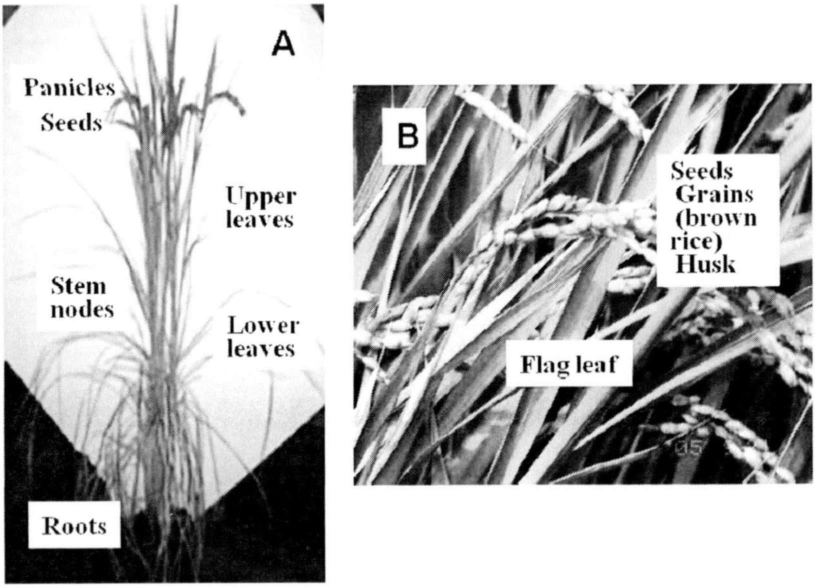


**Figure 1.** Rice plants (cv. Koshihikari) grown in potted soil (**A**) and in a field (**B**) at maturity.

Grain Zn concentrations in rice plants grown in the Philippines were unchanged by Zn fertilization (15 kg Zn·ha$^{-1}$), while this Zn fertilization increased straw Zn concentrations by 43%–95% [11].

When a rice cultivar (Todorokiwase) was grown in a culture solution at 0.01 to 3.0 mg·L$^{-1}$ Cd, the Cd concentrations in the leaf blades greatly increased from 3 to 100 mg·kg$^{-1}$ and those in the grains also increased from 0.5 to 10 mg·kg$^{-1}$[12]. In contrast, when Zn concentrations in the culture solution were increased from 0.05 to 20 mg·L$^{-1}$, Zn concentrations in the leaf blades greatly increased from 50 to 2500 mg·kg$^{-1}$, but those in the grains increased only slightly from 33 to 80 mg·kg$^{-1}$[13]. Recently, Jiang *et al.* [14] reported that when a rice cultivar (Handao297) grown in a nutrient solution containing Zn at 0.15 to 2250 μM, Zn concentrations in the shoots greatly changed from 53 to 1540 mg·kg$^{-1}$, while those in brown rice changed only slightly from 52 to 106 mg·kg$^{-1}$.

These results suggest that specific regulatory mechanisms for each of the three metals may exist between the xylem delivery to stems and leaves and the allocation of the metals to grains. In this review, to determine the regulation of the transport on Zn, Cd, and Fe via the xylem and phloem, we synthesized information of Zn, Cd, and Fe concentrations and their chemical forms in xylem and phloem saps, the localizations of metal transporters, and finally the routes of transport of these metals to the grains.

## 2. UPTAKE AT ROOT-SURFACE MEMBRANES AND RADIAL TRANSPORT TO THE XYLEM

Plant availability of metals from soils is controlled by three steps: (1) soil conditions (upland or flooded soil, soil solution pH); (2) mineralization (ionization and complex formation); and (3) uptake transporters.

As shown in Figure 2, Zn in both drained and flooded soils is largely ions ($Zn^{2+}$), although some Zn may be bound to organic substances, and immobilized as Zn–sulfide (ZnS) in the anaerobic layer [15]. Cadmium in drained acidic soils is ionized as $Cd^{2+}$, while Cd in paddy alkaline soils is present in the forms of $CdCO_3$and humic acid-bound Cd [16]. Cd is immobilized as Cd-sulfide (CdS) and colloids-bound Cd by flooding of soils [17]. Drainage converts CdS to $Cd^{2+}$ and dramatically increases its availability to plants. Fe in acidic soils is ionized as $Fe^{2+}$/$Fe^{3+}$, while in aerobic alkaline soils Fe is immobilized as $Fe(OH)_3$.

As shown in Table 2, the uptake of these metals at root-surface membranes is driven by specific uptake transporters, $Zn^{2+}$, $Cd^{2+}$, and $Fe^{2+}$ commonly by OsIRT1 (rice iron-regulated transporter1) [18,21,23] and $Cd^{2+}$ predominantly by OsNRAMP5 (rice natural resistance-associated macrophage protein5) [19]. The possible uptake of some Zn–phytosiderophores together with the uptake of $Zn^{2+}$ by a Zn-deficiency-tolerant line of rice has been suggested under lowland conditions [32]. Iron ($Fe^{3+}$) in neutral and alkaline soils binds to mineral crystals and organic substances so strongly that such soil ions are barely available to plants and the iron is solubilized by forming a complex with a phytosiderophore, 2′-deoxymugineic acid (DMA) [33], which is excreted by rice roots by OsTOM1 (rice DMA effluxer) [34]. Fe(III)–DMA complexes in the soil solution are taken up by OsYSL15 (rice yellow stripe-like15) [22]. Under flooded conditions, rice plants may absorb both Fe(III)–DMA and $Fe^{2+}$ [23].

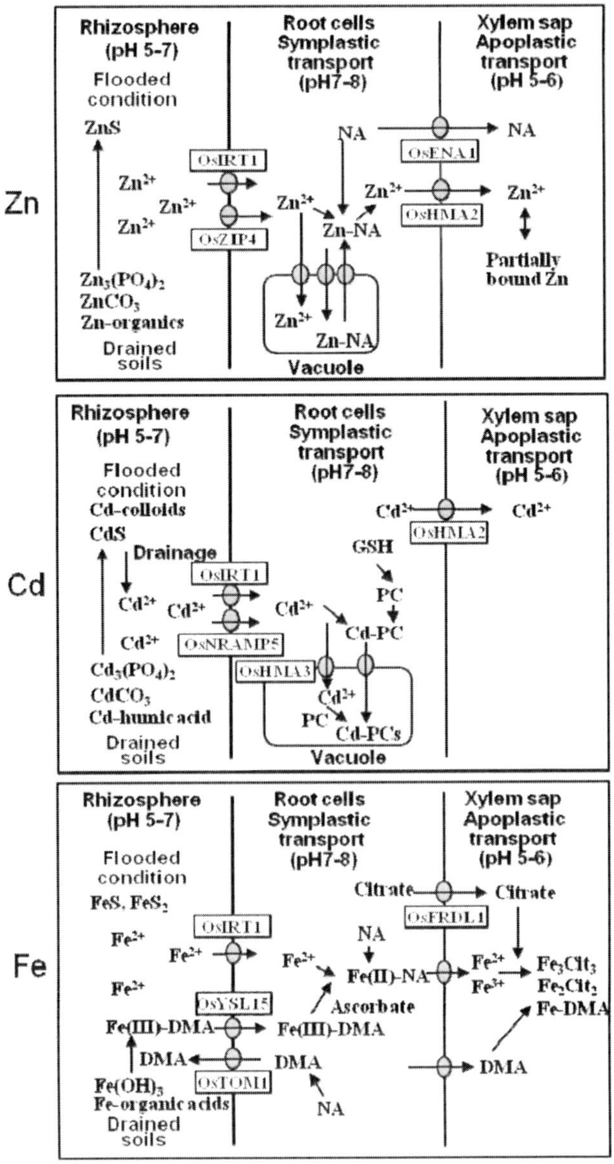


**Figure 2.** Models of uptake and transport of Zn, Cd, and Fe in rice roots. DMA, 2′-deoxymugineic acid; GSH, glutathione; NA, nicotianamine; PC, phytochelatin. Arrows indicate flows of substances and grey ellipses indicates transporters.

**Table 2.** Transporters involved in the acquisition and inter-organ transport of Zn, Cd, and Fe in rice plants.

| Site | Zn | Cd | Fe |
|---|---|---|---|
| Acquisition at root cell membranes | OsIRT1 [1]; OsZIP4.5 [2] | OsNRAMP5 [3]; OsIRT1/OsIRT2 [4] | OsYSL15 [5]; OsIRT1/OsIRT2 [6] |
| Vacuolar import through the tonoplast in root cells | (ZIF1) [7] | OsHMA3 [8] | |
| Xylem loading at root pericycle cells | OsHMA2 [9] | OsHMA2 [5,9] | |
| Xylem-to-phloem transport at nodes | OsHMA2 [10] | OsHMA2 [10] | OsYSL16 [11] |
| Phloem loading after mobilization in leaves | ZIP and YSL families | | OYSL15 [12] |
| Phloem unloading at reproductive organs | | | OsYSL18 [13] |

[1] Lee and An [18]; [2] White and Broadley [4]; [3] Ishikawa *et al.* [19], Sasaki *et al.* [20]; [4] Nakanishi *et al.* [21]; [5] Inoue *et al.* [22]; [6] Ishimaru *et al.* [23]; [7] Haydon *et al.* [24]; [8] Ueno *et al.* [25]; [9] Nocito *et al.* [26], Takahashi *et al.* [27]; [10] Yamaji *et al.* [28]; [11] Kakei *et al.* [29]; [12] Lee *et al.* [30]; [13] Aoyama *et al.* [31].

Zinc ($Zn^{2+}$) and $Fe^{2+}$ in root cell cytosols form complexes with nicotianamine (NA) in the forms of Zn–NA and Fe(II)–NA (Figure 2). Cadmium in the root cell cytosols may be $Cd^{2+}$ ions or complexes with phytochelatins (PCs). Fe(III)–DMA absorbed in the root cell cytosols can be reduced by ascorbate, transforming to Fe(II)-NA [35]. Fe of cytosolic Fe(II)–NA may be excreted to the xylem and makes complexes predominantly with citrate ($Fe_2Cit_2$, $Fe_3Cit_3$) and some with DMA (Fe–DMA) [36].

Root cell vacuoles can function as a storage compartment for metals. Zn–NA in the root cell cytosols is transferred to the vacuoles by the ZIF1 (zinc induced facilitor1) transporter [24]. Cadmium in the cell cytosols may be partly sequestered through the tonoplast as $Cd^{2+}$ by OsHMA3 (rice heavy metal ATPase3) [25] and as Cd-PC complex, presumably by ABCC-type transporters in *Arabidopsis* [37], and both are stored as Cd-PCs in the vacuoles. Enhancement of OsHMA3 activity has been found to increase storage in roots and decrease the transport of Cd to the shoot and the final accumulation of Cd in rice grains [25]. A high rate of root-to-shoot transport and subsequent accumulation in the grains of $^{107}Cd$, which was administered from a culture solution, was observed in OsHMA3-depleted rice lines [38].

OsHMA2, which localizes at the root pericycle, is a major transporter of Zn and Cd for xylem loading [26,27]. The excretion of citrate from the root cells to the xylem is partly operated by OsFRDL1 (rice ferric reductase defective1-like) to enhance Fe-transport in the xylem as Fe(III)–citrate complex [39].

# 3. XYLEM AND PHLOEM TRANSPORT

The concentrations of Zn, Cd, and Fe and their chemical forms in rice xylem and phloem saps from 28- to 33-day-old vegetative plants were analyzed. The phloem sap was collected by a unique and excellent technique using the insect-laser method as described by Kawabe *et al.* [40]. Briefly, the insects used were*Nilaparvata lugens* Stål (brown planthopper). Rice plants at the 8th to 9th leaf-age were transferred to 500 mL plastic bottles, one plant per bottle, and placed in an artificially lit chamber (130 $\mu mol \cdot m^{-2} \cdot s^{-1}$photosynthetically active irradiation, 12 h light and 12 h dark cycle). After the plants' adaptation to the environment over 1 or 2 days, overhead projector film sheet cylinders (3 cm high, 1 cm in diameter) with cotton stoppers on both sides were set on the sheaths of the fully developed leaves, and female insects, that had been forced to fast overnight, were transferred into the cylinders to allow the insects to suck the phloem sap. After 1–3 h, the insects' stylets were cut by a YAG laser (SL129Nd; NEC, Tokyo, Japan) beam. After the phloem sap was collected, shoots were cut with a knife at 2 cm from the root-shoot interface and the exudates (xylem sap) from the cut surfaces were collected.

The Zn concentrations in the xylem and phloem saps under four different Zn concentrations in the culture solution are shown in Figure 3. The Zn concentrations in the xylem sap increased with those in the culture solution, while the Zn concentrations in the phloem sap varied only slightly between 55 and 100 μM. With 0.1 μM culture-solution Cd, the xylem and phloem Cd concentrations were around 20-fold higher than the culture-solution Cd concentrations. Under treatment with 10 μM Cd, xylem sap was not exuded due to wilting. Cd concentrations in the collected phloem sap increased with the medium Cd concentrations (Figure 3). Although the Fe concentrations in the culture solution ranged greatly at 4.5, 9.0, 45 and 90 μM, xylem Fe concentrations remained nearly constant at 12 μM under the lower three culture-solution Fe treatments and 16 μM under the 90 μM treatment (Figure 3). Phloem-sap Fe concentrations, around 50 μM Fe, were not affected by the different Fe treatments.

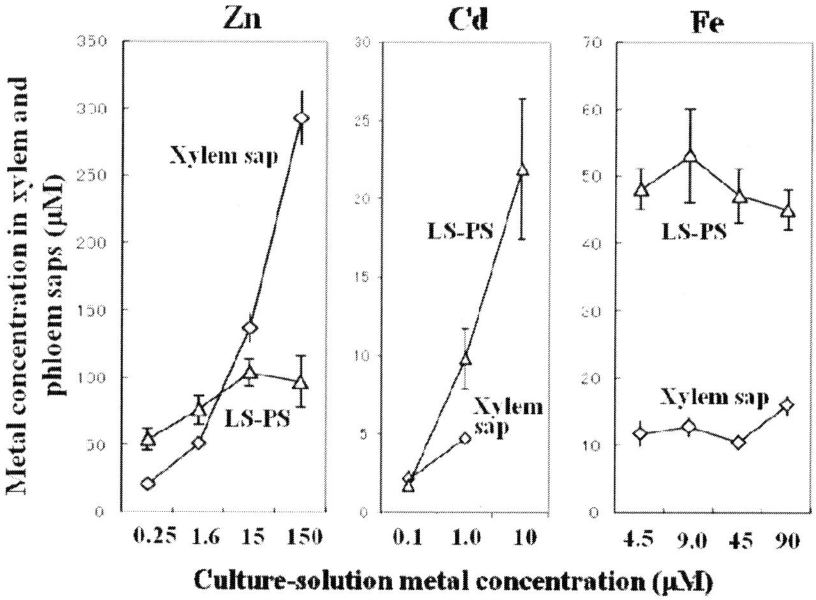


**Figure 3.** Metal concentrations in the xylem and phloem saps of vegetative rice plants under various culture-solution metal concentrations. Phloem sap was collected from the leaf sheaths (LS-PS) of the 7th leaves. Data for Zn and Fe are from Nishiyama [41], and data for Cd are from Mariyo Kato [42].

The chemical forms in xylem and phloem saps from young rice plants are shown in Table 3. Using the phloem and xylem saps collected as described above, chemical forms (speciation) of Zn, Cd, and Fe in such saps were investigated using size-exclusion high performance liquid chromatography (SE-HPLC, Hitachi, Tokyo, Japan), inductively coupled plasma-mass spectrometry (ICP-MS, Yokogawa, Tokyo, Japan), capillary electrophoresis coupled to mass spectrometry (CE-MS, Agilent Technologies, Walbronn, Germany), and electrospray ionization time-of-flight mass spectrometry (ESI-TOF MS, JOC, Tokyo, Japan).

The Zn chemical forms in xylem sap are free ions and Zn partially bound to unidentified chelators [39], while the Zn in phloem sap was dominantly bound to NA [43]. The Cd chemical form in the xylem sap is primarily in free ions (Mariyo Kato [42]), while the Cd in the phloem sap was largely bound to specific proteins although some Cd was bound to low-molecular thiol compounds [44]. The Fe chemical forms in xylem sap were found to be bound largely to citrate (around 65%) and slightly to DMA (around 5%) [36], while the Fe in phloem sap bound to DMA, citric acid, and proteins [43]. Recently, metal species in the xylem and phloem saps from various plants including rice were summarized by Álvarez-Fernández *et al.*[45].

**Table 3.** Chemical forms of Zn, Cd. Fe, and Cu in xylem and phloem saps from rice plants. Metal speciation analyses in xylem and phloem saps were conducted by using SE-HPLC, ICP-MS, CE-MS, and ESI-TOF MS.

| Metal | Chemical Forms in Xylem Sap (pH 6) | Chemical Forms in Phloem Sap (pH 8) |
|---|---|---|
| Zn | Free ions and partially bound [1] | Bound dominantly to NA [2] |
| Cd | Primarily in free ions [3] | Bound largely to specific proteins and slightly to thiol-compounds [4] |
| Fe | Bound largely to citrate (around 65%) and slightly to DMA (around 5%) and some in free ions [5] | Bound to DMA, citrate, and proteins [2] |
| Cu | Bound dominantly to DMA [6] | Bound to NA, histidine and proteins [6] |

[1] Nishiyama [41]; [2] Nishiyama *et al.* [43]; [3] Mariyo Kato [42]; [4] Kato *et al.* [44]; [5] Ariga *et al.* [36]. [6] Ando *et al.* [45].

Changes in copper (Cu) concentrations in xylem and phloem saps and the chemical forms of Cu in rice xylem and phloem saps were investigated by Ando *et al.* [46]. Xylem Cu concentrations were found to range slightly between 5 and 8 μM when culture-solution Cu concentrations ranged from 0.16 to 1.28 μM and the Cu in xylem sap was dominantly bound to DMA. Phloem sap Cu concentrations ranged between 21 and 43 μM and the Cu in phloem sap was bound to NA, histidine and proteins.

Based on the results on variation in metal concentrations (Figure 3) and their chemical forms in xylem and phloem saps (Table 3), the following interesting relationship regarding the regulatory mechanisms that underlie the different changes in the Zn, Cd, Fe, and Cu concentrations in both saps is suggested; if xylem sap contains substantial free metal ions as in the cases of Zn and Cd, its metal concentration increases with increasing culture-solution metal concentration, while if xylem sap contains metal–ligand complexes as in the cases of Fe and Cu, its metal concentration remains nearly constant. If the metals in the phloem saps are definitely bound to ligands as in the cases of Zn–NA, Fe–DMA, and Cu–NA, the metal concentration remains quite constant. The concentration of NA, which may bind Zn and Cu in rice phloem sap, was around 70 μM [43,45], and that of DMA, which may bind Fe in rice phloem sap, was around 150 μM [43]. However, phloem Cd is apparently an exception; phloem concentrations changed with culture-solution and xylem-sap Cd concentrations (Figure 3). The major form of Cd in the phloem saps is protein-bound and the Cd-binding capacity of the proteins may be sufficient to load all Cd in the phloem sap [44].

With respect to the transport of Zn in xylem sap to rapidly growing leaves, Obata and Kitagishi [47] indicate that some Zn ascending via the xylem (transpiration stream) is transferred to the phloem at the vegetative nodes in addition to the Zn which is mobilized from mature leaves (Figure 4). Together this Zn with different origins is terminated to the intercalary meristem to synthesize ribosomes [48]. Such active transport through both routes supports the high Zn accumulation at the meristem, which has been reported to reach 300 mg $Zn{\cdot}kg^{-1}$ dry weight (DW) in the rapidly growing leaf part as compared to 30 mg $Zn{\cdot}kg^{-1}$DW in the mature leaves [49]. Figure 5 shows this unique and quick accumulation of Zn in the early stage of leaves compared to the slow accumulation of Fe and also the early initiation of the decrease after the peak of Zn content, which was one week before reaching the DW peak [49]. The amount of Zn transferred to the phloem via the xylem-to-phloem transfer system seems to be regulated and constant: the transfer rate of Zn from xylem sap is relatively high when the xylem sap Zn concentration is low, and low when the xylem sap Zn concentration is high [50]. The ratio of the Zn deprived by the xylem-to-phloem transfer to that remobilized from the leaves is estimated to be around 3:7 [49]. Partitioning of Cd to the top may be similar to that of Zn and the vegetative nodes may also be the site of the xylem-to-phloem transfer of Cd [51]. $^{115m}$Cd absorbed by roots is partitioned to the dwarf stem and leaves by the pattern of accumulation in the nodal part of the stem, and transport is then predominant to the rapidly growing leaves with little to the mature leaves [52], similar to that of $^{65}$Zn [50]. Recently, preferential movement of $^{109}$Cd and $^{45}$Ca, which were administered to a root–bathing solution as $^{109}CdCl_2$ and $^{45}CaCl_2$, to the newest leaf by transfer to the phloem at the stem, was confirmed by radioisotope imaging [53]. The rate of Fe involved in xylem-to-phloem transfer could be smaller than that of Zn, since the demand-time of Fe is late compared to that of Zn (Figure 5, [49]). It is interesting to note that Fe in rice xylem sap has been found to contain small amounts of Fe–DMA and large amounts of Fe–citrate while the Fe in the xylem sap of barley plants includes a considerable fraction of Fe–mugineic acid (MA) [36]. Barley plants can transfer such xylem sap Fe–MA to the young leaves through the xylem-to-phloem system at nodes as revealed by $^{52}$Fe tracing [54].

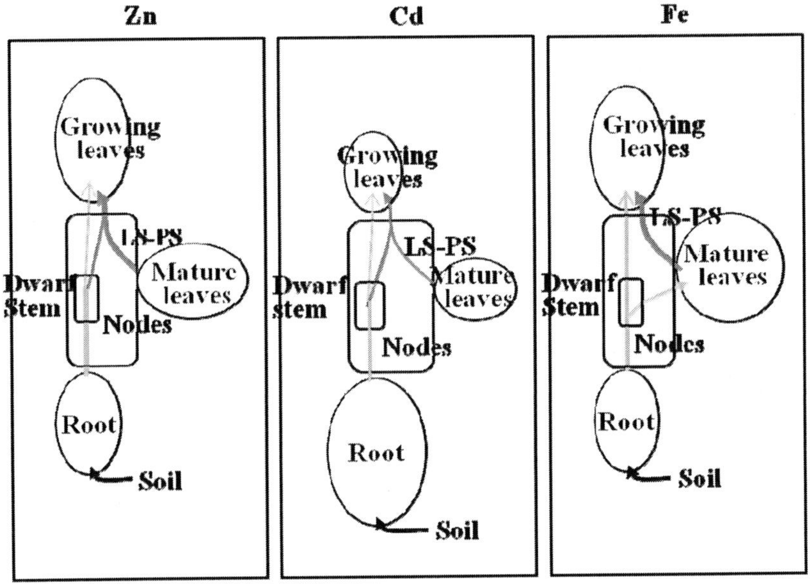


**Figure 4.** Models of the transport of Zn, Cd, and Fe via xylem and phloem in rice plants at the vegetative stage. "Leaves" are leaf blades. "Stem" includes the dwarf culm and leaf sheaths. The green line shows xylem transport. The red line shows phloem transport. Phloem sap was collected from the leaf sheaths (LS-PS). Information is from Yoneyama *et al.* [55]. Important note: At the vegetative nodes of the dwarf stem, Zn and Cd ascending xylem (green line) are transferred to the phloem (red line) via the xylem-to-phloem transfer system at the nodes, while Fe in the xylem (in the form of Fe–citrate) does not pass through this system.

Xylem transfer cells found in vegetative nodes [56,57,58] and localized metal transporters (Table 2) may support the active xylem-to-phloem transfer of xylem sap Zn and Cd.

# 4. ACCUMULATION OF ZN, CD, AND FE IN RICE GRAINS

Phloem and xylem saps were collected from rice plants grown in Cd-contaminated flooded soil. Phloem sap was obtained from leaf sheaths at the 10th and 14th leaf ages and from the uppermost internodes at the grain-filling stage (Figure 6 [55]). Phloem loading after both remobilization from the leaves and stems and xylem-to-

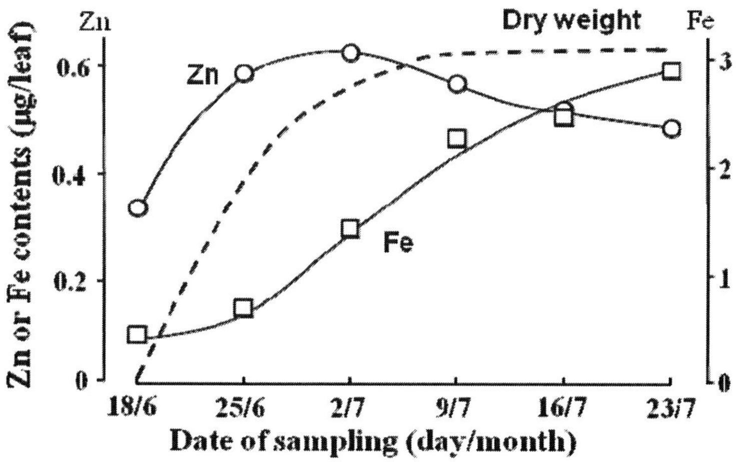


**Figure 5.** Changes in Zn and Fe amounts in the blade of the 10th leaf along with dry weight growth. (Adapted from Obata and Kitagishi [49]). The dry weight of the leaf was drawn arbitrarily as the dry weight at 23/7 had reached the maximum. ○: change in the content of Zn; □: change in the content of Fe. (Adapted from Obata and Kitagishi [49]).

phloem transfer at stem and panicle nodes of the currently ascending fluids may be the source of grain Zn [55,59,60] and Cd [55,61,62], but for Fe the route of remobilization from other organs may be dominant as shown in Figure 7. The contribution of the xylem-to-phloem transfer rate of Zn and probably also of Cd is evident from the high and increased Zn concentration in phloem sap collected at the uppermost internode as compared to that collected from leaf sheaths at the 14th-leaf stage; in contrast, no such increase was observed for Fe (Figure 6). A positron-emitting $^{107}Cd$ imaging study of hydroponically grown rice plants at the panicle-initiation stage suggests the highly preferential transport of currently absorbed Cd to the panicles through the presumed xylem-to-phloem transfer at the nodes (Figure 8) [63]. The presence of xylem transfer cells in the nodes [56] and in the spikelet nodes at the region of the rachilla and pedicle [64,65] and metal transporters, OsHMA2 for Zn and Cd [28] and OsYSL16 (rice yellow stripe-like16) for Fe–DMA [29] although the fraction of Fe–DNA is small [36], may be involved in the active xylem-to-phloem transfer of minerals (at the nodes) currently ascending via the xylem from the roots. The amount of transfer of Zn via the xylem-to-phloem system may be highly regulated at a certain level where there is a large supply of Zn through the xylem, as shown in wheat detached panicles [66]. In contrast, such a restriction may not work in the transport of Cd, since the Cd concentration ascending the xylem is much smaller than that of Zn. Jiang *et al.* [67] demonstrated the efficient transport to the grains and little partitioning to the leaves of $^{65}Zn$ applied to rice plants from a culture solution during the flowering period. Rodda *et al.* [62] estimated that 60% of the final grain Cd could be attributed to remobilization from other tissues and the rest (40%) from uptake during grain maturation. Importantly, mineral transporters for xylem-to-phloem transport at the nodes (OsHMA2, OsYSL16), for the phloem loading at leaves (OsYSL15), and for unloading at panicles (OsYSL18) may play important functions in the regulation of metal transport (Table 2).

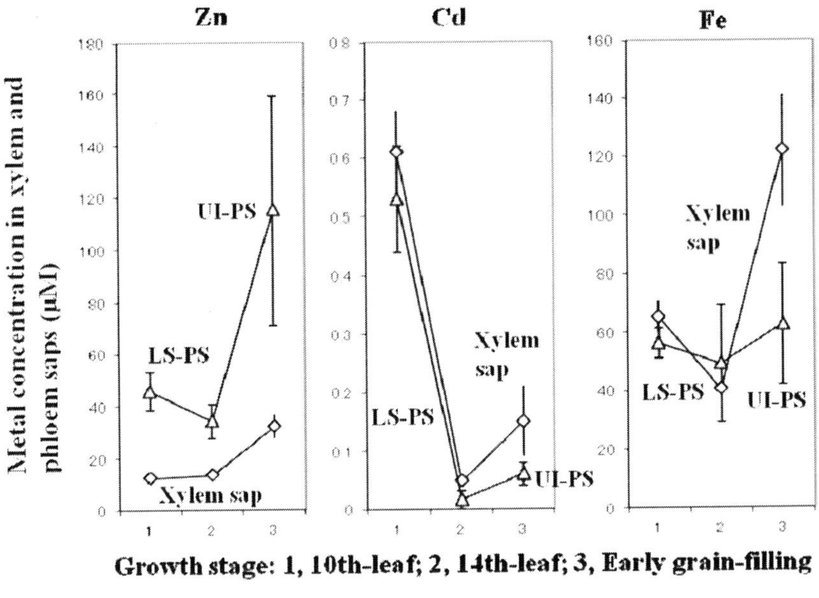


**Figure 6.** Metal concentrations in the xylem and phloem saps obtained from rice plants grown in a flooded Cd-contaminated soil. Phloem sap was collected from the leaf sheaths (LS-PS) of the 9th leaves at 10th-leaf stage and the 13th leaves at 14th-leaf stage, and from the uppermost internodes (UI-PS) at early grain-filling. Data are from Yoneyama *et al.*[55]. ◊: metal concentrations in the xylem sap, Δ: metal concentrations in the phloem sap.

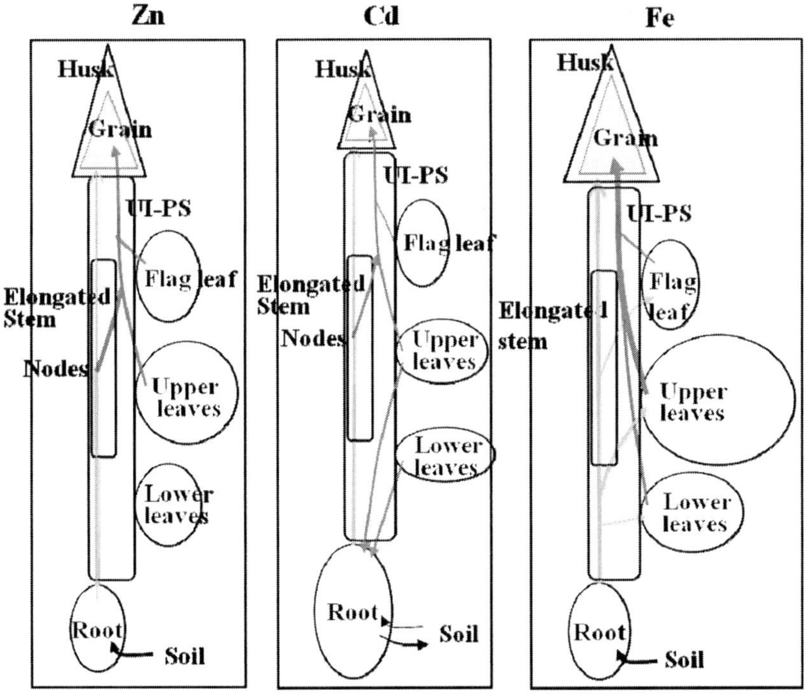


**Figure 7.** Models of the transport of Zn, Cd, and Fe via xylem and phloem in rice plants at grain filling. "Leaves" are Leaf blades. "Stem" includes elongated culm, leaf sheaths, and panicles except husk and grain. Green line shows xylem transport. Red line shows phloem transport. Phloem sap was collected from the uppermost internode (UI-PS). Information is from Yoneyama *et al.* [55]. Important note: At the nodes in the elongated stem, Zn and Cd ascending xylem (green line) are transferred to phloem (red line) via the xylem-to-phloem transfer system, while Fe in the xylem (in the form of Fe–citrate) does not pass through this system.

The deposition of metals in grains is revealed as metal partitioning: Zn and Fe, which combine with phytic acid, are largely accumulated in the aleurone cell layer [4,68] but their concentrations are reduced in white rice by polishing, while a large proportion of Cd is localized at the storage protein (glutelin) in the endosperm [69] and the Cd concentration in white rice is unchanged by polishing.

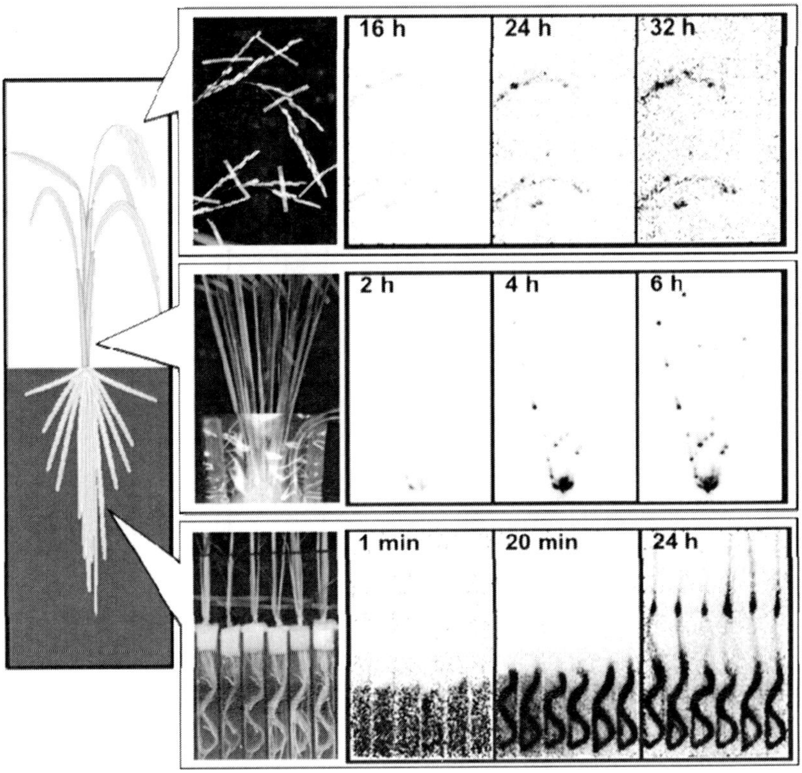


**Figure 8.** Movement of $^{107}Cd$ in rice plants administered from the root–bathing solution visualized with a positron-emitting tracer imaging system (PETIS). Regenerated from the original data of Ishikawa *et al.*[38] and Fujimaki *et al.* [62]. Important note: The images show the uptake and accumulation of $^{107}Cd$ by roots, transport to the shoots accompanying accumulation at the nodes (probably occurring during xylem-to-phloem transport), and final destination in the grains.

As stated in the Introduction section above, the Zn concentration in rice grains is affected only slightly by the availability of culture-solution metals, as compared to the great changes in Zn concentrations in the leaves and stems [13,14]; grain Cd concentrations are easily affected [12]. This observation is strongly related to the regulated and small changes in phloem concentrations of Zn, which may be in the form of Zn–NA complexes. In contrast, Cd loaded into phloem fluids may quickly bind to specific Cd-binding proteins, and those are unsaturated with Cd and sufficiently present relative to Cd, as described by Kato *et al.* [44]. Therefore, there are fewer limitations in the phloem transport of Cd than in Zn phloem transport.

The Fe in phloem sap may be derived largely from remobilization at the leaves (Figure 7, [55]) and probably bind to DMA and some citrate and proteins [43]. Therefore, the amount of Fe transport to the grains may be regulated by ligands and chelators. Schuler *et al.* [70] reported that in *Arabidopsis thaliana*, Fe–citrate in xylem sap may be delivered to the mature leaves and then Fe may be carried to the reproductive organs via the phloem as Fe–NA from the mature leaves. In the case of rice plants, Fe in the xylem is largely bound to citrate with slight binding to DMA [36]. Therefore, a large fraction of xylem Fe may be delivered first to the leaves as Fe–citrate and then to the seeds via the phloem, probably as Fe–DMA. It is possible that small amounts of Fe–DMA in rice xylem sap [36] travel through the xylem-to-phloem transport system at nodes by the OsYSL16 transporter [29]. Foliar application of a solution containing NA in addition to Fe and amino acids to a field-grown rice plant was found to increase the Fe and Zn concentrations in brown rice over those under a treatment with a solution containing Fe and amino acids [71].

## 5. MOLECULAR TECHNOLOGIES TO INCREASE GRAIN FE AND ZN AND TO REDUCE GRAIN CD

Recent attempts at the biofortification of Fe and Zn in rice grains using transgenic techniques have produced interesting results. The introduction of a yeast ferric chelate reductase gene to rice plants induced the enhancement of Fe uptake and an increase in grain yields but had no effect on Fe and Zn concentrations in the grains [72]. In contrast, the over-expression of the barley NA synthase gene *HvNAS1* in rice plants caused an increase in DMA and NA concentrations in roots, shoots, and seeds as well as of Fe, Zn, and Cu concentrations in grains [73]. These results are consistent with the proposed principle that the phloem-sap and grain concentrations of metals may be regulated by making use of the nature of metal-chelating compounds. It is valuable to note that high-NA grain may increase iron-bioavailability to mammals and humans [74,75].

There are three possible ways to reduce Cd content in rice grains: (1) the selection of lines/varieties with low Cd in phloem sap [44]; (2) more sequestration of Cd in the root–cell vacuoles by overexpression of OsHMA3 [25]; and (3) elimination of a Cd-uptake transporter (OsNRAMP5) in the root membranes [19]. Ishikawa *et al.* [19] report that carbon ion beam irradiation produced Cd-deficient rice mutants (Koshihikari-Kan1) with <0.05 mg Cd·kg$^{-1}$ in the grains compared with a mean of 1.1 mg Cd·kg$^{-1}$ in the parent, cultivar Koshihikari (a high eating-quality rice) when plants were grown in Cd-contaminated fields, whereas their Zn and Fe concentrations were less affected (Table 4), and they also developed DNA markers to select cultivars carrying *osnramp5*. In terms of human intake of Cd from Cd-contaminated foods such as rice, its bioavailability and retention in the liver and kidneys are dramatically increased due to the deficiency of Zn, Fe, and Ca in foods [76]. Therefore, biofortification of Zn, Fe and Ca in the grains is highly essential to reduce human Cd intake.

**Table 4.** Concentrations of Zn, Cd and Fe of grains of cultivar Koshihikari (Koshi) and its OsNRAMP5-depleted mutant Koshihikari-Kan1 (Kan1) grown on three Cd-contaminated soils whose irrigation was treated with prolonged drainage after the early-period flooding. Data are means of 5 samples. ND, not detected. Data are from Ishikawa*et al.* [19].

| Field (Soil Cd mg·kg$^{-1}$) | Grain Zn (mg·kg$^{-1}$) | | Grain Cd (mg·kg$^{-1}$) | | Grain Fe (mg·kg$^{-1}$) | |
|---|---|---|---|---|---|---|
| | Koshi | Kan1 | Koshi | Kan1 | Koshi | Kan1 |
| A (1.35) | 48.8 | 36.9 | 0.57 | ND | 21.5 | 16.4 |
| B (1.21) | 34.4 | 31.4 | 1.86 | 0.02 | 14.2 | 15.8 |
| C (0.35) | 50.4 | 37.5 | 0.97 | 0.03 | 15.1 | 14.3 |

# 6. CONCLUSIONS

Zn and Fe are essential nutrients for both plants and humans but Cd is non-essential and toxic if it accumulates at high levels for plants and, more severely, for humans. All three metals are contained in the grains of rice, a staple cereal worldwide. Several studies have reported that Zn and Fe concentrations in rice grains harvested under different levels of soil or hydroponic metals are known to change only within a small range, while grain Cd concentrations show greater changes and easily reach the allowable maximum in polished rice (0.4 mg·kg$^{-1}$) [77]. To gain insight into the mechanisms underlying such different metal contents, we synthesized information about the routes of metal transport and accumulation in rice plants, finding novel regulations involving metal speciation in xylem and phloem saps, metal transporters, and the xylem-to-phloem transport system. Specific metal transporters are involved in uptake in the roots, delivery to the shoots via the xylem-to-phloem transport system, and final transport to the grains via the phloem. Xylem sap Zn is in free ions and partially bound to unidentified chelators and has a highly variable concentration, while phloem sap Zn is dominantly Zn–NA complex with a highly regulated concentration. Xylem sap Cd is primarily in free ions with a variable concentration, while phloem sap Cd is bound to proteins and thiol compounds, and its concentration is dependent on xylem sap Cd. Cd loaded into phloem fluids may quickly bind to specific Cd-binding proteins, those are unsaturated with Cd and sufficiently present relative to Cd. Xylem sap Fe (largely as Fe–citrate) is allocated to all leaves, while phloem Fe is bound to DMA, citrate, and proteins. At grain-filling, Zn and Cd ascending in xylem sap are transferred to the phloem by the xylem-to-phloem transport system operating at stem and panicle nodes, where xylem transfer cells and specific metal transporters are recognized. Grain Fe is largely derived from the leaves by remobilization. Thus, the concentrations of grain Zn and Fe are highly regulated within a small range, while that of grain Cd varies depending on xylem supply. Transgenic techniques to increase tissue and phloem-sap concentrations of NA and DMA are useful to increase grain Zn and Fe concentrations. The elimination of OsNRAMP5 Cd-uptake transporter and the enhancement of root cell vacuolar Cd sequestration reduce uptake and root–to-shoot transport, respectively, resulting in a great reduction of Cd accumulation in grains.

## ACKNOWLEDGMENTS

The authors thank Reiko Nishiyama for her kind supply of information of Zn and Fe concentrations in rice xylem and phloem saps from her Master's thesis [39] and Mariyo Kato for providing her unpublished data of Cd concentrations in xylem and phloem saps as shown in Figure 3.

## AUTHOR CONTRIBUTIONS

Tadakatsu Yoneyama wrote the first draft of the manuscript and organized the tables and figures; Satoru Ishikawa and Shu Fujimaki reviewed the manuscript and added Table 4 and Figure 8, respectively.

## CONFLICTS OF INTEREST

The authors declare no conflicts of interest.

## REFERENCES


1. Nouet, C.; Motte, P.; Hanikenne, M. Chloroplastic and mitochondrial metal homeostasis. Trends Plant Sci. 2011, 16, 395–404.
2. Palmer, C.M.; Guerinot, M.L. Facing the challenges of Cu, Fe and Zn homeostasis in plants. Nat. Chem. Biol. 2009, 5, 333–340.
3. Palmgren, M.G.; Clemens, S.; Williams, L.E.; Krämer, U.; Borg, S.; Schjørring, J.K.; Sanders, D. Zinc biofortification of cereals: Problems and solutions. Trends Plant Sci. 2008, 13, 464–473.
4. White, P.J.; Broadley, M.R. Physiological limits to zinc biofortification of edible crops. Front. Plant Sci.2011, 2, 80.
5. Clemens, S.; Aarts, M.G.M.; Thomine, S.; Verbruggen, N. Plant science: The key to preventing slow cadmium poisoning. Trends Plant Sci. 2012, 18, 92–99.
6. Zimmermann, M.B.; Hurrell, R.F. Improving iron, zinc, vitamin A nutrition through plant biotechnology. Curr. Opin. Biotechnol. 2002, 13, 142–145.
7. Dijkhuizen, M.A.; Wieringa, F.T.; West, C.E. Zinc plus β-carotene supplementation of pregnant women is superior to β-carotene supplementation alone in improving vitamin A status in both mothers and infants. Am. J. Clin. Nutr. 2004, 80, 1299–1307.
8. Fukushima, M.; Ishizaki, A.; Sakamoto, M.; Kobayashi, E. Cadmium concentration in rice eaten by famers in the Jinzu River Basin. Jpn. J. Hyg. 1973, 28, 406–415.
9. Khoshgoftarmanesh, A.H.; Schulin, R.; Chaney, R.L.; Daneshbakhsh, B.; Afyuni, M. Micronutrient-efficient genotypes for crop yield and nutritional quality in sustainable agriculture. A review. Agron. Sustain. Dev. 2010, 30, 83–107.
10. Simmons, R.W.; Pongsakul, P.; Chaney, R.L.; Saiyasitpanich, D.; Klinphoklap, S.; Nobuntou, W. The relative exclusion of zinc and iron from rice grain in relation to rice grain cadmium as compared to soybean: Implications for human health. Plant Soil 2003, 257, 163–170.

11. Wissuwa, M.; Ismail, A.M.; Graham, R.D. Rice grain zinc concentrations as affected by genotype, native soil-zinc availability, and zinc fertilization. Plant Soil 2008, 306, 37–48.

12. Ito, H.; Iimura, K. Absorption of zinc and cadmium by rice plants and their influence on its growth. II. Effect of cadmium. Jpn. J. Soil Sci. Plant Nutr. 1976, 47, 44–48.

13. Ito, H.; Iimura, K. Absorption of zinc and cadmium by rice plants and their influence on its growth. I. Effect of zinc. Jpn. J. Soil Sci. Plant Nutr. 1976, 47, 39–43.

14. Jiang, W.; Struik, P.C.; van Keulen, H.; Zhao, M.; Jin, L.N.; Stomph, T.J. Does increased zinc uptake enhance grain zinc mass concentration in rice? Ann. Appl. Biol. 2008, 153, 135–147.

15. Shiratori, K.; Suzuki, T.; Miyoshi, H. Chemical forms of soil zinc in the salt-rich reclaimed fields, where zinc-deficiency symptoms were observed in rice plants. Jpn. J. Soil Sci. Plant Nutr. 1972, 43, 291–296.

16. Khaokaew, S.; Chaney, R.L.; Landrot, G.; Ginder-Vogel, M.; Sparks, D.L. Speciation and release kinetics of cadmium in an alkaline paddy soil under various flooding periods and draining conditions. Environ. Sci. Technol. 2011, 45, 4249–4255.

17. Hashimoto, Y.; Yamaguchi, N. Chemical speciation of cadmium and sulfur K-edge XANES spectroscopy in flooded paddy soils amended with zerovalent iron. Soil Sci. Soc. Am. J. 2013, 77, 1189–1198.

18. Lee, S.; An, G. Over-expression of OsIRT1 leads to iron and zinc accumulations in rice. Plant Cell Environ. 2009, 32, 408–416.

19. Ishikawa, S.; Ishimaru, Y.; Igura, M.; Kuramata, M.; Abe, T.; Senoura, T.; Hase, Y.; Arao, T.; Nishizawa, N.K.; Nakanishi, H. Ion-beam irradiation, gene identification, and marker-assisted breeding in the development of low-cadmium rice. Proc. Natl. Acad. Sci. USA 2012, 109, 19166–19171.

20. Sasaki, A.; Yamaji, N.; Yokosho, K.; Ma, J.F. Nramp5 is a major transporter responsible for manganese and cadmium uptake in rice. Plant Cell 2012, 24, 2155–2167.

21. Nakanishi, H.; Ogawa, I.; Ishimaru, Y.; Mori, S.; Nishizawa, N.K. Iron deficiency enhances cadmium uptake and translocation mediated by the Fe2+ transporters OsIRT1 and OsIRT2 in rice. Soil Sci. Plant Nutr. 2006, 52, 464–469.

22. Inoue, H.; Kobayashi, T.; Nozoye, T.; Takahashi, M.; Kakei, Y.; Suzuki, K.; Nakazono, M.; Nakanishi, H.; Mori, S.; Nishizawa, N.K. Rice OsYSL15 is an iron-regulated iron(III)-deoxymugineic acid transporter expressed in the roots and is essential for iron uptake in early growth of the seedlings. J. Biol. Chem. 2009, 284, 3470–3479.

23. Ishimaru, Y.; Suzuki, M.; Tsukamoto, T.; Suzuki, K.; Nakazono, M.; Kobayashi, T.; Wada, Y.; Watanabe, S.; Matsuhashi, S.; Takahashi, M.; et al. Rice plants take up iron as an Fe3+-phytosiderophore and as Fe2+. Plant J. 2006, 45, 335–346.

24. Haydon, M.J.; Kawachi, M.; Wirtz, M.; Hillmer, S.; Hell, R.; Krämer, U. Vacuolar nicotianamine has critical and distinct roles under iron deficiency and for zinc sequestration in Arabidopsis. Plant Cell2012, 24, 724–737.

25. Ueno, D.; Yamaji, N.; Kono, I.; Huang, C.F.; Ando, T.; Yano, M.; Ma, J.F. Gene limiting cadmium accumulation in rice. Proc. Natl. Acad. Sci. USA 2010, 107, 16500–16505.

26. Nocito, F.F.; Lancilli, C.; Dendena, B.; Lucchini, G.; Sacchi, G.A. Cadmium retention in rice roots is influenced by cadmium availability, chelation and translocation. Plant Cell Environ. 2011, 34, 994–1008.

27. Takahashi, R.; Ishimaru, Y.; Shimo, H.; Ogo, Y.; Senoura, T.; Nishizawa, N.K.; Nakanishi, H. The OsHMA2 transporter is involved in root-to-shoot translocation of Zn and Cd in rice. Plant Cell Environ. 2012, 35, 1948–1957.

28. Yamaji, N.; Xia, J.; Mitani-Ueno, N.; Yokosho, K.; Ma, J.F. Preferential delivery of zinc to developing tissues in rice is mediated by P-type heavy metal ATPase OsHMA2. Plant Physiol. 2013, 162, 927–939.

29. Kakei, Y.; Ishimaru, Y.; Kobayashi, T.; Yamakawa, T.; Nakanshi, H.; Nishizawa, N.K. OsYSL16 plays a role in the allocation of iron. Plant Mol. Biol. 2012, 79, 583–594.

30. Lee, S.; Chiecko, J.C.; Kim, S.A.; Walker, E.L.; Lee, Y.; Guerinot, M.L.; An, G. Disruption of OsYSL15 leads to inefficiency in rice plants. Plant Physiol. 2009, 150, 786–800.

31. Aoyama, T.; Kobayashi, T.; Takahashi, M.; Nagasaka, S.; Usuda, K.; Kakei, Y.; Ishimaru, Y.; Nakanishi, H.; Mori, S.; Nishizawa, N.K. OsYSL18 is a rice iron(III)-deoxymugineic acid transporter specifically expressed in reproductive organs and phloem of lamina joints. Plant Mol. Biol. 2009, 70, 681–692.

32. Widodo; Broadley, M.R.; Rose, T.; Frei, M.; Pariasca-Tanaka, J.; Yoshihashi, T.; Thomson, M.; Hammond, J.P.; Aprile, A.; Close, T.J.; et al. Response to zinc deficiency of two rice lines with contrasting tolerance is determined by root growth maintenance and organic acid exudation rate, and not by zinc-transport activity. New Phytol. 2010, 186, 400–414.

33. Takagi, S.; Nomoto, K.; Takemoto, S. Physiological aspect of mugineic acid, a possible phytosiderophore of graminaceous plants. J. Plant Nutr. 1984, 7, 469–477.

34. Nozoye, T.; Nagasaka, S.; Kobayashi, T.; Takahashi, M.; Sato, Y.; Uozumi, N.; Nakanishi, H.; Nishizawa, N.K. Phytosiderophore efflux transporters are crucial for iron acquisition in graminaceous plants. J. Biol. Chem. 2011, 286, 5446–5454.

35. Weber, G.; von Wiren, N.; Hayen, H. Investigation of ascorbate-mediated iron release from ferric phytosiderophores in the presence of nicotianamine. Biometals 2008, 21, 503–513.

36. Ariga, T.; Hazama, K.; Yanagisawa, S.; Yoneyama, T. Chemical forms of iron in xylem sap from graminaceous and non-graminaceous plants. Soil Sci. Plant Nutr. 2014, 60, 460–469.

37. Park, J.; Song, W.-Y.; Ko, D.; Eom, Y.; Hansen, T.H.; Schiller, M.; Lee, T.G.; Martinoia, E.; Lee, Y. The phytochelatin transporters AtABCC1 and AtABCC2 mediate tolerance to cadmium and mercury. Plant J. 2012, 69, 278–288.

38. Ishikawa, S.; Suzui, N.; Ito-Tanabata, S.; Ishii, S.; Igura, M.; Abe, T.; Kuramata, M.; Kawachi, N.; Fujimaki, S. Real-time imaging and analysis of differences in cadmium dynamics in rice cultivars (Oryza sativa) using positron-emitting 107Cd trace. BMC Plant Biol. 2011, 11, 172.

39. Yokosho, K.; Yamaji, N.; Ueno, D.; Mitani, N.; Ma, J.F. OsFRDL1 is a citrate transporter required for efficient transformation of iron in rice. Plant Physiol. 2009, 149, 297–305.

40. Kawabe, S.; Fukumorita, T.; Chino, M. Collection of rice phloem sap from stylets of homopterous insects severed by YAG laser. Plant Cell Physiol. 1980, 21, 1319–1327.

41. Nishiyama, R. Zinc Transport via Phloem in Rice Plants. Master thesis, Graduate School of Agricultural and Life Sciences, the University of Tokyo, Tokyo, Japan, 2006.

42. Kato, M. The University of Tokyo, Tokyo, 2006. Unpublished work.

43. Nishiyama, R.; Kato, M.; Nagata, S.; Yanagisawa, S.; Yoneyama, T. Identification of Zn-nicotianamine and Fe-2′-deoxymugineic acid in the phloem sap from rice plants (Oryza sativa L.). Plant Cell Physiol.2012, 53, 381–390.

44. Kato, M.; Ishikawa, S.; Inagaki, K.; Chiba, K.; Hayashi, H.; Yanagisawa, S.; Yoneyama, T. 2010: Possible chemical forms of cadmium and varietal differences in cadmium concentrations in the phloem sap of rice plants (Oryza sativa L.). Soil Sci. Plant Nutr. 2010, 56, 839–847.

45. Álvarez-Fernández, A.; Díaz-Benito, P.; Abadía, A.; Lopez-Millán, A.-F.; Abadía, J. 2014: Metal species involved in long distance metal transport in plants. Front. Plant Sci. 2014, 5, 105.

46. Ando, Y.; Nagata, S.; Yanagisawa, S.; Yoneyama, T. Copper in xylem and phloem from rice (Oryza sativa): The effect of moderate copper concentrations in the growth medium on the accumulation of five essential metals and a speciation analysis of copper-containing compounds. Funct. Plant Biol.2013, 40, 89–100.

47. Obata, H.; Kitagishi, K. Longitudinal distribution pattern of zinc and manganese in leaf with special reference to aging. Jpn. J. Soil Sci. Plant Nutr. 1980, 51, 285–291.

48. Kitagishi, K.; Obata, H.; Kondo, T. Effect of zinc deficiency on 80S ribosome content of meristematic tissues of rice plant. Soil Sci. Plant Nutr. 1987, 33, 423–429.

49. Obata, H.; Kitagishi, K. Accumulation and retranslocation of zinc in a leaf of rice plant with reference to aging. Jpn. J. Soil Sci. Plant Nutr. 1982, 53, 235–240.

50. Kitagishi, K.; Obata, H. Retrieval of zinc from transpiration stream in the nodes of rice plants as affected by the concentration of zinc in culture solution. Rep. Environ. Sci. Mie Univ. 1982, 7, 91–97.

51. Yamaguchi, N.; Ishikawa, S.; Abe, T.; Baba, K.; Arao, T.; Terada, Y. Role of the node in controlling traffic of cadmium, zinc, and manganese in rice. J. Exp. Bot. 2012, 63, 2729–2737.

52. Kitagishi, K.; Obata, H. Distribution of 115mCd in rice plants absorbed by roots at vegetative stage.Rep. Environ. Sci. Mie Univ. 1979, 4, 59–65.

53. Kobayashi, N.I.; Tanoi, K.; Hirose, A.; Nakanishi, T.M. Characterization of rapid intervascular transport of cadmium in

rice stem by radioisotope imaging. J. Exp. Bot. 2013, 64, 507–517.

54. Tsukamoto, T.; Nakanishi, H.; Uchida, H.; Watanabe, S.; Matsuhashi, S.; Mori, S.; Nishizawa, N.K. 2009: 52Fe translocation in barley as monitored by a positron emitting tracer imaging system (PETIS): Evidence for the direct translocation of Fe from roots to young leaves via phloem. Plant Cell Physiol.2009, 50, 48–57.

55. Yoneyama, T.; Gosho, T.; Kato, M.; Goto, S.; Hayashi, H. Xylem and phloem transport of Cd, Zn and Fe into the grains of rice plants (Oryza sativa L.) grown in continuously flooded Cd-contaminated soil.Soil Sci. Plant Nutr. 2010, 56, 445–453.

56. Zee, S.-Y. Transfer cells and vascular tissue distribution in the vegetative nodes of rice. Aust. J. Bot.1972, 20, 41–48.

57. Kawahara, H.; Chonan, N.; Matsuda, T. Studies on morphogenesis in rice plants. 7. The morphology of vascular bundles in the vegetative nodes of the culm. Proc. Crop Sci. Soc. Jpn. 1974, 43, 389–401.

58. Chonan, N.; Kawahara, H.; Matsuda, T. Ultrastructure of elliptical and diffuse bundles in the vegetative nodes of rice. Jpn. J. Crop Sci. 1984, 54, 393–402.

59. Wu, C.-Y.; Lu, L.-L.; Yang, X.-E.; Feng, Y.; Wei, Y.-Y.; Hao, H.-L.; Stoffella, P.J.; He, Z.-L. Uptake, translocation, and remobilization of zinc absorbed at different growth stages by rice genotypes of different Zn densities. J. Agric. Food Chem. 2010, 58, 6767–6773.

60. Nishiyama, R.; Tanoi, K.; Yanagisawa, S.; Yoneyama, T. 2013: Quantification of zinc transport to the grain in rice plants (Oryza sativa L.) at early grain-filling by a combination of mathematical modeling and 65Zn tracing. Soil Sci. Plant Nutr. 2013, 59, 750–755.

61. Tanaka, K.; Fujimaki, S.; Fujiwara, T.; Yoneyama, T.; Hayashi, H. Quantitative estimation of the contribution of the phloem in cadmium transport to grains in rice plants (Oryza sativa L.). Soil Sci. Plant Nutr. 2007, 53, 72–77.

62. Rodda, M.S.; Li, G.; Reid, R.J. The timing of grain Cd accumulation in rice plants: The relative importance of remobilization within the plant and root Cd uptake post-flowering. Plant Soil 2011, 347, 105–114.

63. Fujimaki, S.; Suzui, N.; Ishioka, N.S.; Kawachi, N.; Ito, S.; Chino, M.; Nakamura, S. Tracing cadmium from culture to spikelet: Noninvasive imaging and quantitative characterization of absorption, transport, and accumulation of cadmium in an intact rice plant. Plant Physiol. 2010, 152, 1796–1806.

64. Zee, S.-Y. Vascular tissue and transfer cell distribution in the rice spikelet. Aust. J. Biol. Sci. 1972, 25, 411–414.

65. Kawahara, H.; Matsuda, T.; Chonan, N. Studies on morphogenesis in rice plants. 9. On the structure of vascular bundles and phloem transport in the spikelet. Proc. Crop Sci. Soc. Jpn. 1977, 46, 82–90.

66. Herren, T.; Feller, U. Transfer of zinc from xylem to phloem in the peduncle of wheat. J. Plant Nutr.1994, 17, 1587–1598.

67. Jiang, W.; Struik, P.C.; Lingna, J.; van Keulen, H.; Ming, Z.; Stomph, T.J. Uptake and distribution of root-applied or foliar-applied 65Zn after flowering in aerobic rice. Ann. Appl. Biol. 2007, 150, 383–391.

68. Sperotto, P.A.; Ricachenevsky, F.K.; Waldow, V.A.; Fett, J.P. Iron biofortification in rice: It's a long way to the top. Plant Sci. 2012, 190, 24–39.

69. Moritsugu, M. A study on combination of glutelin with cadmium in rice grain. Ber. Obara Inst. Landwirtsch. Biol. 1964, 12, 251–260.

70. Schuler, M.; Rellán-Álvarez, R.; Fink-Straube, C.; Abadía, J.; Bauer, P. Nicotianamine functions in the phloem-based transport of iron to sink organs in pollen development and pollen tube growth inArabidopsis. Plant Cell 2012, 24, 2380–2400.

71. Yuan, L.; Wu, L.; Yang, C.; Lv, Q. Effects of iron and zinc foliar applications on rice plants and their grain accumulation and grain quality. J. Sci. Food Agric. 2012, 93, 254–261.

72. Ishimaru, Y.; Kim, S.; Tsukamoto, T.; Oki, H.; Kobayashi, T.; Watanabe, S.; Matsuhashi, S.; Takahashi, M.; Nakanishi, H.; Mori, S.; et al. Mutational reconstructed ferric chelate reductase confers enhanced tolerance in rice to iron deficiency in calcareous soil. Proc. Natl. Acad. Sci. USA 2007, 104, 7373–7378.

73. Masuda, H.; Usuda, K.; Kobayashi, T.; Ishimaru, Y.; Kakei, Y.; Takahashi, M.; Higuchi, K.; Nakanishi, H.; Mori, S.; Nishizawa, K.N. Overexpression of the barley nicotianamine synthase gene

HvHAS1increases iron and zinc concentrations in rice grains. Rice 2009, 2, 155–166.

74. Lee, S.; Jeon, U.S.; Lee, S.J.; Kim, Y.-K.; Persson, D.P.; Husted, S.; Schjørring, J.K.; Kakei, Y.; Masuda, H.; Nishizawa, N.K.; et al. Iron fortification of rice seeds through activation of the nicotianamine synthase gene. Proc. Nat. Acad. Sci. USA 2009, 106, 22014–22019.

75. Zheng, L.; Cheng, Z.; Ai, C.; Jiang, X.; Bei, X.; Zheng, Y.; Glahn, R.P.; Welch, R.M.; Miller, D.D.; Lei, X.G.; et al. Nicotianamine, a novel enhancer of rice iron bioavailability to humans. PLoS ONE 2010, 5, e10190.

76. Reeves, P.G.; Chaney, R.L. Bioavailability as an issue in risk assessment and management of food cadmium: A review. Sci. Total Environ. 2008, 398, 13–19.

77. Codex Alimentarius (2014) CODEX STAN 193–1995, General Standard for Contaminants and Toxins in Food and Feed. 1995. Available online: http://www.codexalimentarius.org/download/standards/17/CXS_193e2015.pdf (accessed on 31 March 2015).

10

# ANALYSIS OF METAL ELEMENT DISTRIBUTIONS IN RICE (*ORYZA SATIVA* L.) SEEDS AND RELOCATION DURING GERMINATION BASED ON X-RAY

**Fluorescence Imaging of Zn, Fe, K, Ca, and Mn**

[1] MOE Key Lab of Environmental Remediation and Ecosystem Health, College of Environmental and Resources Science, Zhejiang University, Hangzhou, China

**Abstract**

Knowledge of mineral localization within rice grains is important for understanding the role of different elements in seed development, as well as for facilitating biofortification of seed micronutrients in order to enhance seeds' values in human diets. In this study, the concentrations of minerals in whole rice grains, hulls, brown rice, bran and polished rice were quantified by inductively coupled plasma mass spectroscopy. The in vivo mineral distribution patterns in rice grains and shifts in those distribution patterns during progressive stages of germination were analyzed by synchrotron X-ray microfluorescence. The results showed that half of the total Zn, two thirds of the total Fe, and most of the total K, Ca and Mn were removed by the milling process if the hull and bran were thoroughly polished. Concentrations of all elements were high in the embryo regions even though the local distributions within the embryo varied between elements. Mobilization of the minerals from specific seed locations during germination was also element-specific.

High mobilization of K and Ca from grains to growing roots and leaf primordia was observed; the flux of Zn to these expanding tissues was somewhat less than that of K and Ca; the mobilization of Mn or Fe was relatively low, at least during the first few days of germination

## INTRODUCTION

Micronutrient deficiencies, particularly those involving iron (Fe) and zinc (Zn), are the most prevalent deficiency-related health disorders in the world [1], [2]. Low micronutrient densities in staple foods are generally the major reasons for human micronutrient malnutrition in developing countries [3], [4], [5], [6], [7]. Therefore, biofortification of micronutrient contents in staple foods through agronomic or genetic approaches has attracted increasing interest during the past decades [3], [4], [7], [8]. Rice (*Oryza sativa*L.) is the most important food crop in the world, providing over 21% of the calory intake needs of the world's population and up to 76% for the population of South East Asia [9]. Thus, the enhancement of rice grain micronutrient contents is viewed to be an important goal as part of global strategies for improving the nutritional quality of human diets.

The ability of cereals to supply dietary micronutrients largely depends on their concentrations and bioavailability in the grain. Distribution patterns of micronutrients within the grains are important because a considerable portion of the whole grain generally is removed and lost during processing (milling) before consumption [10] and mineral concentrations often decrease from the outer bran layers toward the endosperm[4]. For instance, in rice grains the mineral elements are highly concentrated in the outer layers [11], with rice bran containing 61% of the total grain mineral fraction [12]. However, most studies of mineral element compartmentation in rice grains have relied on bulk analysis, thus they do not provide detailed information on the distribution of the mineral elements in the different parts of the whole grain [8], [11], [12]. An *in vivo*imaging of mineral elements localization in rice grains should provide clearer indications of possible strategies controlling the bioavailability of important mineral elements (e.g., Zn and Fe) for human health.

Efficient mineral accumulation in seeds is essential for normal germination and establishment of the next vegetative rice plant generation [13]. For instance, Fe demand is high during the reproduction phase of the rice life cycle [14], and the nutrients stored in seed structures are mobilized during germination, suggesting that mineral elements are crucial for seed germination [15]. However, few reports described the details of the mineral element fluxes into the new, growing and differentiating seedling cells and tissues. Thus, a second aim of this study is to describe the germination-associated movements of individual mineral elements from their sites of accumulation in mature rice seeds into seedling plants.

However, the visualization of elements in plant tissues is not readily carried out; the concentrations of micronutrient elements often are quite low and the commonly used methods such as chemical imaging (e.g., [8], [16] generally lack sufficient sensitivity and/or resolution. Trace element analysis requires a technique that has detection limits as low as a few micrograms per gram. Synchrotron-based X-ray microfluorescence (μ-XRF) is a suitable tool for investigating the localization of mineral elements in cells and tissues due to its characteristics of high resolution and sensitivity [17], [18]. For example, μ-XRF has been used to investigate differential metal distribution patterns in wild-type and hyperaccumulating genotypes of *Sedum alfredii* [19], [20], [21]. Recently, spatial unloading of As within grains was also investigated by using SXRF microtomography[22]. In the present study, we used the sensitive μ-XRF technique for analysis of nutritionally relevant metals in different tissues of rice grains and the mobilization of these elements from seeds into developing rice seedling tissues in the early stages of germination.

# MATERIALS AND METHODS

## Plant Materials

The seeds of rice IR68144, kindly supplied by Dr. Glenn Gregorio, the International Rice Research Institute (Manila, The Philippines), were used for this study. IR68144 is a high Zn and Fe density genotype, Fe and Zn in the unpolished rice grains of IR68144 was about 18 and 37 mg $kg^{-1}$, respectively [23]. The seeds of IR68144 were recultivated in a greenhouse, southern China, with standard cultivation practice until harvest.

## Elemental Analysis

Rice grains were dehusked using a roller sheller (Model JLGJ4.5, Taizhou Grain Industry Instrument Corp, Zhejiang Province, China) and damaged kernels were removed with tweezers. A subset of the brown rice kernels was subsequently milled into polished rice and rice bran, the latter consists of aleurone layer plus embryo, using a JNMJ3 rice polisher (Taizhou Grain Industry Instrument Corp, Zhejiang Province,

China). All the rice grains-derived samples (grains, brown rice, bran and polished rice) were milled into powder with a mixer mill (Retsch MM301, German) and oven-dried at 65°C for 72 h. Dried powders (0.1 g) were digested with 4.0 mL of $HNO_3$ (reagent grade) and 1.0 mL of $H_2O_2$ (30%, analytical reagent, Beijing Chemical Works, China) in a screw cap polypropylene sample tube (Corning Incorporated, Corning, NY, USA) using a Hot Block Digestion System (Model SC154, Environmental Express, Mt. Pleasant, SC, USA). The duration of heat digestion is of 0.5 h at 80°C, and 2 h at 125°C. Each digest then was transferred to a 20 ml volumetric flask, made up to volume by water and filtered. The concentrations of elements in the samples (i.e., Ca, Mn, Fe, Zn, and K) were determined using inductively coupled plasma mass spectrometry (ICP-MS; Agilent 7500a, Agilent Technologies, Palo Alto, CA, USA), Standard Reference Materials 1568[a] Rice Flour (National Institute of Staandards & Technology) containing Ca, Fe, K, Mg, Na, Mn, and Zn etc. was used, and the recovery of the elements was 90.2%~108.4% of the certified value during the ICP-MS analysis. All materials were determined in four replicates.

## μ-XRF

### *Sample preparation*

Seeds were grown on agar plates without nutrients, and harvested at 12 h or 48 h after sowing. The rice seeds with or without germination were cut with a cryotome (LEICA, CM1850) into about 200-μm sections at a temperature of −20°C. Briefly, grain samples were frozen using liquid nitrogen, and fixed immediately onto specimen disks using deionized water on a actively cooled (−40°C) specimen quick freezing shelf. The grains were first fractured with the blade longitudinally to obtain a flat surface, by which the grains were then refixed on the specimen disks for final sectioning. The two-step process is important for prevention of seed fracture and pulverization. Sections in good conditions were selected and freeze-dried (−20°C for 3 d).

### *μ-XRF analysis*

Imaging of the distribution of elements (Zn, Fe, K, Ca, and Mn) was carried out using Synchrotron-based X-ray microfluorescence at Beamline 15 U (BL15U), Shanghai Synchrotron Radiation Facility (SSRF), China. The electron energy in the storage ring was 3.5 GeV with a current range from 200 to 300(5) mA. The brilliance of the beam in BL15U was $0.5\times10^{12}$ photons/s/mm$^2$/mrad$^2$/0.1%BW. The microfocused beam of 3.5 μm was provided by a Kirkpatrick-Baez mirror pair (Xradia Inc.) with the sample at 45° to the incident X-ray beam. The fluorescence yield was detected using a 7-element Si (Li) solid state detector, positioned at 90° to the beam line. Dwell time per point was 0.5 s. The step size was set to 10 μm. Scanning areas of the samples were selected and observed using a microscope. BL15U saves full XRF spectrum data at each pixel. Elemental distributions are achieved by windowing on the elements of interest in the XRF spectra. The windows can be applied during data collection or during data analysis since the full XRF spectrum is saved for each pixel. The beam energy was set to 13 Kev during mapping. The fluorescence energies windowed for this investigation were Zn, Fe, K, Ca, and Mn. The fluorescence data are presented as color maps, and pixel brightness is displayed in RGB, with the brightest spots corresponding to the highest element fluorescence.

### Statistical Analysis

All data were statistically analyzed using SPSS (Version 12.0). The figures were made using the software Origin 8.0.

## RESULTS

### Total Concentrations of Minerals in Different Fractions of Rice Grains

The concentrations of Zn, Fe, K, Ca and Mn were determined in different parts of rice grains after separation of whole grains into hulls and brown rice, and then milling the brown rice into bran and polished rice. The polished rice fraction is essentially the rice grain endosperm,and the bran contains most of the embryo and aleurone layer. As shown in Figure 1, the relative concentrations of Zn, Fe and K in the different grain fractions were: bran > hull > whole grain > brown rice > polished rice, whereas the relative concentrations of Mn and Ca were in the order: hull > bran > whole grain > brown rice > polished rice. The whole rice grain was essentially composed of hull, bran (embryo + aleurone layer) and polished rice (endosperm). The concentration of each of these elements in the polished rice (endosperm) was lower than that of the corresponding hull and bran (embryo + aleurone layer). The bran Zn concentration was 3 times the concentrations in the hull and polished rice. Variations in the other elemental concentrations in the different rice fractions were even higher than those for Zn. The Fe and K concentrations in the bran were 7 and 32 times their concentrations in polished rice, respectively. Likewise, the concentrations of Ca and Mn in the hull and bran were 14.3- to 38.5-fold higher than those in the polished rice.

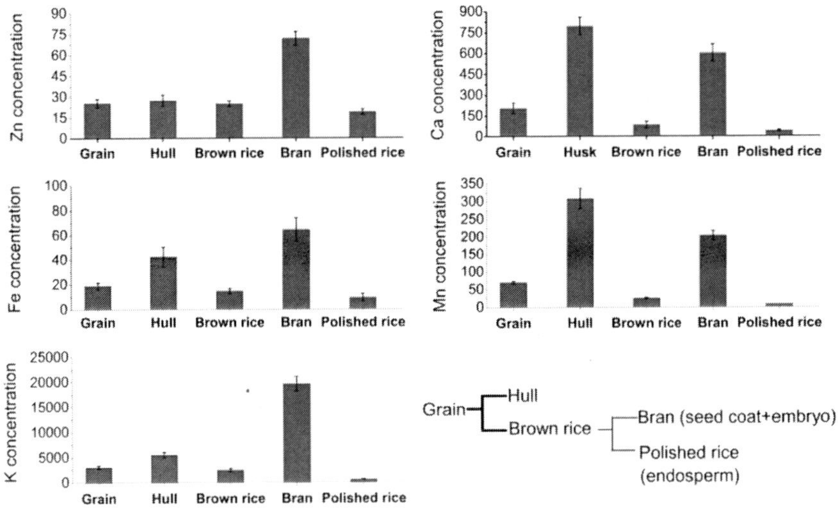


**Figure 1.** Elemental concentrations of rice grains, hull, brown rice, bran, and polished rice.

The percentage distributions of the individual elements (Zn, Fe, K, Ca, and Mn) in the the three rice grain fractions were calculated according to the elemental concentrations and the corresponding weights of the fractions. The average weight percentage for hull, bran and polished rice was 17.9%, 8.3% and 73.8% of the total whole grain weight, respectively (data not shown) and the calculated percentage distributions are shown in Figure 2. More than half of the total Zn presented in the polished rice (endosperm), while Fe was relatively evenly distributed in the hull, bran and polished rice. The element K was preferentially distributed to the bran, followed by the hull, with least in the polished rice. Both Ca and Mn were mainly located in the hull, of 63.8% and 70.8%, respectively. Only 14% of the total Ca and 7% of the total Mn remained in the polished rice.

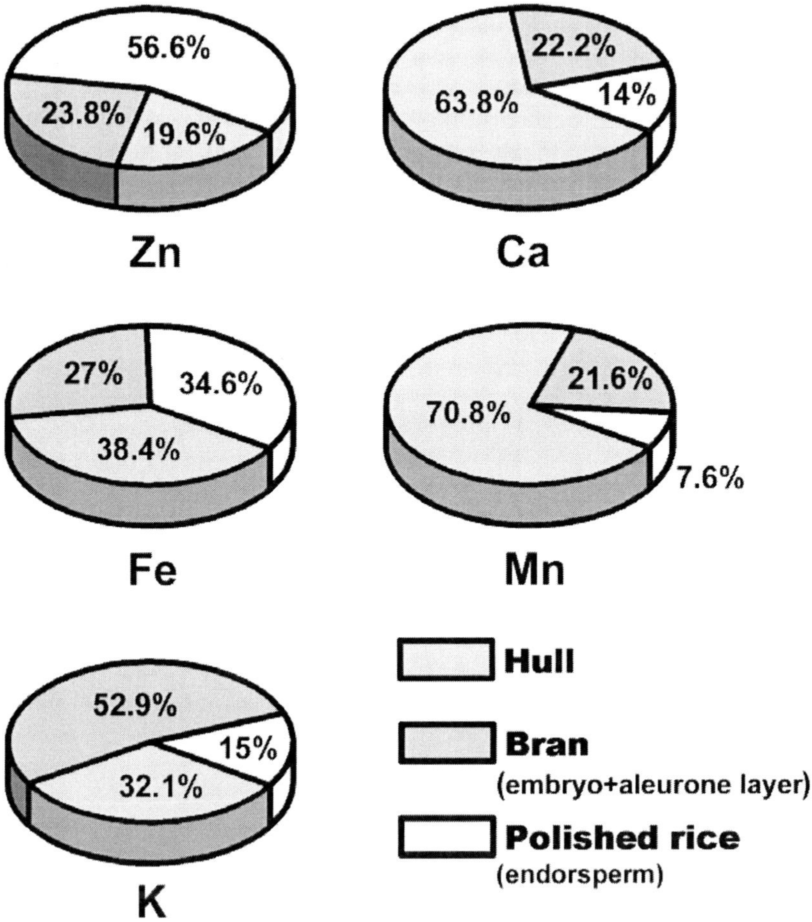


**Figure 2.** Percentage distributions of Zn, Fe, K, Ca, and Mn in different fractions of rice grains.

### In vivo Spatial Imaging of Minerals Distributions in Rice Grains

To investigate the distribution of mineral nutrients in rice grains, micro XRF mapping was performed. The X-ray fluorescence spectrum from a scanning point on the embryo of a rice grain showed clear peaks for K, Ca, Mn, Fe, Cu, and Zn (Fig. 3). The integrated intensity for each element was calculated from the spectrum and normalized by the intensity of the Compton scattering peak. Elemental mapping for the measurement area was obtained from the normalized intensity for each element. The elemental distribution maps of Zn, Fe, K, Ca, and Mn in the scanned areas of different regions of rice grains are presented in Figure 4, together with photographs taken using an optical microscope. Each map indicates the relative distribution of a specific element, and the scales of fluorescence counts vary for each map. The quantitation of the fluorescence yields was normalized by I0 and the dwell time. The normalized X-ray fluorescence intensities were scaled to different color brightness for individual elements, with the brightest spots corresponding to the highest elemental fluorescence.

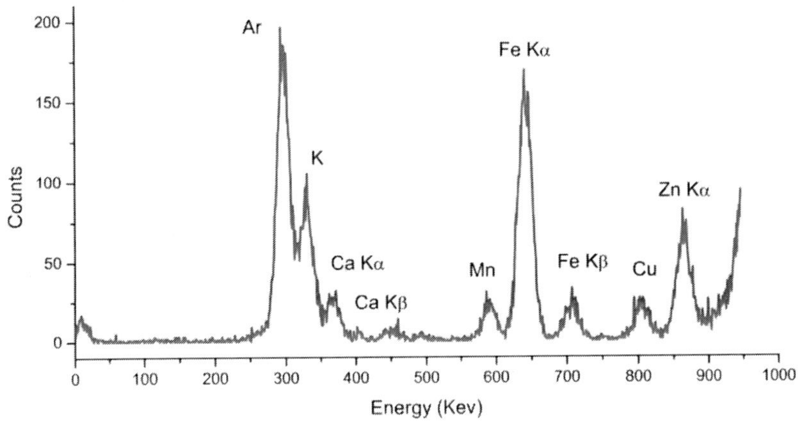


**Figure 3.** Typical synchrotron radiation X-ray fluorescence (SR-XRF) microprobe spectrum in an embryo localized scanning point of rice grain.

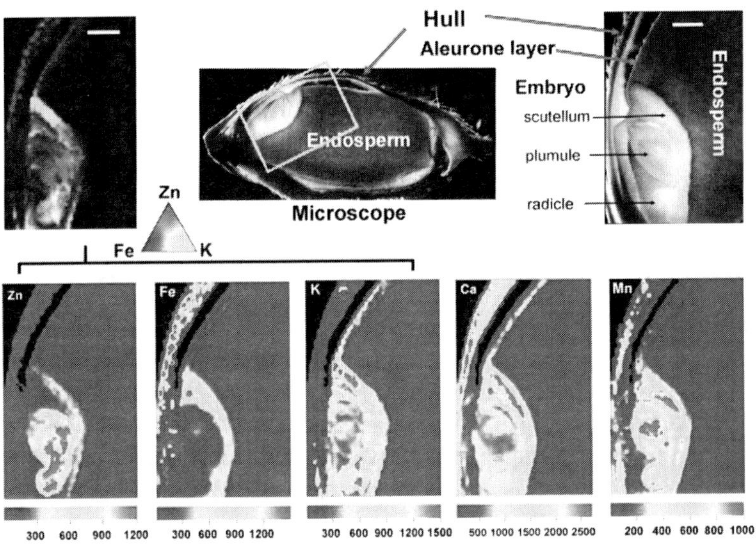


**Figure 4.** μ-XRF elemental maps for Zn, Fe, K, Ca, and Mn in rice grains.

As shown in Figure 4, the *in vivo* scanning maps for Zn, Fe, K, Ca, and Mn in the longitudinal section of the rice grain are consistent with the quantitative elemental distribution results from the ICP-MS analysis. Although the general accumulation of the different mineral elements was low in the endosperm, the distribution patterns varied considerably in the other parts of the rice grain. Concentrations of all the elements were high in the embryo regions even though the local distributions within the different parts of the embryo varied. Zinc was mainly found in the central parts of the embryo (the plumule and radicle), whereas the highest intensity of Fe was observed in the scutellum of embryo and hull, followed by the aleurone layer and the other parts of the embryo. Potassium was highly concentrated in the embryo, particularly in the scutellum. The merged color image for Zn (red), Fe (blue) and K (green) clearly shows the significant differences in their relative distribution patterns within the embryo. Calcium was preferentially distributed to the hull and scutellum, while Mn was mainly localized to the hull and the embryo, the latter including its radicle, plumule and scutellum.

Mobilization of Seed-accumulated Metals during Germination

Changes in the seed distribution patterns of each element at 12 h and 48 h after germination were determined. The changes in element distribution differed for the different elements monitored (Figs. 5 and and6).6). For Zn, Fe, Ca and Mn, the highest concentrations were observed in the rachilla, the short, sterile stem-like structure that bore the spikelets and now remains as part of the hull. However, the greatest concentration of K was in the radicle and plumule regions of the embryo, a localization that is most obvious at 48 h post germination (Fig. 6) when the root and shoot have begun to elongate. Mobilization of Zn, Fe, Ca and Mn to the elongating seedling organs was relatively low at 48 h. While there appeared to be relatively little accumulation of Fe, Zn and Mn in the elongating radical, these elements did accumulate in the elongating shoot tissues. However, there was a clear mobilization of Ca to the radicle, although the movement of Ca into the elongating shoot tissues was greater.

# DISCUSSION

The rice grain consists of four major tissues: the hull, embryo, aleurone layer, and starchy endosperm. The endosperm is the most important grain fraction with respect to human nutrition, as it is the part of the grain primarily consumed in many countries. However, the bulk analysis of mineral element contents in different sections of rice grains (Fig. 1), which agrees well with the more tissue location-specific μ-XRF mapping (Fig. 4), shows very low levels of mineral elements in the endosperm, with considerably more Zn, Fe, K, Ca, and Mn in the embryo, aleurone layer and hull tissues. Taking weight percentage into account, the data for the present study show that 43% of the total Zn, 65% of the total Fe, and 85%~92% of the total K, Ca and Mn were removed by the milling process if the hull and bran tissues (embryo + aleurone layer) were thoroughly removed from the endosperm fraction during polishing (Fig. 2). This is consistent with the previous study on distribution of mineral elements in three different rice cultivars [11]. Thus the removal of husk, embryo and aleurone layer during dehusking and polishing substantially reduces the mineral nutrient value of rice grains. Rice bran has been recognized as an extremely valuable source for nutrients due to its high contents of lipid, protein, vitamin, minerals, and dietary fiber [24]. The present study, therefore, supports the idea that brown rice or germinated brown rice is preferable from a health perspective because it contains more nutritional mineral components than polished rice [25]. It is recently reported that germinated brown

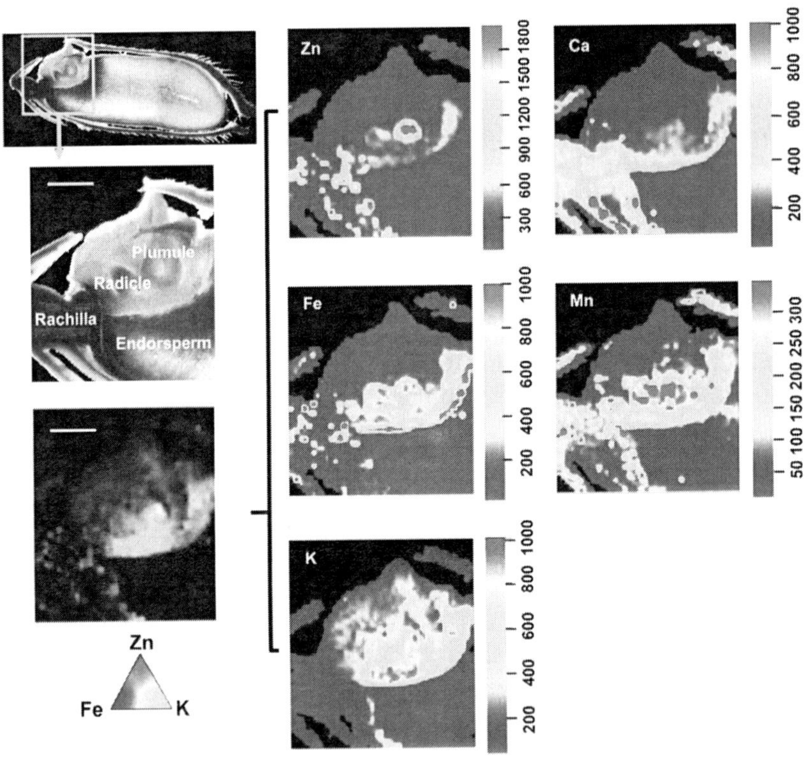


**Figure 5.** μ-XRF elemental maps of rice grains after germination for 12 h.

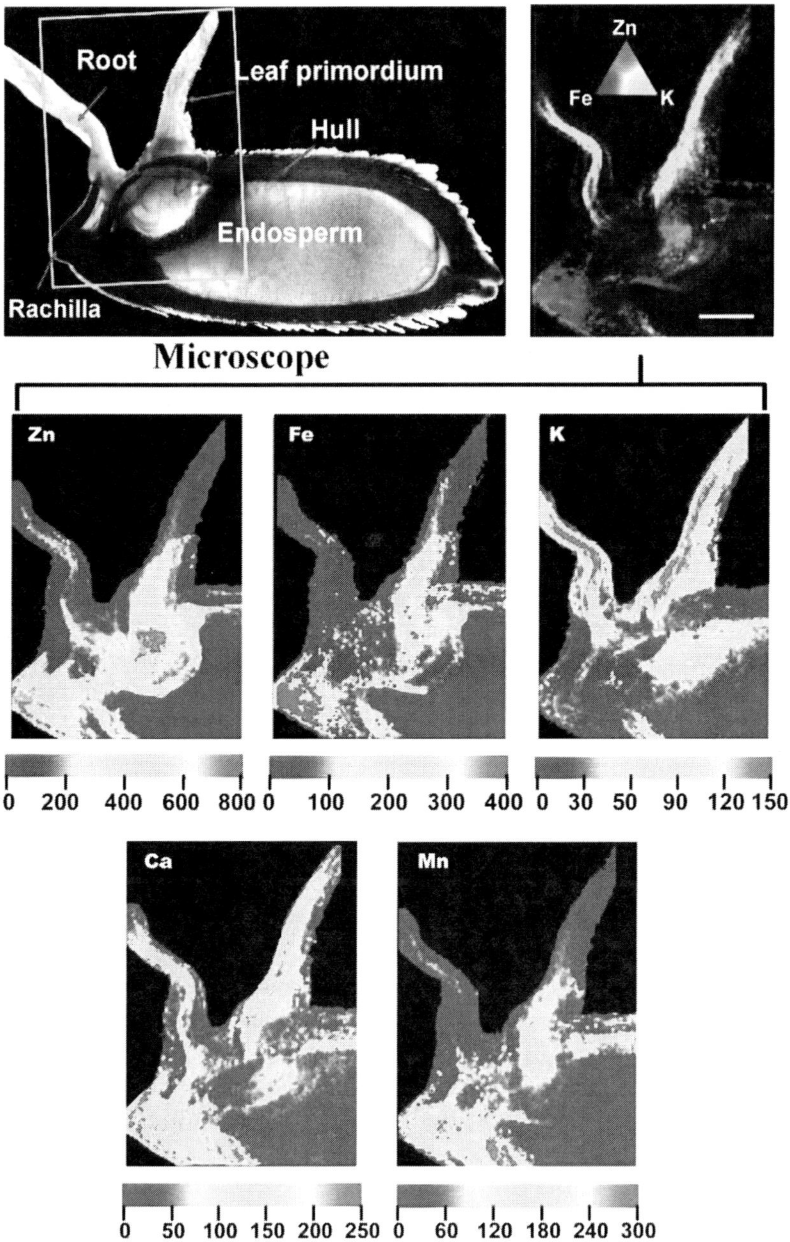


**Figure 6**. µ-XRF elemental maps of early stage rice seedlings after seed germination for 48

rice has become one of the most interesting rice products and gained great attention, particularly in Asian countries, for its high nutritional value [26]. However, cautions should be taken for brown rice or rice bran consumption since rice bran may also be rich in toxic elements such as arsenic [22]. If the traditional practice of eating polished rice is to be continued, our results indicate that enhancement of micronutrient import into the endosperm should have a positive impact on the "mineral nutrient health" of human populations that obtain a lot of their daily calories from cooked rice. If that is so, our data further suggest that the continuing examination of the mechanisms that influence the transfer of mineral elements into the developing maternal tissues and their subsequent accumulation would be a much more important goal than simply increasing the mineral content of whole mature, harvested rice grains. At this time, however, knowledge of the mechanisms involved in mobilization of minerals into the different seed tissues during grain filling is limited.

The filial tissues (aleurone, endosperm, and embryo) of the rice caryopsis are generally isolated from the maternal tissues (e.g., rachilla, hull) by the absence of symplastic continuity [14] or direct vascular connections. For minerals to enter the filial tissues, several transport steps are required. These are, at a minimum: (1) phloem unloading into maternal tissues (i.e., ovule integuments that will develop into the seed coats, and nucellus), (2) efflux from the maternal seed coat cells into the apoplast surrounding the developing fertilized embryo sac, and (3) uptake into the filial tissues [14]. The results from the bulk analysis and μ-XRF mapping in this study showed that mineral nutrients were preferentially localized in the hull (Figs. 1, ,4)4) and rachilla (Fig. 6) except for K and Zn. These observations support the conclusion that the maternal seed tissues are the first mineral storage sites during grain fill. Filling of the seeds is reported to occur through unloading from the phloem into the nucellar tissue followed by uploading into the aleurone layer, and transport into the endosperm [27]. The region of the ovular vascular trace presents on the ventral side of the ovary, which contains both phloem and xylem cells, is the point of entry into the filial tissue (the aleurone and the endosperm) for minerals [22], [27]. Elemental distributions in the outer bran layers are generally not uniform, but largely concentrated in the ovular vascular trace as reported previously [22]. This could also be observed from the images shown in the present study (Figs. 5 and and6).6). Dynamic changes in the distribution of minerals during rice seed development has been reported recently, but the role of OVT has not been determined [28]. Further studies of the transfer of nutrients into the filial tissues are necessarily involve imaging the ovular vascular trace by using transverse sections of grains. Inside the filial tissues of rice grains, our results showed that the minerals were preferentially localized to the embryo and/or aleurone layer (Fig. 4), resulting in higher concentrations of mineral elements present in the bran fraction compared with the polished rice (Fig. 2). The aleurone, which contains phytic acid rich granules, is thought to be a storage reservoir of positively charged metals such as Ca, Mg, K, Zn, and Fe, presumably for support of processes essential for seed germination and growth [29]. It has been reported that metals accumulate preferentially in the protein-rich aleurone and embryo tissues [30]. The embryo, the next generation, is the most important structure in seeds. Thus, from the perspective of the seed's energy economy, it is probably more efficient to store mineral elements needed for enzyme functions, harvesting of light energy, maintenance of turgor as cells grow etc. in the embryo than to use energy for moving these elements from storage locations in the endosperm. Storage of these elements in the endosperm might also expedite the initiation of germination once the appropriate environmental conditions are detected. The μ-XRF mapping data (Fig. 4) support the conclusion that the key mineral nutrients are embryo tissue-localized.

While the embryo represents a high-density site for minerals accumulation, these mineral elements had largely non-overlapping regions of localization within the various regions of the embryo (Fig. 4). In the rice grain embryo, Zn was largely restricted to the plumule and radicle, whereas K, Fe, and Mn were preferentially localized to the scutellum. Distinct locations of elements such as Fe, Mn, and Zn have been observed in embryos of barley grains [10] and Arabidopsis seeds [31], with Fe in provascular strands, Mn on the abaxial sides of the cotyledons, and Zn distributed broadly throughout the embryo. Recently, a confocal 3D μ-XRF spectrometer was applied to rice grains, providing elemental maps for K, Ca, and Fe at different depths in the embryo, these maps indicated different element concentrations at different depths [32]. These distinct distributions of mineral elements possibly result from their various usages during seed germination and growth.

In the present study, we examined changes in the distributions of Zn, Fe, K, Ca, and Mn after the initiation of rice seed germination (Figs. 5 and and6),6), presumably suggesting locations in the embryo tissues where the elements had germination-specific roles to play[33]. During germination the observed shifting patterns of mineral distribution suggested different cellular capacities for element mobilization, as follows: K>Ca>Zn>Mn>Fe (Figs. 5, ,6).6). High concentrations of K and Ca in the newly developed roots and leaf primordium during seed germination were observed (Fig. 6). Both K and Ca are essential plant macronutrients and are of high requirement for proper growth and reproduction of plants. Potassium has an important role in the activation of many growth related enzymes, may be important for allowing growing cells to maintain a turgor pressure in excess of the cell wall yield threshold, and is generally of high mobility in plants. Higher viability and vigor of seeds soaked in K solution has been reported [34]. It is thus not surprising that high remobilization of K occurs during rice seed germination to assure growth of the soil and light-seeking axes. Rapid movement of Ca to the new growing tissues during rice germination, however, contrasts with the general understanding that Ca mobility is relatively limited in plants. Calcium is an important element involved in cell wall structure and cell growth, as well as a central regulator of plant cell signaling [35], serving as an important second messenger involved in signal transduction of many phytohormones, including abscisic acid, which regulates many aspects of plant development including seed germination and seedling growth [36]. The high remobilization of Ca during rice seed germination stage that is inferred from the data in Figures 5 and and6,6, suggests a large requirement of Ca for efficient uses in the highly metabolically active differentiating cells. Zinc is also highly mobile during rice germination, and may be utilized in protein synthesis and functions, membrane structure and functions, gene expression and oxidative stress tolerance in the new growing tissues [16], [37]. Preferential distribution of Zn in the central parts of plumule and radicle suggests a critical role of Zn in either the meristemmatic and/or vascular tissue, which occupy the central axis of these structures. During seed germination, the transport of Zn may be required for a high level of meristemmatic activities. Relatively low remobilization of Fe and Mn were observed in rice grains during germination (Fig. 6). One of possible reasons for the low level of Fe redistribution may be the vacuolar sequestration of the element. Free Fe in the cell prompts the formation of excess reactive oxygen species, which cause damage to subcellular organelles. Fe is stored in vacuoles until it is needed, close to the site of assimilation. The vacuolar storage of Fe in Arabidopsis seeds, mediated by a vasuolar membrane transporter VIT1, is critical for seedling development [31]. Recent studies also showed that functional disruption of vacuolar membrane transporters OsVIT1 and OsVIT2, which highly expressed in flag leaf blade and sheath, leads to increased Fe accumulation in rice seeds[38]. During germination, Fe is required for respiration, and its release from storage vacuoles may occur as a result of a genetic signal that causes upregulation of Fe export proteins such as NRAMP3, which located on the vacuolar membrane to move the metal out of the vacuole for use [39].

Knowledge on these preferential elemental constitutions of the different grain tissues and their remobilization patterns during germination makes the possibility of designing target products with nutritionally optimal constitution more feasible. The result may also be useful in order to optimize various germination procedures (both processes and management strategies) of edible seeds, in order to enhance the nutritional quality of food mixtures based on coarse cereals [40], [41]. However, at present much more work is needed for a better understanding of the important roles of minerals involved in the rice seed development and seed germination.

## ACKNOWLEDGMENTS

This research was carried out at the Shanghai Synchrotron Radiation Facility (SSRF), China. The authors thank all stuff at BL15U, SSRF for technical assistance.

## FUNDING STATEMENT

The work was supported by Normal project from the National Natural Science Foundation of China (30900921, 31000935), and the Fundamental Research Funds for the Central Universities (2012FZA6008). The funders had no role in study design, data collection and analysis, decision to publish, or preparation of the manuscript.

## REFERENCES

1. WHO (2006) Micronutrient deficiencies: Iron deficiency anaemia. Available:http://www.who.int/nutrition/topics/ida/en/index.html
2. WHO (2001) Iron deficiency anaemia: assessment, prevention and control. A guide for programme managers.
3. Cakmak I (2008) Enrichment of cereal grains with zinc: Agronomic or genetic biofortification? Plant and Soil 302: 1–17
4. Cakmak I (2009) Enrichment of fertilizers with zinc: An excellent investment for humanity and crop production in India. Journal of Trace Elements in Medicine and Biology 23: 281–289

5. Gibson RS (2006) Zinc: the missing link in combating micronutrient malnutrition in developing countries. Proceedings of the Nutrition Society 65: 51–60

6. Welch RM, Graham RD (1999) A new paradigm for world agriculture: meeting human needs - Productive, sustainable, nutritious. Field Crops Research 60: 1–10

7. Welch RM, Graham RD (2004) Breeding for micronutrients in staple food crops from a human nutrition perspective. Journal of Experimental Botany 55: 353–364

8. Cakmak I, Kalayci M, Kaya Y, Torun AA, Aydin N, et al. (2010) Biofortification and localization of zinc in wheat grain. Journal of Agricultural and Food Chemistry 58: 9092–9102

9. Fitzgerald MA, McCouch SR, Hall RD (2009) Not just a grain of rice: the quest for quality. Cell 14: 133–139

10. Lombi E, Smith E, Hansen TH, Paterson D, de Jonge MD, et al. (2011) Megapixel imaging of (micro)nutrients in mature barley grains. Journal of Experimental Botany 62: 273–282

11. Wang KM, Wu JG, Li G, Zhang DP, Yang ZW, et al. (2011) Distribution of phytic acid and mineral elements in three indica rice (Oryza sativa L.) cultivars. Journal of Cereal Science 54: 116–121

12. Lamberts L, De Bie E, Vandeputte GE, Veraverbeke WS, Derycke V, et al. (2007)Effect of milling on colour and nutritional properties of rice. Food Chemistry 100: 1496–1503

13. Kranner I, Colville L (2011) Metals and seeds: Biochemical and molecular implications and their significance for seed germination. Environmental and Experimental Botany 72: 93–105

14. Walker EL, Waters BM (2011) The role of transition metal homeostasis in plant seed development. Current Opinion in Plant Biology 14: 318–324

15. Takahashi M, Nozoye T, Kitajima N, Fukuda N, Hokura A, et al. (2009) In vivo analysis of metal distribution and expression of metal transporters in rice seed during germination process by microarray and X-ray Fluorescence Imaging of Fe, Zn, Mn, and Cu. Plant and Soil 325: 39–51

16. Ozturk L, Yazici MA, Yucel C, Torun A, Cekic C, et al. (2006) Concentration and localization of zinc during seed development and germination in wheat. Physiologia Plantarum 128: 144–152

17. West M, Ellis AT, Kregsamer P, Potts PJ, Streli C, et al. (2007) Atomic spectrometry update. X-ray fluorescence spectrometry. Journal of Analytical Atomic Spectrometry 22: 1304–1332

18. Punshon T, Guerinot ML, Lanzirotti A (2009) Using synchrotron X-ray fluorescence microprobes in the study of metal homeostasis in plants. Annals of Botany 103: 665–672

19. Tian SK, Lu LL, Labavitch J, Yang XE, He ZL, et al. (2011) Cellular sequestration of cadmium in the hyperaccumulator plant species Sedum alfredii. Plant Physiology 157: 1914–1925

20. Tian SK, Lu LL, Yang XE, Labavitch JM, Huang YY, et al. (2009) Stem and leaf sequestration of zinc at the cellular level in the hyperaccumulator Sedum alfredii. New Phytologist 182: 116–126

21. Tian SK, Lu LL, Yang XE, Webb SM, Du YH, et al. (2010) Spatial imaging and speciation of lead in the accumulator plant Sedum alfredii by microscopically focused synchrotron X-ray investigation. Environmental Science & Technology 44: 5920–5926

22. Carey A-M, Norton GJ, Deacon C, Scheckel KG, Lombi E, et al. (2011) Phloem transport of arsenic species from flag leaf to grain during grain filling. New Phytologist192: 87–98

23. Sellappan K, Datta K, Parkhi V, Datta SK (2009) Rice caryopsis structure in relation to distribution of micronutrients (iron, zinc, beta-carotene) of rice cultivars including transgenic indica rice. Plant Science (Amsterdam, Netherlands) 177: 557–562

24. Sun G-X, Lu X, Williams PN, Zhu Y-G (2010) Distribution and translocation of selenium from soil to grain and its speciation in paddy rice (Oryza sativa L.).Environmental Science & Technology 44: 6706–6711

25. Wei YY, Shohag MJI, Wang YY, Lu LL, Wu CY, et al.. (2012) Effect of zinc sulfate fortification in germinated brown rice on seed zinc concentration, bioavailability, and seed germination. Journal of Agricultural and Food Chemistry: dx.

26. Patil SB, Khan MK (2011) Germinated brown rice as a value added rice product: A review. Journal of Food Science and Technology-Mysore 48: 661–667

27. Krishnan S, Dayanandan P (2003) Structural and histochemical studies on grain-filling in the caryopsis of rice (Oryza sativa L.). Journal of Biosciences 28: 455–469

28. Iwai T, Takahashi M, Oda K, Terada Y, Yoshida KT (2012) Dynamic changes in the distribution of minerals in relation to phytic acid accumulation during rice seed development. Plant Physiology 160: 2007–2014

29. Meharg AA, Lombi E, Williams PN, Scheckel KG, Feldmann J, et al. (2008)Speciation and localization of arsenic in white and brown rice grains. Environmental Science & Technology 42: 1051–1057

30. Lombi E, Scheckel KG, Pallon J, Carey AM, Zhu YG, et al. (2009) Speciation and distribution of arsenic and localization of nutrients in rice grains. New Phytologist 184: 193–201

31. Kim SA, Punshon T, Lanzirotti A, Li LT, Alonso JM, et al. (2006) Localization of iron in Arabidopsis seed requires the vacuolar membrane transporter VIT1. Science 314: 1295–1298

32. Nakano K, Tsuji K (2006) Development of confocal 3D micro XRF spectrometer and its application to rice grain. Bunseki Kagaku 55: 427–432

33. Ishimaru Y, Bashir K, Nishizawa NK (2011) Zn uptake and translocation in rice plants. Rice 4: 21–27

34. Bam RK, Kumaga FK, Ofori K, Asiedu EA (2006) Germination, vigour and dehydrogenase activity of naturally aged rice (Oryza sativa L.) seeds soaked in potassium and phosphorus salts. Asian Journal of Plant Sciences 5: 948–955

35. Hepler PK (2005) Calcium: A central regulator of plant growth and development.Plant Cell 17: 2142–2155

36. Zhao R, Sun HL, Mei C, Wang XJ, Yan L, et al. (2011) The Arabidopsis Ca(2+)-dependent protein kinase CPK12 negatively regulates abscisic acid signaling in seed germination and post-germination growth. New Phytologist 192: 61–73

37. Cakmak I (2000) Possible roles of zinc in protecting plant cells from damage by reactive oxygen species. New Phytologist 146: 185–205

38. Zhang Y, Xu Y-H, Yi H-Y, Gong J-M (2012) Vacuolar membrane transporters OsVIT1 and OsVIT2 modulate iron translocation between flag leaves and seeds in rice.Plant Journal 72: 400–410

39. Thomine S, Lelievre F, Debarbieux E, Schroeder JI, Barbier-Brygoo H (2003)AtNRAMP3, a multispecific vacuolar metal transporter involved in plant responses to iron deficiency. Plant Journal 34: 685–695

40. Arora S, Jood S, Khetarpaul N (2010) Effect of germination and probiotic fermentation on nutrient composition of barley based food mixtures. Food Chemistry 119: 779–784

41. Omary MB, Fong C, Rothschild J, Finney P (2012) Effects of germination on the nutritional profile of gluten-free cereals and pseudocereals: a review. Cereal Chemistry 89: 1–14

# 11

# CALCIUM SUPPLEMENTATION IMPROVES $NA^+/K^+$ RATIO, ANTIOXIDANT DEFENSE AND GLYOXALASE SYSTEMS IN SALT-STRESSED RICE SEEDLINGS

**Anisur Rahman,[1,2] Kamrun Nahar,[1,3] Mirza Hasanuzzaman,[2,*] and Masayuki Fujita[1]**

*Shabir Hussain Wani, Sher-e-Kashmir University of Agricultural Sciences and Technology, India*

*Sergey Shabala, University of Tasmania, Australia; Rohit Joshi, International Center for Genetic Engineering and Biotechnology, India*

**Abstract**

The present study investigates the regulatory role of exogenous calcium (Ca) in developing salt stress tolerance in rice seedlings. Hydroponically grown 13-day-old rice (Oryza sativa L. cv. BRRI dhan47) seedlings were exposed to 200 mM NaCl alone and combined with 2 mM CaCl2 and 2 mM ethylene glycol tetraacetic acid (EGTA, a Ca scavenger) for 3 days. The salt stress caused growth inhibition, chlorosis and water shortage in the rice seedlings. The salt-induced stress disrupted ion homeostasis through Na+ influx and K+ efflux, and decreased other mineral nutrient uptake. Salt stress caused oxidative stress in seedlings through lipid peroxidation, loss of plasma membrane integrity, higher reactive oxygen species (ROS) production and methylglyoxal (MG) formation. The salt-stressed seedlings supplemented with exogenous Ca recovered from water loss, chlorosis and growth inhibition. Calcium supplementation in the salt-stressed rice seedlings improved ion homeostasis by inhibition of Na+ influx and K+ leakage. Exogenous Ca also improved ROS and MG detoxification by improving the antioxidant defense and glyoxalase systems, respectively. On the other hand, applying EGTA along with salt and Ca again negatively affected the seedlings as EGTA negated Ca activity. It confirms that, the positive responses in salt-stressed rice seedlings to exogenous Ca were for Ca mediated improvement of ion homeostasis, antioxidant defense and glyoxalase system**Keywords:** calcium, methylglyoxal, nutrient homeostasis, osmotic stress, oxidative stress, salinity

## INTRODUCTION

Gradual changes in climate challenges crop production through various abiotic stresses, which become major constraints to crop production due to the unpredictable and complex nature of the environment (Mittler and Blumwald, 2010). Of the environmental factors, salinity is one of the most devastating abiotic stresses because most crop plants are sensitive to salt stress (Hasanuzzaman et al., 2013). Around 20% of irrigated land has been affected by salinity (Pitman and Lauchli, 2002), and it is estimated that salt stress will cause up to 50% loss of cultivable land in the middle of the 21st century (Mahajan and Tuteja, 2005). Plants exposed to higher levels of salinity are affected by both hyperionic and hyperosmotic stress through accumulating $Na^+$ and $Cl^-$ which causes membrane damage, nutrient imbalance, enzymatic inhibition, metabolic dysfunction, photosynthesis inhibition, and hampers other major physiological and biochemical processes that ultimately leads to growth inhibition or death of the plant (Mahajan and Tuteja, 2005;Ahmad and Sharma, 2008; Munns and Tester, 2008; Hasanuzzaman et al., 2012). Higher levels of salt in plant growth medium decrease $K^+$ content and increase $Na^+$ uptake as $Na^+$ causes $K^+$ efflux and triggers K leakage from plant cells. With higher levels of NaCl, Na displaces Ca from membranes, which also increases intracellular Na. As a result, under salt-stress conditions Na content exceeds that of K, resulting in a higher Na/K ratio as well as nutrient imbalance (Cramer et al., 1985; Shabala et al., 2006; Wu and Wang, 2012). In addition, salinity disrupts the antioxidant defense system through overproduction of reactive oxygen species (ROS) including singlet oxygen ($^1O_2$), superoxide radical ($O_2^{\bullet -}$), hydrogen peroxide ($H_2O_2$), and hydroxyl radicals ($OH^\bullet$), which consequently results in oxidative stress (Hasanuzzaman et al., 2013; Mishra et al., 2013). Moreover, salinity accelerates the generation of cytotoxic methylglyoxal (MG) through the glycolysis pathway and causes oxidative damage through degradation of protein synthesis (Yadav et al., 2005; Hasanuzzaman et al., 2014).

Ionic and osmotic homeostasis and ROS and MG detoxification are salt-stress tolerance mechanisms in plants (Wu and Wang, 2012; Nahar et al., 2015a). Some plants produce proline (Pro) or other compatible solutes to maintain the water relationship and stabilize protein and enzyme complexes for ionic and osmotic homeostasis (Iqbal et al., 2015;Reddy et al., 2015). On the other hand, plants normally scavenge over-produced ROS by using non-enzymatic antioxidants (ascorbic acid, AsA; glutathione, GSH; phenolic compounds; alkaloids; non-protein amino acids; and α-tocopherols) and enzymatic antioxidants (superoxide dismutase, SOD; catalase, CAT; ascorbate peroxidase, APX; glutathione reductase, GR; monodehydroascorbate reductase, MDHAR; dehydroascorbate reductase, DHAR; glutathione peroxidase, GPX; and glutathione *S*-transferase, GST; Pang and Wang, 2008; Gill and Tuteja, 2010; Hasanuzzaman et al., 2012). Detoxification of salt-induced overproduced ROS is also maintained by the antioxidant system (Anjum et al., 2014). The salt-induced higher production of MG is detoxified by the glyoxalase system, where the glyoxalase I (Gly I) and glyoxalase II (Gly II) enzymes act together with GSH (Yadav et al., 2005; Nahar et al., 2015a).

Improving ion homeostasis and regulating both the antioxidant and glyoxalase systems are necessary to develop salt-stress tolerance (Hasanuzzaman et al., 2011; Wu and Wang, 2012; Nahar et al., 2015b; Wutipraditkul et al., 2015). As an essential macronutrient, calcium (Ca) plays important roles including stabilizing cell walls and membranes, improving the metabolic processes of other nutrients, regulating enzymatic and hormonal processes, and other essential functions. Calcium also acts as a secondary messenger that mediates many aspects of cell and plant development, as well as the stress-resistance response (White and Broadley, 2003; Jaleel et al., 2007a; Jaleel and Azooz, 2009). In addition, Ca can ameliorate salt-induced $Na^+$ toxicity by blocking non-selective cation channel (NSCC) which are the major pathway of $Na^+$ influx in plant (Demidchik and Tester, 2002; Shabala et al., 2006). Furthermore, supplemental Ca inhibits $K^+$ efflux resulted from $Na^+$-induced plasma membrane depolarization (Cramer et al., 1985; Shabala et al., 2003; Tester and Davenport, 2003; Jaleel et al., 2007b; Shabala and Pottosin, 2014). Moreover, several studies have also revealed that exogenous application of Ca in plant growth medium helps to develop abiotic-stress tolerance by maintaining ion homeostasis (Wu and Wang, 2012), enhancing the antioxidant defense system and other physiological and biochemical attributes (Manivannan et al., 2007; Talukdar, 2012; Srivastava et al., 2014; Ahmad et al., 2015). Considering the above, this research was conducted to investigate maintaining the $Na^+/K^+$ ratio, and the antioxidant defense and glyoxalase systems with Ca supplementation in salt-affected rice seedlings. To the best of our knowledge, this study is the first on Ca-induced salt-stress tolerance through improving ion homeostasis and the antioxidant defense and glyoxalase systems in rice.

## MATERIALS AND METHODS

### Plant Materials and Treatments

Rice (*Oryza sativa* L. cv. BRRI dhan47) seeds were surface sterilized with 70% ethanol for 8–10 min followed by washing several times with sterilized distilled water and soaked in distilled water in a dark place for 48 h. The imbibed seeds were then sown on plastic nets floating on distilled water in 250 ml plastic beakers and kept in the dark at 28 ± 2°C for 72 h. Uniformly germinated seeds were then transferred to a growth chamber (light, 350 μmol photon $m^{-2}$ $s^{-1}$; temperature, 25 ± 2°C; relative humidity, 65–70%) with the same pot providing a diluted (5000 times) commercial hydroponics nutrient solution (Hyponex, Japan). The nutrient solution contained 8% N, 6.43% P, 20.94% K, 11.8% Ca, 3.08% Mg, 0.07% B, 0.24% Fe, 0.03% Mn, 0.0014% Mo, 0.008% Zn, and 0.003% Cu. The nutrient solutions were renewed twice a week. Each pot contained approximately 60 seedlings. Thirteen-day-old rice seedlings were exposed to salt stress (200 mM NaCl) in presence and absence of exogenous Ca (2 mM $CaCl_2$) with nutrient solution to verify the role of Ca under salt-stress conditions. We also applied the Ca scavenger ethylene glycol tetraacetic acid ($C_{14}H_{24}N_2O_{10}$; EGTA; Ammoaghaie and Moghym, 2011) together with NaCl+$CaCl_2$ and alone to determine the role of Ca under salt stress conditions. Control plants were grown in Hyponex solution only. Therefore, our experiment consisted of six treatments as follows: control, 2 mM $CaCl_2$ (Ca), 2 mM EGTA (EGTA), 200 mM NaCl (Salt), 200 mM NaCl+2 mM $CaCl_2$ (Salt+Ca), and 200 mM NaCl+2 mM $CaCl_2$+2 mM EGTA (Salt+Ca+EGTA). The experiment was repeated three times under the same conditions. Data were taken after 3 days of treatment.

### Observation of Salt Toxicity Symptoms and Seedling Growth

Seedling growth and salt toxicity symptoms in rice seedlings were determined by careful observation and measuring fresh weight (FW) and dry weight (DW). For DW, seedlings were oven dried at 70°C for 48 h. Fresh weight and DW were expressed as mg $seedling^{-1}$. Plant height was measured from the base of shoot up to the tip of the longest leaf.

### Determination of Leaf Relative Water Content

Leaf relative water content (RWC) was measured according to Barrs and Weatherley (1962). Leaf laminas were weighed (FW), then placed immediately between two layers of filter paper and immersed in distilled water in a Petri dish for 24 h in a dark place. Turgid weight (TW) was measured after gently removing excess water with a paper towel. Dry weight was measured after 48 h oven drying at 70°C. Finally, RWC was determined using the following formula:

$$RWC\,(\%) = (FW - DW)/(TW - DW) \times 100$$

Determination of Na and Mineral Nutrient Content

Sodium, Ca, and other mineral nutrient content were determined by using an atomic absorption spectrophotometer (Hitachi Z-5000; Hitachi, Japan). Plant samples were oven dried at 70°C for 48 h. The dried samples from the roots and shoots (0.1 g) were ground and digested separately with acid mixture at 70°C for 48 h. The acid mixture consisted of $HNO_3$:$HClO_4$ (5:1 v/v).

### Determination of Chlorophyll Content

Chlorophyll (chl) content was measured according to Arnon (1949) by homogenizing leaf samples (0.5 g) with 10 ml of acetone (80% v/v) followed by centrifuging at 9,000×*g* for 10 min. Absorbance was measured with a UV-vis spectrophotometer at 663 and 645 nm for chl *a* and chl *b* content, respectively. Carotenoid content was also measured spectrophotometrically at wave length 470 nm.

### Determination of Proline Content

Proline content was determined according to Bates et al. (1973). Leaf samples (0.5 g) were homogenized in 5 ml 3% sulfo-salicylic acid and the homogenate was centrifuged at 11,500×*g* for 12 min. Supernatant (1 ml) was mixed with 1 ml glacial acetic acid and 1 ml acid ninhydrin. After 1 h incubation at 100°C, the mixture was cooled. The developed color was extracted with 2 ml toluene and the optical density of the chromophore was observed spectrophotometrically at 520 nm. Proline content was determined by comparing with a standard curve of known concentration of Pro.

### Histochemical Detection of ROS Markers and Membrane Damage

Localization of $O_2^{\bullet -}$ in leaves was detected following Chen et al. (2010) with a slight modification. Leaves were immersed in 0.1%

Nitroblue tetrazolium chloride (NBT) solution and incubated at 25°C (temperature) for incubation. After 12 h, the incubated leaves were immersed in boiling ethanol (90%) for 15 min to decolorize the leaves and to show the dark blue spots produced by the reaction of NBT and $O_2^{\bullet -}$.

Localization of $H_2O_2$ was detected according to the method of Thordal-Christensen et al. (1997) with a minor modification. Leaves were incubated at 25°C in a solution containing 1 mg $ml^{-1}$ 3′,3′-diaminobenzidine (DAB) prepared in HCl acidified (pH 3.8) water. After 12 h of incubation, the leaves were boiled in ethanol (90%) for 15 min to show the reddish brown spots produced by the reaction of $H_2O_2$ and DAB.

Lipid peroxidation in the roots was determined by histochemical staining using Schiff's reagent with a modification of Srivastava et al. (2014). Lipid peroxidation-originated aldehydes were detected after 30 min staining, indicated by pink–red color. The stained roots were rinsed with sulphite solution (0.5% [w/v] $K_2S_2O_5$ in 0.05 M HCl) and dipped in the same solution for 10 min to retain the stained color. The loss of plasma membrane integrity in the roots was measured by histochemical staining using 0.25% aqueous Evan's blue solution with a slight modification of Schützendübel et al. (2001). After 40 min, the roots were rinsed with distilled water and membrane damage was revealed using glycerin.

## Determination of Lipid Peroxidation and Hydrogen Peroxide Levels

The level of lipid peroxidation was measured by estimating malondialdehyde (MDA) following the method of Heath and Packer (1968). Malondialdehyde content was measured by observing the difference in absorbance at 532 nm using an extinction coefficient of 155 $mM^{-1}cm^{-1}$ and expressed as nmol of MDA $g^{-1}$ FW. Hydrogen peroxide content was determined according to Yu et al. (2003) by observing the absorbance at 410 nm using an extinction coefficient of 0.28 $\mu M^{-1}$ $cm^{-1}$.

## Determination of Methylglyoxal Content

Methylglyoxal was measured following the method of Wild et al. (2012) by extracting plant samples in 5% perchloric acid. After centrifuging homogenized leaf tissues at 11,000×*g* for 10 min, the supernatant was decolorized by adding charcoal. The decolorized supernatant was neutralized by adding saturated sodium carbonate and used to estimate MG by adding sodium dihydrogen phosphate and *N*-acetyl-L-cysteine to a final volume of 1 ml. The absorbance was recorded after 10 min at 288 nm and MG content was calculated using a standard curve of known concentration of MG.

### Determination of Ascorbate and Glutathione Redox

Rice leaves (0.5 g) were homogenized in 3 ml ice-cold 5% meta-phosphoric acid containing 1 mM EDTA using a mortar and pestle. The homogenates were centrifuged at 11,500×*g* for 15 min at 4°C and the collected supernatants were used according to the method of Dutilleul et al. (2003) with minor modifications to determine total and reduced AsA. After neutralizing the supernatant with 0.5 M potassium-phosphate (K-P) buffer (pH 7.0), the oxidized fraction was reduced with 0.1 M dithiothreitol. Total and reduced AsA content were assayed spectrophotometrically at 265 nm in 100 mM K-P buffer (pH 7.0) with 1.0 U of ascorbate oxidase (AO). To calculate ascorbate, a specific standard curve of AsA was used. Dehydroascorbate (DHA) was measured using the formula DHA = total AsA – reduced AsA. Reduced glutathione (GSH), oxidized glutathione or glutathione disulfide (GSSG), and total glutathione (GSH + GSSG) were determined according toGriffiths (1980) based on enzymatic recycling. GSH was measured using the formula GSH = Total GSH - GSSG. Glutathione was removed by 2-vinylpyridine derivatization to determine GSSG.

### Determination of Protein

Protein concentration was measured according to Bradford (1976) using bovine serum albumin (BSA) as a protein standard.

### Enzyme Extraction and Assays

Rice leaves (0.5 g) were homogenized in 50 mM ice cold K-P buffer (pH 7.0) containing 100 mM KCl, 1 mM ascorbate, 5 mM β-mercaptoethanol, and 10% (w/v) glycerol using a pre-cooled mortar and pestle. The homogenates were centrifuged two times at 11,500×*g*for 15 min and the supernatants were used to determine protein content and enzyme activity. All procedures were performed at 0–4°C.

Lipoxygenase (LOX, EC: 1.13.11.12) activity was determined according to the method ofDoderer et al. (1992) using linoleic acid as a substrate solution. The increased absorbance was observed at 234 nm and the activity was calculated using an extinction coefficient of 25 $mM^{-1}cm^{-1}$.

Ascorbate peroxidase (APX, EC: 1.11.1.11) activity was determined according to Nakano and Asada (1981) by observing the decreased absorbance at 290 nm for 1 min and using an extinction coefficient of 2.8 $mM^{-1}cm^{-1}$. The reaction buffer solution contained 50 mM K-P buffer (pH 7.0), 0.5 mM AsA, 0.1 mM $H_2O_2$, 0.1 mM EDTA, and enzyme extract.

Monodehydroascorbate reductase (MDHAR, EC: 1.6.5.4) activity was assayed by following the method of Hossain et al. (1984) using an extinction coefficient of 6.2 $mM^{-1}cm^{-1}$.

Dehydroascorbate reductase (DHAR, EC: 1.8.5.1) activity was determined according to the method of Nakano and Asada (1981) by observing the change in absorbance at 265 nm for 1 min using an extinction coefficient of 14 $mM^{-1}cm^{-1}$.

Glutathione reductase (GR, EC: 1.6.4.2) activity was determined according to the method of Foyer and Halliwell (1976) by monitoring the decreased absorbance at 340 nm and using an extinction coefficient of 6.2 $mM^{-1}cm^{-1}$. The reaction mixture solution contained 0.1 M K-P buffer (pH 7.8), 1 mM EDTA, 1 mM GSSG, 0.2 mM NADPH, and enzyme extract.

Glutathione *S*-transferase (GST, EC: 2.5.1.18) activity was measured as described byHossain et al. (2006). The activity was calculated by observing the increased absorbance at 340 nm for 1 min and using an extinction coefficient of 9.6 $mM^{-1}cm^{-1}$. The reaction mixture contained 100 mM Tris-HCl buffer (pH 6.5), 1.5 mM GSH, and 1 mM 1-chloro-2,4-dinitrobenzene (CDNB), and enzyme solution.

Glutathione peroxidase (GPX, EC: 1.11.1.9) activity was determined according to Elia et al. (2003) by monitoring the change in absorbance at 340 nm for 1 min and using an extinction coefficient of 6.62 $mM^{-1}cm^{-1}$. The reaction mixture contained 100 mM K-P buffer (pH 7.5), 1 mM EDTA, 1 mM $NaN_3$, 0.12 mM NADPH, 2 mM GSH, 1 unit GR, 0.6 mM $H_2O_2$, and enzyme solution.

Superoxide dismutase (SOD, EC: 1.15.1.1) activity was measured based on the xanthine-xanthine oxidase system following the method of El-Shabrawi et al. (2010).

Catalase (CAT, EC: 1.11.1.6) activity was measured as described by Hasanuzzaman and Fujita (2011) using an extinction coefficient of 39.4 $mM^{-1}cm^{-1}$.

Glyoxalase I (Gly I, EC: 4.4.1.5) and Glyoxalase II (Gly II, EC: 3.1.2.6) activities were determined as described by Hasanuzzaman and Fujita

(2011) using extinction coefficient of 3.37 $mM^{-1}cm^{-1}$ and 13.6 $mM^{-1}cm^{-1}$, respectively.

### Statistical Analysis

The data were subjected to analysis of variance (ANOVA) and the mean differences were compared by Fisher's LSD using XLSTAT v.2015 software (Addinsoft, 2015). Differences at $P \leq 0.05$ were considered significant.

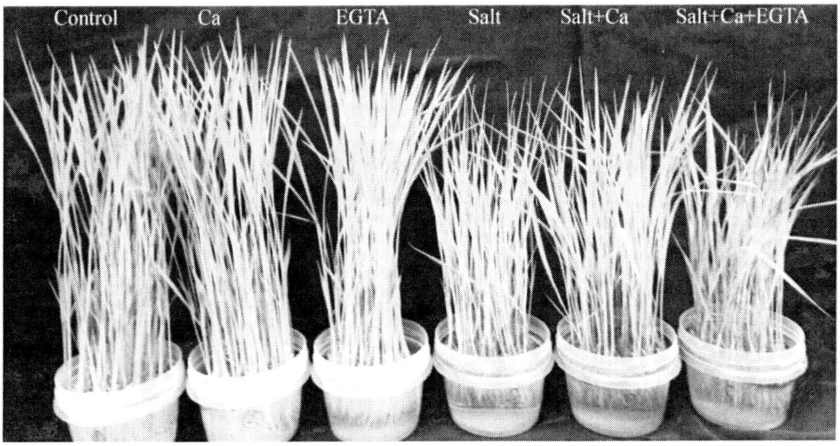


**Figure 1. Phenotypic appearance of rice seedlings under different treatments.** Here, Ca, EGTA and Salt indicate 2 mM $CaCl_2$, 2 mM EGTA, and 200 mM NaCl, respectively.

## RESULTS

### Phenotypic Appearance

Salt stress severely damaged the rice seedlings phenotypically, resulting in the rolling and burning of leaf tips and the yellowing of the whole plant. Supplementation with Ca partially reversed the salt-induced damage and improved the phenotypic appearance of the seedlings. The simultaneous application of Ca and EGTA damaged rice seedlings again phenotypically with the Salt+Ca+EGTA treatment, compared with the Salt+Ca treatment (**Figure Figure11**). However, under non-stress conditions, exogenous Ca and EGTA had no visual effect on the rice seedlings.

## Plant Growth

Salt-induced stress decreased plant growth in terms of plant height, seedling FW and DW (**Table Table11**). Supplementation with Ca to the salt-treated seedlings markedly restored plant growth compared the seedlings treated with salt alone. Applying EGTA to the Salt+Ca+EGTA treatment decreased plant growth again, which indicate that EGTA, as a Ca scavenger, negates the activity of Ca which increases plant growth. However, applying Ca and EGTA without salt stress did not affect plant growth.

**Table 1.** Effect of Ca on growth parameter, leaf relative water content (RWC) and proline content in leaf of rice seedlings under salt stress.

| Treatment | Plant height (cm) | Fresh weight (mg seedling$^{-1}$) | Dry weight (mg seedling$^{-1}$) | Leaf RWC (%) | Proline content (μmol g$^{-1}$ FW) |
|---|---|---|---|---|---|
| Control | $23.3 \pm 0.32^a$ | $151.80 \pm 9.45^a$ | $19.00 \pm 0.46^a$ | $98.37 \pm 0.66^a$ | $0.20 \pm 0.01^b$ |
| Ca | $23.16 \pm 0.24^a$ | $144.10 \pm 7.36^a$ | $18.63 \pm 0.44^a$ | $97.88 \pm 0.25^a$ | $0.21 \pm 0.02^b$ |
| EGTA | $23.26 \pm 0.19^a$ | $142.77 \pm 9.46^a$ | $18.80 \pm 0.50^a$ | $97.57 \pm 0.86^a$ | $0.21 \pm 0.02^b$ |
| Salt | $18.86 \pm 0.13^c$ | $98.33 \pm 5.82^b$ | $14.87 \pm 0.54^b$ | $79.45 \pm 1.51^c$ | $3.73 \pm 0.29^a$ |
| Salt+Ca | $20.10 \pm 0.12^b$ | $136.33 \pm 6.71^a$ | $18.50 \pm 0.78^a$ | $93.08 \pm 1.62^b$ | $0.25 \pm 0.02^b$ |
| Salt+Ca+EGTA | $18.47 \pm 0.32^c$ | $100.67 \pm 8.31^b$ | $15.97 \pm 0.99^b$ | $79.56 \pm 1.52^c$ | $3.61 \pm 0.17^a$ |

*Means (±SD) were calculated from three replicates for each treatment. Values with different letters are significantly different at $P \leq 0.05$ applying the Fisher's LSD test. Here, Ca, EGTA and salt indicate 2 mM $CaCl_2$, 2 mM EGTA, and 200 mM NaCl, respectively.*

## Leaf RWC

Salt stress significantly reduced leaf RWC of the rice seedlings, compared with the control seedlings. Exogenous application of Ca to the salt-stressed seedlings improved RWC compared with the seedlings treated with salt alone. Adding the Ca scavenger EGTA again reduced leaf RWC compared with the Salt+Ca+EGTA treatment (**Table Table11**).

## Proline Content

Treating the rice seedlings with salt considerably increased Pro content compared with the control seedlings, whereas Ca supplementation reduced Pro content compared with the seedlings treated with salt alone. However, applying Ca and EGTA without salt stress did not affect the rice seedlings (**Table Table11**).

## Photosynthetic Pigments

Rice seedlings treated with salt resulted in decreased chl *a*, chl *b*, chl (*a*+*b*) and carotenoid content by 33, 38, 34, and 38%, respectively, compared with control seedlings (**Table Table22**). Exogenous application of Ca to the salt-treated rice seedlings improved chl and carotenoid content compared with the seedlings treated with salt alone, but applying the Ca scavenger decreased chl and carotenoid content again in the Salt+Ca+EGTA treatment.

**Table 2.** Effect of Ca on chl and carotenoid contents in leaf of rice seedlings under salt stress.

| Treatment | chl *a* ($mg\ g^{-1}$ FW) | chl *b* ($mg\ g^{-1}$ FW) | chl (*a*+*b*) ($mg\ g^{-1}$ FW) | Carotenoid ($mg\ g^{-1}$ FW) |
|---|---|---|---|---|
| Control | $2.48 \pm 0.1^{a}$ | $0.73 \pm 0.03^{a}$ | $3.22 \pm 0.08^{a}$ | $0.56 \pm 0.02^{a}$ |
| Ca | $2.42 \pm 0.09^{a}$ | $0.70 \pm 0.04^{ab}$ | $3.11 \pm 0.13^{ab}$ | $0.54 \pm 0.01^{a}$ |
| EGTA | $2.42 \pm 0.1^{a}$ | $0.73 \pm 0.05^{a}$ | $3.14 \pm 0.12^{ab}$ | $0.55 \pm 0.02^{a}$ |
| Salt | $1.66 \pm 0.03^{b}$ | $0.45 \pm 0.02^{c}$ | $2.11 \pm 0.05^{c}$ | $0.35 \pm 0.02^{c}$ |
| Salt+Ca | $2.30 \pm 0.13^{a}$ | $0.66 \pm 0.02^{b}$ | $2.96 \pm 0.14^{b}$ | $0.46 \pm 0.02^{b}$ |
| Salt+Ca+EGTA | $1.71 \pm 0.13^{b}$ | $0.47 \pm 0.01^{c}$ | $2.18 \pm 0.12^{c}$ | $0.36 \pm 0.03^{c}$ |

*Means (±SD) were calculated from three replicates for each treatment. Values with different letters are significantly different at $P \leq 0.05$ applying the Fisher's LSD test. Here, Ca, EGTA and salt indicate 2 mM $CaCl_2$, 2 mM EGTA, and 200 mM NaCl, respectively.*

## $Na^+$ and $K^+$ Homeostasis

A marked increase in $Na^+$ uptake was observed in the shoots of the salt-treated rice seedlings compared with the control seedlings (**Figures 2A,D**). Exogenous Ca reduced the $Na^+$ uptake in the shoots: it was 45% lower in the Salt+Ca treatment compared with the salt-alone treatment. The Ca scavenger EGTA enhanced $Na^+$ uptake again in the Salt+Ca+EGTA treatment, which indicates that EGTA negates the activity of exogenous Ca. The $K^+$ content in the roots and shoots decreased significantly in the salt-affected rice seedlings compared with the non-stressed control seedlings. The lower $K^+$ uptake partially recovered in the Salt+Ca treatment compared with the salt-treated rice seedlings and decreased again in the Salt+Ca+EGTA treatment (**Figures 2B,E**). The ratio of $Na^+/K^+$increased in the roots and shoots in the salt-stressed seedlings and decreased with Ca supplementation (**Figures 2C,F**). However, exogenous application of Ca and EGTA together to the salt-affected seedlings increased the $Na^+/K^+$ ratio in the Salt+Ca+EGTA treatment compared with the Salt+Ca treatment. Under non-stress conditions, Ca and EGTA did not affect on $Na^+$ content, $K^+$ content or their ratio in both the roots and shoots.

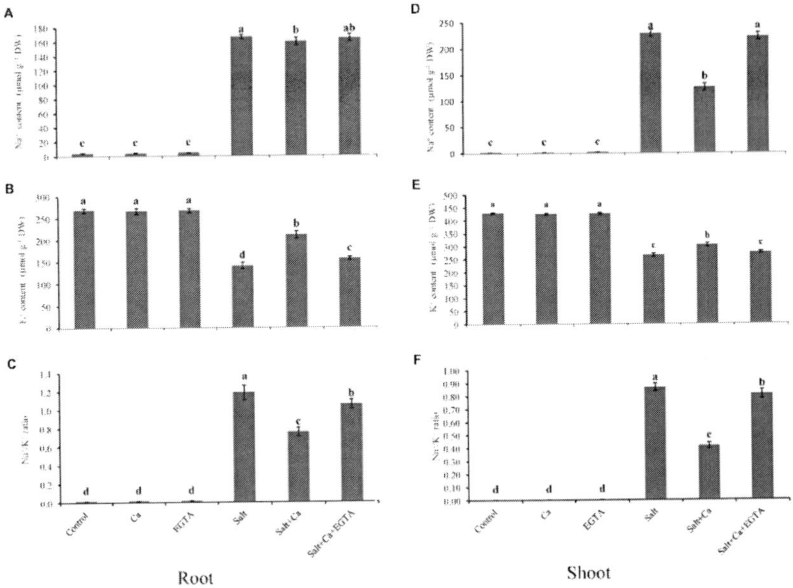


**Figure 2. Effect of Ca on $Na^+$ and $K^+$ contents and their ratio in root (A,B,C) and shoot (D,E,F) of rice seedlings under salt stress.** Here, Ca, EGTA, and Salt indicate 2 mM $CaCl_2$, 2 mM EGTA, and 200 mM NaCl, respectively. Means (±SD) were calculated from ...

## Mineral (Ca, Mg, Mn, and Zn) Nutrient Contents

In the salt-treated rice seedlings, the mineral nutrient content decreased in the roots and shoots compared with the control seedlings. The stress induced by salt decreased the Ca, Mg, Mn, and Zn content in the shoots by 29, 14, 37, and 31%, respectively, compared with the control seedlings. However, Ca supplementation increased the mineral nutrient content (except for Mn) of the shoots in the Salt+Ca treatment compared with the salt-treated rice seedlings. In contrast, the mineral nutrient content in the roots and shoots decreased again with the Salt+Ca+EGTA treatment compared with the Salt+Ca treatment (**Table Table33**). Adding exogenous Ca slightly decreased the Mn content in the roots and shoots under non-stress conditions. However, exogenous application of EGTA to the non-stress control seedlings did not affect on mineral nutrient content except for Ca, where EGTA decreased the Ca content in the roots and shoots.

**Table 3.** Effect of Ca on mineral nutrient contents of rice seedlings under salt stress.

| Treatment | Ca content (μ mol $g^{-1}$ DW) | | Mg content (μ mol $g^{-1}$ DW) | | Mn content (μ mol $g^{-1}$ DW) | | Zn content (μ mol $g^{-1}$ DW) | |
|---|---|---|---|---|---|---|---|---|
| | Root | Shoot | Root | Shoot | Root | Shoot | Root | Shoot |
| Control | $39.47 \pm 1.76^{c}$ | $131.94 \pm 5.81^{b}$ | $69.91 \pm 3.44^{a}$ | $115.17 \pm 2.79^{a}$ | $0.18 \pm 0.01^{a}$ | $0.19 \pm 0.01^{a}$ | $0.16 \pm 0.01^{a}$ | $0.19 \pm 0.01^{a}$ |
| Ca | $57.79 \pm 1.90^{a}$ | $167.51 \pm 5.54^{a}$ | $70.47 \pm 5.14^{a}$ | $113.16 \pm 2.21^{a}$ | $0.15 \pm 0.01^{b}$ | $0.17 \pm 0.01^{b}$ | $0.16 \pm 0.01^{a}$ | $0.19 \pm 0.01^{a}$ |
| EGTA | $35.61 \pm 2.29^{d}$ | $119.36 \pm 3.21^{c}$ | $69.70 \pm 1.99^{a}$ | $113.13 \pm 3.32^{a}$ | $0.18 \pm 0.01^{a}$ | $0.19 \pm 0.01^{a}$ | $0.16 \pm 0.01^{a}$ | $0.18 \pm 0.01^{a}$ |
| Salt | $36.58 \pm 1.01^{cd}$ | $93.34 \pm 2.69^{e}$ | $36.37 \pm 3.09^{d}$ | $99.48 \pm 2.55^{c}$ | $0.13 \pm 0.01^{c}$ | $0.12 \pm 0.01^{c}$ | $0.11 \pm 0.01^{c}$ | $0.13 \pm 0.01^{c}$ |
| Salt+Ca | $47.27 \pm 1.40^{b}$ | $111.57 \pm 1.23^{d}$ | $53.94 \pm 2.91^{b}$ | $108.34 \pm 1.07^{b}$ | $0.14 \pm 0.01^{c}$ | $0.16 \pm 0.01^{b}$ | $0.14 \pm 0.01^{b}$ | $0.16 \pm 0.01^{b}$ |
| Salt+Ca+EGTA | $38.61 \pm 1.71^{cd}$ | $95.56 \pm 1.21^{e}$ | $43.69 \pm 2.92^{c}$ | $102.6 \pm 1.84^{c}$ | $0.12 \pm 0.1^{c}$ | $0.12 \pm 0.01^{c}$ | $0.11 \pm 0.01^{c}$ | $0.13 \pm 0.01^{c}$ |

*Means (±SD) were calculated from three replicates for each treatment. Values with different letters are significantly different at $P \le 0.05$ applying the Fisher's LSD test. Here, Ca, EGTA and Salt indicate 2 mM $CaCl_2$, 2 mM EGTA, and 200 mM NaCl, respectively.*

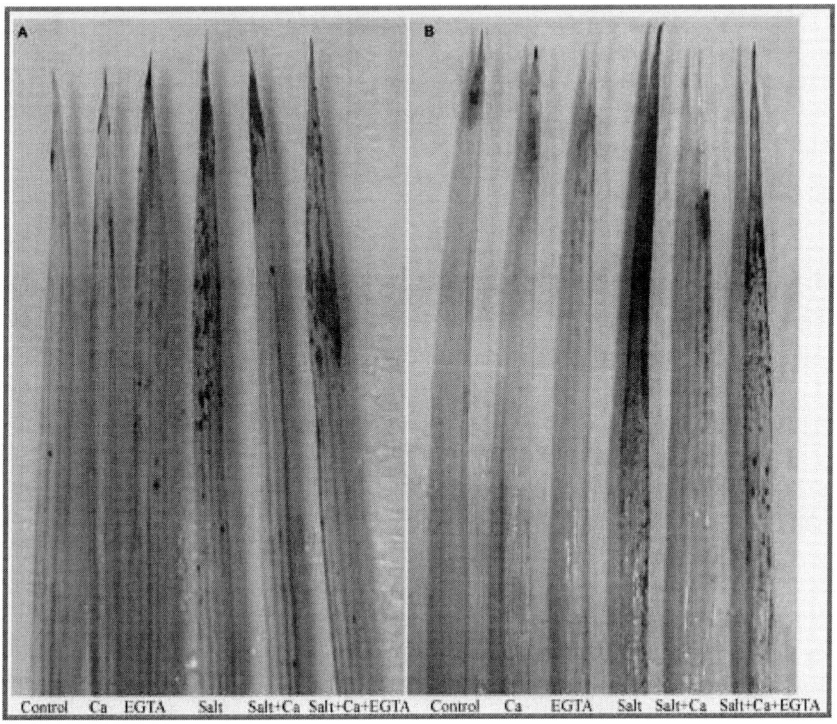


**Figure 3. Histochemical detection of $O_2^{\bullet -}$ (A) and $H_2O_2$ (B) in leaf of rice seedlings under salt stress.** Here, Ca, EGTA and Salt indicate 2 mM $CaCl_2$, 2 mM EGTA, and 200 mM NaCl, respectively.

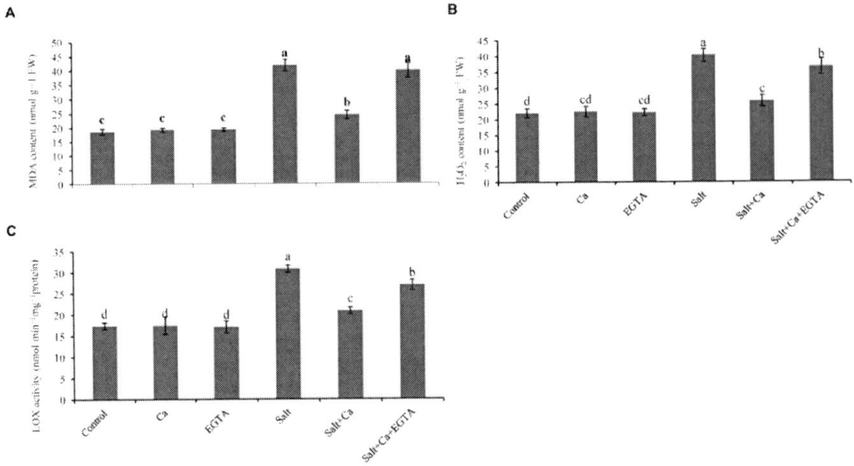


**Figure 4. Effect of Ca on lipid peroxidation (MDA content)(A), $H_2O_2$ content (B) and LOX activity (C) in leaf of rice seedlings under salt stress.** Here, Ca, EGTA and Salt indicate 2 mM $CaCl_2$, 2 mM EGTA, and 200 mM NaCl, respectively. Means (±SD) were calculated...

## ROS Generation, Lipid Peroxidation and Membrane Damage

The salt-induced stress caused overproduction of ROS in the rice seedlings. The increased ROS content resulted in oxidative damage to the rice seedlings leading to increased lipid peroxidation and cell membrane damage. Histochemical staining shows over-production of $O_2^{\bullet-}$ and $H_2O_2$ with dark blue spots and brown spots, respectively, in the salt-treated seedlings (**Figures 3A,B**). Applying Ca to the salt-treated seedlings considerably reduced the spots of $O_2^{\bullet-}$ and $H_2O_2$, compared with salt-alone treatment. Salt exposure also resulted in an increase in $H_2O_2$ level, which was 82% higher compared with the control seedlings (**Figure Figure4B4B**). Adding Ca to the salt-treated seedlings played a positive role in reducing $H_2O_2$ level. However, applying EGTA increased the production of $O_2^{\bullet-}$ (**FigureFigure3A3A**) and $H_2O_2$ (**Figures Figures3B3B** and **4B4B**) again in the Salt+Ca+EGTA treatment as EGTA negated the Ca activity.

The oxidative stress-induced lipid membrane damage was measured using lipid peroxidation in terms of MDA content in the leaves and by histochemical staining of the roots using Schiff's reagent. Membrane damage was also identified by staining the roots with Evan's blue dye and then observing plasma membrane integrity (**Figures 5A,B**). Compared with the control seedlings, a significant rise in MDA content was observed in the leaves of salt-treated rice seedlings (**Figure

**Figure4A4A**). Histochemical staining also showed higher lipid peroxidation indicated by an intense pink–red color and higher loss of plasma membrane integrity indicated by an intense dark blue color in the roots of salt-treated rice seedlings (**Figures 5A,B**). Exogenous application of Ca reduced the membrane damage, indicated by a 42% reduction in MDA content, and a reduction in the intense color formation during histochemical staining of the roots in the Salt+Ca treatment compared with the salt-treated rice seedlings. However, the Ca scavenger EGTA increased membrane damage again in the Salt+Ca+EGTA treatment compared with the Salt+Ca treatment.

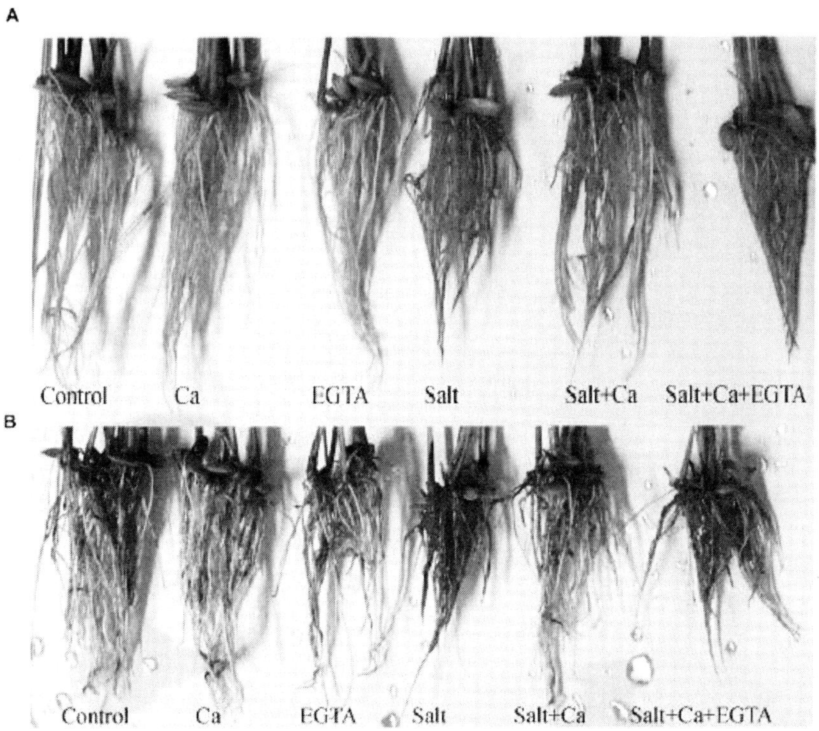


**Figure 5. Histochemical detection of lipid peroxidation (A)and loss of plasma membrane integrity (B) in root of rice seedlings under salt stress.** Here, Ca, EGTA and Salt indicate 2 mM $CaCl_2$, 2 mM EGTA, and 200 mM NaCl, respectively.

### LOX Activity

Lipoxygenase activity increased by 78% in the salt-treated rice seedlings compared with the control seedlings which were decreased with Ca supplementation (**Figure Figure4C4C**). In non-stress conditions, exogenous Ca and EGTA did not affect rice seedlings compared with the control but adding EGTA increased LOX activity again in the Salt+Ca+EGTA treatment.

### Ascorbate and Glutathione Redox System

Treatment of rice seedlings with salt decreased AsA content by 49%, which was partly improved with Ca supplementation in the Salt+Ca treatment (**Figure Figure6A6A**). Applying EGTA to the Salt+Ca+EGTA treatment decreased AsA content again. Dehydroascorbate content increased in the salt-treated rice seedlings and decreased with Ca supplementation (**Figure Figure6B6B**). The ratio of AsA/DHA decreased with salt stress which improved with Ca supplementation in salt-stressed rice seedlings. Applying EGTA in the Salt+Ca+EGTA treatment increased DHA content and decreased AsA/DHA ratio (**Figure Figure6C6C**). However, applying Ca and EGTA to the non-stressed control seedlings did not affect AsA and DHA content or their ratio.

Glutathione and GSSG content significantly increased in the salt-treated rice seedlings compared with the control seedlings (**Figures 6D,E**). The ratio of GSH/GSSG decreased by 42% in the salt-stressed rice seedlings (**Figure Figure6F6F**). Exogenous Ca reduced the GSH and GSSG content but increased the GSH/GSSG ratio in the Salt+Ca treatment compared with salt-stressed rice seedlings. Applying EGTA increased the GSSG content by 55% and decreased the GSH/GSSG ratio by 33% in the Salt+Ca+EGTA treatment compared with the Salt+Ca treatment. However, exogenous Ca and EGTA did not affect the non-stressed control seedlings (**Figures 6E,F**).

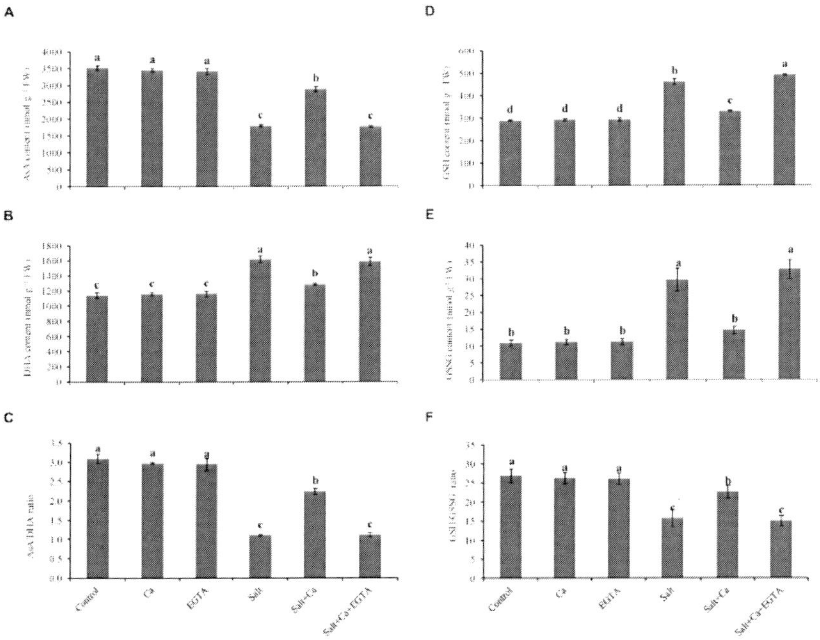


**Figure 6. Effect of Ca on AsA content (A), DHA content (B), AsA/DHA ratio (C), GSH content (D), GSSG content (E), and GSH/GSSG ratio (F) in leaf of rice seedlings under salt stress.** Here, Ca, EGTA and Salt indicate 2 mM $CaCl_2$, 2 mM EGTA, and 200 mM NaCl, respectively. ...

## Activities of Antioxidant Enzymes

Superoxide dismutase activity increased by 24% in the rice seedlings subjected to salt, compared with control. Calcium supplementation further increased SOD activity by 20% in the Salt+Ca treatment compared with the salt-treated rice seedlings. Compared with the Salt+Ca treatment, applying EGTA decreased SOD activity in the Salt+Ca+EGTA treatment. However, in non-stress conditions, exogenous application of Ca and EGTA did not affect SOD activity (**Figure Figure7C7C**).

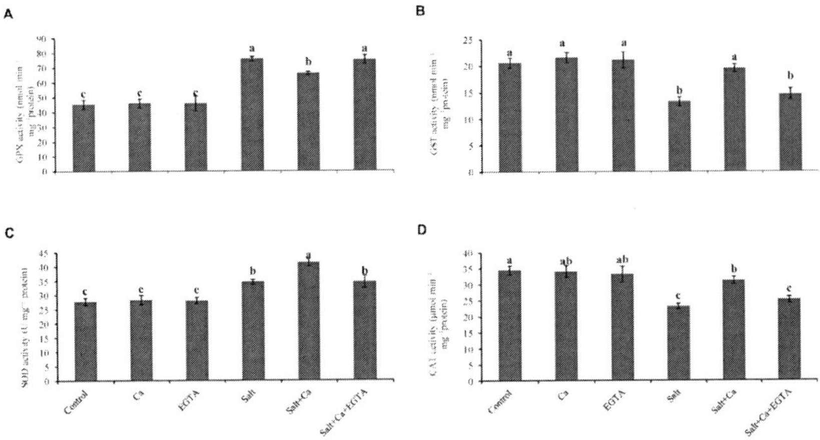

**Figure 7. Effect of Ca on GPX (A), GST (B), SOD (C), and CAT (D) activity in leaf of rice seedlings under salt stress.** Here, Ca, EGTA and Salt indicate 2 mM $CaCl_2$, 2 mM EGTA, and 200 mM NaCl, respectively. Means (±SD) were calculated from three replicates **...**

The rice seedlings, treated with salt had decreased CAT activity by 33% compared with control. In contrast, Ca supplementation increased CAT activity in the salt-treated rice seedlings by 35% compared with the seedlings treated with salt alone. Exogenous Ca and EGTA did not affect CAT activity in the non-stressed control seedlings (**Figure Figure7D7D**).

The rice seedlings exposed to salt stress had increased APX activity compared with control. Exogenous application of Ca decreased APX activity compared with salt-treated rice seedlings. However, exogenous Ca and EGTA did not affect on APX activity under non-stress conditions (**Figure Figure8A8A**).

Salt stress increased MDHAR activity in the rice seedlings compared with the control seedlings. Exogenous Ca further increased MDHAR activity by 25% in the Salt+Ca treated rice seedlings. Applying EGTA decreased MDHAR activity again in the Salt+Ca+EGTA treatment compared with the Salt+Ca treatment (**Figure Figure8B8B**).

Exogenous application of Ca increased DHAR activity in the Salt+Ca-treated rice seedlings compared with salt-treated seedlings. However, exogenous application of EGTA decreased DHAR activity by 15% in the Salt+Ca+EGTA treatment compared with the Salt+Ca treated seedlings (**Figure Figure8C8C**).

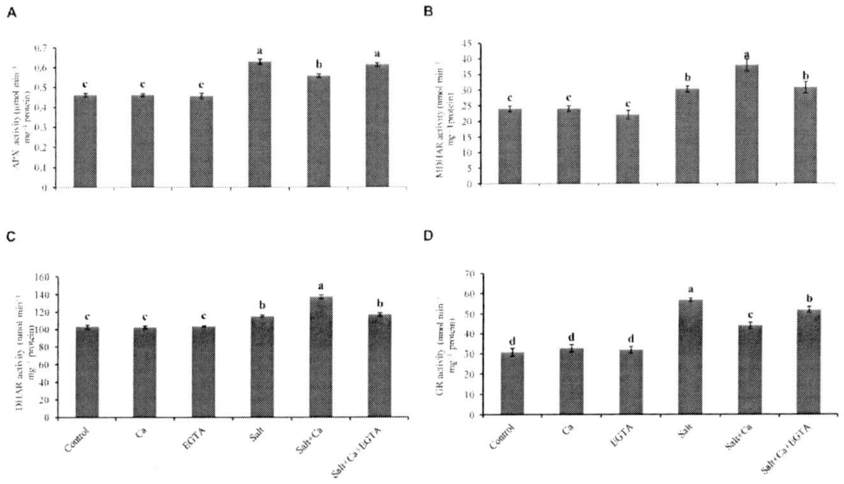


**Figure 8. Effect of Ca on APX (A), MDHAR (B), DHAR (C), and GR (D) activity in leaf of rice seedlings under salt stress.** Here, Ca, EGTA and Salt indicate 2 mM $CaCl_2$, 2 mM EGTA, and 200 mM NaCl, respectively. Means (±SD) were calculated from three replicates **...**

Glutathione reductase activity increased with the Salt and Salt+Ca+EGTA treatment, compared with the control seedlings. In contrast with the salt-treated rice seedlings, Ca supplementation did not increase GR activity in the Salt+Ca treated rice seedlings. Exogenous application of Ca and EGTA did not affect on GR activity in non-stress conditions (**Figure Figure8D8D**).

Compared with the control seedlings, GPX activity increased in the salt-treated seedlings by 67%. Adding Ca decreased GPX activity in Salt+Ca treatment but slightly increased together with EGTA in the Salt+Ca+EGTA treatment (**Figure Figure7A7A**).

Salt stress reduced GST activity in the salt-treated rice seedlings. Compared with the salt-treated rice seedlings, GST activity increased by 47% in the Salt+Ca treatment. Compared with the control seedlings, exogenous Ca and EGTA did not affect on GST activity in non-stress conditions (**Figure Figure7B7B**).

Glyoxalase System

Rice seedlings exposed to salt had sharply increased MG content compared with the non-stressed control seedlings. Adding Ca to the salt-treated rice seedlings reduced MG content by 44% in the Salt+Ca treatment compared with the salt-treated rice seedlings. Applying the Ca scavenger EGTA increased MG content again in the Salt+Ca+EGTA treatment compared with the Salt+Ca treated seedlings. Adding Ca and EGTA to the non-stressed control seedlings did not result in a marked change in MG content compared with the control seedlings (**Figure Figure9C9C**).

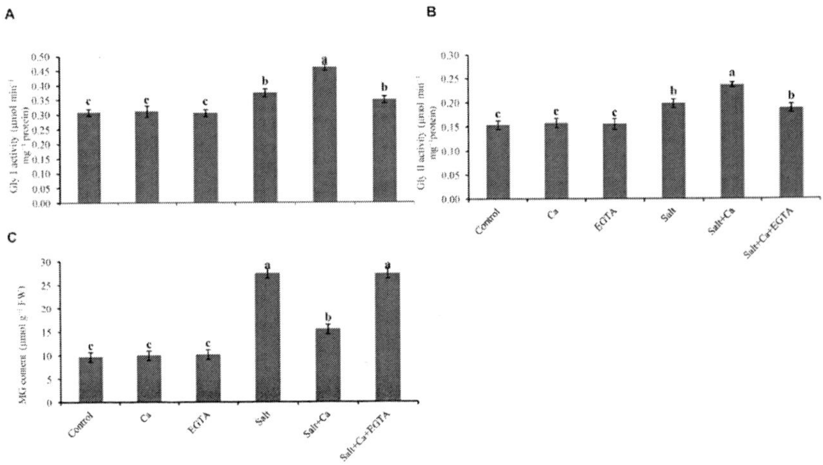


**Figure 9. Effect of Ca on Gly I (A) and Gly II activity (B), and MG content (C) in leaf of rice seedlings under salt stress.** Here, Ca, EGTA and Salt indicate 2 mM $CaCl_2$, 2 mM EGTA, and 200 mM NaCl, respectively. Means (±SD) were calculated from three replicates ...

Glyoxalase I and Gly II activity increased in the salt-treated rice seedlings by 21 and 29%, respectively, compared with the control seedlings. However, exogenous application of Ca further increased Gly I and Gly II activity by 24 and 20%, respectively, in the Salt+Ca treatment, compared with the control seedlings (**Figures 9A,B**).

# DISCUSSION

The immediate and primary response of plants exposed to higher salt is $Na^+$-induced $K^+$efflux (Nedjimi and Daoud, 2009; Anschutz et al., 2014; Bose et al., 2014). In the presence of excess salt in plant growth medium, $Na^+$ influx depolarizes the root plasma membrane which activate guard cell outward rectifying potassium channels (GORK), that provide a pathway for diffusion of $Na^+$ into cell and concomitantly decrease cytosolic $K^+$and increase $Na^+$ content (Blumwald et al., 2000; Demidchik and Tester, 2002). Higher salt in plant growth medium also displaces Ca from membranes, which also increases membrane permeability and intracellular $Na^+$ concentration (Lahaye and Epstein, 1969). Higher $Na^+$ content from salt-induced stress causes disruption of the $Na^+/K^+$ ratio (Simaei et al., 2012) and ion homeostasis (Tuncturk et al., 2008). In this study, salt-induced stress increased $Na^+$ content and decreased $K^+$ content in the shoots and roots of rice seedlings which might be due to entry of higher amount of $Na^+$ into plant by NSCC that caused $K^+$efflux or leakage through NSCC and GORK channel. Higher $Na^+$ accumulation also results in a higher $Na^+/K^+$ ratio, which disrupts ion homeostasis by decreasing Mg, Mn, and Zn contents. Decreased Ca content was also observed in the salt-affected rice seedlings, which might be due to displacement of Ca by $Na^+$. The $Na^+$ influx and $K^+$leakage might be also for higher ROS production that can also activate NSCC (Demidchick and Maathuis, 2007). Similar disruption of ion homeostasis under salt stress conditions was demonstrated in previous studies (Tuncturk et al., 2008; Wu and Wang, 2012). However, it is reported that exogenous Ca promotes membrane stability, ameliorate salt toxicity by decreasing $Na^+$ influx through NSCC and inhibiting $K^+$ efflux through GORK channel in plants (Cramer et al., 1985; Essah et al., 2003; Shabala et al., 2006;Nedjimi and Daoud, 2009; Shabala and Pottosin, 2014). Moreover, exogenous Ca decreases the uptake and transport of $Na^+$ and prevents binding to the cell wall (Kurth et al., 1986; Rubio et al., 2003). In addition, vacuolar and cytosolic Ca block the fast vacuole (FV) channel in voltage dependent and independent manner (Tikhonova et al., 1997) which prevent back leaking of $Na^+$ into vacuole and their transportation into the cell (Shabala, 2013). In our study, exogenous application of Ca improved ion homeostasis by decreasing $Na^+$ uptake, ROS production and increasing mineral nutrient uptake including $K^+$ and Ca. The reduction of $Na^+$ content and improvement of $K^+$ retention might be due to Ca-induced block in NSCC and GORK channel. The reduction of $Na^+$ accumulation was higher in shoot compared with root might be due to Ca-induced block in FV channel which inhibit further transport of $Na^+$ from root to shoot. These results are in agreement with Wu and Wang (2012), who reported that exogenous Ca regulates $K^+/Na^+$homeostasis by decreasing $Na^+$ uptake and increasing $K^+$ and Ca uptake. On the other hand, exogenous Ca along with EGTA could not maintain ion homeostasis in salt-stressed rice seedlings because EGTA negated Ca activity.

Under salt stress conditions higher accumulation of $Na^+$ disrupts ion homeostasis, causes osmotic stress and inhibits growth (Tuncturk et al., 2008; Munns, 2011). Salt-affected rice seedlings showed growth inhibition in terms of plant height, seedling FW and DW, which were restored with Ca supplementation. This mitigation of growth inhibition under salt stress might be due to the improved ion homeostasis with Ca supplementation. This result is consistent with previous findings (Manivannan et al., 2007; Rahman et al., 2015b) in which exogenous Ca restored growth under abiotic-stress conditions.

Since salt stress causes both ionic toxicity and osmotic stress which creates physiological drought due to exosmosis and interruption of water uptake (Munns, 2011). As an osmoprotectant with antioxidant potential, Pro plays a vital role in abiotic-stress tolerance in plants (Hasanuzzaman et al., 2014; Nahar et al., 2016). Rice seedlings exposed to salt showed lower RWC and higher Pro accumulation, which indicated a salt-induced water imbalance and osmotic stress. Similar salt-induced water shortage and Pro accumulation were observed in salt-affected rice seedlings (Hasanuzzaman et al., 2014). However, exogenous Ca restored water loss (indicated by increased RWC) and decreased Pro accumulation in the salt-affected rice seedlings.

Like other abiotic stresses, salt-induced stress destabilizes the pigment protein complex and decreases photosynthetic pigments by increasing the activity of chlorophyllase enzyme and/or overproduction of ROS (Saha et al., 2010; Hasanuzzaman et al., 2014). In our experiment, we observed that Ca supplementation restored chl and carotenoid content of the rice seedlings under salt-stress conditions. The restoration of photosynthetic pigment might be due to lower production of ROS with Ca supplementation under salt-stress conditions. This result is in agreement with the findings of previous studies in which Ca supplementation improved chl and carotenoid content under abiotic-stress conditions (Ahmad et al., 2015; Rahman et al., 2015b).

One of the major effects of salt stress is the production of excess amount ROS and higher lipid peroxidation (Zhu et al., 2004; Hasanuzzaman et al., 2014; Nahar et al., 2015a). Overproduction of ROS under stress causes lipid peroxidation, protein oxidation, enzyme inhibition and eventually leads to cell death (Gill and Tuteja, 2010). Oxidative stress resulting from higher ROS production increases LOX activity and causes lipid peroxidation (Molassiotis et al., 2006). Rice seedlings exposed to salt caused oxidative stress through higher ROS production, lipid peroxidation and LOX activity. However, exogenous Ca applied to the salt-stressed rice seedlings decreased oxidative stress by lowering ROS production, lipid peroxidation and LOX activity, which might be due to Ca-mediated response that is disrupted under salt stress by decreasing Ca uptake. This result is supported by previous studies (Cramer et al., 1985; Nedjimi and Daoud, 2009;Ahmad et al., 2015) in which exogenous Ca re-stabilized Ca-mediated signaling, maintained nutrient homeostasis and reduced oxidative stress. However, exogenous Ca along with EGTA could not reduce ROS production, lipid peroxidation and oxidative stress in the salt-stress induced rice seedlings because EGTA negated Ca activity. This result is in agreement with Ammoaghaie and Moghym (2011) who showed that, EGTA increased stress injury including lipid peroxidation by chelating Ca and expelling its activity.

Non-enzymatic antioxidants, (AsA and GSH), play vital a role in maintaining cellular redox potential for abiotic stress-tolerance by scavenging overproduced ROS (Pang and Wang, 2008; Mahmood et al., 2010). The primary antioxidant, AsA, directly quenches ROS by reacting with it (Gill and Tuteja, 2010) and GSH also plays an important role in scavenging ROS or toxic compounds with the help of the antioxidant enzymes GPX and GST (Szalai et al., 2009). In this study, lower AsA content and AsA/DHA ratio resulting from increased DHA content observed under salt-stress which were facilitated by higher ROS generation. However, exogenous application of Ca increased the AsA content and AsA/DHA ratio and decreased the DHA content with increased MDHAR and DHAR activity. This result is supported by Srivastava et al. (2014), who reported that exogenous Ca restored AsA content under abiotic-stress conditions by stimulating MDHAR activity. Treatment of the rice seedlings with salt increased GSH content with increased GR and decreased GST activity. The level of GSSG also increased due to oxidation of GSH to GSSG during the scavenging of ROS.

The enzymes of AsA-GSH cycle (APX, MDHAR, DHAR, and GR), together with AsA and GSH work against oxidative stress by reducing ROS production and recycling of AsA and GSH (Asada, 1992; Mishra et al., 2013). Ascorbate peroxidase mobilizes $H_2O_2$to $H_2O$ via oxidation of AsA to DHA. Monodehydroascorbate reductase and DHAR regenerate AsA from DHA using NADPH and GSH as electron donors (Mishra et al., 2013). The enzyme GR together with MDHAR and DHAR also regenerates the antioxidant components such as AsA and GSH to maintain redox cellular balance (Srivastava et al., 2014). In the present study, salt-induced stress increased APX, MDHAR, DHAR, and GR activity along with decreased AsA content and increased GSH content. Stimulation of these antioxidant enzyme activities indicates that they are associated with oxidative stress tolerance (Mishra et al., 2013). The increased APX activity might be due to higher $H_2O_2$ content and lower AsA content and increased GR activity due to an increased level of GSH content under salt-stress conditions. This result is consistent with previous findings (Mishra et al., 2013; Hasanuzzaman et al., 2014;Ozfidan-Konakci et al., 2015). However, exogenous Ca applied to the salt-treated rice seedlings further stimulated MDHAR and DHAR activity along with increased AsA content and decreased DHA content. This increased MDHAR and DHAR activities might detoxify $H_2O_2$ by regenerating AsA from DHA. This result is also consistent with previous studies (Talukdar, 2012; Srivastava et al., 2014) in which it was reported that exogenous Ca stimulates MDHAR and DHAR activity under abiotic-stress condition.

Superoxide dismutase is considered a first-line enzymatic defense in controlling ROS, which converts $O_2^{\bullet -}$ to $H_2O_2$ (Mittler, 2002; Gill et al., 2015), and $H_2O_2$ is readily detoxified to $H_2O$ and $O_2$ by CAT (Sanchez-Casas and Klesseg, 1994). The present study showed a significant increase in SOD activity and a decrease in CAT activity under salt-stress conditions which are in agreement with previous reports (Mishra et al., 2013;Wutipraditkul et al., 2015). This increased SOD activity might be due to higher formation of $O_2^{\bullet -}$ and $H_2O_2$ and decreased CAT activity due to higher production of $H_2O_2$, which were increased by salt-induced oxidative stress and supported by previous studies (Mishra et al., 2013; Hasanuzzaman et al., 2014; Nahar et al., 2015a). Exogenous application of Ca stimulated SOD and CAT activity under salt stress and reduced overproduction of $O_2^{\bullet -}$ and $H_2O_2$. Similar results were reported by Srivastava et al. (2014) and Ahmad et al. (2015) who found that exogenous Ca stimulated SOD and CAT activity to reduce ROS under oxidative-stress conditions.

To protect plants from oxidative stress, the enzyme GPX and GST work together to produce less toxic and water-soluble conjugates by catalyzing the binding of different xenobiotics and their electrophilic metabolites (Edwards et al., 2000; Noctor et al., 2002). The salt-induced oxidative stress increased GPX activity but decreased GST activity might be due to higher production of $H_2O_2$ and insufficient detoxification of over-produced $H_2O_2$. This result is supported by Tammam et al. (2011) and Hasanuzzaman et al. (2014), who reported similar GPX and GST activity under salt-induced oxidative stress conditions. Supplementation with Ca in the salt-stressed rice seedlings increased GST activity, which might be playing a role in detoxifying $H_2O_2$. Similar findings were also reported by Rahman et al. (2015b), who showed stimulation of GST activity with Ca supplementation played a role in alleviating oxidative stress by scavenging $H_2O_2$.

Upregulation of the MG detoxification system or glyoxalase system is vital to eliminate overproduced MG, or MG-induced oxidative stress (Yadav et al., 2005). Overexpression of the Gly I and Gly II enzymes increased the tolerance in plants to abiotic stresses (Singla-Pareek et al., 2008). The salt-stressed rice seedlings showed higher MG production along with slight stimulation of Gly I and Gly II activity which is consistent with the findings of Hasanuzzaman et al. (2014). Supplementation of Ca in salt-treated rice seedlings showed decreased

MG production with increased Gly I and Gly II activities. Decreased production of MG is partly due to increased Gly I and Gly II activities. This result is consistent with Nahar et al. (2015b), who showed that upregulation of glyoxalase enzyme activity partially resulted in oxidative-stress tolerance by increasing MG detoxification. This result is also supported by Rahman et al., 2015a,b), who showed that exogenous Ca increased MG detoxification by stimulating glyoxalase enzyme activity under toxic metal-induced oxidative stress.

## CONCLUSION

Considering the above, our results suggest that salinity causes disruption of ion homeostasis, and the antioxidant defense and glyoxalase systems by increasing $Na^+$uptake, ROS production and MG formation, respectively. Exogenous Ca in the salt-treated rice seedlings improved ion homeostasis by decreasing $Na^+$ influx and $K^+$ efflux through NSCC and GORK channel, and increasing nutrient uptake. Exogenous Ca also increased detoxification of overproduced ROS and MG by improving the antioxidant defense and glyoxalase systems under salt stress-conditions. Finally, the rice seedlings with salt-induced oxidative damage recovered with Ca supplementation, which improved ion homeostasis, and the antioxidant defense and glyoxalase systems.

## AUTHOR CONTRIBUTIONS

AR conceived, designed, and performed the experiment and prepared the manuscript. KN actively participated in executing the experiment. MH designed the experiment and analyzed the data. MF conceived, designed, and monitored the experiment.

## CONFLICT OF INTEREST STATEMENT

The authors declare that the research was conducted in the absence of any commercial or financial relationships that could be construed as a potential conflict of interest.

## ACKNOWLEDGMENTS

This research was funded by the Ministry of Education, Culture, Sports, Science and Technology (MEXT), Japan. We thank Mr. Dennis Murphy,

United Graduate School of Agricultural Sciences, Ehime University, Japan for a critical review and editing the English of the manuscript. We also thank Mr. Shahadat Hossain and Mr. Jubayer-Al-Mahmud, Laboratory of Plant Stress Responses, Faculty of Agriculture, Kagawa University, Japan for the critical reading of the manuscript.

## REFERENCES

1. Addinsoft (2015). *XLSTAT V. 2015.1.01: Data Analysis and Statistics Software for Microsoft Excel*. Paris: Addinsoft.

2. Ahmad P., Sarwat M., Bhat N. A., Wani M. R., Kazi A. G., Tran L. P. (2015).Alleviation of cadmium toxicity in *Brassica juncea* L. (Czern. & Coss.) by calcium application involves various physiological and biochemical strategies. *PLoS ONE*10:e0114571

3. Ahmad P., Sharma S. (2008). Salt stress and phyto-biochemical responses of plants.*Plant Soil Environ.* 54 89–99.

4. Ammoaghaie R., Moghym S. (2011). Effect of polyamines on thermotolerance and membrane stability of soybean seedling. *Afr. J. Biotechnol.*

5. Anjum N. A., Aref I. M., Duarte A. C., Pereira E., Ahmad I., Iqbal M. (2014).Glutathione and proline can coordinately make plants with stand the joint attack of metal(loid) and salinity stresses. *Front. Plant Sci.* 5:662 1

6. Anschutz U., Becker D., Shabala S. (2014). Going beyond nutrition: regulation of potassium homeostasis as a common denominator of plant adaptive responses to environment. *J. Plant Physiol.* 171 670–687.

7. Arnon D. T. (1949). Copper enzymes in isolated chloroplasts polyphenol oxidase in*Beta vulgaris*. *Plant Physiol.* 24 1–15.

8. Asada K. (1992). Ascorbate peroxidase-a hydrogen peroxide-scavenging enzymes in plants. *Physiol. Plant* 85 235–241.

9. Barrs H. D., Weatherley P. E. (1962). A re-examination of the relative turgidity technique for estimating water deficits in leaves. *Aust. J. Biol. Sci.* 15 413–428.

10. Bates L. S., Waldren R. P., Teari D. (1973). Rapid determination of free proline for water stress studies. *Plant Soil* 39 205–207.

11. Blumwald E., Aharon G. S., Apse M. P. (2000). Sodium transport in plant cells.*Biochim. Biophys. Acta* 1465 140–151. 10.1016/S0005-2736(00)00135-8

12. Bose J., Rodrigo-Moreno A., Shabala S. (2014). ROS homeostasis in halophytes in the context of salinity stress tolerance. *J. Exp. Bot.* 65 1241–1257.

13. Bradford M. (1976). A rapid and sensitive method for the quantitation of microgram quantities of protein utilizing the principle of protein-dye binding. *Anal. Biochem.*72 248–254.

14. Chen F., Wang F., Wu F., Mao W., Zhang G., Zhou M. (2010). Modulation of exogenous glutathione in antioxidant defense system against Cd stress in the two barley genotypes differing in Cd tolerance. *Plant Physiol. Biochem.* 48 663–672.

15. Cramer G. R., Läuchli A., Polito V. S. (1985). Displacement of $Ca^{2+}$ and $Na^{+}$ form the plasma lemma of root cells. *Plant Physiol.* 79 207–211.

16. Demidchick V., Maathuis F. J. M. (2007). Physiological role of nonselective cation channels in plants: from salt stress to signaling and development. *New Phytol.* 175387–404.

17. Demidchik V., Tester M. (2002). Sodium fluxes through nonselective cation channels in the plasma membrane of protoplasts from *Arabidopsis* roots. *Plant Physiol.* 128 379–387.

18. Doderer A., Kokkelink I., Van der Veen S., Valk B., Schram A., Douma A. (1992).Purification and characterization of two lipoxygenase isoenzymes from germinating barley. *Biochim. Biophys. Acta.* 112 97–104.

19. Dutilleul C., Driscoll S., Cornic G., De Paepe R., Foyer C. H., Noctor G. (2003).Functional mitochondrial complex I is required by tobacco leaves for optimal photosynthetic performance in photo respiratory conditions and during transients.*Plant Physiol.* 131 264–275.

20. Edwards R., Dixon D. P., Walbot V. (2000). Plant glutathione S-transferases: enzymes with multiple functions in sickness and in health. *Trends Plant Sci.* 5 193–198.

21. Elia A. C., Galarini R., Taticchi M. I., Dorr A. J. M., Mantilacci L. (2003).Antioxidant responses and bioaccumulation in *Ictalurus* melas under mercury exposure. *Ecotoxicol. Environ. Saf.* 55 162–167.

22. El-Shabrawi H., Kumar B., Kaul T., Reddy M. K., Singla-Pareek S. L., Sopory S. K. (2010). Redox homeostasis, antioxidant defense, and methylglyoxal detoxification as markers for salt tolerance in Pokkali rice. *Protoplasma* 245 85–96.

23. Essah P. A., Davenport R., Tester M. (2003). Sodium influx and accumulation in*Arabidopsis*. *Plant Physiol.* 133 307–318.

24. Foyer C. H., Halliwell B. (1976). The presence of glutathione and glutathione reductase in chloroplasts: a proposed role in ascorbic acid metabolism. *Planta* 13321–25.

25. Gill S. S., Anjum N. A., Gill R., Yadav S., Hasanuzzaman M., Fujita M., et al. (2015). Superoxide dismutase - mentor of abiotic stress tolerance in crop plants.*Environ. Sci. Pollut. Res.* 22 10375–10394.

26. Gill S. S., Tuteja N. (2010). Reactive oxygen species and antioxidant machinery in abiotic stress tolerance in crop plants. *Plant Physiol. Biochem.* 48 909–930.

27. Griffiths O. W. (1980). Determination of glutathione and glutathione disulphide using glutathione reductase and 2-vinylpyridine. *Anal. Biochem.* 106 207–212.

28. Hasanuzzaman M., Alam M. M., Rahman A., Hasanuzzaman M., Nahar K., Fujita M. (2014). Exogenous proline and glycine betaine mediated upregulation of antioxidant defense and glyoxalase systems provides better protection against salt-induced oxidative stress in two rice (*Oryza sativa* L.) *varieties. Biomed. Res. Int.*2014:757219

29. Hasanuzzaman M., Fujita M. (2011). Selenium pretreatment upregulates the antioxidant defense and methylglyoxal detoxification system and confers enhanced tolerance to drought stress in rapeseed. *Biol. Trace Elem. Res.* 143 1758–1776.

30. Hasanuzzaman M., Hossain M. A., Fujita M. (2011). Nitric oxide modulates antioxidant defense and the methylglyoxal detoxification system and reduces salinity-induced damage of wheat seedlings. *Plant Biotechnol. Rep.* 5 353–365.

31. Hasanuzzaman M., Hossain M. A., Teixeira da Silva J. A., Fujita M. (2012). "Plant responses and tolerance to abiotic oxidative stress: antioxidant defense is a key factor," in *Crop Stress and its Management: Perspectives and Strategies*, eds Bandi V., Shanker A. K., Shanker C., Mandapaka M., editors. (Berlin: Springer; ), 261–316.

32. Hasanuzzaman M., Nahar K., Fujita M. (2013). "Plant response to salt stress and role of exogenous protectants to mitigate salt-induced damages," in *Ecophysiology and Responses of Plants Under Salt Stress*, eds Ahmed P., Azooz M. M., Prasad M. N. V., editors. (New York, NY: Springer; ), 25–87.

33. Heath R. L., Packer L. (1968). Photo peroxidation in isolated chloroplast: I. Kinetics and stoichiometry of fatty acid peroxidation. *Arch. Biochem. Biophys.* 125189–198.

34. Hossain M. A., Nakano Y., Asada K. (1984). Monodehydroascorbate reductase in spinach chloroplasts and its participation in the regeneration of ascorbate for scavenging hydrogen peroxide. *Plant Cell Physiol.* 25 385–395.

35. Hossain M. Z., Hossain M. D., Fujita M. (2006). Induction of pumpkin glutathione S-transferase by different stresses and its possible mechanisms. *Biol. Plant.* 50 210–218.

36. Iqbal N., Shahid U., Khan N. A. (2015). Nitrogen availability regulates proline and ethylene production and alleviates salinity stress in mustard (*Brassica juncea*). *J. Plant Physiol.* 178 84–91.

37. Jaleel C. A., Azooz M. M. (2009). Exogenous calcium alters pigment composition, γ-glutamyl kinase and proline oxidase activities in salt stressed *Withania somnifera.Plant Omics. J.* 2 85–90.

38. Jaleel C. A., Manivannan P., Kishorekumar A., Sankar B., Panneerselvam R. (2007a). Calcium chloride effects on salinity induced oxidative stress, proline metabolism and indole alkaloid accumulation in *Catharanthus roseu*. *Compt. Rend. Biol.* 330 674–683.

39. Jaleel C. A., Manivannan P., Sankar B., Kishorekumar A., Gopi R., Somasundaram R., et al. (2007b). Water deficit stress mitigation by calcium chloride in*Catharanthus roseus*: effects on oxidative stress, proline metabolism and indole alkaloid accumulation. *Colloids Surf. B Biointerfaces* 60 110–116.

40. Kurth E., Cramer G. R., Läuchli A., Epstein E. (1986). Effects of NaCl and CaCl2 on cell production in cotton roots. *Plant Physiol.* 82 1102–1106.

41. Lahaye P. A., Epstein E. (1969). Salt toleration by plants: enhancement with calcium. *Science* 166 395–396.

42. Mahajan S., Tuteja N. (2005). Cold, salinity and drought stresses: an overview.*Arch. Biochem. Biophys.* 444 139–158.

43. Mahmood Q., Ahmad R., Kwak S. S., Rashid A., Anjum N. A. (2010). "Ascorbate and glutathione: protectors of plants in oxidative stress," in *Ascorbate-Glutathione Pathway and Stress Tolerance in Plants*, eds Anjum N. A., Chan M. T., Umar S., editors. (Dordrecht: Springer; ), 209–229.

44. Manivannan P., Jaleel C. A., Sankar B., Somasundaram R., Murali P. V., Sridharan R., et al. (2007). Salt stress mitigation by calcium chloride in *Vigna radiata* (L.) wilczek. *Acta Biol. Cracov Ser. Bot.* 49 105–109.

45. Mishra P., Bhoomika K., Dubey R. S. (2013). Differential responses of antioxidative defense system to prolonged salinity stress in salt-tolerant and salt-sensitive indica rice (*Oryza sativa* L.) *seedlings. Protoplasma* 250 3–19.

46. Mittler R. (2002). Oxidative stress: antioxidants and stress tolerance. *Trends Plant Sci.* 7 405–410.

47. Mittler R., Blumwald E. (2010). Genetic engineering for modern agriculture: challenges and perspectives. *Annu. Rev. Plant Biol.* 61 443–462.

48. Molassiotis A., Sotiropoulos T., Tanou G., Diamantidis G., Therios I. (2006).Boron induced oxidative damage and antioxidant and nucleolytic responses in shoot tips culture of the apple rootstock EM9 (*Malus domestica* Borkh). *Environ. Exp. Bot.* 56 54–62.

49. Munns R. (2011). Plant adaptations to salt and water stress: differences and commonalities. *Adv. Bot. Res.* 57 1–32.

50. Munns R., Tester M. (2008). Mechanism of salinity tolerance. *Annu. Rev. Plant Biol.* 59 651–681.

51. Nahar K., Hasanuzzaman M., Alam M. M., Fujita M. (2015a). Roles of exogenous glutathione in antioxidant defense system and methylglyoxal detoxification during salt stress in mung bean. *Biol. Plant.* 59 745–756.

52. Nahar K., Hasanuzzaman M., Alam M. A., Fujita M. (2015b). Exogenous glutathione confers high temperature stress tolerance in mung bean (*Vigna radiata*L.) by modulating antioxidant defense and methylglyoxal detoxification system.*Environ. Exp. Bot.* 112 44–54.

53. Nahar K., Hasanuzzaman M., Fujita M. (2016). "Roles of osmolytes in plant adaptation to drought and salinity," in *Osmolytes and Plants Acclimation to Changing Environment: Emerging Omics Technologies*, eds Iqbal N., Nazar R., Khan N. A., editors. (New Delli: Springer; ), 37–58. 10.1007/978-81-322-2616-1_4

54. Nakano Y., Asada K. (1981). Hydrogen peroxide is scavenged by ascorbate-specific peroxidase in spinach chloroplasts. *Plant Cell Physiol.* 22 867–880.

55. Nedjimi B., Daoud Y. (2009). Ameliorative effect of CaCl2 on growth, membrane permeability and nutrient uptake in *Atriplex halimus* subsp. schweinfurthii grown at high (NaCl) salinity. *Desalination* 249 163–166.

56. Noctor G., Gomez L., Vanacker H., Foyer C. H. (2002). Interactions between biosynthesis, compartmentation and transport in the control of glutathione homeostasis and signalling. *J. Exp. Bot.* 53 1283–1304.

57. Ozfidan-Konakci C., Yildiztugay E., Kucukoduk M. (2015). Protective roles of exogenously applied gallic acid in *Oryza sativa* subjected to salt and osmotic stresses: effects on the total antioxidant capacity. *Plant Growth Regul.* 75 219–234.

58. Pang C. H., Wang B. S. (2008). "Oxidative stress and salt tolerance in plants," in*Progress in Botany*, eds Lüttge U., Beyschlag W., Murata J., editors. (Heidelberg: Springer; ), 231–245.

59. Pitman M. G., Lauchli A. (2002). "Global impact of salinity and agricultural ecosystems," in *Salinity: Environment–Plants–Molecules*, eds Lauchli A., Luttge U., editors. (Dordrecht: Kluwer; ),

60. Rahman A., Mostofa M. G., Nahar K., Alam M. M., Hasanuzzaman M., Fujita M. (2015a). Calcium mitigates arsenic toxicity in rice seedlings by reducing arsenic uptake and modulating the antioxidant defense and glyoxalase systems and stress markers. *Biomed Res. Int.* 2015:340812

61. Rahman A., Mostofa M. G., Nahar K., Hasanuzzaman M., Fujita M. (2015b).Exogenous calcium alleviates cadmium-induced oxidative stress in rice (*Oryza sativa* L.) seedlings by regulating the antioxidant defense and glyoxalase systems.*Braz. J. Bot.* 1–15.

62. Reddy P. S., Jogeswar G., Rasineni G. K., Maheswari M., Reddy A. R., Varshney R. K., et al. (2015). Proline over-accumulation alleviates salt stress and protects photosynthetic and antioxidant enzyme activities in transgenic sorghum [*Sorghum bicolor* (L.) Moench]. *Plant Physiol. Biochem.* 94 104–113.

63. Rubio F., Flores P., Navarro J. M., Martínez V. (2003). Effects of $Ca^{2+}$, $K^{+}$ and cGMP on $Na^{+}$ uptake in pepper plants. *Plant Sci.* 165 1043–1049.

64. Saha P., Chatterjee P., Biswas A. K. (2010). NaCl pretreatment alleviates salt stress by enhancement of antioxidant defense system and osmolyte accumulation in mungbean (*Vigna radiata* L.*Wilczek). Ind. J. Exp. Biol.* 48 593–600.

65. Sanchez-Casas P., Klesseg D. F. (1994). A salicyclic acid-binding activity and a salicyclic acid-inhibitable catalase activity are present in a variety of plant species.*Plant Physiol.* 106 1675–1679.

66. Schützendübel A., Schwanz P., Teichmann T., Gross K., Langenfeld-Hyser R., Godbold D. L., et al. (2001). Cadmium induced changes in antioxidative systems, hydrogen peroxide content and differentiation in scot pine (*Pinus sylvestris*) roots.*Plant Physiol.* 127 887–892.

67. Shabala S. (2013). Learning from halophytes: physiological basis and strategies to improve abiotic stress tolerance in crops. *Ann. Bot.* 112 1209–1221.

68. Shabala S., Demidchick V., Shabala L., Cuin T. A., Smith S. J., Miller A. J., et al. (2006). Extracellular $Ca^{2+}$ ameliorates NaCl-induced $K^{+}$ loss from *Arabidopsis*root and leaf cells by controlling plasma membrane $K^{+}$ -permeable channels. *Plant Physiol.* 141 1653–1665.

69. Shabala S., Pottosin I. (2014). Regulation of potassium transport in plants under hostile conditions:implications for abiotic and biotic stress tolerance. *Physiol. Plant.*151 257–279.

70. Shabala S., Shabala L., Volkenburgh E. (2003). Effect of calcium on root development and root ion fluxes in salinized barley seedlings. *Funct. Plant Biol.* 30507–514.

71. Simaei M., Khavari-nezad R. A., Bernard F. (2012). Exogenous application of salicylic acid and nitric oxide on the ionic contents and enzymatic activities in NaCl-stressed soybean plants. *Am. J. Plant Sci.* 3 1495–1503.

72. Singla-Pareek S. L., Yadav S. K., Pareek A., Reddy M. K., Sopory S. K. (2008).Enhancing salt tolerance in a crop plant by overexpression of glyoxalase II.*Transgenic Res.* 17 171–180.

73. Srivastava R. K., Pandey P., Rajpoot R., Rani A., Gautam A., Dubey R. S. (2014).Exogenous application of calcium and silica alleviates cadmium toxicity by suppressing oxidative damage in rice. *Protoplasma* 252 959–975.

74. Szalai G., Kellõs T., Galiba G., Kocsy G. (2009). Glutathione as an antioxidant and regulatory molecule in plants under abiotic stress conditions. *Plant Growth Regul.*28 66–80.

75. Talukdar D. (2012). Exogenous calcium alleviates the impact of cadmium induced oxidative stress in *Lens culinaris* medic. through modulation of antioxidant enzyme activities. *J. Crop Sci. Biotechnol.* 15 325–334.

76. Tammam A. A., Fakhry E. M., El-sheekh M. (2011). Effect of salt stress on antioxidant system and the metabolism of the reactive oxygen species in *Dunaliella salina* and *Dunaliella tertiolecta*. *Afr. J. Biotechnol.* 10 3795–3808.

77. Tester M., Davenport R. (2003). $Na^+$ tolerance in higher plants. *Ann. Bot.* 91 503–507.

78. Thordal-Christensen H., Zhang Z., Wei Y., Collinge D. B. (1997). Subcellular localization of $H_2O_2$ in plants, $H_2O_2$ accumulation in papillae and hypersensitive response during barley powdery mildew interaction. *Plant J.* 11 1187–1194.

79. Tikhonova L. I., Potossin I. I., Dietz K., Schonknecht G. (1997). Fast-activating cation channel in barley mesophyll vacuoles inhibition by calcium. *Plant J.* 111059–1070.

80. Tuncturk M., Tuncturk R., Yasar F. (2008). Changes in micronutrients, dry weight and plant growth of soybean (*Glycine max* L. Merrill) cultivars under salt stress. *Afr. J. Biotechnol.* 7 1650–1654.

81. White P. J., Broadley M. R. (2003). Calcium in plants. *Ann. Bot.* 92 487–511.

82. Wild R., Ooi L., Srikanth V., Münch G. (2012). A quick: convenient and economical method for the reliable determination of methylglyoxal in millimolar concentrations: the N-acetyl-L-cysteine assay. *Anal. Bioanal. Chem.* 403 2577–2581.

83. Wu G. Q., Wang S. M. (2012). Calcium regulates $K^+/Na^+$ homeostasis in rice (*Oryza sativa* L.) under saline conditions. *Plant Soil Environ.* 58 121–127.

84. Wutipraditkul N., Wongwean P., Buaboocha T. (2015). Alleviation of salt-induced oxidative stress in rice seedlings by proline and/or glycinebetaine. *Biol. Plant.* 59547–553.

85. Yadav S. K., Singla-Pareek S. L., Reddy M. K., Sopory S. K. (2005).Methylglyoxal detoxification by glyoxalase system: a survival strategy during environmental stresses. *Physiol. Mol. Biol. Plants* 11 1–11.

86. Yu C. W., Murphy T. M., Lin C. H. (2003). Hydrogen peroxide-induces chilling tolerance in mung beans mediated through ABA-independent glutathione accumulation. *Funct. Plant Biol.* 30 955–963.

87. Zhu Z. J., Wei G. Q., Li J., Qian Q. Q., Yu J. Q. (2004). Silicon alleviates salt stress and increases antioxidant enzymes activity in leaves of salt-stressed cucumber (*Cucumis sativus* L.). *Plant Sci.* 167 527–533.

12

# BRASSINOSTEROIDS ARE INVOLVED IN FE HOMEOSTASIS IN RICE (*ORYZA SATIVA* L.)

**Baolan Wang[1], Gen Li[1] and Wen-Hao Zhang[1,2]**

[1] *State Key Laboratory of Vegetation and Environmental Change, Institute of Botany, the Chinese Academy of Sciences, Beijing 100093, P. R. China*

[2] *Research Network of Global Change Biology, Beijing Institutes of Life Sciences, Chinese Academy of Sciences, Beijing, P. R. China*

## ABSTRACT

Brassinosteroids (BRs) are steroid hormones that modulate numerous physiological processes in plants. However, few studies have focused on the involvement of BRs in sensing and responding to the stress of mineral nutrient deficiency. In the present study, we evaluated the roles of BRs in the response of rice (*Oryza sativa*) to iron (Fe) deficiency during Fe uptake, transport, and translocation. Exogenous application of 24-epibrassinolide (EBR) to wild-type (WT) plants exaggerated leaf symptoms of Fe deficiency and suppressed growth. EBR increased and decreased Fe concentrations in roots and shoots, respectively, under both Fe-deficient and Fe-sufficient conditions. Transcripts involved in Fe homeostasis, including Os*IRT1*, Os*YSL15*, Os*YSL2*, Os*NAS1*, and Os*NAS2*, were enhanced by EBR under Fe-deficient conditions. EBR depressed expression of Os*NAS1*, Os*NAS2*, and Os*YSL2* in shoots, and inhibited Fe transport and translocation via the phloem. Rice mutant *d2-1*, which is defective in BR biosynthesis, was more tolerant to Fe deficiency than the WT, and accumulated greater amounts of Fe in roots than the WT under Fe-sufficient conditions. A greater upregulation of Os*IRT1*, Os*YSL15*, Os*YSL2*, Os*NAS1*, and Os*NAS2*in the *d2-1* mutant compared to the WT was found under Fe-sufficient conditions, while expression of these genes in the *d2-1* mutant was lower than in the WT under Fe-deficient conditions. The greater tolerance of the*d2-1* mutant could be partly mitigated by exogenous application of EBR. These novel findings highlight the important role of BR in mediating the response of strategy II plants to Fe deficiency by regulating Fe uptake and translocation in rice.

**Keywords:** Brassinosteroids (BRs) *d2-1* mutant Fe deficiency Fe translocation Fe uptake rice (*Oryza sativa*) strategy II plant.

# INTRODUCTION

Iron (Fe) is one of the essential mineral nutrients required for plant growth and development. Plant growth is often limited by low availability of Fe in soil due to its low solubility, especially in calcareous soils (Romera and Alcántara, 2004). Plants have evolved various strategies to cope with Fe deficiency in soil. These strategies have been classified as strategy I and strategy II, and these exist in non-graminaceous monocots and dicots, and in graminaceous monocots, respectively (Römheld and Marschner, 1986; Kobayashi and Nishizawa, 2012). Increased ferric chelate reductase activity, acidification of the rhizosphere, and upregulation of $Fe^{2+}$transporters (IRTs) are major mechanisms by which strategy I plants maximize their Fe acquisition (Curie and Briat, 2003; Hell and Stephan, 2003; Romera and Alcántara, 2004). In contrast, strategy II plants commonly secrete phytosiderophores (PSs) belonging to the mugineic acid (MA) family from roots to solubilize $Fe^{3+}$ (Kobayashi and Nishizawa, 2012). A gene encoding an $Fe^{3+}$-MA transporter has been isolated from maize mutant*yellow trip 1*, and an $Fe^{3+}$-phytosiderophore uptake transporter was named as Yellow Stripe1 (YS1) (von Wiren *et al.*, 1994;Curie *et al.*, 2001). Secretion of MAs from rice roots to the rhizosphere is mediated by Os*TOM1* (Nozoye *et al.*, 2011), and the resulting $Fe^{3+}$-MA complexes are adsorbed into root cells by yellow-stripe like (YSL) transporters in the plasma membrane (Conte and Walker, 2011). In rice, OsYSL15 is the primary transporter responsible for uptake of $Fe^{3+}$-MA from the rhizosphere (Inoue *et al.*, 2009). Recent studies reveal that, in addition to acquisition of Fe by MA, rice plants also possess the $Fe^{2+}$-transporter system, and two genes encoding $Fe^{2+}$ transporters, Os*IRT1*and Os*IRT2*, have been isolated (Bughio *et al.*, 2002; Ishimaru *et al.*, 2006). Expression of Os*IRT1* and Os*IRT2* is upregulated by Fe deficiency, and mutation in NAAT stimulates the Fe (II) acquisition system in cultures with an abundant $Fe^{2+}$ source, leading to Fe accumulation in rice plants (Cheng *et al.*, 2007).

Iron is transported in complexed forms once it is loaded into the xylem (Conte and Walker, 2011). In *Arabidopsis*, FRD3, which belongs to the multidrug and toxic compound extrusion (MATE) family, is involved in loading of citrate into the xylem (Rogers and Guerinot, 2002; Green and Rogers, 2004; Durrett *et al.*, 2007). *FRD3* is expressed in the root vasculature, and its expression is enhanced by Fe deficiency (Green and Rogers, 2004). Similar to *Arabidopsis*, rice also possesses an *FRD*-like gene (Os*FRDL1*), which encodes a citrate transporter localized at the rice root pericycle cells and mediates the translocation of Fe to the shoot in the form of Fe-citrate complex (Yokosho *et al.*, 2009). A recent study reported that Fe exists as oxo-bridged tri-$Fe^{3+}$, tri-citrate ($Fe_3Cit_3$) complex in the xylem sap of Fe-deficient tomato (Rellán-Álvarez *et al.*, 2010). In addition to citrate, nicotianamine (NA) is another important agent to complex metals in plants. Nicotianamine exists ubiquitously in roots and shoots as well as in the xylem and phloem sap of higher plants, and it can complex $Fe^{2+}$, $Fe^{3+}$, $Mg^{2+}$, and $Zn^{2+}$ (Morrissey and Guerinot, 2009; Conte and Walker, 2011). In rice, nicotianamine is synthesized by NA synthase (NAS) from *S*-adenosylmethionine, and involves long-distance Fe transport (Inoue *et al.*, 2003). OsYSL2 is a rice metal-NA transporter responsible for translocation of Fe and Mn into the grain via the phloem (Koike *et al.*, 2004). Moreover, OsYSL2 can also play roles in the mediation of translocation of Fe from root to shoot (Ishimaru *et al.*, 2010).

A number of phytohormones and messenger molecules such as auxin, ethylene, cytokinins, and nitric oxide (NO) have been reported to be involved in the regulation of Fe deficiency-induced changes in morphological and physiological processes in strategy I plants (Ivanov *et al.*, 2012). In contrast, there is limited information on the role of phytohormones in the response of strategy II plants to Fe deficiency (Wu *et al.*, 2011). As a class of plant polyhydroxysteroids, brassinosteroids (BRs) are ubiquitous in plants (Noguchi *et al.*, 1999). There is emerging evidence demonstrating that BRs play important roles in the response of plants to biotic and abiotic stresses (Sasse, 2003). Our previous studies showed that brassinosteroids are involved in response of cucumber (*Cucumis sativus*) to Fe deficiency by regulating Fe deficiency-induced FRO and Fe translocation from roots to shoots

(Wang *et al.*, 2012). In the present study, we evaluated the role of BRs in the response of strategy II rice plants to Fe deficiency using wild-type rice and the BR-deficient rice mutant *d2-1*. The *d2-1* plants are dwarf mutants resulting from a defect in BR biosynthesis (Hong *et al.*, 2003). The *D2* gene encodes a novel cytochrome P450 classified as CYP90D that is highly similar to the reported BR synthesis enzymes. The D2/CYP90D2 enzyme catalyses the steps from 6-deoxoteasterone to 3-dehydro-6-deoxoteasterone and from teasterone to 3-dehydroteasterone in the late BR biosynthesis pathways (Hong *et al.*, 2003). Our results demonstrate that BR also played an important role in the response of strategy II plant to Fe deficiency by regulating long-distance transport and translocation of Fe via the phloem.

# MATERIALS AND METHODS

Wild-type (WT) rice (*Oryza sativa* L. cv. 'Taichung 65') and *d2-1* mutants derived from Taichung 65 were used. The *d2-1* plants were screened from a mutant library produced by *N*-methyl-*N*-nitrosourea. Hong *et al.* (2003)cloned the *D2* gene by map-based cloning and showed quantitatively that endogenous BR levels in the mutants were much lower than in their counterpart WT plants under normal growth conditions. The seeds were surface sterilized by incubation for 3min in 75% ethanol followed by 10min in 0.1% $HgCl_2$, and were then washed thoroughly with sterile water. The sterilized seeds were soaked in water for 24h in the dark and then transferred to a nylon net floating on water for 1 week. Thereafter, the 7-d-old seedlings were transferred to nutrient solution containing half-strength Kimura B solution. The nutrient solution contained the macronutrients (mM) $(NH_4)_2SO_4$ (0.18), $MgSO_4{\cdot}7H_2O$ (0.27), $KNO_3$ (0.09), Ca $(NO_3)_2{\cdot}4H_2O$ (0.18), and $KH_2PO_4$ (0.09); and micronutrients (μM) $MnCl_2{\cdot}4H_2O$ (0.5), $H_3BO_3$ (3), $(NH_4)_6Mo_7O_{24}{\cdot}4H_2O$ (1), $ZnSO_4{\cdot}7H_2O$ (0.4), and $CuSO_4{\cdot}5H_2O$ (0.2). The solution also contained 50 μM FeEDTA. The pH was adjusted daily to 5.5 and the solution was renewed every 3 d. The hydroponic experiments were carried out in a growth room with a 16-h light (30°C)/8-h dark (22°C) photoperiod, and the relative humidity was kept at ~70%. After 10-d growth, the pre-cultured seedlings were used for the following experiments.

### Measurement of chlorophyll

Ten-d-old WT seedlings pre-cultured in solution containing 50 μM Fe-EDTA were transferred to full-strength Kimura B solution supplemented with 0 μM (Fe-deficient medium) or 100 μM Fe-EDTA

(Fe-sufficient medium) with varying concentrations of 24-epibrassinolide (EBR) (0, 1, 10, 100, and 500nM) for 2 weeks. The EBR was dissolved in a minimal volume of ethanol, and then made up to volume with nutrient solution (Yu *et al.*, 2004). After treatment, foliar chlorophyll concentrations were measured. Newly formed leaves were weighed and then ground with aqueous acetone (80% v/v) and centrifuged at 10 000*g* for 5min. Absorbance (A) readings of the supernatant were recorded at 645 and 663nm. Total chlorophyll concentration (mg $l^{-1}$) was calculated as 8.02A663 + 20.21A645, and expressed as mg chlorophyll $g^{-1}$ fresh weight. Ten-d-old WT and *d2-1*mutant seedlings pre-cultured in solution containing 50 μM Fe-EDTA were transferred to full-strength Kimura B solution supplemented with 0 μM (Fe-deficient medium) or 100 μM Fe-EDTA (Fe-sufficient medium) with or without 100nM EBR for 2 weeks. Foliar chlorophyll concentrations were measured.

## Determination of plant biomass and metal analysis in roots and shoots

Ten-d-old WT and *d2-1* seedlings pre-cultured in solution containing 50 μM Fe-EDTA were transferred to 0 μM (–Fe) and 100 μM (+Fe) Fe-EDTA full-strength Kimura B solution in the absence and presence of 100nM EBR for 2 weeks. After treatments, seedlings were harvested and separated into roots and shoots, then dried for 2 d at 75ºC. After measurements of biomass, root and shoot samples were ground to fine powder and digested with concentrated nitric acid and hydrogen peroxide. The total Fe concentrations were determined by Inductive Coupled Plasma Emission Spectrometry (ICP-OES).

## Expression patterns of genes encoding Fe uptake and translocation proteins

Total RNA was extracted from roots and leaves of rice plants subjected to Fe or EBR treatments for varying periods (1, 3, and 7 d). Total RNA was isolated using RNAiso reagent (Takara) and reverse-transcribed into first-strand cDNA with PrimeScript® RT reagent Kit with gDNA Erager (Takara). Real-time PCR was performed in an optical 96-well plate with an Applied Biosystems SteponeTM Real-Time PCR system. Each reaction contained 7.5 μl of 2 × SYBR Green Master Mix reagent, 0.5 μl of cDNA samples, and 0.6 μl of 10 μM gene-specific primers in a final volume of 15 μl. The thermal cycle used was as follows: 95°C for 10min; and 40 cycles of 95°C for 30 s, 55°C for 30 s, and 72°C for 30 s. All the primers used for quantitative RT-PCR are listed in Supplementary Table S1. The relative quantification method (Delta-Delta cycle threshold) was used to evaluate quantitative variation between the replicates examined. The PCR signals were normalized to those of actin or rice polyubiquitin (RubQ1).

### Analysis of the phloem sap

The protocols described by Corbesier *et al.* (2003) were used for collection of phloem sap. Briefly, newly formed leaves were detached at their petiole bases, and the petioles were recut in medium containing 20mM EDTA-$K_2$(pH 7.5). The leaves collected from each individual plant were placed in a 2ml microcentrifuge tube with their petioles immersed in 1.5ml of 15mM EDTA-$K_2$ (pH 7.5). The tubes were placed in airtight transparent plastic containers in an illuminated growth room for 4h to dissolve the phloem sap in EDTA solution (Corbesier *et al.*, 2003); the atmosphere was water saturated (to prevent uptake of EDTA solution by the leaves). Iron concentration in the collected phloem sap was measured by Inductive Coupled Plasma Mass Spectrometry (ICP-MAS). The leaves were dried at 80°C and weighed.

### Statistical analysis

Analysis of variance was conducted between different treatments. The significant differences between treatments were evaluated by LSD multiple range tests ($P \leq 0.05$) using SAS statistical software.

## RESULTS

### Exogenous application of EBR enhanced leaf symptoms of Fe deficiency

To test whether BR is involved in Fe deficiency-induced changes in physiological processes in rice plants, the effect of exogenous EBR at varying concentrations (0–500nM) on cholorophyll concentrations of rice seedlings grown in Fe-sufficient and Fe-deficient media was studied. Apparent chlorosis was observed in young leaves of rice seedlings grown in Fe-deficient medium for 2 weeks (Fig. 1A), leading to a decrease in cholorophyll concentration (Fig. 1B). Furthermore, the chlorosis became more evident by application of EBR to Fe-deficient seedlings. In contrast, application of EBR had no apparent effect on leaf cholorosis in Fe-sufficient seedlings (Fig. 1A). Accordingly, treatments with EBR led to a significant decrease in chlorophyll concentration of Fe-deficient plants, while the same treatment had no effect on chlorophyll concentration in Fe-sufficient seedlings (Fig. 1B). The reduction in chlorophyll concentration in Fe-deficient seedlings by EBR occurred at a concentration of 1nM, and no further reduction in the chlorophyll concentration was observed when EBR concentration was increased up to 500nM, suggesting that the effect of EBR on the chlorophyll concentration is independent of EBR dose, and that BR may be an important signal during Fe deficiency. Although 1nM EBR can have the negative effect, at >100nM it can partly restore the phenotype of the *d2-1* mutant. Therefore, an EBR concentration of 100nM was used throughout this study, which can partly restore growth of *d2-1* and has no effect on growth of WT plants. Since rice can take up both $Fe^{2+}$- and $Fe^{3+}$-MA, in addition to Fe-EDTA, we also investigated the effects of EBR on plants with different forms of Fe present in the medium ($FeSO_4$, $Fe^{3+}$EDTA, and $FeCl_3$). Similar to FeEDTA, EBR-induced leaf chlorosis was also detected under conditions of deficiency in $FeSO_4$, $Fe^{3+}$EDTA, or $FeCl_3$ in the growth medium (Supplementary Figure S1). These results indicate that the effect of BR on Fe nutrition is independent of Fe species in the growth medium. We therefore focused on the effect of BR on rice plants with FeEDTA in the medium throughout our study.

The involvement of BR in the mediation of Fe deficiency-induced changes in physiological processes was further evaluated using a BR-deficient mutant *d2-1*. Similar to WT plants, Fe deficiency also decreased leaf chlorophyll in the *d2-1* mutant, and exogenous application of EBR enhanced Fe-deficiency-induced leaf chlorosis in young leaves of *d2-1*seedlings (Fig. 2). However, the *d2-1* mutant had a higher chlorophyll concentration than the WT plant, and the magnitude of decrease in chlorophyll concentration by EBR was much greater in WT plants than in*d2-1* mutants under Fe- deficient conditions (Fig. 2), indicating that the WT is more sensitive to EBR than *d2-1* mutant plants under Fe-deficient conditions. In contrast, application of EBR had no apparent effect on foliar chlorophyll concentration in Fe-sufficient *d2-1* mutant seedlings (Fig. 2).

## BR-deficient mutant *d2-1* was less sensitive to Fe deficiency and EBR

In addition to chlorophyll, dry mass of shoots and roots of WT rice seedlings was significantly reduced when they were grown in Fe-deficient medium. A further reduction in dry weight of shoots and roots of Fe-deficient seedlings was found in the presence of EBR in the growth medium, while no effect of EBR on biomass of Fe-sufficient WT seedlings was observed (Fig. 3A, B). Both shoot and root biomass of *d2-*

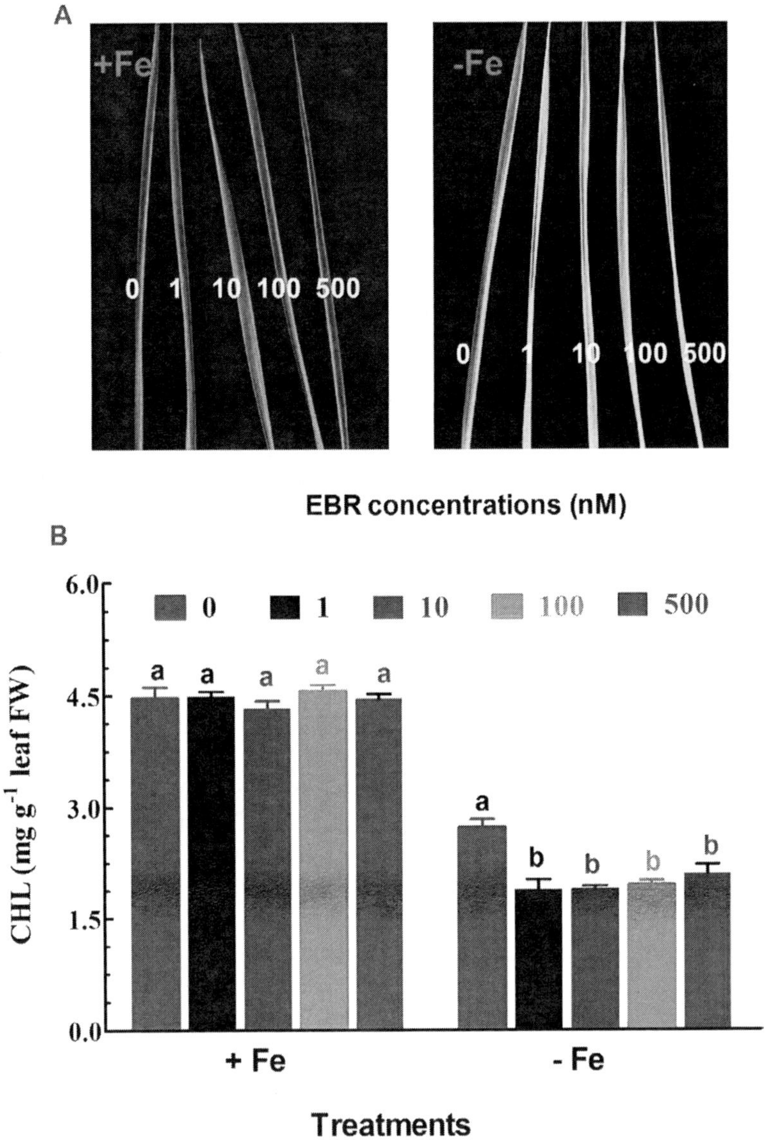


**Figure 1.** Effect of EBR on chlorophyll (CHL). (A) Photographs of 10-d-old WT rice seedlings exposed to Fe-sufficient or Fe-deficient medium with or without different concentrations of EBR (0, 1, 10, 100, and 500nM) for 2 weeks. (B) The chlorophyll concentrations in WT rice leaves were determined following treatment of WT seedlings of –Fe and +Fe plants with different concentrations of EBR (0, 1, 10, 100, and 500nM) for 2 weeks. Data are means ± SE ($n = 4$). Means with different letters are significantly different ($P \leq 0.05$) with regard to treatments.

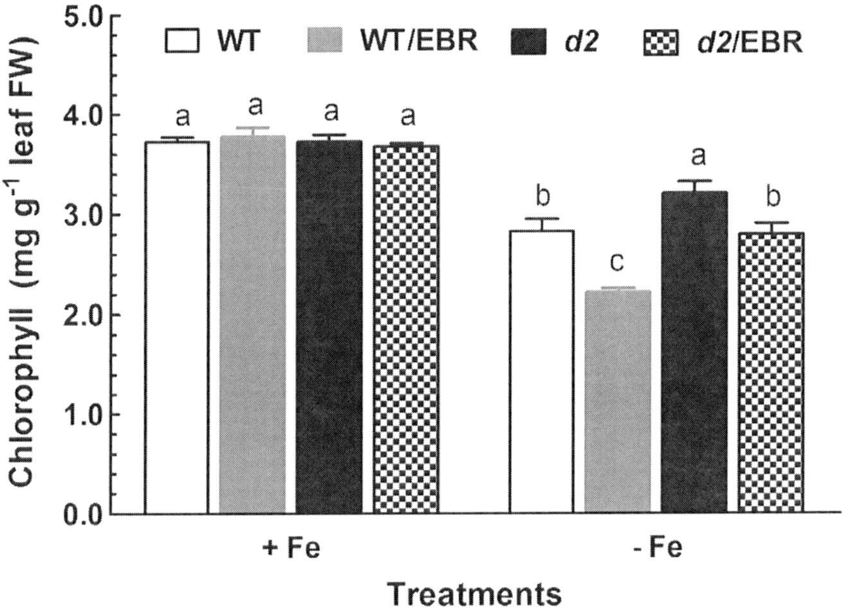


**Figure2.** Effect of EBR on chlorophyll of the WT and *d2-1* mutant. Ten-d-old WT and *d2-1*mutant seedlings were exposed to Fe-sufficient and Fe-deficient medium with or without 100nM EBR for 2 weeks. After treatments, chlorophyll concentration in leaves were determined. Data are means ± SE ($n$ = 4). Means with different letters are significantly different with regard to treatments ($P \leq 0.05$).

*1* mutant was significantly lower than that of WT plants when grown under Fe-sufficient conditions (Fig. 3A, B). In contrast to the WT, an increase in dry weight of the shoots and roots of the *d2-1* mutant was observed under Fe-deficient conditions (Fig. 3B). There was a significant increase in shoot dry weight and a slight increase in root dry weight in the *d2-1* mutant by EBR application under Fe-deficient and Fe-sufficient conditions, respectively (Fig. 3A, B).

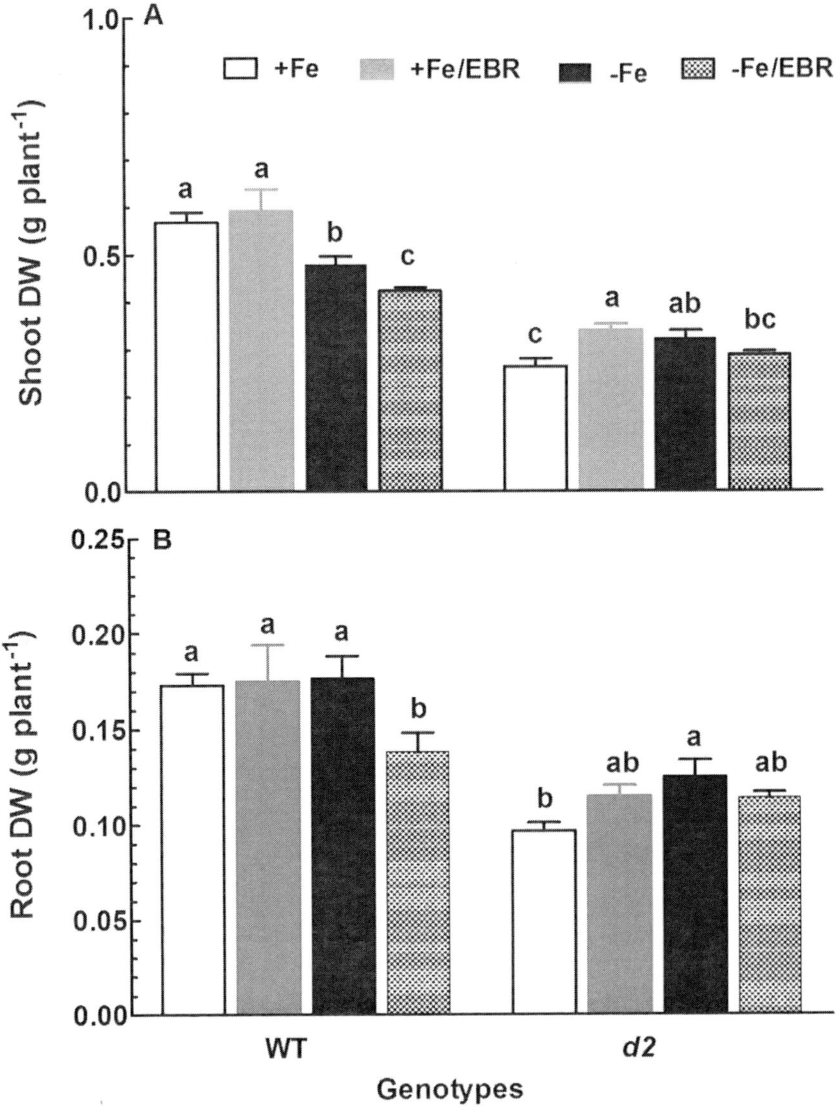


**Figure 3.** Effect of EBR on (A) shoot and (B) root dry weight (DW) of WT and *d2-1* plants. Ten-d-old WT and *d2-1*seedlings were exposed to Fe-sufficient and Fe-deficient medium with or without 100nM EBR for 2 weeks. After treatments, the dry biomass was measured. Data are means ± SE ($n$ = 4). Means with different letters are significantly different ($P \leq 0.05$) within the same genotype.

Exposure of rice seedlings to Fe-deficient medium led to a significant decrease of Fe concentrations in roots and shoots in both the WT and the*d2-1* mutant (Fig. 4). Also, Fe concentrations in roots of the *d2-1* mutant were significantly higher than those of WT plants under both Fe-deficient and Fe-sufficient conditions (Fig. 4B). In contrast to Fe concentrations in roots, concentrations in shoots of *d2-1* plants were higher than those of the WT grown in Fe-deficient medium (Fig. 4A), but no differences in shoot Fe concentrations among WT and *d2-1* under Fe-sufficient conditions were observed (Fig. 4A). Exogenous application of EBR had contrasting effects on Fe concentrations in roots and shoots of WT rice seedlings regardless of Fe supply, such that treatment with EBR led to decreases in Fe concentrations in shoots by 16 and 15% in Fe-sufficient and Fe-deficient seedlings, respectively (Fig. 4A), while there were 35 and 27% increases in root Fe concentrations of both Fe-sufficient and Fe-deficient seedlings when treated with EBR (Fig. 4B). In contrast to WT plants, EBR had no effect on Fe concentrations of *d2-1* in shoots and roots under both Fe-sufficient and Fe-deficient conditions (Fig. 4).

To test whether the EBR-induced changes in Fe concentrations in shoots and roots were specific to Fe, the effect of EBR on other metals concentrations were studied under Fe-sufficient conditions. In contrast to Fe, Mg and Zn concentrations in shoots and roots were not affected by EBR (Supplementary Figure S2). The concentration of Mn in roots was not affected by EBR, but it was significantly increased by EBR in shoots (Supplementary Figure S2). These results suggest that BR has a specific effect on Fe nutrition in shoots and roots of rice.

### Expression patterns of genes related to Fe deficiency in roots

OsIRT1 and OsYSL15 are directly involved in Fe uptake from the rhizosphere (Conte and Walker, 2011). Therefore, we examined the responses of these genes to EBR in WT and *d2* mutants under both Fe-deficient and Fe-sufficient conditions. Upregulation of Os*IRT1* and Os*YSL15* was observed after 1-d treatment with Fe deficiency in both the WT and *d2-1* mutants (Fig. 5A, B). The expression of Os*IRT1* and Os*YSL15*was significantly upregulated by EBR under Fe-sufficient conditions (Fig. 5A, B), and EBR further enhanced the Fe deficiency-induced expression of Os*YSL15* and Os*IRT1* in WT and *d2-1* plants (Fig. 5A, B). Moreover, longer exposure (3 and 7 d) of WT and *d2-1* seedlings

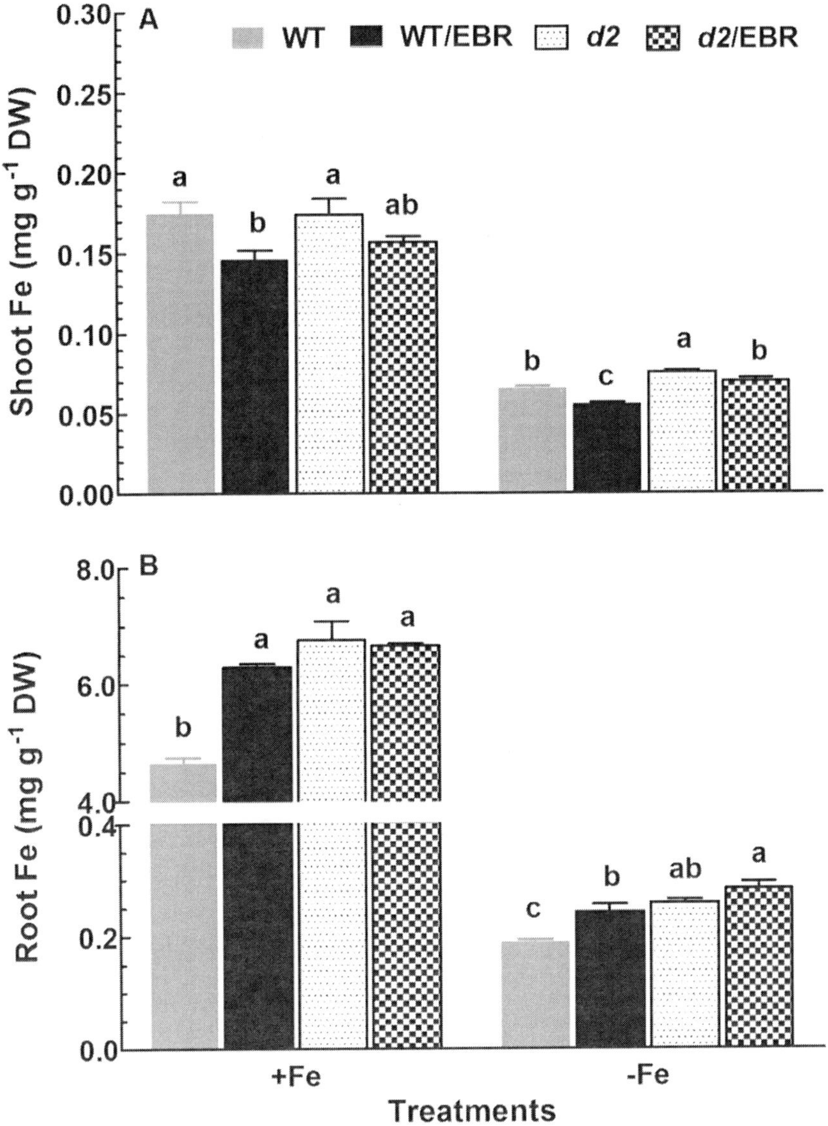


**Figure 4.** Effect of EBR on Fe concentrations in (A) shoots and (B) roots of wild-type and *d2-1* mutant plants. Ten-d-old WT seedlings were exposed to Fe-sufficient and Fe-deficient medium with or without 100nM EBR for 2 weeks. After treatments, Fe concentration was measured. Data are means ± SE ($n$ = 4). Means with different letters are significantly different ($P \leq 0.05$) within the same Fe treatment.

to Fe-deficient medium and EBR also led to upregulation of Os*IRT1* and Os*YSL15* (Fig. 5C–F). However, the magnitude of upregulation of Os*IRT1* and Os*YSL15* by EBR was much greater in WT plants than in *d2-1* mutants under both Fe-sufficient and Fe-deficient conditions. In general, similar effects of EBR and Fe deficiency on expression of Os*IRT1* and Os*YSL15* were observed after treatments with Fe deficiency and EBR for 3 and 7 d (Fig. 5C–F), suggesting that both short- and long-term treatment with Fe deficiency and EBR can alter expression patterns of Os*IRT1* and Os*YSL15*. The expression patterns of Os*IRT1* and Os*YSL15* in WT and *d2-1* mutant plants grown in Fe-sufficient and Fe-deficient media were also compared. Expression levels of Os*IRT1* and Os*YSL5* in *d2-1* mutants were higher than in WT plants grown in Fe-sufficient medium after treatment for 1 and 3 d, and thereafter the mutant and WT plants had comparable expression levels of Os*YSL15* (Fig. 5A–F). Exposure of WT and *d2-1* mutant plants to Fe-deficient medium led to similar changes in expression patterns of Os*IRT1* (Fig. 5 A–F). In contrast to Os*IRT1* expression, the Fe deficiency-induced upregulation of Os*YSL15* expression in *d2-1* mutant plants was less than in WT plants after exposure for 1 and 3 d.

YSL2 and NA have been proposed to mediate long-distance translocation of Fe, and their expression is upregulated under Fe-deficient conditions (Inoue *et al.*, 2003; Ishimaru *et al.*, 2010). Os*FRDL1* encodes a citrate transporter that is localized at the pericycle cells, and is essential for translocation of Fe-citrate complex to the shoot (Yokosho *et al.*, 2009). There were increases in expression levels of Os*YSL2*, Os*NAS1*, and Os*NAS2* in Fe-sufficient WT and *d2-1* plants upon addition of EBR to the medium (Fig. 6A–I). In addition to EBR, exposure of WT and *d2-1* plants to Fe-deficient medium also led to similar increases in expression levels of Os*YSL2*, Os*NAS1*, and Os*NAS2* in terms of magnitude and time course (Fig. 6A–I). In addition, the magnitude of upregulation of Os*YSL2*, Os*NAS1* and Os*NAS2* expression was much greater in WT and *d2-1* mutants challenged by Fe deficiency and EBR together than by treatment with Fe deficiency and EBR alone (Fig. 6A–I), suggesting that Fe deficiency and EBR may have additive effects on the expression of these genes. In contrast to Os*YSL2*, Os*NAS1*, and Os*NAS2*, the expression level of Os*FRDL1* was not responsive to treatments with Fe deficiency and EBR alone or Fe deficiency and EBR together (Fig. 6J–L). Transcript levels of Os*NAS1* and Os*NAS2* in *d2-*

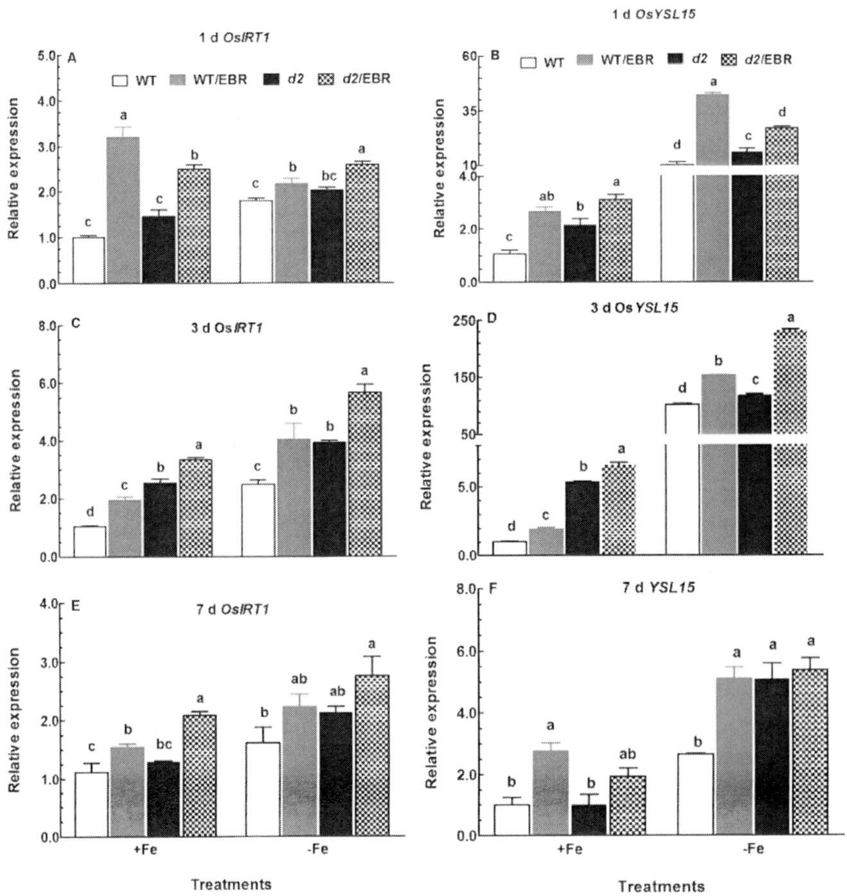


**Figure 5.** Time-course quantitative RT-PCR analysis of Fe uptake-related genes in roots: effect of EBR on Os*IRT1* and Os*YSL15*expression in roots of WT and *d2-1* plants under +Fe and –Fe conditions. Data are means ± SE of three biological replicates. Means with different letters are significantly different within the same gene ($P \leq 0.05$).

*1*plants were generally higher than in the WT under Fe-sufficient conditions (Fig. 6A–I). Treatment with Fe deficiency also induced upregulation of expression of Os*YSL2*, Os*NAS1*, and Os*NAS2* in *d2-1* mutant plants (Fig. 6A–I). However, the magnitude of the upregulation in *d2-1* plants was less than the Fe deficiency-induced upregulation of these genes in WT plants (Fig. 6A–I). No apparent differences in expression levels of Os*FRDL1*between WT and *d2-1* plants under both Fe-sufficient and Fe-deficient conditions were observed (Fig. 6J–L).

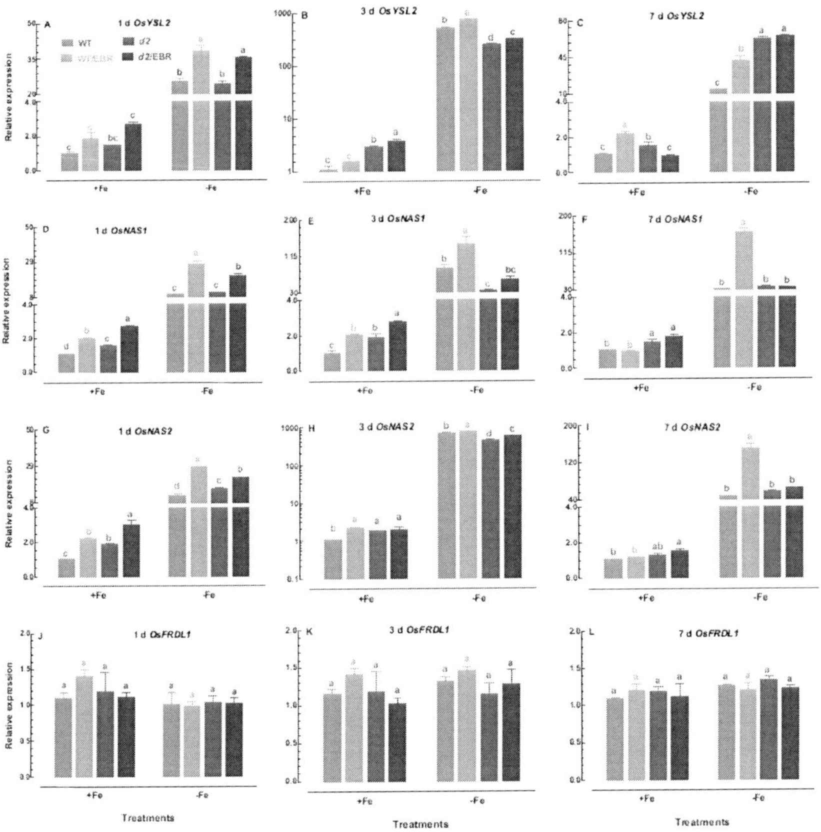


**Figure 6.** Time-course quantitative RT-PCR analysis of Fe translocation related genes in roots: effect of EBR on Os*YSL2*, Os*NAS1*, Os*NAS2*, and Os*FRDL1* expression in roots of WT and *d2-1* plants under +Fe and –Fe conditions. Data are means ± SE of three biological replicates. Means with different letters are significantly different within the same Fe treatment ($P \leq 0.05$). (This figure is available in colour at *JXB* online)

## Expression patterns of transcription factor Os*IRO2* in roots

The rice bHLH protein OsIRO2 is an essential regulator involved in mediation of Fe uptake (Ogo *et al.*, 2007). The expression level of Os*IRO2*was enhanced after addition of EBR to Fe-sufficient medium in both WT and *d2-1* plants (Fig. 7A–C). In addition to EBR, expression of Os*IRO2* was also upregulated by exposure to Fe-deficient medium, and the effect of EBR and Fe deficiency on expression of Os*IRO2* was additive, such that the expression levels were highest in plants exposed to Fe-deficient medium containing EBR (Fig. 7A–C). However, the

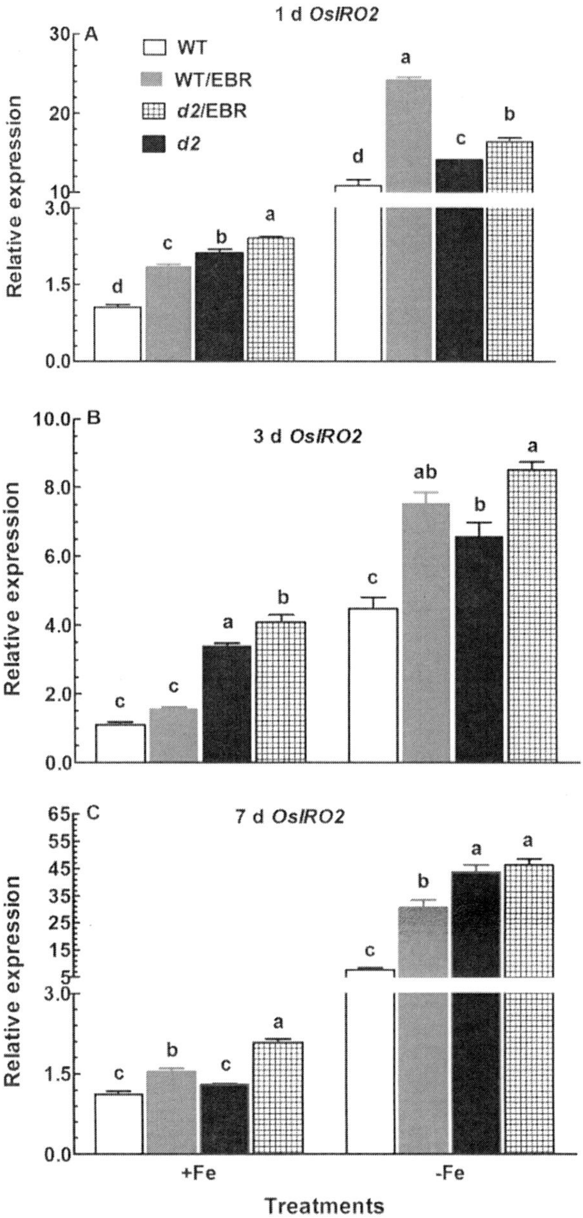


**Figure 7.** Time-course quantitative RT-PCR analysis of Os*IRO2*in roots: effect of EBR on Os*IRO2* expression in roots of WT and *d2-1* plants under +Fe and –Fe conditions. Data are means ± SE of three biological replicates. Means with different letters are significantly different within the same Fe treatments ($P \leq 0.05$).

magnitude of the upregulation by EBR in *d2-1* plants was less than in WT plants under both Fe-sufficient and Fe-deficient conditions. The abundance of Os*IRO2* transcript was higher in *d2-1* plants than in WT plants under Fe-sufficient conditions after 1 and 3 d of treatment, and became comparable after 7-d exposure to Fe-deficient medium (Fig. 7A–C).

### Expression patterns of Os*YSL2*, Os*NAS1*, and Os*NAS2* in shoots

OsYSL2 is a critical Fe-nicotianamine transporter involved in the translocation of Fe, especially in shoots and endosperms (Ishimaru *et al.*, 2010). The responsiveness of Os*YSL2* in shoots of WT and *d2-1* mutants to EBR under Fe-sufficient and Fe-deficient conditions was monitored. The expression level of Os*YSL2* was suppressed by addition of EBR to the Fe-sufficient medium for 1 and 7 d in both WT and *d2-1* plants (Fig. 8A–C). In contrast, exposure of WT and *d2-1* seedlings to Fe-deficient medium led to a sustained upregulation of Os*YSL2* (Fig. 8A–C). Treatment of Fe-deficient seedlings with EBR led to a suppression of Os*YSL2* expression at all experimental stages, such that the expression level was lower in plants exposed to Fe-deficient medium with EBR than in plants exposed to Fe-deficient medium without EBR (Fig. 8A–C). The expression level of Os*YSL2*in *d2-1* plants was slightly higher than in the WT under Fe-sufficient conditions (Fig. 8A–C).

It has been demonstrated that NA is essential for Fe mobilization from the vasculature into the interveinal tissues, and that loss of NA leads to leaf chlorosis (Morrissey and Guerinot, 2009). In the present study, we tested the expression patterns of Os*NAS1* and Os*NAS2* in shoots under varying conditions. The expression levels Os*NAS1* was not affected by EBR from 1 to 7 d in WT plants, but the expression level of Os*NAS2* was suppressed by addition of EBR to Fe-sufficient medium for 1 and 3 d in WT plants (Fig. 8D–I). Treatments of EBR inhibited both Os*NAS1* and Os*NAS2* expression in *d2-1* plants at 1 and 7d under Fe-sufficient conditions (Fig. 8D–I). Similar to Os*YSL2*, treatment of Fe-deficient seedlings of WT plants with EBR led to suppression of Os*NAS1* and Os*NAS2* at all experimental stages (Fig. 8D–I). The expression level of Os*NAS1* and Os*NAS2* was depressed by EBR in *d2-1* mutants at 1 and 7 d under Fe-deficient conditions (Fig. 8D–I). The expression level of Os*NNAS1* and OsNAS2 in *d2-1* plants was slightly higher than in WT under Fe-sufficient conditions (Fig. 8D–I).

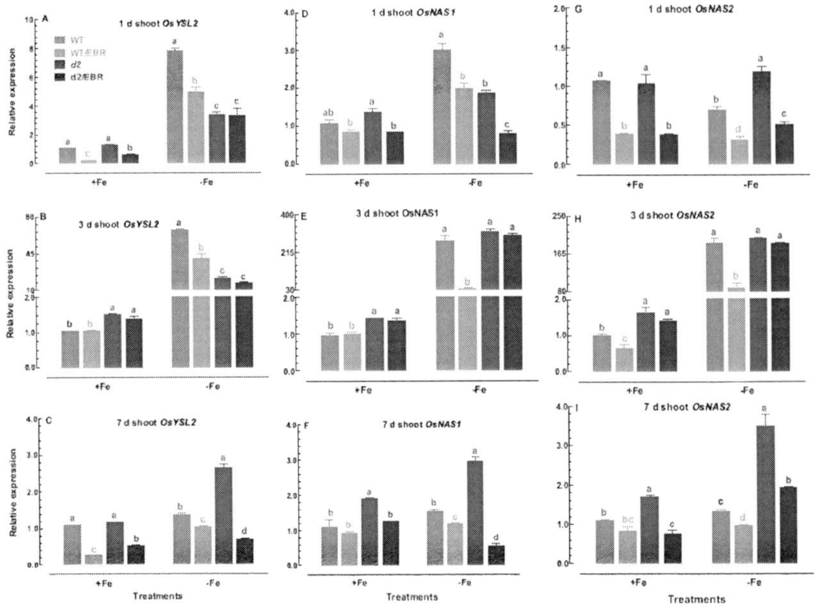


**Figure 8.** Time-course quantitative RT-PCR analysis of Os*YSL2*, Os*NAS1*, and Os*NAS2* in shoots: Effect of EBR on Os*YSL2* expression in shoots of WT and *d2-1* plants under +Fe and –Fe conditions. Data are means ± SE of three biological replicates. Means with different letters are significantly different within the same Fe treatment ($P \leq 0.05$). (This figure is available in colour at *JXB* online)

## Fe concentrations in the phloem sap

OsYSL2 is a metal-NA transporter responsible for translocation of Fe in the phloem of rice (Koike *et al.*, 2004). To test whether the EBR-induced inhibition of Os*YLS2* expression can affect transport or translocation of Fe in the phloem, Fe concentrations in the phloem sap were measured. Fe concentrations in the phloem of the WT were significantly reduced in the presence of EBR under Fe-sufficient conditions (Fig. 9). In contrast, Fe concentrations in the phloem of Fe-sufficient *d2-1* plants were not changed by EBR. Little Fe could be detected in the phloem sap when rice plants were grown in Fe-deficient medium in the absence and presence of EBR (Fig. 9). These results indicate that EBR inhibits the translocation of Fe via the phloem.

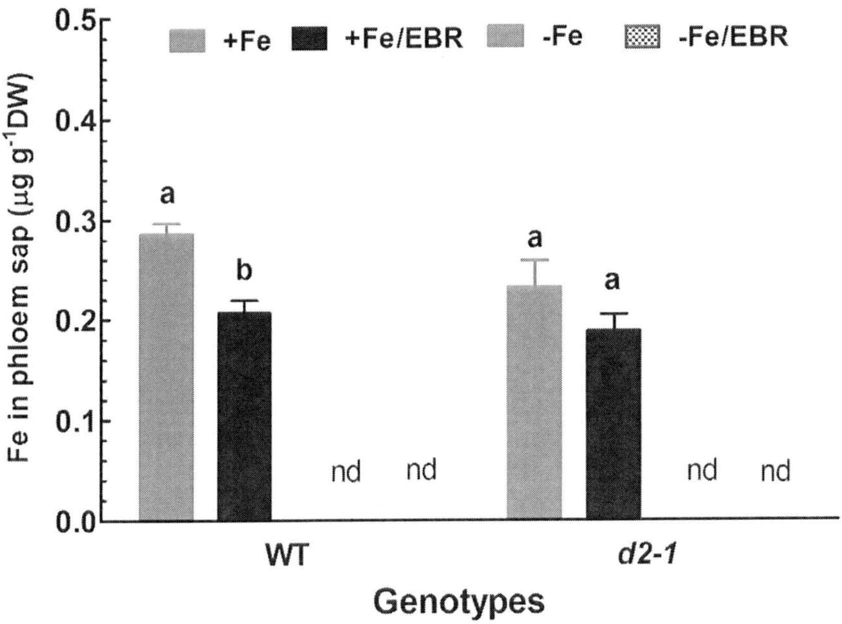


**Figure 9.** Effect of EBR on Fe concentration in phloem sap of the WT and *d2-1* mutant. Ten-d-old WT and d2-1 seedlings were exposed to Fe-sufficient and Fe -deficient medium with or without 100nM EBR for 2 weeks. After treatments, phloem sap was collected and Fe concentration was measured. Data are means ± SE ($n$ = 4). Means with different letters are significantly different within the same genotype ($P \leq 0.05$).

**Expression patterns of genes related to BR biosynthesis and signal transduction**

To dissect the network associated with BR-dependent Fe uptake and translocation, the response of BR biosynthesis and signalling to Fe deficiency was examined at the transcriptional level in shoots and roots. The expression levels of *WRARF* and *D2*, which encode proteins involved in BR biosynthesis (Hong *et al.*, 2002; Hong *et al.*, 2003), and *BRI1*, which encodes a BR receptor (Morinaka *et al.*, 2006), were substantially suppressed after exposure to Fe-deficient medium for 1 d (Fig. 10A–C). The expression levels of *WRARF* and *D2* in Fe-deficient and Fe-sufficient seedlings became comparable after exposure to Fe-deficient medium for 3 and 7 d (Fig. 10B, C). The Fe deficiency-induced suppression of *BRI1* was also observed after 3 d of exposure to Fe-deficient medium, but the expression level became comparable to that in Fe-sufficient plants after exposure to Fe-deficient medium for 7 d (Fig. 10B, C). In contrast, expression of the three genes in roots was relatively constant after exposure to Fe-deficient medium up to 7 d (Fig. 10D–F). These results suggest that both BR biosynthesis and signal transduction in shoots may be closely regulated by Fe status in plants.

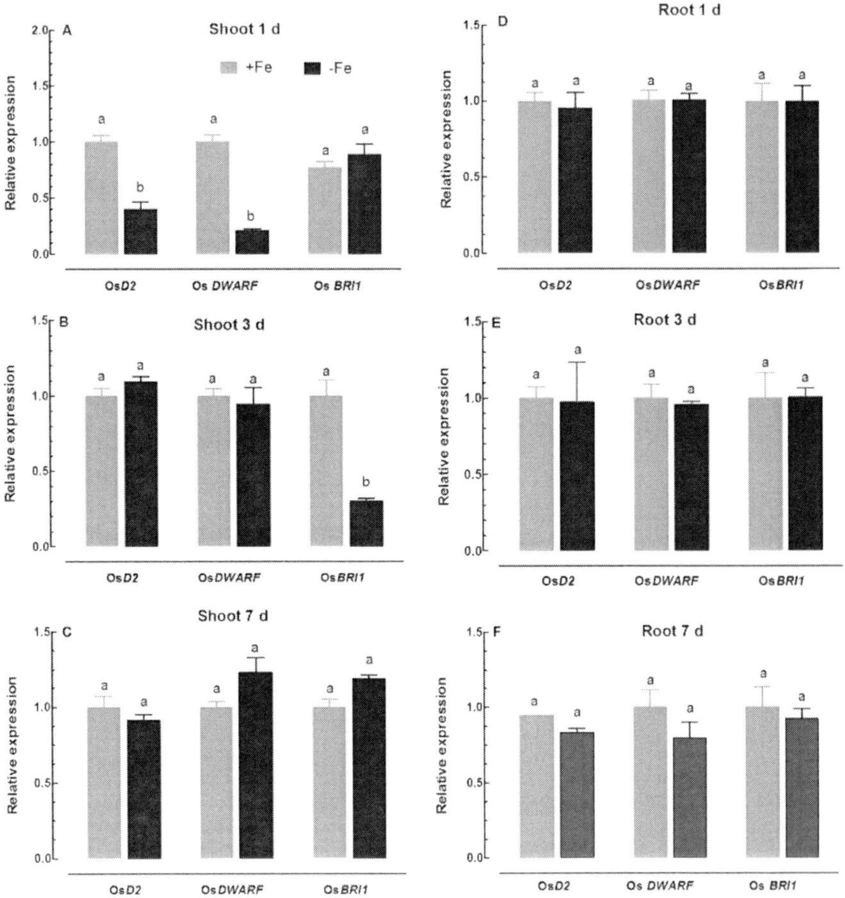


**Figure 10.** Time-course quantitative RT-PCR analysis of genes related to BR biosynthesis and signal transduction in shoots and roots: effect of Fe deficiency on Os*D2*,Os*DWARF*, and Os*BRI1*expression in shoots (A, B, and C) and roots (D, E, and F) of WT plants. Data are means ± s.e. of three biological replicates. Means with different letters are significantly different within the same gene ($P \leq 0.05$)

# DISCUSSION

There is increasing evidence demonstrating the involvement of BR in the mediation of abiotic stress responses (Sasse, 2003). However, few studies have investigated the role of BR in the response of plants to deficiency in mineral nutrients. Our previous studies revealed that BR is involved in the response of cucumber, a strategy I plant, to Fe deficiency by negatively regulating Cs*FRO1*, Cs*IRT1*, and Fe translocation from roots to shoots (Wang *et al.*, 2012). Since the mechanisms by which Fe uptake and translocation differ between strategy I and II plants, different mechanisms may account for the effect of BR on their Fe acquisition. In the present study, we demonstrate that BR may also play a role in the regulation of the response of rice plants, a strategy II plant, to Fe deficiency using wild-type and BR-deficient mutant *d2-1*. We further show that an exogenous application of EBR rendered WT plants more sensitive to Fe deficiency by interfering with Fe homeostasis, and that the effect is specific to Fe. Rice mutant *d2-1*, which is deficient in endogenous BR levels due to disruption of BR biosynthesis, exhibited enhanced tolerance to Fe-deficiency, and the increased tolerance could be partly reversed by EBR complementation. These results suggest that BR is involved in the response of strategy II plants to Fe deficiency. Two mutant lines, *d2-1* and *d2-2*, were originally generated by Hong *et al.* (2003). The *d2-1* mutant exhibits more severe phenotypes than the *d2-2* mutant, and the two types of plant are allelic (Hong *et al.*, 2003). Therefore, the results obtained from the *d2-1* mutant would not undermine our conclusion.

Exogenous application of EBR to WT rice seedlings enhanced Fe deficiency-induced leaf chlorosis (Fig. 1), but the BR-deficient mutant *d2-1* was more tolerant to Fe deficiency than WT plants (Fig. 2). The growth rate was lower in the *d2-1* mutant than in WT plants, which may lead to a lower nutrient demand in the *d2-1* mutant. To test whether the enhanced tolerance of *d2-1* plants to Fe deficiency is not caused by their lower growth rate, we measured other mineral nutrients and compared the response of *d2-1* and *d61-2* to Fe deficiency. The *d61-2* mutation was caused by loss of function of OsBRI1, a putative BR receptor (Hong *et al.*, 2003), and *d61-2* mutants exhibit reduced growth compared to WT plants under normal growth conditions (Morinaka *et al.*, 2006). In contrast to increased Fe concentrations in *d2-1*, there were no differences in Mg and K concentrations in shoots and roots between WT and *d2-1* under Fe-sufficient conditions (data not shown). Our data also showed that *d2-1*and *d61-2* exhibited similar shoot dry weight under Fe-deficient conditions, but *d61-2* was more sensitive to Fe deficiency than *d2-1* in terms of chlorophyll concentration, shoot dry weight, and shoot Fe concentrations (Supplementary Figure S3). These results suggest that the enhanced tolerance to Fe deficiency of the *d2-1* mutant may not simply be accounted for by its reduced growth rate, and that BR may be specifically involved in Fe uptake, transport, and translocation processes in rice. OsIRT1 and OsYSL15 are directly involved in Fe uptake from the rhizosphere in rice (Conte and Walker, 2011). Our results showing that Fe deficiency significantly enhanced expression of Os*IRT1* and Os*YSL15* (Fig. 5) are in agreement with those reported in the literature. Expression of Os*IRT1* and Os*YSL15* in the *d2-1* mutant was higher than in WT plants under Fe-sufficient conditions (Fig. 5), which may underpin the higher Fe accumulation in roots of the *d2-1* mutant than in roots of WT plants. After uptake, Fe is transported in the complexed forms once it is loaded into the xylem (Conte and Walker, 2011). OsFRDL1, a citrate transporter localized at the rice root pericycle cells, is necessary for efficient translocation of Fe-citrate complex to shoots (Yokosho *et al.*, 2009). Expression of Os*FRDL1* was relatively insensitive to Fe deficiency and EBR (Fig. 6). A similar insensitivity of Os*FRDL1* to Fe deficiency has been reported in the literature (Yokosho *et al.*, 2009). Although citrate plays an important role in long-distance transport of Fe in rice, knockout of Os*FRDL1* results in mild defects in Fe homeostasis compared with the severe phenotype of the*Arabidopsis frd3* mutant (Kobayashi and Nishizawa, 2012), suggesting that alternative chelators may exist in rice to mediate transport of Fe in the xylem. In addition to citrate, NA levels have a significant effect on metal homeostasis (Morrissey and Guerinot, 2009). Overexpression of NAS in tobacco and *Arabidopsis* increases NA levels in shoots, resulting in increased Fe in the shoots (Takahashi *et al.*, 2003; Kim *et al.*, 2005). However, it is unclear whether these changes are the result of greater root to shoot translocation facilitated by NA or increased metal uptake in the roots driven by the creation of new Fe sinks in the shoot (Morrissey and Guerinot, 2009). In rice, YSL2 and NA have been proposed to mediate long-distance translocation of Fe and/or are responsible for the phloem transport of Fe in shoots (Inoue *et al.*, 2003; Koike *et al.*, 2004; Ishimaru*et al.*, 2010). In our study, we found that expression of Os*YSL2*, Os*NAS1*, and Os*NAS2* in shoots was significantly depressed by EBR treatment (Fig. 8), and that Fe concentrations in phloem sap of WT plants were also decreased by EBR application (Fig. 9). EBR treatment may decrease shoot NA and inhibit Fe translocation from roots to shoots or decrease the Fe sink in shoots. The suppression of shoot Os*YSL2* may suppress the unloading of Fe from the phloem to mesophyll cells and lead to a low Fe concentration in protoplasts of leaf mesophyll cells and enhanced leaf chlorosis. The lowered shoot Fe by BR feedbacks to roots enhanced the expression of many genes involved in Fe homeostasis, leading to Fe accumulation in roots, but decreased biomass and Fe of shoots.

Os*IRO2* is an essential transcription factor modulating Fe uptake and translocation in rice plants (Kobayashi and Nishizawa, 2012). Expression of Os*IRO2* is often upregulated upon exposure to Fe-deficient medium, thus activating the expression of genes responsible for Fe homeostasis in roots (Ogo *et al.*, 2007, 2011). Our results are in agreement with those reported in the literature. Moreover, our results showed that EBR significantly enhanced Os*IRO2* expression in both Fe-sufficient and Fe-deficient WT rice plants (Fig. 7), which may account for the EBR-induced upregulation of Fe homeostasis-related genes, such as Os*YSL15*, Os*NAS1*, and Os*NAS2* (Fig. 6). Similar to EBR application, a higher expression of Os*IRO2* and genes related to Fe homeostasis was observed by BR deficiency in the *d2-1* mutant (Fig. 6). Root Fe and expression levels of genes related to Fe homeostasis in the WT and *d2-1* mutant were increased or upregulated by exogenous EBR application and endogenous BR defects, respectively, but the mechanisms may be different. Expression of Os*IRT1* and Os*YSL15* in *d2-1* mutants was higher in *d2-1* than in WT plants under Fe-sufficient conditions (Fig. 5), which may account for the higher Fe uptake and accumulation in roots of *d2-1* mutants than in roots of WT plants. In addition to efficient Fe-uptake systems of roots in *d2-1*, the expression of genes related to Fe transport and translocation in shoots of *d2-1* was also higher than that in WT plants (Fig. 8). Thus, BR-deficient mutant *d2-1* had comparable shoot Fe concentrations with WT plants under Fe-sufficient conditions (Fig. 4A), suggesting that, for the *d2-1*mutant, upregulation of genes associated with Fe homeostasis may account for the higher Fe concentrations in shoots. These may provide an explanation for the greater tolerance of *d2-1* to Fe deficiency than WT plants. The efficient uptake and translocation of Fe may make the *d2-1*mutant more tolerant to Fe deficiency and less responsive to EBR treatment, as evidenced by less suppression of plant biomass and Fe concentrations in the *d2-1* mutant than the WT when grown in Fe-deficient medium, and lower expression levels of genes associated with Fe uptake and translocation at early stages of Fe deficiency. Unlike the *d2-1*mutant, exogenous EBR suppressed the expression of genes related to Fe transport and translocation in shoots (Fig. 8), leading to reductions in shoot Fe concentrations of WT plants (Fig. 4). Decreased shoot Fe concentration by EBR enhanced leaf chlorosis, which may feed back to the root and activate the expression of Fe homeostasis-related genes, thus leading to Fe accumulation in roots. The symptoms in rice seedlings treated with exogenous BR are comparable to those in *Arabidopsis* mutant*frd3*, including leaf chlorosis, constitutive expression of genes associated with

Fe uptake, and low Fe level in the plastid, even under Fe-sufficient conditions (Rogers and Guerinot, 2002).

Exogenous application of BRs has been shown to improve stress tolerance by activating the BR signal transduction pathway and BR-regulated expression of stress-related genes (Kagale *et al.*, 2007). In the present study, we found that Fe concentrations in shoots were negatively regulated by BRs, but the signal transduction pathways remain to be dissected. In rice, Os*D2* and Os*DWARF* are responsible for biosynthesis of BRs, and Os*BRI1* is a receptor for BR (Yamamuro *et al.*, 2000; Hong et al., 2002,2003). Under salt and drought stress, expression of salt- and drought-responsive genes is rapidly altered by BR (Kagale *et al.*, 2007). Also, expression of the BR receptor gene in rice can be modified within several hours by treatment with IAA (Sakamoto *et al.*, 2013). These indicate that plants can be quickly responsive to environmental and hormonal cues by modulating BR signalling cascades. Expression of Os*D2*, Os*DWARF*, and Os*BRI1* in roots of WT plants was not responsive to Fe deficiency (Fig. 10D–F). In contrast, expression of Os*D2* and Os*DWARF* in shoots was markedly suppressed by exposure to Fe-deficient medium for 1 d, while the Fe deficiency-induced inhibition of Os*BRI1* expression occurred after 3-d exposure to Fe-deficient medium (cf. Fig. 10). These results imply that BRs may be involved in regulation of Fe transport and translocation from roots to shoots, but the underlying mechanisms remain to be elucidated. In rice, the regulatory network involving Os*IDEF1*, Os*IDEF2*, and Os*IRO2* in response to Fe deficiency has been elucidated (Kobayashi *et al.*, 2007; Ogo *et al.*, 2008; Kobayashi *et al.*, 2009, 2012; Kobayashi and Nishizawa, 2012). Based on the information and our results, a putative working model is proposed to illustrate the possible role of BR in regulating the response of rice plants to Fe deficiency (Fig. 11). The iron deficiency signal transmits from shoot to root, and activates transcription factors Os*IDEF1* and Os*IRO2*, which in turn modulates the downstream targets involved in Fe homeostasis at the transcriptional level, leading to Fe uptake and accumulation in roots. In contrast, Fe deficiency inhibited BR biosynthesis, and the reduced endogenous BRs may facilitate Fe transport and translocation from roots to shoots. The exogenous application of EBR to rice seedlings would suppress the transport and translocation of Fe from roots to shoots, thus leading to a more severe phenotype of Fe deficiency in shoots and strengthen Fe deficiency signal. The enhanced signal of Fe deficiency will further upregulate downstream genes involved in Fe homeostasis, and lead to Fe uptake and accumulation in roots. BRs negatively regulated Fe transport and translocation from root to shoot in rice seedlings, but the mechanisms are not clear. Therefore, future research focusing on the interaction of BR with Fe transport and translocation in strategy II plants is warranted.

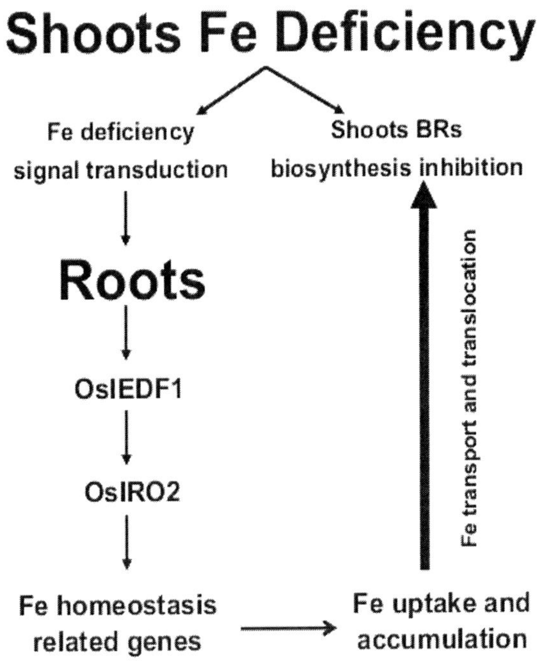


**Figure 11.** A putative working model to illustrate the possible role of BR in regulating the response of rice plants to Fe deficiency. Pathways possibly responsible for Fe uptake or transport and translocation from roots to shoots are separated. Shoot Fe deficiency could induce signal transduction from shoots to roots, and activate Fe mobilization and uptake by roots. On the other hand, Fe deficiency could decrease BR levels in shoots and inhibit Fe transport and translocation from roots to shoots.

In conclusion, our results highlight the importance of BR as a signalling molecule involved in mediating the response of rice plants to Fe deficiency. More specifically, we demonstrate that BR plays a negatively regulatory role in control of transport and translocation from roots to shoots, thus indirectly modulating Fe mobilization and acquisition by possibly regulating Os*IRO2*.

## FUNDING

This work was supported by the Natural Science Foundation of China (31101594) and State Key Laboratory of Vegetation and Environmental Change.

## ACKNOWLEDGEMENTS

We thank Dr Tomoaki Sakamoto for the gift of *d2-1* and *d61-2* mutants. We thank the editor and anonymous reviewers for their constructive suggestions on the previous version of the manuscript.

## REFERENCES

1. Bughio N, Yamaguchi H, Nishizawa NK, Nakanishi H, Mori S. 2002. Cloning an iron-regulated metal transporter from rice. Journal of Experimental Botany 53, 1677–1682.
2. Cheng L, Wang F, Shou H, et al. 2007. Mutation in nicotianamine aminotransferase stimulated the Fe (II) acquisition system and led to iron accumulation in rice. Plant Physiology 145, 1647–1657.
3. Conte SS, Walker EL. 2011. Transporters contributing to iron trafficking in plants. Molecular Plant 4, 464–476.
4. Corbesier L, Prinsen E, Jacqmard A, Lejeune P, Van Onckelen H, Perilleux C, Bernier G. 2003. Cytokinin levels in leaves, leaf exudate and shoot apical meristem of Arabidopsis thaliana during floral transition. Journal of Experimental Botany 54, 2511–2517.
5. Curie C, Briat JF. 2003. Iron transport and signaling in plants. Annual Review of Plant Biology 54, 183–206.
6. Curie C, Panaviene Z, Loulergue C, Dellaporta SL, Briat JF, Walker EL. 2001. Maize yellow stripe1 encodes a membrane protein directly involved in Fe(III) uptake. Nature 409, 346–349.
7. Durrett TP, Gassmann W, Rogers EE. 2007. The FRD3-mediated efflux of citrate into the root vasculature is necessary for efficient iron translocation. Plant Physiology 144, 197–205.
8. Green L, Rogers EE. 2004. FRD3 controls iron localization in Arabidopsis. Plant Physiology 136, 2523–2531.

9. Hell R, Stephan UW. 2003. Iron uptake, trafficking and homeostasis in plants. Planta 210, 541–551.

10. Hong Z, Ueguchi-Tanaka M, Shimizu-Sato S, et al. 2002. Lossof-function of a rice brassinosteroid biosynthetic enzyme, C-6 oxidase, prevents the organized arrangement and polar elongation of cells in the leaves and stem. The Plant Journal 32, 495–508.

11. Hong Z, Ueguchi-Tanaka M, Umemura K, Uozu S, Fujioka S, Takatsuto S, Yoshida S, Ashikari M, Kitano H, Matsuoka M. 2003. A rice brassinosteroid-deficient mutant, ebisu dwarf (d2), is caused by loss of function of a new member of cytochrome P450. The Plant Cell 15, 2900–2910.

12. Inoue H, Higuchi K, Takahashi M, Nakanishi H, Mori S, Nishizawa NK. 2003. Three rice nicotianamine synthase genes, OsNAS1, OsNAS2, and OsNAS3 are expressed in cells involved in long-distance transport of iron and differentially regulated by iron. The Plant Journal 36, 366–381.

13. Inoue H, Kobayashi T, Nozoye T, Takahashi M, Kakei Y, Suzuki K, Nakazono M, Nakanishi H, Mori S, Nishizawa NK. 2009. Rice OsYSL15 is an iron-regulated iron(III)-deoxymugineic acid transporter expressed in the roots and is essential for iron uptake in early growth of the seedlings. The Journal of Biological Chemistry 284, 3470–3479.

14. Ishimaru Y, Masuda H, Bashir K, Inoue H, Tsukamoto T, Takahashi M, Nakanishi H, Aoki N, Hirose T, Ohsugi R, Nishizawa NK. 2010. Rice metal-nicotianamine transporter, OsYSL2, is required for the long-distance transport of iron and manganese. The Plant Journal 62, 379–390.

15. Ishimaru Y, Suzuki M, Tsukamoto T, et al. 2006. Rice plants take up iron as an Fe3+-phytosiderophore and as Fe2+. The Plant Journal 45, 335–346.

16. Ivanov R, Brumbarova T, Bauer P. 2012. Fitting into the harsh reality: regulation of iron-deficiency responses in dicotyledonous plants. Molecular Plant 5, 27–42.

17. Kagale S, Divi UK, Krochko JE, Keller WA, Krishna P. 2007. Brassinosteroid confers tolerance in Arabidopsis thaliana and Brassica napus to a range of abiotic stresses. Planta 225, 353–364.

18. Kim S, Takahashi M, Higuchi K, Tsunoda K, Nakanish H, Yoshimura E, Mori S, Nishizawa NK. 2005. Increased

nicotianamine biosynthesis confers enhanced tolerance of high levels of metals, in particular nickel, to plants. Plant Cell Physiology 46, 1809–1818.

19. Kobayashi T, Itai RN, Aung MS, Senoura T, Nakanishi H, Nishizawa NK. 2012. The rice transcription factor IDEF1 directly binds to iron and other divalent metals for sensing cellular iron status. The Plant Journal 69, 81–91.

20. Kobayashi T, Itai RN, Ogo Y, Kakei Y, Nakanishi H, Takahashi M, Nishizawa NK. 2009. The rice transcription factor IDEF1 is essential for the early response to iron deficiency, and induces vegetative expression of late embryogenesis abundant genes. The Plant Journal 60, 948–961.

21. Kobayashi T, Nishizawa NK. 2012. Iron uptake, translocation, and regulation in higher plants. Annual Review of Plant Biology 63, 132–152.

22. Kobayashi T, Ogo Y, Itai RN, Nakanishi H, Takahashi M, Mori S, Nishizawa NK. 2007. The transcription factor IDEF1 regulates the response to and tolerance of iron deficiency in plants. Proceedings of the National Academy of Sciences, USA 104, 19150–19155.

23. Koike S, Inoue H, Mizuno D, Takahashi M, Nakanishi H, Mori S, Nishizawa NK. 2004. OsYSL2 is a rice metal-nicotianamine transporter that is regulated by iron and expressed in the phloem. The Plant Journal 39, 415–424.

24. Morinaka Y, Sakamoto T, Inukai Y, Agetsuma M, Kitano H, Ashikari M, Matsuoka M. 2006. Morphological alteration caused by brassinosteroid insensitivity increases the biomass and grain production of rice. Plant Physiology 141, 924–931.

25. Morrissey J, Guerinot L. 2009. Iron uptake and transport in plants: the good, the bad, and the ionome. Chemical Reviews 109, 4553–4567.

26. Noguchi T, Fujioka S, Choe S, Takatsuto S, Yoshida S, Yuan H, Feldmann KA, Tax FE. 1999. Brassinosteroid-insensitive dwarf mutants of Arabidopsis accumulate brassinosteroids. Plant Physiology 121, 743–752.

27. Nozoye T, Nagasaka S, Kobayashi T, Takahashi M, Sato Y, Sato Y, Uozumi N, Nakanishi H, Nishizawa NK. 2011. Phytosiderophore efflux transporters are crucial for iron acquisition in graminaceous plants. The Journal of Biological Chemistry 286, 5446–5454.

# INDEX

28. Ogo Y, Itai RN, Kobayashi T, Aung MS, Nakanishi H, Nishizawa NK. 2011. OsIRO2 is responsible for iron utilization in rice and improves growth and yield in calcareous soil. Plant Molecular Biology 75, 593–605.

29. Ogo Y, Itai RN, Nakanishi H, Kobayashi T, Takahashi M, Mori S, Nishizawa NK. 2007. The rice bHLH protein OsIRO2 is an essential regulator of the genes involved in Fe uptake under Fe-deficient conditions. The Plant Journal 51, 366–377.

30. Ogo Y, Kobayashi T, Itai R N, Nakanishi H, Kakei Y, Takahashi M, Toki S, Mori S, Nishizawa NK. 2008. A novel NAC transcription factor, IDEF2, that recognizes the iron deficiency-responsive element 2 regulates the genes involved in iron homeostasis in plants. The Journal of Biological Chemistry 283, 13407–13417.

31. Rellán-Álvarez R, Giner-Martínez-Sierra J, Orduma J, Orera I, Rodríguez-Castrillón JA, García-Alonso JI, Abadia J, ÁlvarezFernández A. 2010. Identification of a tri-iron (III), tri-citrate complex

## B



## C



## G



## H



## I



## K



## M

# Pediatric and Adolescent Medicine

## Vol. 10

Series Editors

*D. Branski* *Jerusalem*
*W. Kiess* *Leipzig*

KARGER

# Diabetes in Childhood and Adolescence

Volume Editors

*F. Chiarelli* *Chieti*
*K. Dahl-Jørgensen* *Oslo*
*W. Kiess* *Leipzig*

40 figures, 1 in color, and 40 tables, 2005

KARGER

Basel · Freiburg · Paris · London · New York ·
Bangalore · Bangkok · Singapore · Tokyo · Sydney

**Prof. Francesco Chiarelli**
Clinica Pediatrica
Ospedale Policlinico Chieti
Chieti, Italy

**Prof. Knut Dahl-Jørgensen**
Diabetes Research Centre
Pediatric Department
Ullevål University Hospital Oslo
Oslo, Norway

**Prof. Wieland Kiess**
Universitätsklinik und Poliklinik
für Kinder und Jugendliche
Universität Leipzig, Leipzig, Germany

Library of Congress Cataloging-in-Publication Data

Diabetes in childhood and adolescence / volume editors, F. Chiarelli, K. Dahl-Jørgensen, W. Kiess.
p. ; cm. – (Pediatric and adolescent medicine, ISSN 1017-5989 ; v. 10)
Includes bibliographical references and index.
ISBN 3-8055-7766-4 (hard cover : alk. paper)
1. Diabetes in children. 2. Diabetes in adolescence.
[DNLM: 1. Diabetes Mellitus–Adolescent. 2. Diabetes Mellitus–Child. WK 810 D5375235 2005] I. Chiarelli, F. (Francesco) II. Dahl-Jørgensen, K. (Knut) III. Kiess, W. (Wieland) IV. Series.
RJ420.D5D533 2005
618.92′462–dc22
2005003110

Bibliographic Indices. This publication is listed in bibliographic services, including Current Contents® and Index Medicus.

Drug Dosage. The authors and the publisher have exerted every effort to ensure that drug selection and dosage set forth in this text are in accord with current recommendations and practice at the time of publication. However, in view of ongoing research, changes in government regulations, and the constant flow of information relating to drug therapy and drug reactions, the reader is urged to check the package insert for each drug for any change in indications and dosage and for added warnings and precautions. This is particularly important when the recommended agent is a new and/or infrequently employed drug.


www.karger.com
Printed in Switzerland on acid-free paper by Reinhardt Druck, Basel
ISSN 1017–5989
ISBN 3–8055–7766–4

## Contents

# Preface

Diabetes mellitus is one of the most frequent chronic diseases affecting children and adolescents. Next to obesity it is the most common metabolic disorder in childhood and adolescence. The number of young children being diagnosed with type 1 diabetes is increasing worldwide. An epidemic of type 2 diabetes already at a young age is being observed in most societies around the world.

This book aims to increase physicians' knowledge and understanding of diabetes in childhood and adolescence as well as to summarize the most recent scientific discoveries related to diabetes. Leading experts from the USA, Europe and Israel have gathered to provide a state-of-the-art summary of today's knowledge in the field of pediatric and adolescent diabetes. Several chapters deliver insight into the basic understanding of which factors contribute to or prevent the development of diabetes in young people. For example, Achenbach and colleagues outline the basic concepts underlying the autoimmune pathogenesis of type 1 diabetes. Knip from Helsinki summarizes the global knowledge on the etiopathogenesis of type 1 diabetes and reports on the very extensive experience and scientific contributions from his group in Finland. Other contributions provide tools for the clinician to manage the care of the child and adolescent with diabetes. For instance, continuous subcutaneous insulin infusion regimens are nicely developed by the group of Phillip in Tel Aviv and the management of diabetic ketoacidosis in a child or adolescent is taught by Brink from Boston. Diabetes complications occur even at a young age and may be prevented. This fact is acknowledged in a number of excellent chapters such as the ones by Bittner and coworkers on retinopathy, Chiarelli and coworkers on nephropathy, Dahl-Jørgensen and coworkers on macrovascular disease, or Donaghue on autonomic and peripheral neuropathy. In addition, knowledge from the latest scientific studies on the molecular biology of diabetes is also presented. For example, Cucca from Cagliari outlines the most recent advances in the genetics of type 1 diabetes. The contribution by Polak's group from Paris reviews our knowledge on neonatal diabetes and the underlying genetics. In addition, Falqui from Milan describes the potential implications of gene therapy and islet transplantation for the future cure of diabetes.

The editors would like to extend their gratitude and appreciation to the authors who are all world authorities in their field. To have worked with them has made this project both a great joy and a success. In addition, the understanding, patience, great care and enthusiasm with which the publisher, Dr. Thomas Karger and his team have supported this book are gratefully acknowledged.

*Francesco Chiarelli,* Chieti
*Knut Dahl-Jørgensen,* Oslo
*Wieland Kiess,* Leipzig

Chiarelli F, Dahl-Jørgensen K, Kiess W (eds): Diabetes in Childhood and Adolescence.
Pediatr Adolesc Med. Basel, Karger, 2005, vol 10, pp 1–27

# Etiopathogenetic Aspects of Type 1 Diabetes

*Mikael Knip*

Hospital for Children and Adolescents, University of Helsinki, Helsinki, and
Department of Paediatrics, Tampere University Hospital, Tampere, Finland

Type 1 diabetes is perceived as a chronic immune-mediated disease with a subclinical prodromal period characterized by selective loss of insulin-producing β-cells in the pancreatic islets in genetically susceptible subjects. The most important genes contributing to disease susceptibility are located in the HLA class II locus on the short arm of chromosome 6 [1]. Nevertheless, only a relatively small proportion, i.e. less than 10%, of genetically susceptible individuals progress to clinical disease. This implies that additional factors are needed to trigger and drive β-cell destruction in genetically predisposed subjects. Clinical type 1 diabetes represents end-stage insulitis, and it has been estimated that at the time of diagnosis only 10–20% of the insulin-producing β-cells are still functioning. Environmental factors have been implicated in the pathogenesis of type 1 diabetes both as triggers and potentiators of β-cell destruction [2–4], although the contribution of any individual exogenous factor has not been definitely proven so far.

## Natural History of Type 1 Diabetes

The clinical presentation of type 1 diabetes is preceded by an asymptomatic period of variable duration [5]. Aggressive β-cell destruction may lead to disease manifestation within a few months in young children, while in other individuals the process will continue for years, in some cases even for more than 10 years, before the eventual presentation of clinical disease.

The appearance of diabetes-associated autoantibodies is the first detectable sign of emerging β-cell autoimmunity. There are four disease-related

**Table 1.** Environmental factors implicated in the pathogenesis of type 1 diabetes

| |
|---|
| *Dietary factors* |
| Cow's milk proteins |
| Casein |
| Bovine serum albumin |
| β-Lactoglobulin |
| Bovine insulin |
| Gluten and other plant proteins |
| Fats |
| Nitrate and nitrite |
| Coffee, tea |
| Deficiency of zinc |
| Vitamin D deficiency |
| Frequent intake of solid foods rich in carbohydrate and protein |
| *Viral infections* |
| Mumps |
| Rubella |
| Cytomegalovirus |
| Enteroviruses |
| Retroviruses |
| Rotavirus |
| Ljunganvirus |
| *Standard of hygiene and vaccinations* |
| Toxins |
| Alloxan |
| Streptozotocin |
| N-nitroso compounds |
| Bafilomycin A1 |
| Growth |
| Infant growth |
| Childhood growth |
| *Psycosocial factors* |
| *Latitude and temperature* |
| *Antenatal and perinatal risk* |

anecdotal reports suggesting a low incidence of type 1 diabetes in people from countries with a low protein intake, Elliott and Martin [37] were the first to report that manipulation of the protein component in the diet of BB rats affects the natural history of autoimmune diabetes: feeding rats a semi-synthetic amino acid diet from the onset of weaning led to a considerable reduction in the incidence of diabetes from 52% on milk protein supplementation to 15%. Subsequent studies by the Toronto group confirmed that the effect of CM proteins is established during a relatively narrow, early phase in the postnatal (weaning) period [38]. The prevention of diabetes by a synthetic diet in which CM proteins were replaced by a purified casein hydrolysate before weaning has subsequently been confirmed in the NOD mouse [39, 40].

The main differences in protein composition between cow's and human milk are that (i) the protein concentration is higher in CM, principally due to the larger casein content; (ii) the main whey protein component in CM is β-lactoglobulin (BLG), which is not an endogenous component in human milk, and (iii) the primary serum albumin amino acid sequence differs from that of human and rodents in a small, circumscribed area [41]. An additional intriguing fact is that there is a three amino acid difference between bovine insulin present in CM and human insulin.

The association between CM consumption and the incidence of type 1 diabetes in children has been dealt with in two ecological studies. Scott [42] reported in 1990 a close correlation ($r = 0.86$) between the per capita consumption of unfermented milk proteins in the whole population and the incidence of diabetes, and Dahl-Jørgensen et al. [43] confirmed one year later the same trend using incidence data from children aged 0–14 years and validated registries from the Diabetes Epidemiology Research International Study Group (1978–1985), the correlation coefficient being 0.96. Studies like these are prone to various biases but can serve as background information to hypotheses linking type 1 diabetes to exposure to CM. Data from three population-based case-control studies on CM intake prior to diagnosis of type 1 diabetes are conflicting: Dahlquist et al. [44] found in a Swedish series a lower frequency of milk intake among diabetic children, whereas in New South Wales, Australia the CM intake had been higher in prediabetic children than in the controls [45]. In our Finnish nationwide 'Childhood Diabetes in Finland' (DiMe) study, we observed that a high consumption of CM in childhood was associated with a more frequent appearance of diabetes-associated autoantibodies in initially unaffected siblings of children with type 1 diabetes [46]. There was also an almost significant association between high CM consumption and progression to clinical type 1 diabetes.

An inverse correlation between the duration of breastfeeding and type 1 diabetes in childhood was first observed in a Scandinavian study about 20 years ago [47]. This association has been confirmed in several but not all studies from various countries [3]. In a Finnish population-based study, the duration of exclusive breastfeeding and age at start of supplementary feeding with regular CM-based formulas were both related to an increased risk for type 1 diabetes [48]. In comparison with controls matched for sex and age, young diabetic children had been more often predominantly breast-fed for less than 6 months and exclusively breastfed for less than 3 months. In addition, a greater proportion of the affected children had received supplementary CM-based formula over the first 3 months of life. These findings have been confirmed subsequently in a larger series of diabetic children [49]. A multivariate analysis of the total series of Finnish children with type 1 diabetes indicated that early CM exposure was a more important risk factor than short breastfeeding [50].

Two meta-analyses have been performed with the aim to critically review and summarize the clinical evidence for the possible role of a short duration of breastfeeding or early CM exposure in the pathogenesis of type 1 diabetes. Gerstein [51] analyzed in 1994, 13 case-control studies and found that the risk of diabetes was 1.4 times higher in children who were breast-fed for less than 3 months and 1.6 times higher in those exposed to CM before the age of 3 months. The author concluded that early CM exposure might be an important determinant of subsequent type 1 diabetes. Norris and Scott [52] reported quite similar risk ratios, 1.2 and 1.6, respectively, but stressed that the increased risk of type 1 diabetes associated with any of the infant diet exposures is low. They pointed out that retrospectively collected infant diet data might have their limitations due to possible recall bias and different response rates for cases and controls. The above-mentioned risk ratios most likely underestimate the association between type 1 diabetes and early CM exposure, however. Firstly, the breastfeeding data did not reflect exclusive breastfeeding in most studies. Secondly, controls for these studies were drawn from the general population, and such controls will include a majority of individuals not genetically susceptible to type 1 diabetes.

Four birth cohort studies have reported preliminary findings on the relationship between infant feeding patterns and emergence of type 1 diabetes-associated autoantibodies [53–56]. The findings of these studies are consistent in showing no association of breastfeeding or age at introduction of supplementary milk feeding with emergence of up to three autoantibodies. However, the Finnish DIPP study explored also the possible association between infant feeding and emergence of all four predictive autoantibody reactivities [54]. Short exclusive breastfeeding and early introduction of supplementary milk feeding were related to an increased risk of developing all four autoantibodies and IA-2A, which represent the strongest predictive marker of clinical type 1 diabetes among the four individual autoantibody reactivities [57]. It should be noted that all prospective studies reported so far have been clearly underpowered to detect such low risk ratios (about 1.5) that have been reported for early exposure to CM proteins in case-control studies.

### Immune Responses to CM Proteins in Patients with Newly Diagnosed Type 1 Diabetes

Savilahti et al. [58] reported in 1988 that children with newly diagnosed type 1 diabetes had significantly higher levels of serum IgA antibodies to CM and BLG, and IgG antibodies to BLG than age-matched controls. The authors inferred that the pattern of CM consumption is altered in children who will develop type 1 diabetes, the immunological reactivity to CM proteins is enhanced, or the permeability of their intestines to CM proteins is increased. The initial finding has been confirmed in the nationwide 'Childhood Diabetes in Finland' study, comprising 706 children with newly diagnosed type 1 diabetes, 456 nondiabetic siblings and 105 unrelated age-matched controls below 7 years of age [59]. Dahlquist et al. [60] and Saukkonen et al. [61] reported from the Swedish nationwide case-control study that most CM antibody levels tended to be increased in diabetic children when compared with controls, the difference being significant for IgA antibodies to CM, bovine serum albumin (BSA) and BLG. The differences in these antibodies were more pronounced among young children. In a multiple logistic regression analysis, the authors observed that IgA antibodies to BLG were significantly associated with an increased risk of diabetes at young age independent of islet cell antibody status and of early weaning to CM-based formula. The authors concluded that in genetically susceptible children early exposure to BLG might be one trigger of the autoimmune process leading to the development of type 1 diabetes.

The humoral immunity to various CM proteins has subsequently been studied in children and adults with type 1 diabetes by many groups as reviewed by Åkerblom and Knip [3]. A majority of these studies have reported increased antibody levels to one or more protein components in CM. An enhanced humoral immune response to CM proteins seems to be specific for type 1 diabetes, since elevated levels have not been generally observed in other autoimmune diseases. The active immune response has been reported to be restricted to CM proteins, since patients with newly diagnosed type 1 diabetes have not been shown to have increased antibody levels to other dietary antigens, such as ovalbumin or gliadin [58, 61].

Observations on the cellular immunity to CM proteins are of potential interest, as all pathogenetic models of type 1 diabetes ascribe a crucial role to T cells as actively involved in β-cell destruction. The published data on T cell responses to CM proteins are controversial. Enhanced T cell responses have been reported to BSA, the ABBOS fragment of BSA (amino acids 152–168), BLG and β-casein [see 3]. These observations have not been consistently confirmed in other studies, however.

### Possible Mechanisms Involved in the β-Cell Lesion Related to CM Proteins

Several mechanisms have been proposed to explain how CM proteins may be related to β-cell damage. The BSA hypothesis, according to which structural homology between BSA and an islet protein p69 leads to a misdirected immune response against p69, was introduced in 1992 by Karjalainen et al. [62]. Another hypothesis is based on the observation that digestion of bovine β-casein results in a bioactive peptide, β-casomorphin-7, with immunosuppresive activity [63]. A third alternative is that subjects who develop type 1 diabetes have a dysregulated mucosal immune response predisposing to autoimmune diabetes [64, 65].

Recently Vaarala et al. [66, 67] suggested that early feeding with CM-based formulas leads to immunisation to bovine insulin that differs structurally from human insulin in three amino acid positions (amino acids 8 and 10 in the A-chain and amino acid 30 in the B-chain). Infants fed with CM-based formulas had significantly higher IgG antibodies to bovine insulin than breast-fed infants at the age of 3 months. No such difference was seen any more between these two groups at the age of 12 and 18 months, but as a matter of fact the antibody levels decreased in both groups reflecting the induction of oral tolerance to bovine insulin. There were, however, 11 deviant infants, who developed signs of β-cell autoimmunity over their first 2 years of life, and whose IgG class antibodies to bovine insulin increased continuously during longitudinal follow-up. Infants fed a CM-based formula have also been shown to have a higher T cell response to bovine insulin at the age of 3 months than exclusively breastfed infants [68]. These observations suggest that the immune response initially induced by bovine insulin may later be diverted into autoaggressive immunity against the β-cells in a few unfortunate individuals. This hypothesis goes along with other observations suggesting that immunization to insulin plays a key role in the autoimmune process leading to the loss of pancreatic β-cells and the development of type 1 diabetes. Insulin is the only known β-cell-specific autoantigen in type 1 diabetes and insulin autoantibodies are frequently detected in young children with newly diagnosed disease [69, 70]. In prospective birth-cohort studies insulin autoantibodies appear most frequently as the first sign of β-cell autoimmunity [10, 71], indicating that insulin may be the primary or one of the primary autoantigens in human type 1 diabetes.

Regardless of the mechanism the only strategy to definitely assess the prevailing controversy whether early exposure to dietary complex proteins, being CM proteins in more than two thirds of all infants, is a risk factor for type 1 diabetes in man is to perform a dietary intervention trial [72]. Therefore such a trial (Trial to Reduce IDDM in Genetically at Risk, TRIGR) has been initiated in May 2003 as an international multicenter study after the study design had been tested in two pilot series. The objective of the second pilot study was to explore whether weaning to a highly hydrolyzed casein hydrolysate over the first 6–8 months of life will decrease the cumulative incidence of diabetes-associated autoantibodies by the age of 2 years. The intervention resulted in an almost significant reduction in the range of 40–60% in the cumulative incidence of the various diabetes-associated autoantibodies by the age of 2 years except for antibodies to glutamic acid decarboxylase [73]. Subsequent observation up to a maximum age of 7 years has revealed a significant difference in the seroconversion rate to ICA positivity or positivity for at least one autoantibody reactivity between the casein hydrolysate group and the control group [Akerblom et al., submitted].

Other Dietary Factors

Some experimental studies indicate that gluten may be diabetogenic [40, 74]. Two recent prospective studies have indicated that early exposure to cereals may increase the risk of seroconversion to positivity for diabetes-associated autoantibodies [55, 56]. The American report suggested that both early (before the age of 4 months) and late exposure (at the age of 7 months or later) to cereals were associated with an increased risk of β-cell autoimmunity, while the German study implied that an increased risk was related to exposure to cereals before the age of 3 months. In addition, the American survey indicated that both gluten-containing and non-gluten-containing cereals conferred an increased risk for β-cell autoimmunity. Neither of the studies reported any data on the amount of cereals the infants were exposed to at various ages. Early exposure to cereals is in conflict with the infant nutrition recommendations in most developed countries and occurs only rarely. Accordingly, one may ask whether early exposure to cereals is a proxy of other baby care practices predisposing to type 1 diabetes.

Two small-scale pilot studies have been performed in family members testing positive for diabetes-associated autoantibodies to assess whether gluten elimination modifies the natural course of β-cell autoimmunity. In the German trial seven autoantibody-positive first-degree relatives were placed on a gluten-free diet for a period of 12 months followed by gluten re-exposure over the subsequent 12 months [75]. The autoantibody titers did not change significantly during the gluten-free intervention period or during the re-exposure period. Seventeen family members testing positive for at least two diabetes-associated autoantibodies were put on a gluten-free diet for 6 months in an Italian trial [76] and then again on a normal diet for another 6 months. There were no significant changes in the autoantibody titers during the intervention period or during the subsequent 6 months. The first-phase insulin response to intravenous glucose increased in 12 of 14 subjects tested during the gluten-free period and decreased in 10 of 13 retested family members during the re-exposure period. Accordingly, this trial indicated that a gluten-free diet has no effect on the signs of β-cell autoimmunity in first-degree relatives of affected patients, but such a diet may increase the endogenous insulin secretion in family members at increased risk of type 1 diabetes.

Studies in BB rats have suggested a diabetogenic effect of soy protein [77, 78], and Fort et al. [79] reported that children progressing to type 1 diabetes had been given soy-based formulas in infancy more often than the controls. Recently, a protein with a high amino acid sequence homology with a wheat storage globulin was identified, and antibodies to this molecule were detected both in diabetic BB rats and a few patients with newly diagnosed type 1 diabetes [80]. No consistent data are available on the possible role of dietary fats in the development of autoimmune diabetes [3].

A significant correlation between the incidence of type 1 diabetes and the national coffee consumption per person has been reported in an ecological study [81]. Later surveys have indicated that the maternal coffee consumption during pregnancy does not affect the risk of diabetes in the offspring [82, 83]. A Swedish study found that a high groundwater zinc concentration was associated with a significantly reduced risk for type 1 diabetes, and the authors concluded that zinc deficiency may lead to type 1 diabetes [84].

A European multicenter study observed that vitamin D supplementation in early childhood was associated with a decreased risk of type 1 diabetes [85]. A Finnish birth cohort study reported subsequently that regular or irregular vitamin D supplementation in infancy is associated with a reduced risk of type 1 diabetes later in childhood, while a suspicion of rickets was linked with an increased disease risk [86]. These observations are theoretically interesting from that point of view that vitamin D has been shown to prevent experimental thyroiditis [87] and autoimmune diabetes in the NOD mouse [88].

*Viral Infections*

Viral infections have been implicated in the etiology of type 1 diabetes for more than 100 years. More recently, several studies have been published showing that certain viruses, such as enteroviruses are capable of inducing diabetes in experimental animals, and seroepidemiological studies have indicated their role in human Type 1 diabetes as well [3, 89]. Viruses may act by at least two possible mechanisms, either via a direct cytolytic effect, or by triggering an autoimmune process leading gradually to β-cell destruction [90]. The role of molecular mimicry in diabetes-associated autoimmune responses has been indicated by the observations of structural and functional homology between viral structures and β-cell antigens. Persistent or slow virus infections, like in the congenital rubella syndrome and cytomegalovirus infections (CMV), may also be important in the induction of the autoimmune response. The role of viral infections in the etiopathogenesis of human type 1 diabetes has been elucidated by serological and epidemiological studies, and case histories [91].

Enteroviruses

Enteroviruses (EV) belong to the picornavirus family comprising small, naked icosahedral RNA viruses. The EV subfamily consists of four subgroups: polioviruses, coxsackie B viruses (CBV), coxsackie A viruses (CAV) and echoviruses, and includes more than 60 distinct serotypes. There are both epidemiological, serological and biological indications suggesting that EV may be involved in the pathogenesis of type 1 diabetes [89, 92, 93]. Infections with different serotypes are common, starting in infancy. The virus frequently causes viremia and spreads to many organs including the pancreas. Most of these infections are mild and subclinical.

The role of EV in the pathogenesis of type 1 diabetes have been strengthened over the last 10–20 years, one reason being methodological developments in the diagnosis of EV infections and an other the insight that the diabetic disease process starts months and years before the clinical presentation of the disease requiring prospective studies to identify potential triggers and boosters of the process. Gamble and Taylor [94] reported in 1969 parallel changes in the seasonal variation in the incidence of type 1 diabetes and in the frequency of CBV infections. A series of serological case-control studies have shown an increased prevalence of elevated levels of CBV antibodies in patients with newly diagnosed type 1 diabetes [92, 93]. There are, however, also contradictory results, since some other reports have been unable to find any difference between patients with diabetes and controls [95, 96] or even demonstrated decreased levels of CBV antibodies in patients [97].

The first serological studies measured neutralizing EV antibodies that are good markers of infection immunity but poor indicators of a recent infection, if the analyses do not include IgM antibodies. More recent studies have assessed the occurrence of recent or current EV infections by quantifying IgM antibodies with μ-antibody capture methods based on enzyme or radioimmunoassays. With such a methodology patients with newly diagnosed type 1 diabetes were found to have increased IgM class antibodies against EV suggesting an excess of recent infections [see 98]. A Swedish group detected IgM class antibodies to CBV in 40% of children with newly diagnosed type 1 diabetes and in none of the controls [99]. The majority of those, who had IgM class antibodies at the diagnosis of diabetes, had experienced previously an EV infection caused by a different serotype, indicated by IgG class antibodies [100]. As increased IgM titres reflect an ongoing or recent infection, Fohlman and Friman [100] concluded that these observations suggest that successive infections by different CBV and other EV increase the risk of manifestation of overt diabetes in genetically susceptible individuals. Such a process fits well into the 'Copenhagen model' for the pathogenesis of type 1 diabetes, i.e. the multiple hit hypothesis [101].

The use of polymerase chain reaction (PCR) methodology has enabled viruses to be detected by molecular methods from serum, whole blood or mononuclear cells, thus circumventing the indirect approach through antibody-based analyses. An additional advantage is that these methods can be extended to delineate virus nucleotide sequences. There are studies from four different countries, showing an increased frequency of EV detected with PCR from the peripheral circulation in subjects with newly diagnosed type 1 diabetes [102–107]. The prevalence of EV mRNA varied from 27 to 64% among the patients and from 0 to 5% among the control subjects. Altogether 33% of the patients with newly diagnosed type 1 diabetes had detectable EV mRNA compared to 3% of the controls verifying an increased frequency of EV viremia at the time of clinical presentation of type 1 diabetes.

Finnish prospective studies have repeatedly shown an increased frequency of EV infections among prediabetic subjects compared to unaffected controls and an unequivocal temporal association between EV infections and the appearance of the first diabetes-associated autoantibodies [108–112]. The latter observation strongly indicates that EV are capable of triggering β-cell autoimmunity. There are two prospective studies from Germany and Colorado, USA, showing no association between EV infections and β-cell autoimmunity [113, 114]. Those studies are, however, hampered by limitations due to long sampling intervals and a narrow methodological arsenal. Short sampling intervals (optimally 3 months or less) are critical, when the aim is to assess the temporal association between EV infections and seroconversion to positivity for diabetes-associated autoantibodies.

Two studies from Northern Europe have indicated that maternal enteroviral infections during pregnancy may be associated with later development of type 1 diabetes in the offspring. Dahlquist et al. [115] analyzed maternal sera taken at delivery and observed the closest relation between IgM to CBV 3 and type 1 diabetes in the children. A Finnish survey tested sera obtained at the end of the first trimester and showed the strongest association between CBV 5 and type 1 diabetes in offspring under the age of 3 years at diagnosis but not in those older than 3 [108]. A more recent Finnish study in a larger cohort of pregnant women did not, however, support the earlier observation that EV infections during the first trimester is associated with an increased risk of type 1 diabetes in the offspring [116].

Taken together, most cross-sectional studies in patients with newly diagnosed type 1 diabetes support the hypothesis that EV can precipitate clinical disease in subjects with signs of β-cell autoimmunity. Data from prospective studies suggest that EV may trigger β-cell autoimmunity and boost existing β-cell autoimmunity.

The tropism phenomenon (the characteristics of a virus to infect a particular tissue or cell type), in which the attachment of virus to the viral receptors on cell surface is a central feature, is thought to explain why some variants of EV are diabetogenic and others are not [100]. It has been proposed that pancreatic β-cell tropic variants of CBV are present in the general population and that they are able to induce β-cell damage in susceptible individuals [117]. In vitro studies have shown that EV are capable of infecting β-cells and inducing functional impairment and cell death [118, 119]. Such a capacity seems to be shared by a wide range of serotypes, but the extent of the cellular lesions appears to be characteristic of individual virus strains. Recent studies have shown that EV mRNA can be detected in pancreatic islets of patients affected by type 1 diabetes [120, 121]. These findings raise the possibility that patients with type 1 diabetes may have a chronic EV infection in their pancreatic islets.

Other Viruses

Gundersen [122], in his classical study of 1927, reported an increase in the number of cases with type 1 diabetes 2–4 years after a mumps epidemic. Subsequently, there have been numerous case reports describing a temporal relationship between mumps and clinical onset of diabetes [3]. In epidemiological studies peaks in the incidence of childhood type 1 diabetes have been observed 2–4 years after mumps epidemics. Serological evidence of an association between mumps infection and type 1 diabetes has been difficult to obtain due to the long interval between the infection and the clinical manifestation of type 1 diabetes. A Finnish study reported decreased IgG class mumps antibody titers in children with newly diagnosed type 1 diabetes compared with those in controls, the finding being interpreted as indicative of an abnormal immunological response to mumps infection [123]. Interestingly, in patient series collected earlier, when natural mumps was still common in Finland, IgG class mumps virus antibodies were not decreased, and IgA antibodies were elevated in diabetic children. This decline in mumps antibody levels may reflect the elimination of cases with mumps-induced type 1 diabetes by the MMR vaccine.

Diabetes has been observed in 10–20% of patients with the congenital rubella syndrome (CRS) with a latent period of 5–25 years [see 3]. A recent study showed, however, that signs of humoral β-cell autoimmunity are extremely rare among patients with the CRS, indicating that CRS-associated diabetes may be caused by other than autoimmune mechanisms [124].

The human cytomegalovirus (CMV) can be transmitted before birth, like the rubella virus, either transplacentally or at conception from an infected parent carrying the CMV genome in his or her genomic DNA. CMV infections may also be transmitted prenatally or postnatally through close contact or breast milk. CMV has been implicated in the development of type 1 diabetes by a case report of an infant with congenital CMV infection who presented with diabetes at the age of 13 months [125]. In a Swedish prospective study 16,474 newborn infants were screened for congenital CMV infections by virus isolation from the urine, and 76 infants were found to be infected. Only 1 of 73 infected individuals (1.4%) manifested type 1 diabetes, when observed up to the age of 7 years or more, whereas 38 of 19,483 controls (0.2%) became affected by diabetes [126]. This observation suggests that congenital CMV infection is not a major trigger of type 1 diabetes.

Hiltunen et al. [109] found comparable levels of CMV IgG and IgM antibodies in children with newly diagnosed type 1 diabetes and in control children, while the patients had higher IgA antibodies than the controls. The latter observation may reflect reactivated or persistent CMV infections in children with recent-onset diabetes. No association was observed between ICA and CMV antibodies. Neither could any differences be seen in the CMV antibodies in early pregnancy between mothers whose offspring later presented with clinical type 1 diabetes and control mothers. During prospective follow-up of unaffected siblings of children with diabetes no seroconversions could be detected in CMV antibodies, and no changes could be seen in CMV antibodies in relation to seroconversion to positivity for ICA or progression to clinical diabetes in the siblings. Accordingly no evidence was found in favor of the hypothesis that primary CMV infections *in utero* or in childhood could promote or precipitate type 1 diabetes. If CMV infections play a role in the pathogenesis of this disease, it must be limited to a very small proportion of cases.

The human genome contains numerous retroviral sequences, a majority of which is non-infectious. Endogenous retroviruses exist as viral DNA integrated into the genome of every cell in the host, and they are transmitted vertically to the next generation via germ-line DNA. Retroviruses have been associated with autoimmune diabetes in animal models such as the NOD mouse [128]. Retroviruses have not been consistently shown to be involved in the development of human type 1 diabetes, although insulin autoantibodies (IAA) from patients with type 1 diabetes and unaffected first-degree relatives have been observed to cross-react with the retroviral antigen p73 [129], indicating that IAA-positive sera contain antibodies that recognize both insulin and p73.

Honeyman et al. [130] reported a few years ago molecular homology between the VP7 protein of rotavirus and T cell epitopes in the protein tyrosine phosphatase related IA-2 molecule and in the 65-kDa isoform of glutamic acid decarboxylase. In a prospective study of infants genetically predisposed to type 1 diabetes they observed that the appearance of diabetes-associated autoantibodies was associated with significant rises in rotavirus antibodies, indicating that rotavirus infections may induce β-cell autoimmunity in genetically susceptible infants [131]. A Finnish prospective study showed that about 16% of infants and young children with HLA-conferred susceptibility to type 1 diabetes experienced a rotavirus infection during the 6-month window preceding the detection of the first diabetes-associated autoantibodies, whereas 15% of the control subjects matched for gender, birth date, delivery hospital and HLA genotype had signs of a rotavirus infection during the corresponding time period [132]. That observation does not support the role of rotavirus infections as triggers of β-cell autoimmunity.

A Swedish group has recently reported that the development of autoimmune diabetes in captured wild bank voles is associated with the Ljungan virus, a novel picornavirus isolated from bank voles [133]. The authors reported also that young children with newly diagnosed type 1 diabetes had increased titres of Ljungan virus antibodies and implicated that bank voles may play a role as a zoonotic reservoir and vector for a potentially diabetogenic virus in man.

*Other Environmental Factors*

As listed in table 1 there are a series of other environmental factors that have been proposed to be involved in the pathogenesis of type 1 diabetes. Some new developments in this area deserve to be mentioned. An Australian study reported in 2001 that bafilomycin A1, a macrolide antibiotic produced by *Streptomyces* species ubiquitous in soil, may induce glucose intolerance and pancreatic islet disruption in mice [134]. Tuberous vegetables, potatoes and beets in particular, may be infested by such *Strepomyces* species and thereby humans could be exposed to high concentrations of bafilomycin A1. The potential diabetogenicity of this compound is open in man, however.

Increased weight gain in infancy has repeatedly been reported to be a risk factor for type 1 diabetes later in childhood [3]. A Finnish study showed that those children who presented with type 1 diabetes had been not only heavier but also taller in infancy [135]. Increased height and weight later in childhood turned as well out to be definite risk factors for type 1 diabetes [136]. Accelerated linear growth and weight gain results in an enhanced β-cell load and increasing insulin resistance. It has been shown experimentally that active β-cells are more prone to cytokine-induced damage than resting cells. This suggests that rapid growth induces β-cell stress. According to the accelerator hypothesis presented by Wilkin [137] a few years ago, insulin resistance is an important factor affecting the rising incidence of both type 1 and type 2 diabetes, the only differences between these two forms of diabetes being the pace of progression to overt disease and the fact that those who present with type 1 diabetes carry genetic susceptibility to autoimmunity.

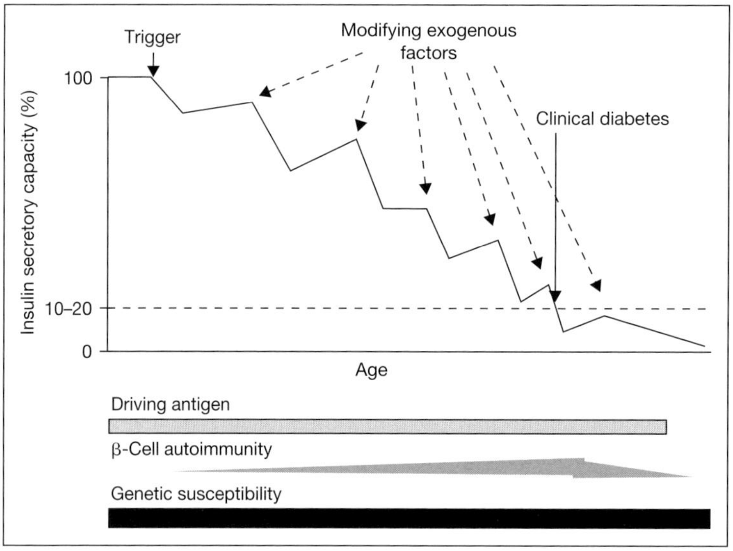


*Fig. 2.* Progression from genetic susceptibility to overt type 1 diabetes. The disease process is triggered by an exogenous factor, driven by another environmental determinant, and modified by a series of environmental factors in individuals with increased genetic diabetes susceptibility.

## A Pathogenetic Model of Type 1 Diabetes

A series of observations suggest that β-cell autoimmunity may be triggered by an environmental culprit at any age, although a majority of the processes appear to start early in childhood [5]. Figure 2 presents a pathogenetic model of type 1 diabetes according to which the genetic disease susceptibility allows the initiation of a β-cell destructive process resulting in the presentation of clinical type 1 diabetes in some unfortunate individuals. What might be the most likely environmental trigger of β-cell autoimmunity? Based on present knowledge a critically timed diabetogenic EV infection is the most likely candidate. Initiation of the process does not necessarily lead to progression to clinical disease, however. According to the hypothesis favored by this author there is a need for a driving exogenous antigen playing the same role as gluten in celiac disease. Bovine insulin present in most CM-based products could be such a driving antigen, high exposure to the antigen resulting in a progressive destructive process. A Finnish study have shown that a high CM consumption (more than two glasses of milk/day) is associated with an increased risk of seroconversion to autoantibody positivity and progression to clinical type 1 diabetes in initially non-diabetic siblings of affected children [46] supporting the idea that a CM component could be the driving dietary antigen in type 1 diabetes. In addition there are most likely a series of environmental factors modifying the fate and pace of the β-cell destructive process. Such factors may include e.g. non-specific infections, weight gain, linear growth, and vitamin D deficiency. This hypothesis holds that progression to clinical diabetes requires the combination of genetic disease susceptibility, a critically timed diabetogenic EV infection and high exposure to dietary bovine insulin. If any of these determinants is missing or any of the exogenous factors inappropriately timed the risk of type 1 diabetes is minimal even in the presence of the other predisposing elements. Such a model can also explain why only about 10% of those with HLA-conferred genetic susceptibility to type 1 diabetes do progress to overt disease.

## Conclusions

The identification of exogenous factors triggering and boosting β-cell destruction offers potentially means for intervention aimed at the prevention of type 1 diabetes. Therefore, it is important to pursue studies on the role of environmental factors in the pathogenesis of type 1 diabetes. Environmental modification offers likely the most powerful strategy for effective prevention of this disease, since such an approach can target the whole population or at least that proportion of the population carrying increased genetic disease susceptibility and would therefore prevent both sporadic and familial type 1 diabetes, if successful. This consideration is crucial, since the sporadic cases comprise 83–98% of all children with newly diagnosed diabetes according to a comparative European survey [138]. The preliminary results of the second pilot study of the TRIGR project, suggesting that it is possible to manipulate the spontaneous appearance of β-cell autoimmunity by dietary modification early in life in high-risk individuals, represent the first indication that environmental modification may affect the natural history of preclinical type 1 diabetes.

The scientific challenges in the near future are to define the most likely environmental culprits and boosters of β-cell autoimmunity and to delineate how exogenous factors affect the natural history of type 1 diabetes in the preclinical phase. A new consortium comprising six prospective birth cohort studies, the German BABYDIAB Study, the American Diabetes Autoimmunity Study in the Young (DAISY) and the Finnish DIPP Study among others, and observing risk individuals from birth through signs of β-cell autoimmunity to clinical disease provides an optimal setting for successful explorative work. This TEDDY (Triggers and Environmental Determinants in Diabetes of the

Young) consortium has been funded by the National Institute of Diabetes, Digestive and Kidney Diseases (NIDDK) for a 5-year period (2003–2007), and has started to recruit participating families in the fall 2004. We have also to keep our eyes and minds open for potential protective environmental factors, since family studies have shown that all high risk individuals do not progress to clinical diabetes within a foreseeable period of time [139, 140].

## References


1 Ilonen J, Sjöroos M, Knip M, Veijola R, Simell O, Åkerblom HK, Paschou P, Bozas E, Havarini B, Malamitsi-Puchner A, Thymelli J, Vazeou A, Bartsocas CS: Estimation of genetic risk for type 1 diabetes. Am J Med Genet 2002;115:30–36.

2 Dahlquist G: Environmental risk factors in human type 1 diabetes: An epidemiological perspective. Diabetes Metab Rev 1995;11:37–46.

3 Åkerblom HK, Knip M: Putative environmental factors in type 1 diabetes. Diabetes Metab Rev 1998;14:31–67.

4 Åkerblom HK, Vaarala O, Hyöty H, Ilonen J, Knip M: Environmental factors in the etiology of type 1 diabetes. Am J Med Genet 2002;115:18–29.

5 Knip M: Natural course of preclinical type 1 diabetes. Horm Res 2002;57(suppl 1):6–11.

6 Knip M: Can we predict type 1 diabetes in the general population? Diab Care 2002;25:623–625.

7 Bingley PJ, Bonifacio E, Williams AJK, Genovese S, Bottazzo GF, Gale EAM: Prediction of IDDM in the general populations: Strategies based on combinations of autoantibody markers. Diabetes 1995;46:1701–1710.

8 LaGasse JM, Brantley MS, Leech NJ, Rowe RE, Monks S, Palmer JP, Nepom GT, McCulloch DK, Hagopian WA: Successful prospective prediction of type 1 diabetes in schoolchildren by multiple defined autoantibodies: Eight year follow-up of the Washington State Diabetes Prediction Study. Diab Care 2002;25:505–511.

9 Ziegler A-G, Hummel M, Schenker M, Bonifacio E: Autoantibody appearance and risk for development of childhood diabetes in offspring of parents with type 1 diabetes: The 2-year analysis of the German BABYDIAB Study. Diabetes 1999;48:460–468.

10 Kimpimäki T, Kupila A, Hämäläinen A-M, Kukko M, Kulmala P, Savola K, Simell T, Muona P, Ilonen J, Simell O, Knip M: The first signs of β-cell autoimmunity appear in infancy in genetically susceptible children from the general population: The Finnish Type 1 Diabetes Prediction and Prevention Study. J Clin Endocrinol Metab 2001;86:4782–4788.

11 Kimpimäki T, Kulmala P, Savola K, Kupila A, Korhonen S, Simell T, Ilonen J, Simell O, Knip M: Natural history of beta-cell autoimmunity in young children with increased genetic susceptibility to type 1 diabetes recruited from the general population. J Clin Endocrinol Metab 2002;87:4572–4579.

12 Kupila A, Muona P, Ronkainen M, Simell T, Erkkilä S, Arvilommi P, Korhonen S, Kimpimäki T, Sjöroos M, Ilonen J, Knip M, Simell O: Genetic risk determines the emergence of diabetes-associated autoantibodies in young children. Diabetes 2002;51:646–651.

13 Mrena S, Savola K, Kulmala P, Åkerblom HK, Knip M, the Childhood Diabetes in Finland Study Group: Natural course of preclinical type 1 diabetes in siblings of affected children. Acta Paediatr 2003;92:1403–1410.

14 Kimpimäki T, Kulmala P, Savola K, Vähäsalo P, Reijonen H, Ilonen J, Åkerblom HK, Knip M, the Childhod Diabetes in Finland Study Group: Disease-associated autoantibodies as surrogate markers of type 1 diabetes in young children at increased genetic risk. J Clin Endocrinol Metab 2000;85;1126–1130.

15 Sabbah E, Savola K, Ebeling T, Kulmala P, Vähäsalo P, Salmela P, Knip M: Genetic, autoimmune, and clinical characteristics of childhood- and adult-onset Type 1 diabetes mellitus. Diab Care 2000;23:1326–1332.

16 Williams AJK, Bingley PJ, Moore WPT, Gale EAM, ENDIT Screening Group: Islet autoantibodies, nationality and gender: A multinational screening study in first-degree relatives of patients with type I diabetes. Diabetologia 2002;45:217–223.
17 Cavan D, Bain S, Barnett A: The genetics of type 1 (insulin-dependent) diabetes mellitus. J Med Genet 1992;29:441–446.
18 Friday RP, Trucco M, Pietropaolo M: Genetics of type 1 diabetes mellitus. Diabetes Nutr Metab 1999;12:3–26.
19 Davies JL, Kawaguchi Y, Bennett ST, Copeman JB, Cordell HJ, Pritchard LE, Reed PW, Gough SCL, Jenkins SC, Palmer SM, Balfour KM, Rowe BR, Farrall M, Barnett AH, Bain SC, Todd JA: A genome-wide search for human type 1 diabetes susceptibility genes. Nature 1994;371:130–136.
20 Hashimoto L, Habita C, Beressi JP, Delepine M, Besse C, Cambon-Thomsen A, Deschamps I, Rotter JL, Djoulah S, James MR, Froguel P, Weissenbach J, Lathrop GM, Julier C: Genetic mapping of a susceptibility locus for insulin-dependent diabetes mellitus on chromosome 11q. Nature 1994;371:161–164.
21 Concannon P, Gogolin-Ewens KJ, Hinds DA, Wapelhorst P, Morrison VA, Dtirling B, Mitra M, Farmer J, Williams SR, Cox NJ, Bell GI, Risch N, Spielman RS: A second-generation screen of the human genome for susceptibility to insulin-dependent diabetes mellitus. Nat Gen 1998;19:213–214.
22 Cox NJ, Wapelhorst B, Morrison VA, Johnson L, Pinchuk L, Spielman RS, Todd JA, Concannon P: Seven regions of the genome show evidence of linkage to type 1 diabetes in a consensus analysis of 767 multiplex families. Am J Hum Genet 2001;69:820–830.
23 European Consortium for IDDM Genome Studies: A genomewide scan for type 1-diabetes susceptibility in Scandinavian families: Identification of new loci with evidence of interactions. Am J Hum Genet 2001;69:1301–1313.
24 Ueda H, Howson JM, Esposito L, et al: Association of the T-cell regulatory gene CTLA4 with susceptibility to autoimmune disease. Nature 2003;423:506–511.
25 Wen L, Wong FS, Tang J, Chen NY, Altieri M, David C, Flavell R, Scherwin R: In vivo evidence for the contribution of human histocompatibility leukocyte antigen (HLA)-DQ molecules to the development of diabetes. J Exp Med 2000;191:97–104.
26 Kennedy GC, German MS, Rutter WJ: The minisatellite in the diabetes susceptibility locus IDDM2 regulates insulin transcription. Nat Genet 1995;9:293–298.
27 Pugliese A, Zeller M, Fernandez A Jr, Zalcberg LJ, Bartlett RJ, Ricordi C, Pietropaolo M, Eisenbarth GS, Bennett ST, Patel DD: The insulin gene is transcribed in the human thymus and transcription levels correlated with allelic variation at the INS VNTR-IDDM2 susceptibility locus for type 1 diabetes. Nat Genet 1997;15:293–297.
28 Vafiadis P, Bennett ST, Todd JA, Nadeau J, Grabs R, Goodyer CG, Wickramasinghe S, Colle E, Polychronakos C: Insulin expression in human thymus is modulated by INS VNTR alleles at the IDDM2 locus. Nat Genet 1997;15:289–292.
29 Vafiadis P, Bennett ST, Colle E, Grabs R, Goodyer CG, Polychronakos C: Imprinted and genotype-specific expression of genes at the IDDM2 locus in pancreas and leucocytes. J Autoimmun 1996;9:397–403.
30 Barnett AH, Eff C, Leslie RDG, Pyke DA: Diabetes in identical twins. A study of 200 pairs. Diabetologia 1981;20:87–93.
31 Kaprio J, Tuomilehto J, Koskenvuo M, Romanov K, Reunanen A, Eriksson J, Stengård J, Kesäniemi YA: Concordance for type 1 (insulin-dependent) and type 2 (non-insulin-dependent) diabetes mellitus in a population-based cohort of twins in Finland. Diabetologia 1992;35:1060–1067.
32 The EURODIAB ACE Study Group: Variation and trends in incidence of childhood diabetes in Europe. Lancet 2000;355:873–876.
33 Gale EA: The rise of childhood type 1 diabetes in the 20th century. Diabetes 2002;51:3353–3361.
34 Helgason T, Jonasson MR: Evidence for a food additive as a cause of ketosis-prone diabetes. Lancet 1981;ii:716–720.
35 Helgason T, Ewen SWB, Ross IS, Stowers JM: Diabetes produced in mice by smoked/cured mutton. Lancet 1982;ii:1017–1022.
36 Scott FW, Trick KD: Dietary modification of spontaneous diabetes in the BB Wistar rat. Proc Canad Fed Biol Soc 1983;26:222.

37 Elliott RB, Martin JM: Dietary protein: A trigger of insulin-dependent diabetes in the BB rat? Diabetologia 1984;26:297–299.
38 Daneman D, Fishman L, Clarson C, Martin JM: Dietary triggers of insulin-dependent diabetes in the BB rat. Diabetes Res 1987;5:93–97.
39 Elliott RB, Reddy SN, Bibby NJ, Kida K: Dietary prevention of diabetes in the non-obese diabetic mouse. Diabetologia 1988;31:62–64.
40 Coleman DL, Kuzava JE, Leiter EH: Effect of diet on incidence of diabetes in nonobese diabetic mice. Diabetes 1990;39:432–436.
41 Martin JM, Trink B, Daneman D, Dosch H-M, Robinson B: Milk proteins in the etiology of insulin-dependent diabetes mellitus. Ann Med 1991;23:447–452.
42 Scott FW: Cow milk and insulin-dependent diabetes mellitus: Is there a relationship? Am J Clin Nutr 1990;51:489–491.
43 Dahl-Jørgensen K, Joner G, Hanssen KF: Relationship between cow's milk consumption and incidence of IDDM in childhood. Diabetes Care 1991;14:1081–1083.
44 Dahlquist GG, Blom L, Persson L-Å, Sandström AIM, Wall SGI: Dietary factors and the risk of developing insulin dependent diabetes in childhood. Br Med J 1990;300:1302–1306.
45 Verge CF, Howard NJ, Irwig L, Simpson JM, Mackerras D, Silink M: Environmental factors in childhood IDDM: A population-based case-control study. Diabetes Care 1994;17: 1381–1389.
46 Virtanen SM, Hyppönen E, Läärä E, Vähäsalo P, Kulmala P, Savola K, Räsänen L, Knip M, Åkerblom HK, the Childhood Diabetes in Finland Study Group: Cow's milk consumption, disease associated autoantibodies and type 1 diabetes mellitus: A follow-up study in siblings of diabetic children. Diabetic Med 1998;15:730–738.
47 Borch-Johnsen K, Joner G, Mandrup-Poulsen T, Christy M, Zachau-Christiansen B, Kastrup K, Nerup J: Relation between breast-feeding and incidence rates of insulin-dependent diabetes mellitus. A hypothesis. Lancet 1984;ii:1083–1086.
48 Virtanen SM, Räsänen L, Aro A, Lindström J, Sippola H, Lounamaa R, Toivanen L, Tuomilehto J, Åkerblom HK, the Childhood Diabetes in Finland Study Group: Infant feeding in Finnish children <7 yr of age with newly diagnosed IDDM. Diabetes Care 1991;14:415–417.
49 Virtanen SM, Räsänen L, Aro A, Ylönen K, Lounamaa R, Tuomilehto J, Åkerblom HK, the Childhood Diabetes in Finland Study Group: Feeding in infancy and the risk of Type 1 diabetes mellitus in Finnish children. Diab Med 1992;9:815–819.
50 Virtanen SM, Räsänen L, Ylönen K, Aro A, Clayton D, Langholz B, Pitkäniemi J, Savilahti E, Lounamaa R, Tuomilehto J, Åkerblom HK, the Childhood Diabetes in Finland Study Group: Early introduction of dairy products associated with increased risk for insulin-dependent diabetes mellitus in Finnish children. Diabetes 1993;42:1786–1790.
51 Gerstein HM: Cow's milk exposure and type 1 diabetes mellitus: A critical overview of the clinical literature. Diab Care 1994;17:3–19.
52 Norris JM, Scott FW: A meta-analysis of infant diet and insulin-dependent diabetes mellitus: Do biases play a role. Epidemiology 1996;7:87–92.
53 Couper JJ, Steele C, Beresford S, Powell T, McCaul K, Pollard A, Gellert S, Tait B, Harrison LC, Colman PG: Lack of association between duration of breast-feeding or introduction of cow's milk and development of islet autoimmunity. Diabetes 1999;48:2145–2149.
54 Kimpimäki T, Erkkola M, Korhonen S, Kupila A, Virtanen SM, Ilonen J, Simell O, Knip M: Short exclusive breast-feeding predisposes young children with increased genetic risk of type 1 diabetes to progressive beta-cell autoimmunity. Diabetologia 2001;44;63–69.
55 Norris JM, Barriga K, Klingensmith G, Hoffman M, Eisenbarth GS, Erlich HA, Rewers M: Timing of initial cereal exposure in infancy and risk of islet autoimmunity. JAMA 2003;290: 1713–1720.
56 Ziegler A-G, Schmid S, Huber D, Hummel M, Bonifacio E: Early infant feeding and risk of developing type 1 diabetes-associated autoantibodies. JAMA 2003;290:1721–1728.
57 Decochez K, De Leeuw IH, Keymeulen B, Mathieu C, Rottiers R, Weets I, Vandemeulebroucke E, Truyen I, Kaufman L, Shuit FC, Pipeleers D, Gorus FK, the Belgian Diabetes Registry: IA-2 antibodies predict impending type I diabetes in siblings of patients. Diabetologia 2002;45: 1658–1666.

58 Savilahti E, Åkerblom HK, Tainio V-M, Koskimies S: Children with newly diagnosed insulin dependent diabetes mellitus have increased levels of cow's milk antibodies. Diabetes Res 1988;7:137–140.
59 Savilahti E, Saukkonen TT, Virtala ET, Tuomilehto J, Åkerblom HK, the Childhood Diabetes in Finland Study Group: Increased levels of cow's milk and β-lactoglobulin antibodies in young children with newly diagnosed IDDM. Diab Care1993;16:984–989.
60 Dahlquist G, Savilahti E, Landin-Olsson M: An increased level of antibodies to beta-lactoglobulin is a risk determinant for early-onset type 1 (insulin-dependent) diabetes mellitus independent of islet cell antibodies and early introduction of cow's milk. Diabetologia 1992;35: 980–984.
61 Saukkonen T, Savilahti E, Vaarala O, Virtala ET, Tuomilehto J, Åkerblom HK, the Childhood Diabetes in Finland Study Group: Children with newly diagnosed IDDM have increased levels of antibodies to bovine serum albumin but not to ovalbumin. Diabetes Care 1994;17: 970–976.
62 Karjalainen J, Martin JM, Knip M, Ilonen J, Robinson BH, Savilahti E, Åkerblom HK, Dosch H-M: A bovine albumin peptide as a possible trigger of insulin-dependent diabetes mellitus. N Engl J Med 1992;327:302–307.
63 Elliott RB, Harris DP, Hill JP, Bibby NJ, Wasmuth HE: Type I (insulin-dependent) diabetes mellitus and cow milk: Casein variant consumption. Diabetologia 1999;42:292–296.
64 Vaarala O, Saukkonen T, Savilahti E, Klemola T, Åkerblom HK: Development of immune response to cow's milk proteins in infants receiving cow's milk or hydrolyzed formula. J Allergy Clin Immunol 1995;96:917–923.
65 Paronen J, Klemetti P, Kantele JM, Savilahti E, Perheentupa J, Åkerblom HK, Vaarala O: Glutamate decarboxylase-reactive peripheral blood lymphocytes from patients with IDDM express gut-specific homing receptor $\alpha_4\beta_7$-integrin. Diabetes 1997;46:583–588.
66 Vaarala O, Paronen J, Otonkoski T, Åkerblom HK: Cow milk formula feeding induces antibodies to insulin in children: A link between cow milk and insulin-dependent diabetes mellitus. Scand J Immunol 1998;47:131–135.
67 Vaarala O, Knip M, Paronen J, Hämäläinen A-M, Muona P, Väätäinen M, Ilonen J, Simell O, Åkerblom HK: Cow milk formula feeding induces primary immunization to insulin in infants at genetic risk for type 1 diabetes. Diabetes 1999;48:1389–1394.
68 Paronen J, Knip M, Savilahti E, Virtanen SM, Ilonen J, Åkerblom HK, Vaarala O, the Finnish TRIGR Study Group: The effect of cow milk exposure and maternal type 1 diabetes: Cellular and humoral immunization to dietary insulin in infants at genetic risk for type 1 diabetes. Diabetes 2000;49:1657–1665.
69 Arslanian SA, Becker DJ, Rabin B, Atchison R, Eberhardt M, Cavender D, Dorman J, Drash AL: Correlates of insulin autoantibodies in newly diagnosed children with insulin-dependent diabetes before insulin therapy. Diabetes 1985;32:926–930.
70 Karjalainen J, Knip M, Mustonen A, Ilonen J, Åkerblom HK: Relation between insulin antibody and complement-fixing islet cell antibody at clinical diagnosis of IDDM. Diabetes 1986;35:620–622.
71 Ziegler AG, Hummel M, Schenker M, Bonifacio E: Autoantibody appearance and risk for development of childhood diabetes in offspring of parents with type 1 diabetes: The 2-year analysis of the German BABYDIAB Study. Diabetes 1999;48:460–468.
72 Åkerblom HK, Savilahti E, Saukkonen TT, Paganus A, Virtanen SM, Teramo K, Knip M, Ilonen J, Karjalainen J, Vaarala O, Reunanen A: The case for elimination of cow's milk in early infancy in the prevention of type 1 diabetes: The Finnish experience. Diabetes Metab Rev 1993;9: 269–278.
73 Åkerblom HK, Virtanen SM, Hämäläinen AM, Ilonen J, Savilahti E, Vaarala O, Reunanen A, Teramo K, Knip M: Emergence of diabetes associated autoantibodies in the nutritional prevention of IDDM (TRIGR) project. Diabetes 1999;480(suppl 1):A45.
74 Scott FW, Sarwar G, Cloutier HE: Diabetogenicity of various protein sources in the diet of the diabetes-prone BB rat; in Camerini-Davalos RA, Cole HS (eds): Prediabetes. New York, Plenum Press 1988, pp 277–285.
75 Hummel M, Bonifacio E, Naserke HE, Ziegler AG: Elimination of dietary gluten does not reduce titers of type 1 diabetes-associated autoantibodies in high-risk subjects. Diab Care 2002;25: 1111–1116.

76 Pastore MR, Bazzigaluppi E, Belloni C, Arcovio C, Bonifacio E, Bosi E: Six months of gluten-free diet do not influence autoantibody titers, but improve insulin secretion in subjects at high risk for type 1 diabetes. J Clin Endocrinol Metab 2003;88:162–165.
77 Atkinson MA, Winter WE, Skordis N, Beppu H, Riley WM, MacLaren NK: Dietary protein restriction reduces the frequency and delays the onset of insulin dependent diabetes in BB rats. Autoimmunity 1988;2:11–220.
78 Hoorfar J, Scott FW, Cloutier HE: Dietary plant materials and development of diabetes in the BB rat. J Nutr 1991;121:908–916.
79 Fort P, Lanes R, Dahlem S, Recker B, Weyman-Daum M, Pugliese M, Liftshitz F: Breast feeding and insulin-dependent diabetes mellitus in children. J Am Coll Nutr 1986;5:439–441.
80 MacFarlane AJ, Burghardt KM, Kelly J, Simell T, Simell O, Altosaar I, Scott FW: A type 1 diabetes-related protein from wheat (*Triticum aestivum*): A cDNA clone of a wheat storage globulin, Glb1, linked to islet damage. J Biol Chem 2003;278:54–63.
81 Tuomilehto J, Tuomilehto-Wolf E, Virtala E, LaPorte R: Coffee consumption as trigger for insulin dependent diabetes mellitus in childhood. Br Med J 1990;300:642–643.
82 Soltesz G, Jeges S, Dahlquist G, Hungarian Childhood Diabetes Epidemiology Study Group: Non-genetic risk determinants for type 1 (insulin-dependent) diabetes mellitus in childhood. Acta Paediatr 1994;83:730–735.
83 Virtanen SM, Räsänen L, Aro A, Ylönen K, Lounamaa R, Åkerblom HK, Tuomilehto J, the Childhood Diabetes in Finland Study Group: Is children's or parents' coffee or tea consumption associated with the risk for type 1 diabetes mellitus in children? Eur J Clin Nutr 1994;48: 279–285.
84 Haglund B, Ryckenberg K, Selinus O, Dahlquist G: Evidence of a relationship between childhood-onset type 1 diabetes and low groundwater concentration of zinc. Diabetes Care 1996;19:873–875.
85 The EURODIAB Substudy 2 Study Group: Vitamin D supplement in early childhood and risk of type I (insulin-dependent) diabetes mellitus. Diabetologia 1999;42:51–54.
86 Hyppönen E, Läärä E, Järvelin MR, Virtanen SM. Intake of vitamin D and risk of type 1 diabetes: A birth cohort study. Lancet 2001;358:1500–1504.
87 Fournier C, Gepner P, Sadouk M, Charriere J: In vivo beneficial effects of cyclosporin A and 1,25-dihydroxyvitamin $D_3$ on the induction of experimental autoimmune thyroiditis. Clin Immunol Immunopathol 1990;54:53–63.
88 Mathieu C, Waer M, Laureys J, Rutgeerts O, Nouillon R: Prevention of type 1 diabetes in NOD mice by 1,25-dihydoxyvitamin $D_3$. Diabetologia 1994;37:552–558.
89 Hyöty H, Taylor KW: The role of viruses in human diabetes. Diabetologia 2002;45:1353–1361.
90 Yoon J-W: Role of viruses in the pathogenesis of IDDM. Ann Med 1991;23:437–445.
91 Szopa TM, Titchener PA, Portwood ND, Taylor KW: Diabetes mellitus due to viruses: Some recent developments. Diabetologia 1993;36:687–695.
92 Barrett-Connor E: Is insulin-dependent diabetes mellitus caused by Coxsackie B infection? A review of the epidemiologic evidence. Rev Infect Dis 1985;7:207–215.
93 Banatvala JE: Insulin-dependent (juvenile-onset, type 1) diabetes mellitus. Coxsackie B viruses revisited. Prog Med Virol 1987;34:33–54.
94 Gamble DR, Taylor KW: Seasonal incidence of diabetes mellitus. Br Med J 1969;iii:631–633.
95 Orchard TJ, Atchison RW, Becker D, Rabin B, Eberhardt M, Kuller LH, LaPorte RE, Cavender D: Coxsackie infection and diabetes. Lancet 1983;ii:631.
96 Mertens T, Grüneklee D, Eggers HJ: Neutralizing antibodies against Coxsackie B viruses in patients with recent onset of type 1 diabetes. Eur J Pediatr 1983;140:293–294.
97 Palmer JP, Cooney MK, Ward RH, Hansen JA, Brodsky JB, Ray CG, Crossley JR, Asplin CM, Williams RH: Reduced Coxsackie antibody titers in type 1 (insulin-dependent) diabetic patients presenting during an outbreak of Coxsackie B3 and B4 infection. Diabetologia 1982;22:426–429.
98 Graves PM, Norris JM, Pallansch MA, Gerling IC, Rewers M: The role of enteroviral infections in the development of IDDM: Limitations of current approaches. Diabetes 1997;46:161–168.
99 Frisk G, Fohlman J, Kobbah M, Ewald U, Tuvemo T, Diderholm H, Friman G: High frequency of Coxsackie-B-virus-specific IgM in children developing type 1 diabetes during a period of high diabetes morbidity. J Med Virol 1985;17:219–227.
100 Fohlman J, Friman G: Is juvenile diabetes a viral disease? Ann Med 1993;25:569–574.

101 Nerup J, Mandrup-Poulsen T, Mølvig J, Helqvist S, Wogensen L, Egeberg J: Mechanisms of pancreatic beta-cell destruction in type 1 diabetes. Diabetes Care 1988;11(suppl 1):16–23.
102 Clements GB, Galbraith DN, Taylor KW: Coxsackie B virus infection and onset of childhood diabetes. Lancet 1995;346:221–223.
103 Andreoletti L, Hober D, Hober-Vandenberghe C, Belaich S, Vantyghem MC, Lefebvre J, Wattre P: Detection of coxsackie B virus RNA sequences in whole blood samples from adult patients at the onset of type I diabetes mellitus. J Med Virol 1997;52:121–127.
104 Nairn C, Galbraith DN, Taylor KW, Clements GB: Enterovirus variants in the serum of children at the onset of type 1 diabetes mellitus. Diab Med 1999;16:509–513.
105 Chehadeh W, Weill J, Vantyghem MC, Alm G, Lefebvre J, Wattre P, Hober D: Increased level of interferon-alpha in blood of patients with insulin-dependent diabetes mellitus: Relationship with coxsackievirus B infection. J Infect Dis 2000;181:1929–1939.
106 Yin H, Berg AK, Tuvemo T, Frisk G: Enterovirus RNA is found in peripheral blood mononuclear cells in a majority of type 1 diabetic children at onset. Diabetes 2002;51:1964–1971.
107 Craig ME, Howard NJ, Silink M, Rawlinson WD: Reduced frequency of HLA DRB1*03-DQB1*02 in children with type 1 diabetes associated with enterovirus RNA. J Infect Dis 2003;187:1562–1570.
108 Hyöty H, Hiltunen M, Knip M, Laakkonen M, Vähäsalo P, Karjalainen J, Koskela P, Roivainen M, Leinikki P, Hovi T, Åkerblom HK, the Childhood Diabetes in Finland Study Group: A prospective study of the role of Coxsackie B and other enterovirus infections in the pathogenesis of IDDM. Diabetes 1995;44:652–657.
109 Hiltunen M, Hyöty H, Knip M, Ilonen J, Reijonen H, Vähäsalo P, Roivainen M, Leinikki P, Hovi T, Åkerblom HK, the Childhood Diabetes in Finland Study Group: ICA seroconversion in children is temporally associated with enterovirus infections. J Infect Dis 1997;175:554–560.
110 Lönnrot M, Salminen K, Knip M, Savola K, Kulmala P, Leinikki P, Hyypiä T, Åkerblom HK, Hyöty H, the Childhood Diabetes in Finland Study Group: Enterovirus RNA in serum is a risk factor for beta-cell autoimmunity and clinical type 1 diabetes: A prospective study. J Med Virol 2000;61:214–220.
111 Lönnrot M, Korpela K, Knip M, Ilonen J, Simell O, Korhonen S, Savola K, Muona P, Simell T, Koskela P, Hyöty H: Enterovirus infection as a risk factor for β-cell autoimmunity in a prospectively observed birth cohort: The Finnish Diabetes Prediction and Prevention (DIPP) Study. Diabetes 2000;49:1314–1318.
112 Salminen K, Sadeharju K, Lönnrot M, Vähäsalo P, Ilonen J, Simell O, Knip M, Hyöty H: Enterovirus infections are associated with the induction of beta-cell autoimmunity in a prospective birth cohort study. J Med Virol 2003;69:91–98.
113 Fuchtenbusch M, Irnstetter A, Jager G, Ziegler AG: No evidence for an association of coxsackie virus infections during pregnancy and early childhood with development of islet autoantibodies in offspring of mothers or fathers with type 1 diabetes. J Autoimmun 2001;17:333–340.
114 Graves PM, Rotbart HA, Nix WA, Pallansch MA, Erlich HA, Norris JM, Hoffman M, Eisenbarth GS, Rewers M: Prospective study of enteroviral infections and development of beta-cell autoimmunity: Diabetes autoimmunity study in the young (DAISY). Diab Res Clin Pract 2003;59: 51–61.
115 Dahlquist CG, Ivarsson S, Lindberg B, Forsgren M: Maternal enteroviral infection during pregnancy. Diabetes 1995;44:408–413.
116 Viskari HR, Roivainen M, Reunanen A, Pitkaniemi J, Sadeharju K, Koskela P, Hovi T, Leinikki P, Vilja P, Tuomilehto J, Hyöty H: Maternal first-trimester enterovirus infection and future risk of type 1 diabetes in the exposed fetus. Diabetes 2002;51:2568–2571.
117 Szopa TM, Ward T, Dronfield DM, Portwood ND, Taylor KW: Coxsackie B4 viruses with the potential to damage beta cells of the islets are present in clinical isolates. Diabetologia 1990;33: 325–328.
118 Roivainen M, Rasilainen S, Ylipaasto P, Nissinen R, Ustinov J, Bouwens L, Eizirik DL, Hovi T, Otonkoski T: Mechanisms of coxsackievirus-induced damage to human pancreatic beta-cells. J Clin Endocrinol Metab 2000;85:432–440.
119 Roivainen M, Ylipaasto P, Savolainen C, Galama J, Hovi T, Otonkoski T: Functional impairment and killing of human beta cells by enteroviruses: The capacity is shared by a wide range of

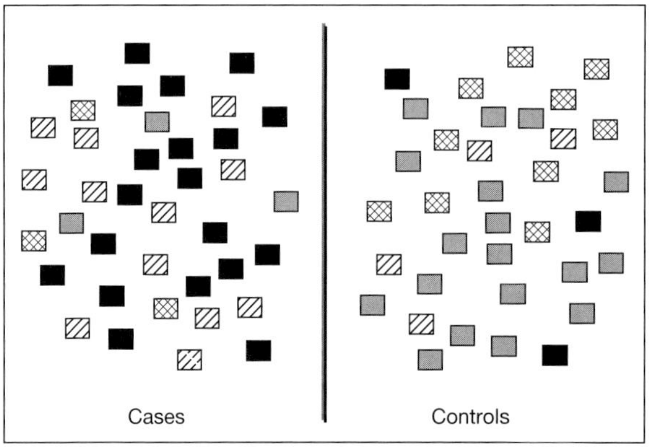


*Fig. 3.* Schematic representation of association studies using a case-control design. This method assesses for significant difference in the allelic frequencies between independent patients and independent controls from the same source population. In this example, the alleles indicated with black and diagonal patterned rectangles are positively associated with the disease (because they are more common in the patients) while the alleles represented by hatch and tinted rectangles are negatively associated (because they are more common in the controls).

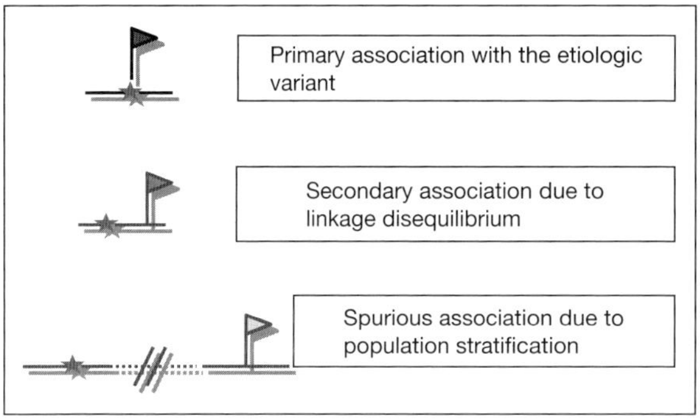


*Fig. 4.* Schematic representation of the main mechanisms underlining the association of a given polymorphism with a given trait.

the test variant with the primary-associated mutation. This underlines a key concept: association on its own does not imply causation; (3) the association is spurious in that it is due to confounding by population admixture or stratification. In mixed populations, any trait present more frequently in a given ethnic group will be apparently associated with any allele more common in that group. The problem of population stratification in case-control analyses can be reduced to some extent at the design stage by a careful selection of the control group or by

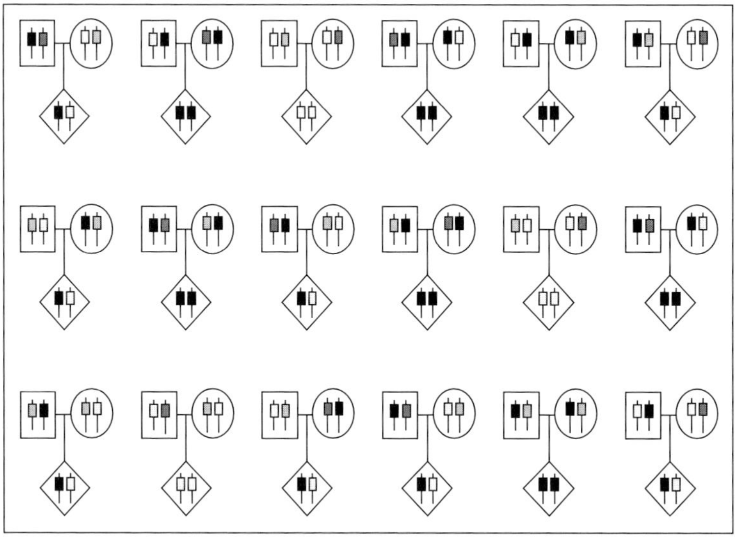

*Fig. 5.* Schematic representation of association studies using the Transmission Disequilibrium Test (TDT). This test evaluates the observed transmission of a given allele from heterozygous parents to affected children versus the random expectations of 50% in the absence of disease association. In this example, the alleles indicated with black and light grey rectangles are positively associated with the disease (because they are transmitted more often than 50% to affected children) while the alleles represented by dark grey and medium grey rectangles are negatively associated (because they are transmitted less often than 50% to affected children).

using genetically isolated populations, for instance the Sardinian population [24]. However, this could be difficult and even in populations that are regarded as 'homogenous', such as the Finnish one, there is clear evidence of population substructure [25]. In mixed populations it is advised to use family-association tests like the haplotype relative risk, the family-based control, or the transmission disequilibrium test (TDT) methods (fig. 5) [26–28]. Regardless of the tests used, association analyses require a much denser map of marker variants but have higher statistical power and provide a much higher mapping resolution than linkage analysis (fig. 6). Association analyses could be applied using direct and indirect experimental designs. The direct approach is named candidate gene-approach. This strategy utilizes knowledge of the pathophysiology of the disorder and tests variants of a gene which because of its function might be directly involved in the etiology of the disease. The indirect approach is often referred to as LD mapping and is used to infer the location of unknown disease genes simply by virtue of their correlated appearance with surrounding markers. This latter design exploits the LD, or non-random association of alleles at closely linked loci, in genomic

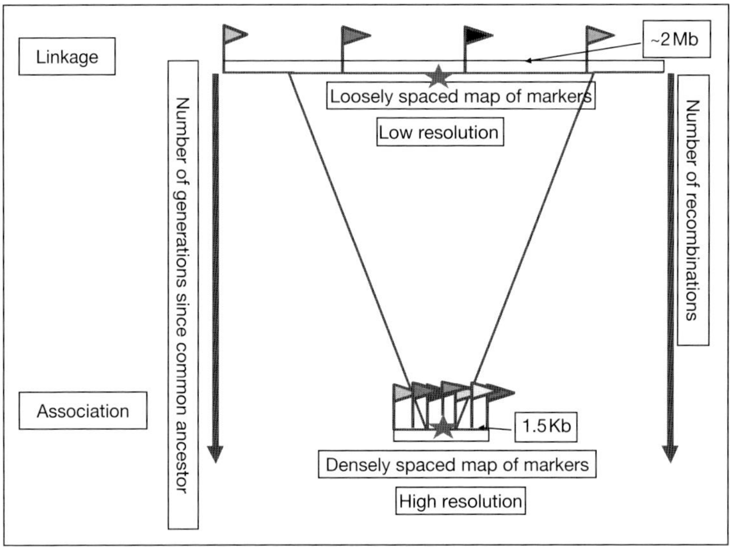


*Fig. 6.* Schematic representation of the main differences between linkage and association studies. Both studies base their mapping capacity on the observed recombinations whose numbers depend on the number of generations since the common ancestor of the patients. In linkage analysis, the number of recombinations is relatively low because this type of study is based on the analysis of contemporary meioses that have occurred in 1 or 2 generations. In association analysis, the number of recombinations is very high because this type of study exploits the historical recombinations that have occurred in the history of the assessed population. Consequently, linkage analysis has low resolving power and uses a loosely-spaced map of markers while association analysis affords high resolving power and utilizes a densely-spaced map of markers.

regions of interest. In effect, the LD affects gene mapping in two ways. While at the initial detection level LD facilitates the localization effort, once a gene effect has been identified within a chromosome interval, LD complicates precise resolution by pointing out not only the etiological variant, but also everything else that shows a correlated inheritance with it. Indeed, in this post-detection phase the main task is the deconstruction of LD. As expected for both steps of this LD-based approach, the allelic association in a chromosome region is heavily influenced by the allele-specific LD patterns of the various marker alleles with the disease allele [29]. Several factors make these LD patterns somewhat unpredictable. Indeed, evidence exists that LD is influenced by chromosome region-specific variables, notably by the presence of hot spots for recombination and by population-demographic variables as well as by functional constraints and specific selective forces [30]. For instance, it has been shown that small and demographically stable populations tend to have higher degrees of LD than large, rapidly expanding populations [30] and that across the genome there are areas of extensive LD, named LD blocks, punctuated by intervening regions of equilibrium [31]. One additional, critical issue in the LD-mapping approach appears to be the potential discrepancy between marker and disease allele frequencies [32]. The current available data supports the view that common markers should be preferred in order to optimize the chances of finding both common disease alleles with small relative risks, as well as rare ones with large relative risks. Irrespectively, by the frequency of the marker alleles there is full agreement that the marker density in the critical region must be very high [29, 32, 33]. This, on one hand would ensure initial detection by virtue of the strong LD between the markers employed in the map and the causal variant and, on the other hand, would provide the combinations of markers essential to solve LD around the etiological variant itself. In this respect, marker informativity, that is, the distribution of marker alleles on disease-associated chromosomes, is the critical parameter. This distribution could vary considerably between two populations. An allele at a marker locus could be in LD with the causal allele at the disease locus in one population but not in another [29]. This underscores the importance of performing and of cross-comparing the LD- mapping curves in different human groups; an approach named trans-racial analysis [34]. Consistent results at the level of a given polymorphism reinforce evidence for disease causality. Considering the unpredictable nature of the forces that influence LD [30], the re-sequencing of the exons and of the functionally-relevant regions of the genes of interest, further improves the chance of detecting disease association and of finding the causal polymorphism [33].

Technical aspects aside, however, there are also potentially serious problems in the interpretation of the results of association studies. These are represented essentially by the low statistical power of many studies and by the multiple testing issue.

The statistical power is the chance of detecting a given genetic effect assuming that it exists. It should always be computed at the beginning of a study. In effect, the power critically depends on the number of individuals studied as well as on the magnitude of the genetic effects and on the frequencies of the causal alleles at the disease locus. In indirect LD mapping studies, one should also consider the decrease in statistical power due to both the potentially incomplete LD and discrepancy in the allele frequencies between marker and disease alleles. Considering that the vast majority of susceptibility alleles involved in T1D and in other complex traits carry small genetic effects (classically odds ratios lower than 2 and in many cases lower than 1.5), the chance of success of such analyses essentially depends on the use of very large sample sets, in the order of thousands of individuals and on the disease gene architecture in the population examined.

The second problem to be critically evaluated in interpreting the results of association studies is represented by the multiple testing issue. This is becoming increasingly important and arises because of the large number of genetic markers typed in association studies. Classical procedures that correct the inflation of false positive results due to the great number of tests performed include the Bonferroni adjustment in which the observed p values are multiplied by the number of tests performed. However, considering that the number of tests performed by researchers surmounts those carried out in a single study and also taking into account the bias towards the publication of positive results, genome-wide significance levels have been established and proposed to reduce the false positive rate. A level of significance corresponding to a p value of $10^{-8}$ would be necessary to be confident that the result is not a false positive [35]. Prior evidence of linkage or strong functional evidence lowers this threshold p value from $10^{-8}$ to $10^{-5}$ [35].

Finally, an emerging issue that will become of great relevance in the future, when more disease loci will be identified, is represented by the analysis of the gene-gene interactions. Two main statistical models of multilocus interaction, named respectively multiplicative and additive, were originally described by Risch [36] and subsequently discussed by Cordell [37, 38]. Briefly, in the multiplicative model the probability of developing disease due to genotypes at one locus increases or decreases by a factor (the multiplicative factor) that is constant (i.e. it does not vary according to genotype variation and relative risks provided by the other locus). In the additive model, the probability of developing disease due to genotypes at one locus does not increase or decrease by a constant factor but increases or decreases by a constant amount. The multiplicative model was originally proposed by Risch [36] as an epistatic model, in which loci and biological pathways are not independent in contrast with the additive model that was described as a nonepistatic model in which the biological pathways involved in the disease are thought to be separate. However, it has been pointed out that this interpretation may be unrealistically simplistic [37, 38] and that both the current statistical models could be inadequate to illustrate the underlying biological complexity of a multifactorial disease [39, 40].

## Detection and Fine Mapping of *IDDM1* within the MHC/HLA Region

Numerous studies have provided a convincing case that the MHC/HLA region contains the major genetic component of T1D predisposition and protection (*IDDM1*). The MHC region of human chromosome 6p21.31 contains a densely-packed array of 224 genes in 3.6 Mb of DNA (fig. 7) and the fine

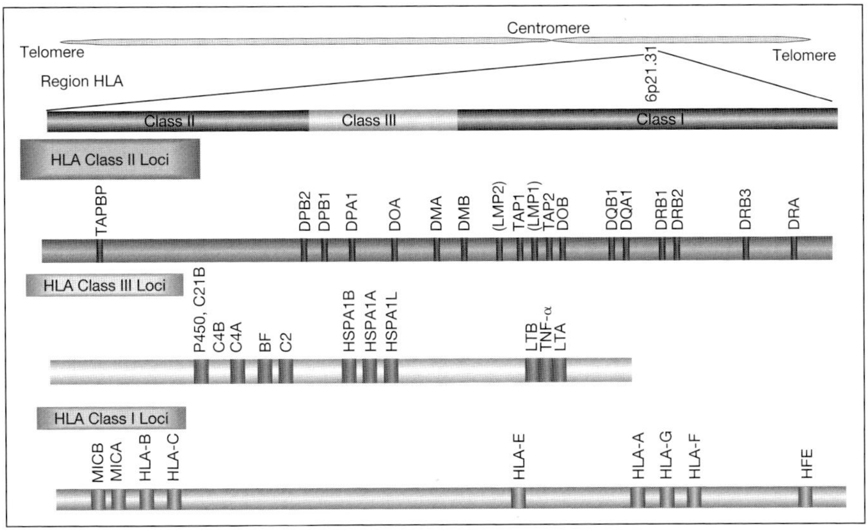


***Fig. 7.*** Schematic representation of the HLA region on chromosome 6p21.

dissection of *IDDM1* required a long series of allelic association mapping studies. These experiments, which began in 1973, have been hampered by technical limitations related to the genetic maps available at the infancy of molecular genetics and by the complex multiallelic and multilocus nature of *IDDM1*. Indeed, it is now evident that *IDDM1* is not one, but several polymorphisms showing very strong LD between each other.

The earliest demonstration that genes in the HLA region are involved in the inherited risk of T1D was detected more than thirty years ago by association studies using a candidate gene approach and a case-control study design [9–11]. The first associations of T1D with HLA antigens involved the HLA class I alleles B8 and B15 [9–11]. These observations were subsequently substantiated by linkage analysis in families with multiple cases [41]. Further analyses revealed that associations of the DR3 and DR4 alleles of the *HLA-DRB1* locus were significantly stronger than those at the class I loci. In addition, HLA-DR2 and -DR5 alleles were decreased in frequency in patients compared to controls, implying that these alleles are associated with alleles of the disease loci that encode protection from or resistance to T1D [27, 42]. With the cloning of class II loci, restriction fragment length polymorphism analysis revealed that the *HLA-DQB1* locus was even more strongly associated with T1D than *DRB1* [43–45]. In 1987, Todd and colleagues identified within the second exon of the *DQB1* locus a critical polymorphism at position DQB57, splitting to some extent positively associated and negatively associated *DQB1* alleles [46]. This was the first evidence of a 'single nucleotide polymorphism' (SNP) detected in a complex multifactorial disease. In the same year, the HLA class I A2 allotype crystal structure predicted the central structural role of β 57 in the peptide-binding site [47]. However, the $DQ^{\beta 57}$ correlation was not complete [48] and a role for DR was also indicated [49] and confirmed [50–52]. Furthermore, a trans-racial analysis of Afro-Caribbean and European-derived samples suggested that polymorphism of exon 2 of *HLA-DQA1* might also be implicated in susceptibility/resistance [34]. Contrast this long series of experiments providing complicated results with the recent advances in the *IDDM1* mapping strategies, which allow demonstration in just a short space of time that the association of the HLA region with T1D is in fact dominated by variation at the *DRB1* and *DQB1* loci [29, 53]. It is also clear that these HLA class II loci do not fully account for the association of the whole HLA/MHC region with the disease. The presence of extended haplotypes identical at the DR, DQ loci but differently associated with the disease [54] indicated that other genes in the HLA/MHC further influence the disease risk. For instance, it has been found that specific variants of the *HLA-DPB1* locus, or other variants in close LD with them, are associated with T1D independently of DR-DQ variants [55–57]. Furthermore, additional polymorphisms as yet unidentified, outside the exon 2 sequences of the DR/DQ/DP loci but within the HLA region act as additional risk modifiers. For example, it has been shown that distinct DR3 haplotypes, defined by the presence of three HLA markers at the *DMB* and *DOB* genes and the microsatellite locus *TNFc* in the first intron of the *TNF*-β gene, were associated at a different extent in Sardinian type 1 diabetic families, leading to the estimate that about 40% of DR3 haplotypes are in fact not predisposing to T1D in the Sardinian population [30]. In another example, heterogeneity within DRB1*04 haplotypes, using a case-control design, has been reported from Finland, with the causative variant(s) in LD with *HLA-B* [58]. Also, the microsatellite marker *D6S2223* at the telomeric end of the HLA region marks significant heterogeneity in the association of DR3 haplotypes with T1D in Norwegian and UK families [59]. In all three of these examples, different HLA haplotypes carry different degrees of disease predisposition despite having identical *HLA-DRB1* and *-DQB1* exon 2 sequences. The strong albeit irregular LD present in the HLA region has hampered the identification of the non-DR/DQ etiological variants [30, 59]. Thus, these studies, while indicating the presence of additional HLA risk modifiers, did not provide conclusive evidence about their nature. In the future, it will be essential to compare the critical haplotypes in different populations in order to define the sequence of mutational events which decreased (or increased) the predisposition conferred by the ancestral HLA haplotypes.

*Table 1*. Association of the DRB1-DQA1-DQB1 haplotypes with type 1 diabetes

| DR serological type | *DRB1* | *DQA1* | *DQB1* | *TID risk* |
|---|---|---|---|---|
| *High* | | | | |
| DR4 | 0405 | 0301 | 0302 | ++++++ |
| DR4 | 0401 | 0301 | 0302 | ++++++ |
| DR3 | 0301 | 0501 | 0201 | ++++ |
| DR4 | 0404 | 0301 | 0302 | ++++ |
| DR4 | 0402 | 0301 | 0302 | ++++ |
| *Intermediate* | | | | |
| DR4 | 0405 | 0301 | 0201 | + |
| DR8 | 08 | 0401 | 0402 | + |
| DR6 | 1302 | 0102 | 0604 | + |
| DR9 | 0901 | 0301 | 0303 | + |
| DR1 | 01 | 0101 | 0501 | ± |
| DR2AZH | 1601 | 0102 | 0502 | ± |
| *Low* | | | | |
| DR4 | 0401 | 0301 | 0301 | – |
| DR7 | 0701 | 0201 | 0201 | – |
| DR4 | 0405 | 0501 | 0301 | – |
| DR4 | 0403 | 0301 | 0302 | – |
| DR4 | 0406 | 0301 | 0302 | – |
| DR6 | 1301 | 0103 | 0603 | – – |
| DR10 | 1001 | 0101 | 0501 | – – |
| DR6 | 1303–5 | 0501 | 0301 | – – |
| *Very low* | | | | |
| DR5 | 11–12 | 0501 | 0301 | – – – – |
| DR2 | 1501 | 0102 | 0602 | – – – – – |
| DR7 | 0701 | 0201 | 0303 | – – – – – |
| DR6 | 1401 | 01 | 0503 | – – – – – |

## Association of the HLA Class II *DRB1-DQA1-DQB1* Variants with Type 1 Diabetes

The genetic data demonstrate the existence of a continuum of association from high-risk to low-risk *DRB1-DQA1-DQB1* variants. In particular, the three-locus *DRB1-DQA1-DQB1* haplotypes can be ranked into four main groups based on their association with the disease (table 1) [60]:

(1) Positively associated, e.g. DR4 (DRB1*0405/*0401-DQA1*0301-DQB1*0302), DR3 (DRB1*0301-DQA1*0501-DQB1*0201). Note that

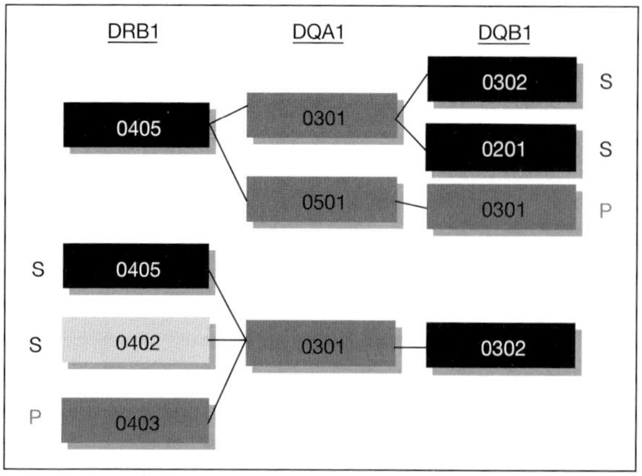


***Fig. 8.*** Schematic representation of the different 'splits' of the DR4 haplotypes observed in the Sardinian population. In the upper part of the figure: 'Splits' of the DRB1*0405. In the lower part of the figure: 'Splits' of the DQA1*03, DQB1*0302 haplotypes. S = Susceptibility haplotype; P = protective haplotype.

within this grouping the DR4 (DRB1*0405 and *0401) haplotypes are significantly more predisposing than the DR3 haplotype [60].

(2) Neutral, e.g. DR8 (DRB1*08-DQA1*0401-DQB1*0402), DR9 (DRB1* 0901-DQA1*0301-DQB1*0303), DR6 (DRB1*1302-DQA1* 0102-DQB1*0604), DR2AZH (DRB1*1601-DQA1*0102-DQB1*0502).

(3) Negatively associated with moderate significance, e.g. DR6 (DRB1*1301-DQA1*0103-DQB1*0603), DR7 (DRB1*0701-DQA1*0201-DQB1* 0201).

(4) Strongly negatively associated, e.g. DR5 (DRB1*11/12-DQA1*0501-DQB1*0301), DR2 (DRB1*1501-DQA1*0102-DQB1*0602), DR7 (DRB1*0701-DQA1*0201-DQB1*0303), DR14 (DRB1* 1401-QA1*01-DQB1*0503), which were either never or hardly ever transmitted from the parents to diabetic children.

The presence of DR4 haplotypes with several splits at the *DQB1* and *DRB1* loci in the Sardinian population offered a valuable opportunity for an unambiguous analysis of the effect of *DRB1* and *DQB1* loci in conferring T1D risk [51, 52, 60] (fig. 8). Haplotype analysis suggests that whether a particular *DQB1* allele confers diabetes risk depends on the nature of the allele at the *DRB1* locus on the same haplotype and vice versa. In fact, among the various *DRB1-DQB1* allelic combinations a single dose of a protective *DRB1* or *DQB1* allele (for example, DQB1*0301 or DRB1*0403) is sufficient to provide protection from T1D, while susceptibility requires a combination of

*DRB1* and *DQB1* permissive alleles (for example, DQB1*0302 and DR1*0405). Thus, the presence of only one protective allele at either locus results in a haplotype that is not associated or protective overall. Interestingly, in the Japanese the DQB1*0302 allele is not associated with T1D [61] simply because the vast majority of the DR4-DQB1*0302 haplotypes of the background population carry the DRB1*0403 or the DRB1*0406 protective alleles. These two alleles are structurally and functionally related; they differ only at codon 37 of the *DRB1* second exon [62]. However, the DQB1*0302 variant is strongly and significantly associated with T1D in the Japanese population when on a DR8 haplotype. The individual predisposing effect of DQB1*0302 is not apparent because the associated DR8-DQB1*0302 haplotype is very rare (1%) while DRB1*0403/06-DQB1*0302 protective haplotypes are quite frequent (18%) in the general Japanese population [62]. The above illustrates the complexity of disease association and of the difficulties created in genetic analysis of multifactorial disease by interactions between different loci and modes of transmission of disease susceptibility.

The complexity of the HLA class II association with T1D is further underlined by the presence of important genotype effects. This implies that the relative predisposition of an allele and haplotype is influenced by the allele and haplotype present on the other chromosome and, therefore, by the complete mating type. In general, the presence of only one protective haplotype on either chromosome results in a genotype that is neutrally or negatively associated overall. More specifically, genotypes positive for protective haplotypes like the (DR2) DRB1*1501-DQA1*0102-DQB1*0602 are negatively associated with, and hence strongly protective against, the disease, no matter what the haplotype present on the other chromosome is. Other haplotypes, such as DR5 (DRB1*11–12-DQA1*0501-DQB1*0301) or DR7 (DRB1*0701-DQA1*0201-DQB1*0201), which individually conferred less marked degrees of protection (table 1), generate genotypes that are only protective in the absence of the predisposing DR4-DQB1*0302 haplotype on the other chromosome. Both DR5-DQB1*0301 and DR7-DQB1*0201 are neutrally associated when the highly predisposing DR4-DQB1*0302 haplotype is present on the other chromosome. Taken together, the available data support the dominant-like effect of protection and suggest that the association of the HLA class II molecules with T1D is largely determined by the whole HLA class II genotype.

The genotype effects in T1D also include the presence of preferential pairing of predisposing haplotypes as T1D risk factors. This means that there is evidence that some combinations of haplotypes, for instance DR3 and DR4, form genotypes (DR3/4) that confer a higher risk than would be expected under a multiplicative model (in which the genotype relative risk for an individual with a given genotype, in our case DR3/4, takes the form of the product of the individual haplotype relative risks). Additionally, in T1D, DR3/4 is increased in frequency in most patient populations over the frequency expected by Hardy-Weinberg equilibrium [63]. Taken together, these genetic data might suggest the presence of interactions between molecules encoded within the DR3 and DR4 haplotypes. In fact, a possible explanation for these interactions involves the formation of heterodimers in trans, for instance DQA1*0501- DQB1*0302 (in which DQA1*0501 is carried by DR3 and DQB1*0302 is carried by DR4) with increased T1D risk [64]. This would be due to peptide-binding properties of these particular DQ molecules and their direct functional activity in the development of the disease. However, the heterodimer model cannot be a fully adequate explanation because the DR3/4 trans-effect in disease risk is more evident in some populations than in others while the DQ heterodimers formed in DR3/4 are identical in different populations.

Interestingly, some studies have attempted to analyze the association of the various HLA class II haplotypes with the human T1D after removing the main predisposing DR3/DR4 molecules [65]. In this sub-group of patients, the neutral-permissive alleles were apparently the most predisposing. These analyses mirror what happens in populations, such as the Japanese, in which the highly predisposing European haplotypes are absent and the disease is extremely rare. Haplotypes that appear predisposing in Asian populations are only neutral in European populations, consistent with the overall risk they bestow on Asian populations [61, 66]. Importantly, these data suggest that an HLA-presenting molecule is a necessary factor for disease occurrence. This molecule is most likely encoded by the alleles most positively associated with the disease but in their absence other molecules, with a lower probability, can invoke the same response. Indeed, the risk of developing the disease will be different in the different HLA categories, as the disease prevalence is different in diverse populations.

## Amino Acids, Mechanisms and Lessons from Animal Models of Type 1 Diabetes

Binding of peptides is a complex property of the MHC class II molecules. It involves the joint ability of particular peptide-binding pockets, formed by specific amino-acids of the MHC class II exon 2-encoded domains, to accommodate and display to the T cell receptors (TCRs) of CD4-T lymphocytes linear stretches of 12–20 amino acids derived from self and foreign peptides. Residue variation of the various MHC alleles is critical to determine the specificity of such interactions. In order to pinpoint which amino acid residues in the peptide-binding site of the MHC molecules are determining resistance and susceptibility to T1D, we must first know the underlying relative associations of the various DR-DQ haplotypes. Next, we have to compare haplotypes with significant differences in disease predisposition and differing only at one or few residues. Finally, we need to assess the functional relevance of the putative causal residues and evaluate in which mechanistic context they may act. Owing to the difficulty of studying mechanisms in the immune system in humans, particularly in the generation and maintenance of tolerance, murine model systems have been developed and provide important insights into these distal mechanisms. There is a mouse strain, the non-obese diabetes (NOD) mouse, which spontaneously develops a form of autoimmune diabetes closely resembling human T1D. The NOD mouse possesses a unique MHC class II haplotype ($H2^{g7}$) [67, 68] which carries a null IEa gene (IE is the murine orthologue of DR), and encodes an IA β chain (IA is the murine orthologue of DQ) carrying serine at position 57 instead of the more common aspartic acid. Studies of congenic NOD mice expressing non-NOD MHC haplotypes and of NOD mice expressing $IE\alpha^{d}$, modified $IA\beta^{g7}$, $IA\alpha^{k}/IA\beta^{k}$, or $IA\beta^{d}$ transgenes, have proved that both isotypes of class II molecules are directly involved in disease predisposition and protection [69–73].

The crystal structures of both the human DQ (α1*0301, β1*0302) and murine $IA\beta^{g7}$ allotypes have been resolved and revealed marked similarities in critical positions of the peptide-binding pockets of these molecules [74–76]. These conserved inter-species structural features between T1D predisposing class II molecules contrasted with equally conserved similarities between the predicted structures of human and mouse protective molecules [60]. The data provide evidence for a joint action of the first, fourth and ninth class II peptide-binding pockets (P1, P4 and P9) in disease susceptibility and resistance with a main role for P9. The peptide-binding pocket P9 of the predisposing DQ/IA allotypes is more capacious than the corresponding predicted pocket of the protective/neutral allotypes. Consequently, in P9 the predisposing molecules might have a preference for large acidic residues (Asp, Glu) although they could also bind with lower affinity medium to large-sized hydrophobic residues [60]. It is likely that in this position, all the protective molecules bind preferentially medium-sized, non-charged residues such as Ser or Ala but also Gly, Thr, Gln. DQ $Asp^{\beta57}$ is the critical residue in P9. Its carboxylate group forms a salt bridge with $Arg^{\alpha76}$ that stabilizes the heterodimer and determines the affinity of the peptide binding [74–76].

This conservation of structure within and across species indicates that not only is it likely that similar peptides are involved in T1D etiology in mice and humans, but also that the mechanisms distal to class II-peptide-T cell receptor interaction are shared. In particular, the strong protective effect of specific human HLA alleles and haplotypes mirrors that of certain mouse dominantly protective H2-A molecules, such as H2-Ab. In NOD mice, T lymphocytes carrying a highly diabetogenic, H2-$A^{g7}$ restricted, transgenic TCR undergo negative selection in the thymus of class II heterozygous ($H2^{g7/b}$, $H2^{g7/q}$, $H2^{g7/k}$, $H2^{g7/nbl}$) NOD mice, by engaging the non diabetogenic class II molecules on thymic-bone-marrow-derived T cells [77]. These NOD mice carrying on one chromosome the predisposing H-$2^{g7}$ haplotype and on the other one, specific class II haplotypes, were diabetes resistant. Moreover, the degree of insulitis directly correlated with the degree of thymocyte deletion [77]. These results suggest that the HLA/MHC-encoded protection is most likely related to an active role of the MHC protective molecules in the pathway of peptide presentation, probably via thymic clonal deletion of autoreactive T cells. This view is also supported by the observation that the loss of the autoreactive phenotype, observed in the NOD/ NOD.H2k-congenic F1 mice is not due to insufficient H2-Ag7 expression, since (NOD.MHC-null/NOD) F1 mice, which were hemizygous for H2-Ag7, had the autoreactive T cell phenotype [78]. Thus, the requirement for MHC homozygosity (or double heterozygosity for predisposing variants) in autoimmune diabetes is not simply related to the need of expressing a given number of predisposing molecules on the cell surface. The disease resistance might be directly proportional to the efficiency in the binding of the same diabetogenic peptide by these HLA molecules in the thymus. The HLA-predisposing molecules might determine a positive, but not a negative thymic selection of the diabetogenic T cell clones, possibly because of intermediate affinity complexes with the diabetogenic peptide and the pathogenetic TCRs. In the periphery, the T cell clones that escape the thymic deletion could be able to recognize the diabetogenic peptide in specific conditions such us those related to exposition of cryptic epitopes, high expression or post-translational modification of the critical auto-antigens. It is also likely that, in agreement with another mouse transgenic model [79], regulatory T cells positively selected in the thymus might also contribute to the protection conferred by specific HLA class II haplotypes. The two mechanisms: negative selection of diabetogenic T cells in the thymus and positive selection of T cells with suppressive activity might not be mutually exclusive. For instance, it is possible that 'appropriate' MHC-controlled thymic selection, would also bias the T cells that were not deleted in the thymus toward regulatory/suppressive responses in the periphery, resulting in a more sophisticated, multipoint regulatory mechanism against autoimmunity. These events in the thymus could affect both the CD4 and CD8 T cell repertoires [80, 81].

A major unsolved question remains the role and relative importance of the DR and DQ molecules in the disease process. While in the case of the DQ alleles, the relationship between genetic association and structural features of the molecules appears satisfactory, it is more difficult, DR4 subtypes aside, to find a common structural denominator which differentiates the DR molecules encoded within predisposing haplotypes from those detected in the protective ones. As stated above, the clearest genetic evidence of the *DRB1* effect in human T1D comes from the analysis of the DR4 subtypes and from the presence of a *DRB1* allele, DRB1*0403, which is able to override the predisposition conferred by the high risk DQA1*03-DQB1*0302 haplotype. How can the DRB1*0403 allele confer protection from T1D? Interestingly, the predicted structure of the protective molecules $IA^b$, DR ($\alpha$1*0101, $\beta$*0403) and DQ ($\alpha$1*0501, $\beta$1*0301) showed significant similarities, particularly in P4 and P9 [60]. It is, therefore, possible that in the thymus or in the periphery the protection bestowed by these *DRB1* alleles is related to the same pathway of peptide presentation involving the *DQB1* alleles. It remains to be established if other *DRB1* alleles, such as the DRB1*0405, DRB1*0401 and DRB1*0301, might have some direct role in the disease process, for instance, by promoting the positive selection and the peripheral restriction of autoreactive T cell clones. Also, from the available data it is not clear whether the decrease in risk of the predisposing DQB1*0201 allele within the DR7 haplotype is related to the *DRB1* locus itself or to the DQA1*0201 allele present on this haplotype or to another unknown component within the haplotype.

### The Association of the VNTR (*IDDM2*) in the *INS* Promoter Region with Type 1 Diabetes

A second T1D disease locus, *IDDM2*, has been detected [12] and subsequently mapped [82–84] to a polymorphic minisatellite VNTR locus in the *INS* promoter region on chromosome 11p15.5. Indeed, allelic association and functional studies have shown that within *IDDM2*, the VNTR locus itself in the *INS* promoter region is likely to represent the etiologic polymorphism [4, 7, 82, 84–88]. Differences in length occur in three discrete classes of VNTR alleles. The shorter class of alleles, named class I, is positively associated with T1D, while the longer class of alleles, named class III, is negatively associated. An intermediate-sized class of alleles named class II has been detected in African samples and is extremely rare in European-derived samples. A large body of studies supports the direct involvement of *INS*-VNTR variation in T1D. Experimental evidence suggests that the VNTR may bind transcriptional regulatory proteins depending on the sequence of the particular VNTR allele [89]. The *INS*-VNTR locus affects expression of the insulin gene and its precursors in the thymus. This is consistent with a model in which either positive selection or negative selection of autoreactive T cell clones against epitopes from preproinsulin (PPI) play a key role in the disease process [85–88]. A two- to threefold decrease in the amount of the PPI in the thymus caused by *INS*-VNTR class I alleles can explain their positive association with the disease [85, 86, 88]. This model was greatly strengthened by the discovery that mutations in the transcription factor AIRE (autoimmune regulator) cause autoimmune disease in humans, including T1D [4, 5] and in mice [7] by lowering the expression of peripheral antigens such as PPI in the thymus. However, interpreting the biological mechanisms underlying the *INS-IDDM2* associations with T1D only in terms of the effects of the products of these genes in the thymus is oversimplistic. Indeed, the functional consequences of *INS-VNTR* variation in T1D susceptibility and protection might include extra-thymic immunological and metabolic effects.

### *IDDM1* and *IDDM2:* Gene-Gene Interactions

The two unequivocally-established disease loci, *HLA-DRB1/DQB1 (IDDM1)* and *INS*-VNTR(*IDDM2*) offer one of the few current opportunities to evaluate gene-gene interactions in a complex, multifactorial disorder. In fact, the interaction of the HLA and *INS* loci has been evaluated in different studies but there has been uncertainty, both in the results obtained and the nomenclature used. Julier et al. [82], using a French sample set initially reported evidence of linkage and association of the disease with *INS*-VNTR allelic variation only in *HLA*-DRB1*04-positive patients. This observation supported an etiopathological pathway restricted to a specific HLA-class II allotype/preproinsulin peptide complex. However, subsequent reports based on the analysis of UK and German samples showed not only that the *INS*-VNTR-encoded susceptibility was independent from *HLA*-DRB1*04 but also that, consistent with the multiplicative model of gene-gene interaction, genotype variation at both loci occurred independently of each other [90, 91]. Still, other studies, in Belgian [92] and Finnish sample sets [93], reported that the predisposing *INS* class I alleles might have less [40, 93] or no effect [92] in individuals with high-risk HLA genotypes, compared to intermediate and low-risk HLA genotypes. The uncertainty present in the literature is illustrated by the conflicting way in which the results of previous studies have been reported; the joint action of HLA and *INS* has variously been described as being multiplicative [94, 95], additive [96], providing evidence of interaction [94, 97] and exhibiting no interaction [95, 96]. Two recent studies in Sardinian and Finnish samples [39, 40] shed some light onto this controversial issue. These studies, in agreement with some previous work [90, 91], proved that the

*INS* genotype significantly influences T1D risk in all HLA genotype risk categories. However, confirming earlier observations suggesting a heterogeneity in the relative effects of *INS* [92, 93] they also provided convincing evidence that the *INS*-predisposing genotype is significantly less frequent in high-risk HLA genotype positive patients than in those with HLA intermediate and low-risk categories. Thus, these results highlighted a particular feature in the interactions between *INS* and HLA: the effects of *INS* on T1D risk are detectable in all of the HLA genotype risk categories but at the same time these effects are less pronounced in individuals carrying HLA high-risk genotypes. When these data were evaluated in the context of the statistical models of gene-gene interaction, the additive model was rejected. However, the multiplicative model is also inadequate in explaining the gene-gene interaction and does not reflect the complexity of the molecular interaction of the protein products of the *INS* and HLA class II genes [39]. Indeed, a powerful and robust case-only analysis showed that the distribution of the *IDDM2* genotypes was significantly uneven, and not constant as expected under the multiplicative model, in the different genotype categories at *IDDM1* [39]. These fluctuations from a pure mathematical model observed in Sardinia and in Finland are not surprising if we consider that any statistical model tends to be inherently oversimplistic and thus can capture only a small portion of the biological complexity of a trait.

Taking the experimental functional/mechanistic observations into account, the *IDDM1-IDDM2* joint genetic data could be explained by a stepwise progression in the strength of binding of the MHC protein products with a self peptide that determines different windows of T cell avidity for the MHC-self peptide complexes in the thymus. More specifically, the observed genetic results are consistent with an MHC-self peptide-TCR biological model. In this model, the affinity and specificity of different MHC class II allotypes for a preproinsulin-derived peptide and the levels of this peptide in the thymus during the generation of self-tolerance, act jointly to influence positive selection, T regulatory cell selection and negative selection. However, as highlighted by several studies, the HLA-class II/peptide-preproinsulin interaction is only one of many factors in the editing of T cell antigen receptor specificities in the thymus. The overall avidity of the interaction might involve several additional molecules such as CD80, CD86, CD54, CTLA-4, CD28 and LYP. Furthermore, the HLA-*INS* interactions in T1D might include peripheral immunological and metabolic effects and might also be influenced by environmental factors, which could vary in different populations. The complex and unpredictable nature of these variables might help to explain the contradictory results obtained in analyzing the *IDDM1* and *IDDM2* interactions in different studies from diverse populations.

## Other Non *IDDM1-IDDM2* Loci

The HLA (*IDDM1*) and *INS* (*IDDM2*) variants cannot completely explain the familial clustering and the inherited risk of T1D [13, 14]. The existence of non-HLA variants which regulate inflammation and which are involved in T1D is consistent with experimental work in animal models of autoimmune diabetes. Several quantitative trait loci influencing susceptibility to T1D have been mapped in the NOD mouse [98–101]. The mode of inheritance of the susceptibility to T1D observed in these mouse animal models suggests that the MHC genes are important, as are the non-MHC genes, but neither the MHC or the non-MHC genes alone are sufficient to cause the disease [102–104].

A number of whole genome linkage scans have also been performed in human T1D but they have given, overall, weak and conflicting results. For instance, a combined analysis on 767 UK and USA affected sib-pair families (ASP), showed that after *HLA*/*IDDM1*, the 2 loci exhibiting the highest Maximum Likelihood Score (MLS) were *IDDM2* on chromosome 11p15 and the marker D16S3098 on chromosome 16q22-q24 [105]. Another whole-genome scan of 408 Scandinavian ASP families subsequently reported no significant evidence for sharing in the D16S3098 region. In this Scandinavian study, even *IDDM2*, which is an unequivocally established disease locus, was undetected on the unstratified data and only upon sub-grouping the data by HLA was significant sharing at *IDDM2* seen [106]. These results illustrate the difficulties of detecting (or replicating the detection of) linkage for genes of low to moderate effects using affected sib-pair-based strategies. These limitations are mainly related to the limited statistical power to detect disease genes with small genetic effects using linkage strategies. In reality, the previous genome scans have been of great importance to better define the disease model: they indicated that *IDDM1*/MHC is the only locus with major genetic effects in T1D. Other genes must be involved to explain the inheritance of T1D in humans and in mouse experimental models but they provide modest individual contributions to familial clustering and to the inherited disease risk. Further complications in the detection of T1D genes might be caused by interlocus and allelic heterogeneity, interactions between different disease variants and interactions between disease variants and environmental factors.

Some of these limitations, in particular those related to the statistical power of the study, could be alleviated by further increasing the number of ASP families. However, the detection of non-MHC genes using linkage strategies appears problematic. It is becoming evident that association-based methods both within gene regions of potential interest, because their protein products could affect pathways relevant to T1D etiology, and at the genome-wide level must be employed. For instance, using a candidate gene-region approach, polymorphisms of the cytotoxic T lymphocyte antigen *CTLA-4* gene on chromosome 2q33 have been found to be associated with T1D, Graves' disease and autoimmune hypothyroidism [15]. In humans, a change located in 279 base pairs distal to the major polyadenylation cleavage site of the mRNA correlated with the relative mRNA levels of the alternative full length and soluble splice forms of *CTLA-4* and with disease resistance. Likewise, in the mouse model of T1D, a variant of *CTLA-4* exon 2 has been discovered that correlated with suppression of the splicing of the mRNA of a ligand-independent isoform and protection from disease [15]. These data illustrate that subtle inherited variation in negative regulation affects the fine balance between immunity and harmful tissue destruction. These results also show the power of positional genetics, especially when the human and mouse genes are pursued together. They suggest that polymorphisms that affect transcript regulation could be a rich source of the population variation underlying common disease. *CTLA-4* is a crucial negative regulatory molecule of the T cell antigen receptor-signalling pathway. This is hardly surprising, since T1D is an autoimmune disorder caused by autoreactive T cells. The involvement of this immune-pathway in T1D is also indicated by the recent observation of an association of variation at the *PTPN22* locus on chromosome 1p13. Indeed, *PTPN22* encodes a lymphoid protein tyrosine kinase (LYP) that is important in negative control of T cell activation and in T cell development. Bottini and colleagues first reported evidence that a non-synonymous single nucleotide polymorphism (SNP) at nucleotide 1858 in codon 620 (Arg620Trp) in *PTPN22* was associated with T1D in two independent case-control collections from North America and Sardinia [16]. These results were subsequently replicated by Smyth and colleagues who provided massive statistical support for the involvement of variation at the *PTPN22* locus in two large independent sets of T1D families and case-control samples, respectively [17]. We can conclude that *PTPN22* is an unequivocally established T1D locus. Interestingly, there is also evidence for an association of Trp620 with Graves' disease [17] as well as with rheumatoid arthritis [107] and systemic lupus erythematosus [108]. Thus, taken together, these results indicate a more general association of both the *CTLA-4* and *PTPN22* loci with autoimmune disease. The existence of variants with a central role in general autoimmunity is consistent with the observation that T1D occurs more frequently in the patients and in the families of the patients with other autoimmune disorders, such as autoimmune thyroid disease, rheumatoid arthritis, celiac disease and multiple sclerosis (MS) [14, 109, 110]. Interestingly, it has been shown that shared disease associations due to variants at the HLA class II *DRB1-DQB1* loci provide only a partial explanation for the observed increased prevalence of T1D in Sardinian MS patients [110].

Taken all together these data suggest that variation at other non-HLA class II loci contribute significantly to the inheritance, and in some cases to the co-inheritance, of T1D and other autoimmune disorders.

## Conclusions

During the last few years, the identification of genetic variants involved in the inherited risk of T1D has considerably improved our understanding of the factors causing this autoimmune disease. Despite this progress, the genes underlying T1D are still only partially known and the environmental component that perforce must be involved in the disease process remains largely speculative. A more comprehensive knowledge of the disease-causing variants and of their functional consequences in immunity and in β-cell autoimmunity will expand our understanding of the causal factors, lead to more accurate estimates of the disease risk in unaffected people and underpin research into new preventive treatments. Furthermore, identification of the major susceptibility and protective variants should permit large prospective studies of genetically-susceptible individuals and ultimately the identification of key environmental factors. The sequencing of the human genome and subsequent efforts to characterize genetic variation has created an unprecedented opportunity to relate genes with phenotypes via large-scale SNP association studies. We anticipate that these studies performed in informative populations and in large and statistically well-powered sample sets will have a major positive impact in the quest to prevent this common multifactorial disease.

## Acknowledgements

We thank John Todd, Antonio Cao and Mauro Congia, for continuous help and support and Rebecca Lewis for editorial assistance.

## References

1 Wildin RS, Ramsdell F, Peake J, Faravelli F, Casanova JL, Buist N, Levy-Lahad E, Mazzella M, Goulet O, Perroni L, Bricarelli FD, Byrne G, McEuen M, Proll S, Appleby M, Brunkow ME: X-linked neonatal diabetes mellitus, enteropathy and endocrinopathy syndrome is the human equivalent of mouse scurfy. Nat Genet 2001;27:18–20.

2 Fontenot JD, Gavin MA, Rudensky AY: Foxp3 programs the development and function of CD4+CD25+ regulatory T cells. Nat Immunol 2003;4:330–336.

3 Khattri R, Cox T, Yasayko SA, Ramsdell F: An essential role for Scurfin in CD4+CD25+ T regulatory cells. Nat Immunol 2003;4:337–342.

4 Consortium TF-GA: An autoimmune disease, APECED, caused by mutations in a novel gene featuring two PHD-type zinc-finger domains. The Finnish-German APECED Consortium. Autoimmune Polyendocrinopathy-Candidiasis-Ectodermal Dystrophy. Nat Genet 1997;17:399–403.
5 Nagamine K, Peterson P, Scott HS, Kudoh J, Minoshima S, Heino M, Krohn KJ, Lalioti MD, Mullis PE, Antonarakis SE, Kawasaki K, Asakawa S, Ito F, Shimizu N: Positional cloning of the APECED gene. Nat Genet 1997;17:393–398.
6 Medzhitov R, Janeway CA Jr: Decoding the patterns of self and nonself by the innate immune system. Science 2002;296:298–300.
7 Anderson MS, Venanzi ES, Klein L, Chen Z, Berzins SP, Turley SJ, von Boehmer H, Bronson R, Dierich A, Benoist C, Mathis D: Projection of an immunological self shadow within the thymus by the aire protein. Science 2002;298:1395–1401.
8 Brunkow ME, Jeffery EW, Hjerrild KA, Paeper B, Clark LB, Yasayko SA, Wilkinson JE, Galas D, Ziegler SF, Ramsdell F: Disruption of a new forkhead/winged-helix protein, scurfin, results in the fatal lymphoproliferative disorder of the scurfy mouse. Nat Genet 2001;27:68–73.
9 Singal DP, Blajchman MA: Histocompatability antigens, lymphocytotoxic antibodies and tissue antibodies in patients with diabetes mellitus. Diabetes 1973;22:429–432.
10 Cudworth A, Woodrow J: HLA system and diabetes mellitus. Diabetes 1974;24:345–349.
11 Nerup J, Platz P, Andersen OO, Christy M, Lyngsoe J, Poulsen JE, Ryder LP, Nielsen LS, Thomsen M, Svejgaard A: HLA antigens and diabetes mellitus. Lancet 1974;ii:864–866.
12 Bell GI, Horita S, Karam JH: A polymorphic locus near the human insulin gene is associated with insulin-dependent diabetes mellitus. Diabetes 1984;33.
13 Risch N: Assessing the role of HLA-linked and unlinked determinants of disease. Am J Hum Genet 1987;40:1–14.
14 Vyse TJ, Todd JA: Genetic analysis of autoimmune disease. Cell 1996;85:311–318.
15 Ueda H, Howson JM, Esposito L, et al: Association of the T-cell regulatory gene CTLA4 with susceptibility to autoimmune disease. Nature 2003;423:506–511.
16 Bottini N, Musumeci L, Alonso A, Rahmouni S, Nika K, Rostamkhani M, MacMurray J, Meloni GF, Lucarelli P, Pellecchia M, Eisenbarth GS, Comings D, Mustelin T: A functional variant of lymphoid tyrosine phosphatase is associated with type I diabetes. Nat Genet 2004; 36:337–338.
17 Smyth D, Cooper JD, Collins JE, Heward JM, Franklyn JA, Howson JM, Vella A, Nutland S, Rance HE, Maier L, Barratt BJ, Guja C, Ionescu-Tirgoviste C, Savage DA, Dunger DB, Widmer B, Strachan DP, Ring SM, Walker N, Clayton DG, Twells RC, Gough SC, Todd JA: Replication of an association between the lymphoid tyrosine phosphatase locus (LYP/PTPN22) with type 1 diabetes, and evidence for its role as a general autoimmunity locus. Diabetes 2004;53: 3020–3023.
18 Green A: The EURODIAB studies on childhood diabetes 1988–1999. Europe and diabetes. Diabetologia 2001;44(suppl 3):B1–B2.
19 Karvonen M, Viik-Kajander M, Moltchanova E, Libman I, LaPorte R, Tuomilehto J: Incidence of childhood type 1 diabetes worldwide. Diabetes Mondiale (DiaMond) Project Group. Diab Care 2000;23:1516–1526.
20 Muntoni S, Fonte M, Marietti G, Bizzarri C, Crino' A, Ciampalini P, Multari G, Stuppa M, Matteoli M, Lucentini L, Sebastiani L, Visalli N, Pozzilli P, Boscherini B, Muntoni S: Incidence of insulin-dependent diabetes mellitus among Sardinian-heritage children born in Lazio region, Italy. Lancet 1997;349:160–162.
21 Olmos P, A'Hern R, Heaton DA, Millward BA, Risley D, Pyke DA, Leslie RD: The significance of the concordance rate for type 1 (insulin-dependent) diabetes in identical twins. Diabetologia 1988;31:747–750.
22 Kyvik KO, Green A, Beck-Nielsen H: Concordance rates of insulin dependent diabetes mellitus: A population based study of young Danish twins. Br Med J 1995;311:913–917.
23 Evans DM, Cardon LR: Guidelines for genotyping in genomewide linkage studies: Single-nucleotide-polymorphism maps versus microsatellite maps. Am J Hum Genet 2004;75:687–692.
24 Lampis R, Morelli L, Congia M, Macis MD, Mulargia A, Loddo M, De Virgiliis S, Marrosu MG, Todd JA, Cucca F: The inter-regional distribution of HLA class II haplotypes indicates the suitability of the Sardinian population for case-control association studies in complex diseases. Hum Mol Genet 2000;9:2959–2965.

25 Kittles RA, Perola M, Peltonen L, Bergen AW, Aragon RA, Virkkunen M, Linnoila M, Goldman D, Long JC: Dual origins of Finns revealed by Y chromosome haplotype variation. Am J Hum Genet 1998;62:1171–1179.
26 Falk CT, Rubinstein P: Haplotype relative risks: An easy reliable way to construct a proper control sample for risk calculations. Ann Hum Genet 1987.
27 Thomson G, Robinson WP, Kuhner MK, Joe S, MacDonald MJ, Gottschall JL, Barbosa J, Rich SS, Bertrams J, Baur MP, Partanen J, Tait BD, Schober E, Mayr WR, Ludvigsson J, Lindblom B, Farid NR, Thompson C, Deschamps I: Genetic heterogeneity, modes of inheritance, and risk estimates for a joint study of Caucasians with insulin-dependent diabetes mellitus. Am J Hum Genet 1988;43:799–816.
28 Spielman RS, McGinnis RE, Ewens WJ: Transmission test for linkage disequilibrium: The insulin gene region and insulin-dependent diabetes mellitus (IDDM). Am J Hum Genet 1993;52:506–516.
29 Zavattari P, Lampis R, Mulargia A, Loddo M, Angius E, Todd JA, Cucca F: Confirmation of the DRB1-DQB1 loci as the major component of IDDM1 in the isolated founder population of Sardinia. Hum Mol Genet 2000;9:2967–2972.
30 Zavattari P, Deidda E, Whalen M, Lampis R, Mulargia A, Loddo M, Eaves I, Mastio G, Todd JA, Cucca F: Major factors influencing linkage disequilibrium by analysis of different chromosome regions in distinct populations: Demography, chromosome recombination frequency and selection. Hum Mol Genet 2000;9:2947–2957.
31 Gabriel SB, Schaffner SF, Nguyen H, Moore JM, Roy J, Blumenstiel B, Higgins J, DeFelice M, Lochner A, Faggart M, Liu-Cordero SN, Rotimi C, Adeyemo A, Cooper R, Ward R, Lander ES, Daly MJ, Altshuler D: The structure of haplotype blocks in the human genome. Science 2002; 296:2225–2229.
32 Zondervan KT, Cardon LR: The complex interplay among factors that influence allelic association. Nat Rev Genet 2004;5:89–100.
33 Wang WY, Todd JA: The usefulness of different density SNP maps for disease association studies of common variants. Hum Mol Genet 2003;12:3145–3149.
34 Todd JA, Mijovic C, Fletcher J, Jenkins D, Bradwell AR, Barnett AH: Identification of susceptibility loci for insulin-dependent diabetes mellitus by trans-racial gene mapping. Nature 1989;338: 587–589.
35 Dahlman I, Eaves IA, Kosoy R, Morrison VA, Heward J, Gough SC, Allahabadia A, Franklyn JA, Tuomilehto J, Tuomilehto-Wolf E, Cucca F, Guja C, Ionescu-Tirgoviste C, Stevens H, Carr P, Nutland S, McKinney P, Shield JP, Wang W, Cordell HJ, Walker N, Todd JA, Concannon P: Parameters for reliable results in genetic association studies in common disease. Nat Genet 2002; 30:149–150.
36 Risch N: Linkage strategies for genetically complex traits. II. The power of affected relative pairs. Am J Hum Genet 1990;46:229–241.
37 Cordell HJ, Todd JA, Hill NJ, Lord CJ, Lyons PA, Peterson LB, Wicker LS, Clayton DG: Statistical modeling of interlocus interactions in a complex disease: Rejection of the multiplicative model of epistasis in type 1 diabetes. Genetics 2001;158:357–367.
38 Cordell HJ: Epistasis: What it means, what it doesn't mean, and statistical methods to detect it in humans. Hum Mol Genet 2002;11:2463–2468.
39 Motzo C, Contu D, Cordell HJ, Lampis R, Congia M, Marrosu MG, Todd JA, Devoto M, Cucca F: Heterogeneity in the magnitude of the insulin gene effect on HLA risk in type 1 diabetes. Diabetes 2004;53:3286–3291.
40 Laine AP, Hermann R, Knip M, Simell O, Akerblom HK, Ilonen J: The human leukocyte antigen genotype has a modest effect on the insulin gene polymorphism-associated susceptibility to type 1 diabetes in the Finnish population. Tissue Antigens 2004;63:72–74.
41 Cudworth AG, Woodrow JC: Evidence for HL-A-linked genes in 'juvenile' diabetes mellitus. Br Med J 1975;iii:133–135.
42 Wolf E, Spencer KM, Cudworth AG: The genetic susceptibility to type 1 (insulin-dependent) diabetes: Analysis of the HLA-DR association. Diabetologia 1983;24:224–230.
43 Owerbach D, Lernmark A, Platz P, Ryder LP, Rask L, Peterson PA, Ludvigsson J: HLA-D region b-chain DNA endonuclease fragments differ between HLA-DR identical healthy and insulin-dependent diabetic individuals. Nature 1983;303:815–817.

44 Michelsen B, Lernmark A: Molecular cloning of a polymorphic DNA endonuclease fragment that associates insulin-dependent diabetes mellitus with HLA-DQ. J Clin Invest 1987;79: 1144–1152.
45 Festenstein H, Awad J, Hitman GA, Cutbush S, Groves AV, Cassell P, Ollier W, Sachs JA: New HLA DNA polymorphisms associated with autoimmune diseases. Nature 1986;322:64–67.
46 Todd JA, Bell JI, McDevitt HO: HLA-DQ beta gene contributes to susceptibility and resistance to insulin-dependent diabetes mellitus. Nature 1987;329:599–604.
47 Bjorkman PJ, Saper MA, Samraoui B, Bennett WS, Strominger JL, Wiley DC: Structure of the human class I histocompatibility antigen, HLA-A2. Nature 1987;329:506–512.
48 Erlich HA, Bugawan TL, Scharf S, Nepom GT, Tait B, Griffith RL: HLA-DQ beta sequence polymorphism and genetic susceptibility to IDDM. Diabetes 1990;39:96–103.
49 Sheehy MJ, Scharf SJ, Rowe JR, Neme de Gimenez MH, Meske LM, Erlich HA, Nepom BS: A diabetes-susceptible HLA haplotype is best defined by a combination of HLA-DR and -DQ alleles. J Clin Invest 1989;83:830–835.
50 Erlich HA, Zeidler A, Chang J, Shaw S, Raffel LJ, Klitz W, Beshkov Y, Costin G, Pressman S, Bugawan T, et al: HLA class II alleles and susceptibility and resistance to insulin dependent diabetes mellitus in Mexican-American families. Nat Genet 1993;3:358–364.
51 Cucca F, Muntoni F, Lampis R, Frau F, Argiolas L, Silvetti M, Angius E, Cao A, De Virgiliis S, Congia M: Combinations of specific DRB1, DQA1, DQB1 haplotypes are associated with insulin-dependent diabetes mellitus in Sardinia. Hum Immunol 1993;37:85–94.
52 Cucca F, Lampis R, Frau F, Macis D, Angius E, Silvetti M, Chessa M, Frongia P, Masile P, Cao A, De Virgiliis S, Congia M: The distribution of DR4 haplotypes in Sardinia suggests a primary association of insulin dependent diabetes mellitus with DRB1 and DQB1 loci. Hum Immunol 1995;43:301–308.
53 Herr M, Dudbridge F, Zavattari P, Cucca F, Guja C, March R, Campbell RD, Barnett AH, Bain SC, Todd JA, Koeleman BP: Evaluation of fine mapping strategies for a multifactorial disease locus: Systematic linkage and association analysis of IDDM1 in the HLA region on chromosome 6p21. Hum Mol Genet 2000;9:1291–1301.
54 Robinson WP, Barbosa J, Rich SS, Thomson G: Homozygous parent affected method for detecting disease predisposing variants: Application to insulin diabetes mellitus. Genetic Epidemiology 1993;10:273–288.
55 Erlich HA, Rotter JI, Chang JD, Shaw SJ, Raffel LJ, Klitz W, Bugawan TL, Zeidler A: Association of HLA-DPB1*0301 with IDDM in Mexican-Americans. Diabetes 1996;45:610–614.
56 Noble AJ, Valdes AM, Cook M, Klitz W, Thomson G, Erlich HA: The role of HLA class II genes in insulin-dependent diabetes mellitus: Molecular analysis of 180 Caucasian, multiplex families. Am J Hum Genet 1996;59:1134–1148.
57 Cucca F, Dudbridge F, Loddo M, Mulargia AP, Lampis R, Angius E, De Virgiliis S, Koeleman BP, Bain SC, Barnett AH, Gilchrist F, Cordell H, Welsh K, Todd JA: The HLA-DPB1-associated component of the IDDM1 and its relationship to the major loci HLA-DQB1, -DQA1, and -DRB1. Diabetes 2001;50:1200–1205.
58 Nejentsev S, Gombos Z, Laine AP, Veijola R, Knip M, Simell O, Vaarala O, Akerblom HK, Ilonen J: Non-class II HLA gene associated with type 1 diabetes maps to the 240-kb region near HLA-B. Diabetes 2000;49:2217–2221.
59 Lie BA, Todd JA, Pociot F, Nerup J, Akselsen HE, Joner G, Dahl-Jorgensen K, Ronningen KS, Thorsby E, Undlien DE: The predisposition to type 1 diabetes linked to the human leukocyte antigen complex includes at least one non-class II gene. Am J Hum Genet 1999;64:793–800.
60 Cucca F, Lampis R, Congia M, Angius E, Nutland S, Bain SC, Barnett AH, Todd JA: A correlation between the relative predisposition of MHC class II alleles to type 1 diabetes and the structure of their proteins. Hum Mol Genet 2001;10:2025–2037.
61 Todd JA, Fukui Y, Kitagawa T, Sasazuki T: The A3 allele of the HLA-DQA1 locus is associated with susceptibility to type 1 diabetes in Japanese. Proc Natl Acad Sci USA 1990;87: 1094–1098.
62 Awata T, Kuzuya T, Matsuda A, Iwamoto Y, Kanazawa Y: Genetic analysis of HLA class II alleles and susceptibility to type 1 (insulin-dependent) diabetes mellitus in Japanese subjects. Diabetologia 1992;35:419–424. [Published erratum appears in Diabetologia 1992;35:906.]

63 Cucca F, Todd J: HLA/MHC: Genes, molecules and function; in Browning M, McMichael A (eds): HLA Susceptibility to Type 1 Diabetes: Methods and Mechanisms. Oxford, BIOS Scientific Publishers, 1996.
64 Koeleman BP, Lie BA, Undlien DE, Dudbridge F, Thorsby E, de Vries RR, Cucca F, Roep BO, Giphart MJ, Todd JA: Genotype effects and epistasis in type 1 diabetes and HLA-DQ trans dimer associations with disease. Genes Immun 2004;5:381–388.
65 Undlien DE, Kockum I, Ronningen KS, Lowe R, Saanjeevi CB, Graham J, Lie BA, Akselsen HE, Lernmark A, Thorsby E: HLA associations in type 1 diabetes among patients not carrying high-risk DR3-DQ2 or DR4-DQ8 haplotypes. Tissue Antigens 1999;54:543–551.
66 Sheehy MJ: HLA and insulin-dependent diabetes: A protective perspective. Diabetes 1992;41: 123–129.
67 Hattori M, Buse JB, Jackson RA, Glimcher L, Dorf ME, Minami M, Makino S, Moriwaki K, Kuzuya H, Imura H, et al: The NOD mouse: Recessive diabetogenic gene in the major histocompatibility complex. Science 1986;231:733–735.
68 Acha-Orbea H, McDevitt HO: The first external domain of the nonobese diabetic mouse class II I-A beta chain is unique. Proc Natl Acad Sci USA 1987;84:2435–2439.
69 Nishimoto H, Kikutani H, Yamamura K, Kishimoto T: Prevention of autoimmune insulitis by expression of I-E molecules in NOD mice. Nature 1987;328:432–434.
70 Lund T, O'Reilly L, Hutchings P, Kanagawa O, Simpson E, Gravely R, Chandler P, Dyson J, Picard JK, Edwards A, et al: Prevention of insulin-dependent diabetes mellitus in non-obese diabetic mice by transgenes encoding modified I-A beta-chain or normal I-E alpha-chain. Nature 1990;345:727–729.
71 Miyazaki T, Uno M, Uehira M, Kikutani H, Kishimoto T, Kimoto M, Nishimoto H, Miyazaki J, Yamamura K: Direct evidence for the contribution of the unique I-ANOD to the development of insulitis in non-obese diabetic mice. Nature 1990;345:722–724.
72 Slattery RM, Kjer-Nielsen L, Allison J, Charlton B, Mandel TE, Miller JF: Prevention of diabetes in non-obese diabetic I-Ak transgenic mice. Nature 1990;345:724–726.
73 Singer SM, Tisch R, Yang XD, McDevitt HO: An Abd transgene prevents diabetes in nonobese diabetic mice by inducing regulatory T cells. Proc Natl Acad Sci USA 1993;90:9566–9570.
74 Lee KH, Wucherpfennig KW, Wiley DC: Structure of a human insulin peptide-HLA-DQ8 complex and susceptibility to type 1 diabetes. Nat Immunol 2001;2:501–507.
75 Corper AL, Stratmann T, Apostolopoulos V, Scott CA, Garcia KC, Kang AS, Wilson IA, Teyton L: A structural framework for deciphering the link between I-Ag7 and autoimmune diabetes. Science 2000;288:505–511.
76 Latek RR, Suri A, Petzold SJ, Nelson CA, Kanagawa O, Unanue ER, Fremont DH: Structural basis of peptide binding and presentation by the type I diabetes-associated MHC class II molecule of NOD mice. Immunity 2000;12:699–710.
77 Schmidt D, Verdaguer J, Averill N, Santamaria P: A mechanism for the major histocompatibility complex-linked resistance to autoimmunity. J Exp Med 1997;186:1059–1075.
78 Ridgway WM, Ito H, Fasso M, Yu C, Fathman CG: Analysis of the role of variation of major histocompatibility complex class II expression on nonobese diabetic (NOD) peripheral T cell response. J Exp Med 1998;188:2267–2275.
79 Luhder F, Katz J, Benoist C, Mathis D: Major histocompatibility complex class II molecules can protect from diabetes by positively selecting T cells with additional specificities. J Exp Med 1998;187:379–387.
80 Serreze DV, Holl TM, Marron MP, Graser RT, Johnson EA, Choisy-Rossi C, Slattery RM, Lieberman SM, DiLorenzo TP: MHC class II molecules play a role in the selection of autoreactive class I-restricted CD8 T cells that are essential contributors to type 1 diabetes development in nonobese diabetic mice. J Immunol 2004;172:871–879.
81 Morgan DJ, Nugent CT, Raveney BJ, Sherman LA: In a transgenic model of spontaneous autoimmune diabetes, expression of a protective class II MHC molecule results in thymic deletion of diabetogenic CD8+ T cells. J Immunol 2004;172:1000–1008.
82 Julier C, Hyer RN, Davies J, Merlin F, Soularu P, Briant L, Cathelineau G, Deschamps I, Rotter JI, Froguel P, Boitard C, Bell JI, Lathrop GM: Insulin-IGF2 region on chromosome 11p encodes a gene implicated in HLA-DR4-dependent diabetes susceptibility. Nature 1991;354:155–159.

83 Bennett ST, Lucassen AM, Gough SC, Powell EE, Undlien DE, Pritchard LE, Merriman ME, Kawaguchi Y, Dronsfield MJ, Pociot F, et al: Susceptibility to human type 1 diabetes at *IDDM2* is determined by tandem repeat variation at the insulin gene minisatellite locus. Nat Genet 1995; 9:284–292.
84 Barratt BJ, Payne F, Lowe CE, Hermann R, Healy BC, Harold D, Concannon P, Gharani N, McCarthy MI, Olavasen MG, McCormack R, Guja C, Ionescu-Tirgoviste C, Undlien D, Ronningen K, Gillespie KM, Tuomilehto-Wolf E, Tuomilehto J, Bennett ST, Clayton D, Cordell H, Todd JA: Remapping the insulin gene/IDDM2 locus in type 1 diabetes. Diabetes 2004;53:in press.
85 Pugliese A, Zeller M, Fernandez A, Zalcberg LJ, Bartlett RJ, Ricordi C, Pietropaolo M, Eisenbarth GS, Bennett ST, Patel DD: The insulin gene is transcribed in the human thymus and transcription levels correlated with allelic variation at the INS VNTR-IDDM2 susceptibility locus for type 1 diabetes. Nat Genet 1997;15:293–297.
86 Vafiadis P, Bennett ST, Todd JA, Nadeau J, Grabs R, Goodyer CG, Wickramasinghe S, Colle E, Polychronakos C: Insulin expression in human thymus is modulated by INS VNTR alleles at the IDDM2 locus. Nat Genet 1997;15:289–292.
87 Chentoufi AA, Polychronakos C: Insulin expression levels in the thymus modulate insulin-specific autoreactive T-cell tolerance: The mechanism by which the IDDM2 locus may predispose to diabetes. Diabetes 2002;51:1383–1390.
88 Chentoufi AA, Palumbo M, Polychronakos C: Proinsulin expression by Hassall's corpuscles in the mouse thymus. Diabetes 2004;53:354–359.
89 Kennedy C, German M, Rutter W: The minisatellite in the diabetes susceptibility locus IDDM2 regulates insulin transcription. Nat Genet 1995;9:293–298.
90 Bain SC, Prins JB, Hearne CM, Rodrigues NR, Rowe BR, Pritchard LE, Ritchie RJ, Hall JR, Undlien DE, Ronningen KS, et al: Insulin gene region-encoded susceptibility to type 1 diabetes is not restricted to HLA-DR4-positive individuals. Nat Genet 1992;2:212–215.
91 Walter M, Albert E, Conrad M, Keller E, Hummel M, Ferber K, Barratt BJ, Todd JA, Ziegler AG, Bonifacio E: IDDM2/insulin VNTR modifies risk conferred by IDDM1/HLA for development of Type 1 diabetes and associated autoimmunity. Diabetologia 2003;46:712–720.
92 van der Auwera B, Schuit F, Lyaruu I, Falorni A, Svanholm S, Vandewalle CL, Gorus FK: Genetic susceptibility for insulin-dependent diabetes mellitus in Caucasians revisited: The importance of diabetes registries in disclosing interactions between HLA-DQ- and insulin gene-linked risk. Belgian Diabetes Registry. J Clin Endocrinol Metab 1995;80:2567–2573.
93 Metcalfe KA, Hitman GA, Fennessy MJ, McCarthy MI, Tuomilehto J, Tuomilehto-Wolf E: In Finland insulin gene region encoded susceptibility to IDDM exerts maximum effect when there is low HLA-DR associated risk. DiMe (Childhood Diabetes in Finland) Study Group. Diabetologia 1995;38:1223–1229.
94 Cordell HJ, Todd JA, Bennett ST, Kawaguchi Y, Farral M: Two locus maximum lod score analysis of a multifactorial trait: Joint consideration of IDDM2 and IDDM4 with IDDM1 in type I diabetes. Am J Hum Genet 1995;57:920–934.
95 Dizier MH, Babron MC, Clerget-Darpoux F: Interactive effect of two candidate genes in a disease: Extension of the marker-association-segregation chi(2) method. Am J Hum Genet 1994;55: 1042–1049.
96 She JX, Bui MM, Tian XH, Muir A, Wakeland EK, Zorovich B, Zhang LP, Liu MC, Thomson G, Maclaren NK: Additive susceptibility to insulin-dependent diabetes conferred by HLA-DQB1 and insulin genes. Autoimmunity 1994;18:195–203.
97 Cordell HJ, Wedig GC, Jacobs KB, Elston RC: Multilocus linkage tests based on affected relative pairs. Am J Hum Genet 2000;66:1273–1286.
98 Encinas JA, Lees MB, Sobel RA, Symonowicz C, Greer JM, Shovlin CL, Weiner HL, Seidman CE, Seidman JG, Kuchroo VK: Genetic analysis of susceptibility to experimental autoimmune encephalomyelitis in a cross between SJL/J and B10.S mice. J Immunol 1996;157:2186–2192.
99 Sundvall M, Jirholt J, Yang HT, Jansson L, Engstrom A, Pettersson U, Holmdahl R: Identification of murine loci associated with susceptibility to chronic experimental autoimmune encephalomyelitis. Nat Genet 1995;10:313–317.
100 Todd JA, Aitman TJ, Cornall RJ, Ghosh S, Hall JRS, Hearne CM, Knight AM, Love JM, McAleer MA, Prins J-B, Rodrigues N, Lathrop GM, Pressey A, DeLarato N, Peterson LB,

Wicker LS: Genetic analysis of autoimmune type 1 diabetes mellitus in mice. Nature 1991;351: 542–547.
101 Ghosh S, Palmer SM, Rodrigues NR, Cordell HJ, Hearne CM, Cornall RJ, Prins JB, McShane P, Lathrop GM, Peterson LB, et al: Polygenic control of autoimmune diabetes in nonobese diabetic mice. Nat Genet 1993;4:404–409.
102 Wicker LS, Todd JA, Peterson LB: Genetic control of autoimmune diabetes in the NOD mouse. Ann Rev Immunol 1995;13:179–200.
103 Fritz RB, Skeen MJ, Chou CH, Garcia M, Egorov IK: Major histocompatibility complex-linked control of the murine immune response to myelin basic protein. J Immunol 1985;134:2328–2332.
104 Baker D, Rosenwasser OA, O'Neill JK, Turk JL: Genetic analysis of experimental allergic encephalomyelitis in mice. J Immunol 1995;155:4046–4051.
105 Cox NJ, Wapelhorst B, Morrison VA, Johnson L, Pinchuk L, Spielman RS, Todd JA, Concannon P: Seven regions of the genome show evidence of linkage to type 1 diabetes in a consensus analysis of 767 multiplex families. Am J Hum Genet 2001;69:820–830.
106 Nerup J, Pociot F: A genomewide scan for type 1-diabetes susceptibility in Scandinavian families: Identification of new loci with evidence of interactions. Am J Hum Genet 2001;69: 1301–1313.
107 Begovich AB, Carlton VE, Honigberg LA, et al: A missense single-nucleotide polymorphism in a gene encoding a protein tyrosine phosphatase (PTPN22) is associated with rheumatoid arthritis. Am J Hum Genet 2004;75:330–337.
108 Kyogoku C, Langefeld CD, Ortmann WA, Lee A, Selby S, Carlton VE, Chang M, Ramos P, Baechler EC, Batliwalla FM, Novitzke J, Williams AH, Gillett C, Rodine P, Graham RR, Ardlie KG, Gaffney PM, Moser KL, Petri M, Begovich AB, Gregersen PK, Behrens TW: Genetic association of the R620W polymorphism of protein tyrosine phosphatase PTPN22 with human SLE. Am J Hum Genet 2004;75:504–507.
109 Tait KF, Marshall T, Berman J, Carr-Smith J, Rowe B, Todd JA, Bain SC, Barnett AH, Gough SC: Clustering of autoimmune disease in parents of siblings from the Type 1 diabetes Warren repository. Diabet Med 2004;21:358–362.
110 Marrosu MG, Motzo C, Murru R, Lampis R, Costa G, Zavattari P, Contu D, Fadda E, Cocco E, Cucca F: The co-inheritance of type 1 diabetes and multiple sclerosis in Sardinia cannot be explained by genotype variation in the HLA region alone. Hum Mol Genet 2004;13:2919–2924.

Francesco Cucca, MD
Dipartimento di Scienze Biomediche e Biotecnologie
University of Cagliari, Via Jenner, IT–09121 Cagliari (Italy)
Tel. +39 070 6095681, Fax +39 070 6095558, E-Mail fcucca@mcweb.unica.it

Chiarelli F, Dahl-Jørgensen K, Kiess W (eds): Diabetes in Childhood and Adolescence.
Pediatr Adolesc Med. Basel, Karger, 2005, vol 10, pp 57–71

# Autoimmunity in Type 1 Diabetes mellitus

*Peter Achenbach, Anette-G. Ziegler*

Diabetes Research Institute and 3rd Medical Department,
Hospital München-Schwabing, Munich, Germany

Over the last three decades, evidence has accumulated that type 1 diabetes mellitus is an autoimmune disease or at least has a major autoimmune component [1, 2]. The presence of insulitis, a strong linkage between type 1 diabetes development and certain alleles of the major histocompatibility complex (MHC), autoantibodies that react with islet antigens, and the ability to prevent the loss of residual β-cell function in recent-onset type 1 diabetes patients by immunosuppression or immunomodulatory therapies support the autoimmune nature of the disease [3–6].

## Autoantibodies

Autoantibodies can be very reproducibly detected in autoimmune diseases and are useful markers for diagnosis, pathogenesis and prediction. In type 1 diabetes, the best-studied autoantibodies (and, respectively, best characterized major autoantigens) are antibodies to insulin [7], the 65-kDa isoform of glutamic acid decarboxylase (GAD65) [8], and the protein tyrosine phosphatase (PTP)-related molecules IA-2 (ICA512) and IA-2β (phogrin) [9–12]. All of these major type 1 diabetes autoantigens are related to the secretory apparatus of β-cells: insulin is stored in β-cell secretory granules, IA-2 and IA-2β are intrinsic membrane proteins of β-cell secretory granules [10, 13], and GAD65 is a membrane-associated protein of β-cell synaptic-like microvesicles [14]. Apart from these, other autoantigens (GLIMA, Carboxypeptidase H, ICA69, Jun B, SOX13, sulphatides, etc.) [reviewed in 15] have been suggested to be involved in type 1 diabetes pathogenesis but their relevance has not been confirmed in large studies or in the case of GLIMA, the target molecule has not been identified so that their measurement remains too cumbersome for large-scale studies [16].

### T Cells

T cell reactivity against islet autoantigens and their corresponding peptides has been extensively studied in the nonobese diabetic (NOD) mouse [15, 17, 18]. T cell clones have been generated from islet infiltrates, pancreatic lymph nodes, and spleen of prediabetic NOD mice, and shown to be either diabetogenic or diabetes-protective in transfer experiments [19]. Moreover, transgenic NOD mice expressing T cell receptors (TCRs) that target naturally occurring β-cell autoantigens have become available during the last decade greatly facilitating studies on the pathogenic mechanisms of autoimmune diabetes [20]. Furthermore, immune tolerance can be induced to some of the autoantigens resulting in protection of NOD mice from β-cell destruction [21–25].

Human T cell responses, however, are far more difficult to detect reproducibly due to the small number of β-cell-specific T lymphocytes in the peripheral blood of type 1 diabetes patients or preclinical subjects [26]. Using proliferation assays human T cell responses have been described to a long list of target peptides on several molecules, including GAD65, IA-2, (pro)insulin and others [15, 27–29], but these responses could often also be detected in control subjects [30]. More recently, new methods such as ELISpot assay, tetramer analysis, determination of supernatant cytokine production, and the use of antibodies to block co-stimulation have been introduced to identify qualitative differences between autoreactive T cell responses in patients versus control subjects [31–33]. The results are promising and in some but not all cases suggest that responses in control subjects are more likely to have a regulatory phenotype [32] or a non-memory phenotype [33]. Further efforts in improving qualitative and quantitative measurement of T cell autoreactivity, therefore, will be important if the cellular autoimmune response is to provide useful markers of prediction and disease monitoring.

### Autoantibodies and T Cells in Type 1 Diabetes Pathogenesis

An inflammatory cellular infiltrate (insulitis) consisting predominantly of CD8+ T and CD4+ T lymphocytes and variable numbers of B lymphocytes, macrophages, dendritic cells, and natural killer cells is present inside and around the pancreatic islets at and prior to diabetes onset [34, 35]. In mouse models of autoimmune diabetes, it has been shown that both CD4+ and CD8+ T lymphocytes are required for disease development and, therefore, type 1 diabetes is generally considered to be a T cell-mediated disease [26]. B lymphocytes must also have a critical role in disease development in the mouse since models of B lymphocyte-deficient mice do not develop diabetes or insulitis [36]. In man, a pathogenetic role for T cells is likely but the evidence is largely anecdotal. Convincing evidence comes from transplant studies in identical twins, in which the transplant of pancreas segments from the unaffected twin to the diabetic twin resulted in a CD8+ T cell predominant insulitis in the graft and the rapid loss of graft function [37]. A role for B lymphocytes is less convincing. A single case of type 1 diabetes in a child who lacked functional B lymphocytes indicates that B lymphocytes are not strictly necessary for the development of type 1 diabetes [38].

The influence of islet autoantibodies in the pathogenesis of type 1 diabetes has also been examined. In the NOD mouse, removal of maternally transmitted immunoglobulin prevented spontaneous diabetes in the offspring, suggesting that fetal exposure to antibodies including islet autoantibodies increased diabetes risk [39]. In contrast to the mouse, the BABYDIAB study has found that offspring from mothers with type 1 diabetes have a decreased risk to develop islet autoimmunity if they receive maternally transmitted GAD or IA-2 autoantibodies from their mothers during pregnancy, suggesting that fetal exposure to GAD and/or IA-2 autoantibodies protects from the future development of islet autoantibodies and diabetes [40]. Consistent with this observation is the overall decreased risk to develop islet autoimmunity and diabetes in offspring of mothers with type 1 diabetes compared with that of offspring of fathers with type 1 diabetes and nondiabetic mothers also suggesting that exposure to autoimmunity during pregnancy may be advantageous in type 1 diabetes [41–43].

## Standardization of Autoantibody Measurements

The identification and molecular cloning of defined islet antigens resulted in the rapid development of autoantibody assays that now have been established in specialized laboratories worldwide, and that are validated in international workshops organized by the Immunology of Diabetes Society (IDS) and the Centers for Disease Control (CDC) [44]. For autoantibodies to GAD (GADA) and IA-2 (IA-2A), there is high concordance between laboratories, and a WHO standard for worldwide comparison of antibody levels is available. Radio-binding assays and some ELISA can provide both high sensitivity and specificity. The performance of assays in the IDS/CDC-based international workshops, however, should be ascertained prior to use. For autoantibodies to insulin (IAA), there is less consensus between laboratories than for GADA and IA-2A. This is due to the requirement of assays that can reproducibly detect low titers of IAA. Only few assays, all radiobinding assays have sufficient sensitivity and specificity to be considered useful for measuring IAA in preclinical type 1 diabetes. Again, performances in the international workshops should be checked. New assays and assays that measure new antibodies can also be validated in these workshops [44].

### Diagnosis of Type 1 Diabetes through Islet Autoantibody Determination

The measurement of islet autoantibodies to help distinguish between type 1 and type 2 diabetes has become increasingly important in recent years. It is now well established, first that type 2 diabetes is increasing in frequency in childhood and adolescence, second that the typical type 1 diabetes phenotype of acute onset and leanness is now a spectrum that includes an increasing number of obese patients and patients with subacute presentation at diagnosis, and third that a proportion of adults who present with diabetes have autoimmunity and actually have type 1 diabetes. Ten percent of UKPDS patients who were clinically diagnosed as having type 2 diabetes tested positive for GADA [45] and 17% of women with insulin requiring gestational diabetes (White class B) in the German Gestational Diabetes Study had GADA at delivery and developed insulin-dependent diabetes postpartum [46]. Measurement of islet autoantibodies at diabetes diagnosis, therefore, will be useful in overweight children, lean adults and women with gestational diabetes who require insulin during pregnancy. The most sensitive antibodies to be measured for purposes of distinguishing between type 1 and type 2 diabetes are GADA in adults and a combination of GADA and insulin antibodies in young children [47]. Over 80% of patients with newly diagnosed type 1 diabetes have GADA, 70% have IA-2A, and around 60% have IAA [48, 49]. The prevalence of IAA is largely age dependent and around 90% of children diagnosed before age 5 years are IAA-positive [50]. It is unclear whether the lower frequency of IAA found after adolescence is because these patients never developed insulin autoimmunity or because IAA have been lost during the preclinical phase of the disease.

Testing of cytoplasmic islet cell antibodies (ICA) on frozen sections of human pancreas tissue by immunofluorescence has largely been replaced by radioimmunoassay or ELISA detection of antibodies to GAD and IA-2 but has its relevance in rare cases as this method allows the detection of antibodies to unidentified islet antigens which can be helpful for diagnosis in the few subjects who are negative for antibodies to the major islet antigens insulin, GAD, and IA-2.

### Natural History of Islet Autoantibody Appearance

Islet autoimmunity can precede the development of clinical type 1 diabetes by many years [2]. Eisenbarth [51] has proposed a model of the natural history of type 1 diabetes where the development of the disease is characterized in stages, starting with genetic susceptibility (stage 1), the triggering event for the initiation of β-cell autoimmunity (stage 2), the progressive loss of glucose-stimulated insulin release (stage 3), and finally the clinical manifestation of diabetes (stage 4). To test this model in patients developing type 1 diabetes several groups have initiated prospective studies from birth to determine when islet autoantibodies first appear, which genetic and environmental factors influence their development, and which characteristics of islet autoantibodies are most associated with progression to diabetes. The German BABYDIAB study [52] started in 1989 and follows the offspring of mothers and/or fathers with type 1 diabetes up to the age of 15 years. The Finnish Type 1 Diabetes Prediction and Prevention project (DIPP) [53] started in 1994 and follows newborn infants with increased genetic risk in close intervals for up to 10 years. The American Diabetes Autoimmunity Study in the Young (DAISY) [54] follows newborns at genetically increased type 1 diabetes risk from the general population and relatives of patients with type 1 diabetes since 1994, and the Australian BabyDiab study [55] follows newborns that have a first-degree relative with type 1 diabetes.

### First Appearance and Spreading of Humoral Islet Autoimmunity

The BABYDIAB study has demonstrated that children developing type 1 diabetes in early childhood (less than 10 years of age) have the first signs of islet autoimmunity very early in life, the majority by 2 years of age [56, 57]. Moreover, children who have islet autoantibodies by age 2 years have a 50% risk of developing type 1 diabetes before puberty. Around 4% of the offspring of parents with type 1 diabetes in the BABYDIAB study and around 6% of genetically at risk infants from the general population in the Finnish DIPP study developed islet autoantibodies by age 2 years (fig. 1) [57, 58]. IAA are usually the first autoantibodies detected early in infancy. The early appearance of IAA is usually followed by autoantibodies to other β-cell antigens such as

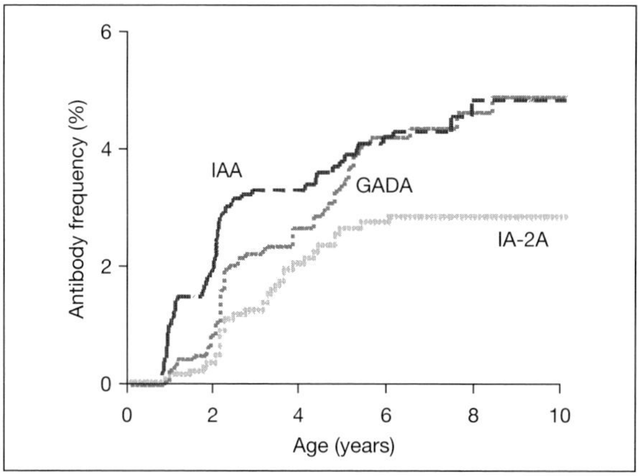


***Fig. 1.*** Life-table islet autoantibody frequencies for IAA, GADA, and IA-2A in offspring of parents with type 1 diabetes. Autoantibody-positive events correspond to samples taken at approximately 9 months and 2, 5 and 8 years of age. Adapted from Hummel et al. [57].

GAD, IA-2 or IA-2β [56–60]. Autoantibodies do not exclusively develop before age 2 years, but the characteristics of islet autoimmunity that develops later in childhood are different to those of early appearance islet autoimmunity. In general, children developing autoantibodies after age 2 years are less frequently IAA-positive and often GADA-positive, they infrequently develop multiple islet autoantibodies, and do not progress rapidly to type 1 diabetes [57].

Spreading of autoimmunity is not only observed between antigens but also within one antigen, indicating maturation of the autoimmune response during the course of β-cell destruction. With respect to GADA, spreading of autoantibody reactivity against the middle region of GAD65 to other epitopes located at the COOH-terminus or NH2-terminus is relatively frequent in young children [61]. Initial IA-2A reactivity is directed against epitopes found on the IA-2 molecule and spreading to IA-2β occurs together with an expansion of the autoimmune response to IA-2 [62].

Once islet autoantibodies appear, they usually persist, although significant fluctuations in antibody titer can be observed during the prediabetic phase [57, 58, 63–65]. Of the three islet antibodies discussed, IAA are reported to be the least persistent [58, 66] and not all children who develop IAA subsequently develop multiple islet autoantibodies and diabetes. The BABYDIAB study has recently identified a 'marker' to distinguish type 1-diabetes-relevant IAA from IAA which either do not persist or are not associated with progression to multiple islet autoantibodies and diabetes [67]. The affinity of IAA has been found to vary considerably between IAA-positive children. IAA are persistent and there is progression to multiple islet autoantibodies in children who develop high-affinity IAA responses, whereas children who remain positive only for IAA or become islet autoantibody negative usually have lower-affinity IAA [67].

Another reason why IAA, and indeed GADA or IA-2A, may not persist is because they are maternally transferred from the mother with type 1 diabetes. Islet autoantibodies pass the placenta [59, 68]. Depending on the titer of antibodies in the mother, maternal insulin antibodies persist in the circulation of the child for 1 year and maternal GADA for up to 18 months [64, 69]. As a consequence, if antibodies are detected in a child early in life, it is important – for the correct assignment of diabetes risk – to distinguish whether these antibodies are indeed de novo-produced antibodies of the child or rather antibodies acquired from the mother. Antibody titer and different immunoglobulin subclasses may help distinguishing between maternal and nonmaternal autoantibodies in some cases [64].

### Progression to Diabetes – Predictive Value of Islet Autoantibodies

Predicting the risk for the development of type 1 diabetes is important for the identification of individuals that might profit from inclusion in interventional trials aiming to prevent the onset of disease.

In type 1 diabetes, disease development is associated with persistent, high-titer, high-affinity autoantibodies to more than one antigen [67, 70]. Each of these qualities increases the likelihood that the detection of autoantibodies in a subject has identified preclinical disease. Transient autoantibody positivity is rarely associated with the development of type 1 diabetes, and repeat positivity in a second sample is therefore an essential part of risk assessment. The magnitude of the autoimmune response is also likely to be an indicator of the severity of β-cell destruction, and therefore type 1 diabetes risk (fig. 2). Magnitude can be measured by titer and by the breadth or range of autoantigen targets. It has been shown that diabetes risk is highest in individuals with more than one islet autoantibody [56–58, 70–76] and in individuals with a high-titer ICA [77, 78], or with high-titer IAA or IA-2A responses [70]. High-titer responses are also often associated with reactivity against more than one epitope or antigen and with more than one IgG subclass. In a recent analysis of autoantibody-positive relatives followed for up to 15 years, the highest risks for type 1 diabetes were associated with high-titer IAA and IA-2A responses, with the appearance of antibody subclasses IgG2, IgG3, and/or IgG4 of IA-2A and

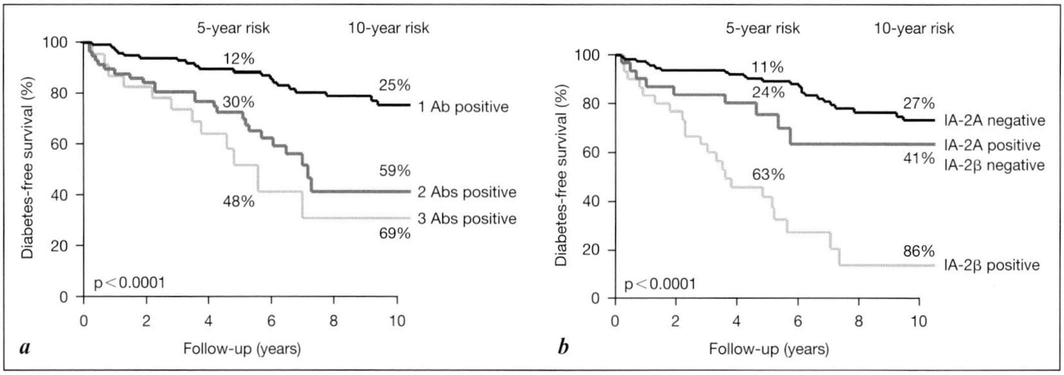


***Fig. 2.*** Cumulative risk of diabetes in first-degree relatives of patients with type 1 diabetes in relation to islet autoantibody number (***a***), and autoantibody reactivity to IA-2 and IA-2β (***b***). Adapted from Achenbach et al. [70].

IAA, and antibodies to the IA-2-related molecule IA-2β [70]. Using various combinations of these islet autoantibody characteristics, it was possible to stratify type 1 diabetes risk from less than 10% to around 90% within 5 years [70]. These data also indicate that there is a hierarchy in the diabetes risk associated with the different islet autoantibodies. Autoantibodies to IA-2 are associated with a higher type 1 diabetes risk than autoantibodies to GAD or IAA [70, 79, 80], and within IA-2A-positive subjects, those with IA-2A reacting against IA-2β have a higher diabetes risk than those who are IA-2β antibody negative [70, 79].

The risk for developing type 1 diabetes can also be stratified on the basis of how early islet autoantibodies developed [57]. Progression to diabetes is significantly faster in individuals who have islet autoantibodies already within the first year of life than in individuals with islet autoantibodies at age 2 or 5 years [57]. Of interest from both the viewpoints of risk assessment and pathogenesis, autoantibodies that appear very early can differ in their binding characteristics as compared to autoantibodies that appear later. For example, IAA that appear in the first 1 or 2 years of life are of higher affinity than IAA that first develop later in childhood. Children with high-affinity IAA are more likely to progress to type 1 diabetes than those who have lower affinity IAA [67]. High-affinity IAA differ to lower affinity IAA in their insulin-binding characteristics in a manner consistent with distinct epitope recognition, and in contrast to the lower-affinity IAA (which often do not bind proinsulin), the epitope associated with high-affinity IAA is also expressed on the proinsulin molecule [67]. In summary, type 1 diabetes risk can be stratified using a variety of autoantibody characteristics which in turn can be used in different combinations to select subjects of defined diabetes risk for intervention trials.

### Genetic Control of Islet Autoantibodies

In Caucasians, type 1 diabetes is strongly associated with HLA DR3-DQ2 and DR4-DQ8 haplotypes [81–83]. Islet autoantibodies differ in their association with these haplotypes. GADA are more frequent in patients with HLA DR3-DQ2 [83, 84], whereas IAA and IA-2A are more frequent in patients with HLA DR4-DQ8 [60, 83–86]. Patients without these haplotypes are often islet autoantibody negative [58, 85, 86]. These haplotypes can also be used to identify children who are most likely to develop islet autoantibodies. Results from the BABYDIAB study, the DIPP study, and the DAISY study consistently show that children carrying high risk HLA genotypes have a higher risk for early and more frequent development of islet autoantibodies in infancy [58, 85–87]. Among BABYDIAB offspring, risk of developing islet autoantibodies by age 2 years is 20% in those who have the high risk DR3-DQ2/DR4-DQ8 and DR4-DQ8/DR4-DQ8 genotypes compared with 2.7% in offspring without these genotypes [85]. A second genetic susceptibility locus has been mapped by a variable number of tandem repeat (VNTR) in the insulin gene (*INS*) promotor region (*IDDM2*) [88]. Risk has been suggested to be conferred by different expression of the insulin protein in the thymus leading to defective central tolerance to the insulin molecule [89–91]. In accordance with this, IAA are less frequent in patients or relatives who have the type 1 diabetes protective *INS* VNTR class I/III or III/III genotypes [83, 87].

### Future Aspects

Childhood type 1 diabetes mellitus is associated with autoimmunity that initiates early in life. Using sophisticated measurements of islet autoantibodies we are able to predict type 1 diabetes, and trace its natural history (fig. 3). We have little idea, however, of the etiologic mechanisms that trigger autoimmunity and promote progression to disease, nor do we have ready access to the autoreactive T cells within the pancreas that are responsible for disease or an ability to quantify and characterize these cells. Advances in these areas are necessary if we are to fully understand the autoimmune pathogenesis of type 1 diabetes. An international initiative sponsored by the National Institutes of Health (NIH) has recently commenced an ambitious study (The Environmental Determinants of

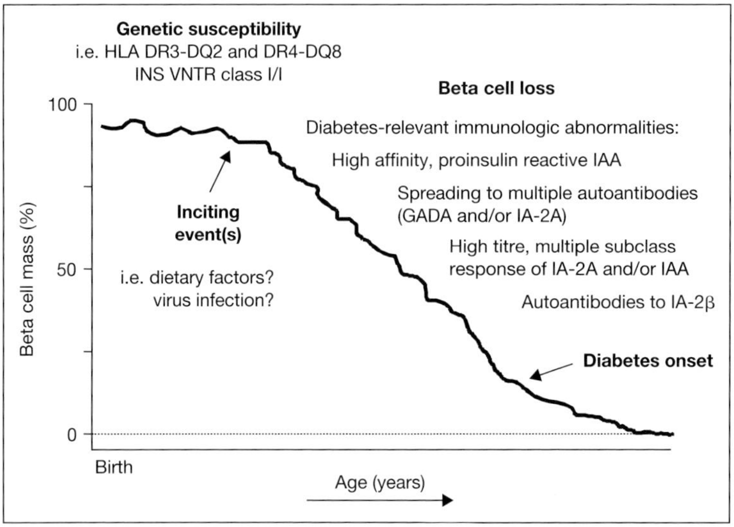


*Fig. 3.* Model of the natural history of type 1 diabetes mellitus. Islet autoimmunity is triggered in genetically at-risk subjects by a currently unknown event, and β-cell mass is lost over an individually variable time period after the inciting event has occurred. First diabetes-relevant immunologic abnormalities can be detected very early in the autoimmune process. The magnitude of the autoimmune response to islet antigens – reflecting the severity of β-cell destruction – can predict rapid progression to clinical type 1 diabetes.

Diabetes in the Young – TEDDY – study) to address the early pathogenetic mechanisms operating in islet autoimmunity (www.teddystudy.org).

## References

1 Bach JF: Insulin-dependent diabetes mellitus as an autoimmune disease. Endocr Rev 1994;15: 516–542.
2 Atkinson MA, Eisenbarth GS: Type 1 diabetes: New perspectives on disease pathogenesis and treatment. Lancet 2001;358:221–229.
3 Notkins AL: Immunologic and genetic factors in type 1 diabetes. J Biol Chem 2002;277: 43545–43548.
4 Stiller CR, Dupre J, Gent M, Jenner MR, Keown PA, Laupacis A, Martell R, Rodger NW, von Graffenried B, Wolfe BM: Effects of cyclosporine immunosuppression in insulin-dependent diabetes mellitus of recent onset. Science 1984;223:1362–1367.
5 Silverstein J, Maclaren N, Riley W, Spillar R, Radjenovic D, Johnson S: Immunosuppression with azathioprine and prednisone in recent-onset insulin-dependent diabetes mellitus. N Engl J Med 1988;319:599–604.
6 Herold KC, Hagopian W, Auger JA, Poumian-Ruiz E, Taylor L, Donaldson D, Gitelman SE, Harlan DM, Xu D, Zivin RA, Bluestone JA: Anti-CD3 monoclonal antibody in new-onset type 1 diabetes mellitus. N Engl J Med 2002;346:1692–1698.

7 Palmer JP, Asplin CM, Clemons P, Lyen K, Tatpati O, Raghu PK, Paquette TL: Insulin antibodies in insulin-dependent diabetics before insulin treatment. Science 1983;222:1337–1339.
8 Baekkeskov S, Aanstoot HJ, Christgau S, Reetz A, Solimena M, Cascalho M, Folli F, Richter-Olesen H, De Camilli P, Camilli PD: Identification of the 64K autoantigen in insulin-dependent diabetes as the GABA-synthesizing enzyme glutamic acid decarboxylase. Nature 1990;347: 151–156.
9 Lan MS, Lu J, Goto Y, Notkins AL: Molecular cloning and identification of a receptor-type protein tyrosine phosphatase, IA-2, from human insulinoma. DNA Cell Biol 1994;13:505–514.
10 Wasmeier C, Hutton JC: Molecular cloning of phogrin, a protein-tyrosine phosphatase homologue localized to insulin secretory granule membranes. J Biol Chem 1996;271:18161–18170.
11 Rabin DU, Pleasic SM, Shapiro JA, Yoo-Warren H, Oles J, Hicks JM, Goldstein DE, Rae PM: Islet cell antigen 512 is a diabetes-specific islet autoantigen related to protein tyrosine phosphatases. J Immunol 1994;152:3183–3188.
12 Lu J, Li Q, Xie H, Chen ZJ, Borovitskaya AE, Maclaren NK, Notkins AL, Lan MS: Identification of a second transmembrane protein tyrosine phosphatase, IA-2beta, as an autoantigen in insulin-dependent diabetes mellitus: Precursor of the 37-kDa tryptic fragment. Proc Natl Acad Sci USA 1996;93:2307–2311.
13 Solimena M, Dirkx R Jr, Hermel JM, Pleasic-Williams S, Shapiro JA, Caron L, Rabin DU: ICA 512, an autoantigen of type I diabetes, is an intrinsic membrane protein of neurosecretory granules. EMBO J 1996;15:2102–2114.
14 Reetz A, Solimena M, Matteoli M, Folli F, Takei K, De Camilli P: GABA and pancreatic beta-cells: Colocalization of glutamic acid decarboxylase (GAD) and GABA with synaptic-like microvesicles suggests their role in GABA storage and secretion. EMBO J 1991;10:1275–1284.
15 Lieberman SM, DiLorenzo TP: A comprehensive guide to antibody and T-cell responses in type 1 diabetes. Tissue Antigens 2003;62:359–377.
16 Roll U, Turck CW, Gitelman SE, Rosenthal SM, Nolte MS, Masharani U, Ziegler AG, Baekkeskov S: Peptide mapping and characterisation of glycation patterns of the glima 38 antigen recognised by autoantibodies in type I diabetic patients. Diabetologia 2000;43:598–608.
17 Tisch R, McDevitt H: Insulin-dependent diabetes mellitus. Cell 1996;85:291–297.
18 Achenbach P, Kelemen K, Wegmann DR, Hutton JC: Spontaneous peripheral T-cell responses to the IA-2beta (Phogrin) autoantigen in young nonobese diabetic mice. J Autoimmun 2002;19: 111–116.
19 Bergman B, Haskins K: Autoreactive T-cell clones from the nonobese diabetic mouse. Proc Soc Exp Biol Med 1997;214:41–48.
20 Yang Y, Santamaria P: Dissecting autoimmune diabetes through genetic manipulation of non-obese diabetic mice. Diabetologia 2003;46:1447–1464.
21 Daniel D, Wegmann DR: Protection of nonobese diabetic mice from diabetes by intranasal or subcutaneous administration of insulin peptide B-(9–23). Proc Natl Acad Sci USA 1996;93:956–960.
22 Yoon JW, Yoon CS, Lim HW, Huang QQ, Kang Y, Pyun KH, Hirasawa K, Sherwin RS, Jun HS: Control of autoimmune diabetes in NOD mice by GAD expression or suppression in beta cells. Science 1999;284:1183–1187.
23 Zhang ZJ, Davidson L, Eisenbarth G, Weiner HL: Suppression of diabetes in nonobese diabetic mice by oral administration of porcine insulin. Proc Natl Acad Sci USA 1991;88:10252–10256.
24 Tian J, Atkinson MA, Clare-Salzler M, Herschenfeld A, Forsthuber T, Lehmann PV, Kaufman DL: Nasal administration of glutamate decarboxylase (GAD65) peptides induces Th2 responses and prevents murine insulin-dependent diabetes. J Exp Med 1996;183:1561–1567.
25 Elias D, Markovits D, Reshef T, van der Zee R, Cohen IR: Induction and therapy of autoimmune diabetes in the non-obese diabetic (NOD/Lt) mouse by a 65-kDa heat shock protein. Proc Natl Acad Sci USA 1990;87:1576–1580.
26 Roep BO: The role of T-cells in the pathogenesis of type 1 diabetes: From cause to cure. Diabetologia 2003;46:305–321.
27 Endl J, Otto H, Jung G, Dreisbusch B, Donie F, Stahl P, Elbracht R, Schmitz G, Meinl E, Hummel M, Ziegler AG, Wank R, Schendel DJ: Identification of naturally processed T cell epitopes from glutamic acid decarboxylase presented in the context of HLA-DR alleles by T lymphocytes of recent onset IDDM patients. J Clin Invest 1997;99:2405–2415.

28 Peakman M, Stevens EJ, Lohmann T, Narendran P, Dromey J, Alexander A, Tomlinson AJ, Trucco M, Gorga JC, Chicz RM: Naturally processed and presented epitopes of the islet cell autoantigen IA-2 eluted from HLA-DR4. J Clin Invest 1999;104:1449–1457.
29 Alleva DG, Crowe PD, Jin L, Kwok WW, Ling N, Gottschalk M, Conlon PJ, Gottlieb PA, Putnam AL, Gaur A: A disease-associated cellular immune response in type 1 diabetics to an immunodominant epitope of insulin. J Clin Invest 2001;107:173–180.
30 Roep BO, Atkinson MA, van Endert PM, Gottlieb PA, Wilson SB, Sachs JA: Autoreactive T cell responses in insulin-dependent (type 1) diabetes mellitus. Report of the first international workshop for standardization of T cell assays. J Autoimmun 1999;13:267–282.
31 Schloot NC, Meierhoff G, Karlsson Faresjo M, Ott P, Putnam A, Lehmann P, Gottlieb P, Roep BO, Peakman M, Tree T: Comparison of cytokine ELISpot assay formats for the detection of islet antigen autoreactive T cells. Report of the third immunology of diabetes society T-cell workshop. J Autoimmun 2003;21:365–376.
32 Arif S, Tree TI, Astill TP, Tremble JM, Bishop AJ, Dayan CM, Roep BO, Peakman M: Autoreactive T cell responses show proinflammatory polarization in diabetes but a regulatory phenotype in health. J Clin Invest 2004;113:451–463.
33 Viglietta V, Kent SC, Orban T, Hafler DA: GAD65-reactive T cells are activated in patients with autoimmune type 1a diabetes. J Clin Invest 2002;109:895–903.
34 Bottazzo GF, Dean BM, McNally JM, MacKay EH, Swift PG, Gamble DR: In situ characterization of autoimmune phenomena and expression of HLA molecules in the pancreas in diabetic insulitis. N Engl J Med 1985;313:353–360.
35 Itoh N, Hanafusa T, Miyazaki A, Miyagawa J, Yamagata K, Yamamoto K, Waguri M, Imagawa A, Tamura S, Inada M, et al: Mononuclear cell infiltration and its relation to the expression of major histocompatibility complex antigens and adhesion molecules in pancreas biopsy specimens from newly diagnosed insulin-dependent diabetes mellitus patients. J Clin Invest 1993;92: 2313–2322.
36 Serreze DV, Chapman HD, Varnum DS, Hanson MS, Reifsnyder PC, Richard SD, Fleming SA, Leiter EH, Shultz LD: B lymphocytes are essential for the initiation of T cell-mediated autoimmune diabetes: Analysis of a new ‘speed congenic’ stock of NOD.Ig mu null mice. J Exp Med 1996;184:2049–2053.
37 Sibley RK, Sutherland DE, Goetz F, Michael AF: Recurrent diabetes mellitus in the pancreas iso- and allograft: A light and electron microscopic and immunohistochemical analysis of four cases. Lab Invest 1985;53:132–144.
38 Martin S, Wolf-Eichbaum D, Duinkerken G, Scherbaum WA, Kolb H, Noordzij JG, Roep BO: Development of type 1 diabetes despite severe hereditary B-lymphocyte deficiency. N Engl J Med 2001;345:1036–1040.
39 Greeley SA, Katsumata M, Yu L, Eisenbarth GS, Moore DJ, Goodarzi H, Barker CF, Naji A, Noorchashm H: Elimination of maternally transmitted autoantibodies prevents diabetes in nonobese diabetic mice. Nat Med 2002;8:399–402.
40 Koczwara K, Bonifacio E, Ziegler AG: Transmission of maternal islet antibodies and risk of autoimmune diabetes in offspring of mothers with type 1 diabetes. Diabetes 2004;53:1–4.
41 Yu L, Chase HP, Falorni A, Rewers M, Lernmark A, Eisenbarth GS: Sexual dimorphism in transmission of expression of islet autoantibodies to offspring. Diabetologia 1995;38:1353–1357.
42 Warram JH, Krolewski AS, Gottlieb MS, Kahn CR: Differences in risk of insulin-dependent diabetes in offspring of diabetic mothers and diabetic fathers. N Engl J Med 1984;311: 149–152.
43 Pociot F, Norgaard K, Hobolth N, Andersen O, Nerup J: A nationwide population-based study of the familial aggregation of type 1 (insulin-dependent) diabetes mellitus in Denmark. Danish Study Group of Diabetes in Childhood. Diabetologia 1993;36:870–875.
44 Bingley PJ, Bonifacio E, Mueller PW: Diabetes antibody standardization program: First assay proficiency evaluation. Diabetes 2003;52:1128–1136.
45 Turner R, Stratton I, Horton V, Manley S, Zimmet P, Mackay IR, Shattock M, Bottazzo GF, Holman R: UKPDS 25: Autoantibodies to islet-cell cytoplasm and glutamic acid decarboxylase for prediction of insulin requirement in type 2 diabetes. UK Prospective Diabetes Study Group. Lancet 1997;350:1288–1293.

46 Fuchtenbusch M, Ferber K, Standl E, Ziegler AG: Prediction of type 1 diabetes postpartum in patients with gestational diabetes mellitus by combined islet cell autoantibody screening: A prospective multicenter study. Diabetes 1997;46:1459–1467.
47 Bingley PJ, Bonifacio E, Ziegler AG, Schatz DA, Atkinson MA, Eisenbarth GS: Proposed guidelines on screening for risk of type 1 diabetes. Diabetes Care 2001;24:398.
48 Bonifacio E, Bingley PJ: Islet autoantibodies and their use in predicting insulin-dependent diabetes. Acta Diabetol 1997;34:185–193.
49 Williams AJ, Bingley PJ, Bonifacio E, Palmer JP, Gale EA: A novel micro-assay for insulin autoantibodies. J Autoimmun 1997;10:473–478.
50 Vardi P, Ziegler AG, Mathews JH, Dib S, Keller RJ, Ricker AT, Wolfsdorf JI, Herskowitz RD, Rabizadeh A, Eisenbarth GS, et al: Concentration of insulin autoantibodies at onset of type I diabetes. Inverse log-linear correlation with age. Diabetes Care 1988;11:736–739.
51 Eisenbarth GS: Type I diabetes mellitus. A chronic autoimmune disease. N Engl J Med 1986; 314:1360–1368.
52 Ziegler AG, Hillebrand B, Rabl W, Mayrhofer M, Hummel M, Mollenhauer U, Vordemann J, Lenz A, Standl E: On the appearance of islet associated autoimmunity in offspring of diabetic mothers: A prospective study from birth. Diabetologia 1993;36:402–408.
53 Kupila A, Muona P, Simell T, Arvilommi P, Savolainen H, Hamalainen AM, Korhonen S, Kimpimaki T, Sjoroos M, Ilonen J, Knip M, Simell O: Feasibility of genetic and immunological prediction of type I diabetes in a population-based birth cohort. Diabetologia 2001;44:290–297.
54 Rewers M, Norris JM, Eisenbarth GS, Erlich HA, Beaty B, Klingensmith G, Hoffman M, Yu L, Bugawan TL, Blair A, Hamman RF, Groshek M, McDuffie RS Jr: Beta-cell autoantibodies in infants and toddlers without IDDM relatives: Diabetes autoimmunity study in the young (DAISY). J Autoimmun 1996;9:405–410.
55 Honeyman MC, Coulson BS, Stone NL, Gellert SA, Goldwater PN, Steele CE, Couper JJ, Tait BD, Colman PG, Harrison LC: Association between rotavirus infection and pancreatic islet autoimmunity in children at risk of developing type 1 diabetes. Diabetes 2000;49:1319–1324.
56 Ziegler AG, Hummel M, Schenker M, Bonifacio E: Autoantibody appearance and risk for development of childhood diabetes in offspring of parents with type 1 diabetes: The 2-year analysis of the German BABYDIAB Study. Diabetes 1999;48:460–468.
57 Hummel M, Bonifacio E, Schmid S, Walter M, Knopff A, Ziegler AG: Brief communication: Early appearance of islet autoantibodies predicts childhood type 1 diabetes in offspring of diabetic parents. Ann Intern Med 2004;140:882–886.
58 Kimpimaki T, Kulmala P, Savola K, Kupila A, Korhonen S, Simell T, Ilonen J, Simell O, Knip M: Natural history of beta-cell autoimmunity in young children with increased genetic susceptibility to type 1 diabetes recruited from the general population. J Clin Endocrinol Metab 2002;87: 4572–4579.
59 Roll U, Christie MR, Fuchtenbusch M, Payton MA, Hawkes CJ, Ziegler AG: Perinatal autoimmunity in offspring of diabetic parents. The German Multicenter BABY-DIAB study: Detection of humoral immune responses to islet antigens in early childhood. Diabetes 1996;45:967–973.
60 Kimpimaki T, Kupila A, Hamalainen AM, Kukko M, Kulmala P, Savola K, Simell T, Keskinen P, Ilonen J, Simell O, Knip M: The first signs of beta-cell autoimmunity appear in infancy in genetically susceptible children from the general population: The Finnish Type 1 Diabetes Prediction and Prevention Study. J Clin Endocrinol Metab 2001;86:4782–4788.
61 Bonifacio E, Lampasona V, Bernasconi L, Ziegler AG: Maturation of the humoral autoimmune response to epitopes of GAD in preclinical childhood type 1 diabetes. Diabetes 2000;49:202–208.
62 Naserke HE, Ziegler AG, Lampasona V, Bonifacio E: Early development and spreading of autoantibodies to epitopes of IA-2 and their association with progression to type 1 diabetes. J Immunol 1998;161:6963–6969.
63 Savola K, Laara E, Vahasalo P, Kulmala P, Akerblom HK, Knip M: Dynamic pattern of disease-associated autoantibodies in siblings of children with type 1 diabetes: A population-based study. Diabetes 2001;50:2625–2632.
64 Naserke HE, Bonifacio E, Ziegler AG: Prevalence, characteristics and diabetes risk associated with transient maternally acquired islet antibodies and persistent islet antibodies in offspring of parents with type 1 diabetes. J Clin Endocrinol Metab 2001;86:4826–4833.

65 Bonifacio E, Scirpoli M, Kredel K, Fuchtenbusch M, Ziegler AG: Early autoantibody responses in prediabetes are IgG1 dominated and suggest antigen-specific regulation. J Immunol 1999; 163:525–532.
66 Colman PG, Steele C, Couper JJ, Beresford SJ, Powell T, Kewming K, Pollard A, Gellert S, Tait B, Honeyman M, Harrison LC: Islet autoimmunity in infants with a type I diabetic relative is common but is frequently restricted to one autoantibody. Diabetologia 2000;43:203–209.
67 Achenbach P, Koczwara K, Knopff A, Naserke H, Ziegler AG, Bonifacio E: Mature high affinity immune responses to (pro)insulin anticipate the autoimmune cascade leading to type 1 diabetes. J Clin Invest 2004;114:589–597.
68 Martikainen A, Saukkonen T, Kulmala PK, Reijonen H, Ilonen J, Teramo K, Koskela P, Knip M, Akerblom HK: Disease-associated antibodies in offspring of mothers with IDDM. Diabetes 1996;45:1706–1710.
69 Hamalainen AM, Ronkainen MS, Akerblom HK, Knip M: Postnatal elimination of transplacentally acquired disease-associated antibodies in infants born to families with type 1 diabetes. The Finnish TRIGR Study Group. Trial to Reduce IDDM in the Genetically at Risk. J Clin Endocrinol Metab 2000;85:4249–4253.
70 Achenbach P, Warncke K, Reiter J, Naserke HE, Williams AJ, Bingley PJ, Bonifacio E, Ziegler AG: Stratification of type 1 diabetes risk on the basis of islet autoantibody characteristics. Diabetes 2004;53:384–392.
71 Bingley PJ, Christie MR, Bonifacio E, Bonfanti R, Shattock M, Fonte MT, Bottazzo GF, Gale EA: Combined analysis of autoantibodies improves prediction of IDDM in islet cell antibody-positive relatives. Diabetes 1994;43:1304–1310.
72 Verge CF, Gianani R, Kawasaki E, Yu L, Pietropaolo M, Jackson RA, Chase HP, Eisenbarth GS: Prediction of type I diabetes in first-degree relatives using a combination of insulin, GAD, and ICA512bdc/IA-2 autoantibodies. Diabetes 1996;45:926–933.
73 Kulmala P, Savola K, Petersen JS, Vahasalo P, Karjalainen J, Lopponen T, Dyrberg T, Akerblom HK, Knip M: Prediction of insulin-dependent diabetes mellitus in siblings of children with diabetes. A population-based study. The Childhood Diabetes in Finland Study Group. J Clin Invest 1998;101:327–336.
74 Krischer JP, Cuthbertson DD, Yu L, Orban T, Maclaren N, Jackson R, Winter WE, Schatz DA, Palmer JP, Eisenbarth GS: Screening strategies for the identification of multiple antibody-positive relatives of individuals with type 1 diabetes. J Clin Endocrinol Metab 2003;88:103–108.
75 LaGasse JM, Brantley MS, Leech NJ, Rowe RE, Monks S, Palmer JP, Nepom GT, McCulloch DK, Hagopian WA: Successful prospective prediction of type 1 diabetes in schoolchildren through multiple defined autoantibodies: An 8-year follow-up of the Washington State Diabetes Prediction Study. Diabetes Care 2002;25:505–511.
76 Maclaren N, Lan M, Coutant R, Schatz D, Silverstein J, Muir A, Clare-Salzer M, She JX, Malone J, Crockett S, Schwartz S, Quattrin T, DeSilva M, Vander Vegt P, Notkins A, Krischer J: Only multiple autoantibodies to islet cells (ICA), insulin, GAD65, IA-2 and IA-2beta predict immune-mediated (type 1) diabetes in relatives. J Autoimmun 1999;12:279–287.
77 Bonifacio E, Bingley PJ, Shattock M, Dean BM, Dunger D, Gale EA, Bottazzo GF: Quantification of islet-cell antibodies and prediction of insulin-dependent diabetes. Lancet 1990;335:147–149.
78 Bingley PJ: Interactions of age, islet cell antibodies, insulin autoantibodies, and first-phase insulin response in predicting risk of progression to IDDM in ICA+ relatives: The ICARUS data set. Islet Cell Antibody Register Users Study. Diabetes 1996;45:1720–1728.
79 Christie MR, Genovese S, Cassidy D, Bosi E, Brown TJ, Lai M, Bonifacio E, Bottazzo GF: Antibodies to islet 37k antigen, but not to glutamate decarboxylase, discriminate rapid progression to IDDM in endocrine autoimmunity. Diabetes 1994;43:1254–1259.
80 Decochez K, De Leeuw IH, Keymeulen B, Mathieu C, Rottiers R, Weets I, Vandemeulebroucke E, Truyen I, Kaufman L, Schuit FC, Pipeleers DG, Gorus FK: IA-2 autoantibodies predict impending type I diabetes in siblings of patients. Diabetologia 2002;45:1658–1666.
81 Todd JA, Bell JI, McDevitt HO: HLA-DQ beta gene contributes to susceptibility and resistance to insulin-dependent diabetes mellitus. Nature 1987;329:599–604.
82 Redondo MJ, Eisenbarth GS: Genetic control of autoimmunity in type I diabetes and associated disorders. Diabetologia 2002;45:605–622.

83 Graham J, Hagopian WA, Kockum I, Li LS, Sanjeevi CB, Lowe RM, Schaefer JB, Zarghami M, Day HL, Landin-Olsson M, Palmer JP, Janer-Villanueva M, Hood L, Sundkvist G, Lernmark A, Breslow N, Dahlquist G, Blohme G: Genetic effects on age-dependent onset and islet cell autoantibody markers in type 1 diabetes. Diabetes 2002;51:1346–1355.
84 Sabbah E, Savola K, Kulmala P, Reijonen H, Veijola R, Vahasalo P, Karjalainen J, Ilonen J, Akerblom HK, Knip M: Disease-associated autoantibodies and HLA-DQB1 genotypes in children with newly diagnosed insulin-dependent diabetes mellitus (IDDM). The Childhood Diabetes in Finland Study Group. Clin Exp Immunol 1999;116:78–83.
85 Schenker M, Hummel M, Ferber K, Walter M, Keller E, Albert ED, Janka HU, Kastendiek C, Sorger M, Louwen F, Ziegler AG: Early expression and high prevalence of islet autoantibodies for DR3/4 heterozygous and DR4/4 homozygous offspring of parents with type I diabetes: The German BABYDIAB study. Diabetologia 1999;42:671–677.
86 Yu J, Yu L, Bugawan TL, Erlich HA, Barriga K, Hoffman M, Rewers M, Eisenbarth GS: Transient anti-islet autoantibodies: Infrequent occurrence and lack of association with 'genetic' risk factors. J Clin Endocrinol Metab 2000;85:2421–2428.
87 Walter M, Albert E, Conrad M, Keller E, Hummel M, Ferber K, Barratt BJ, Todd JA, Ziegler AG, Bonifacio E: IDDM2/insulin VNTR modifies risk conferred by IDDM1/HLA for development of type 1 diabetes and associated autoimmunity. Diabetologia 2003;46:712–720.
88 Bennett ST, Lucassen AM, Gough SC, Powell EE, Undlien DE, Pritchard LE, Merriman ME, Kawaguchi Y, Dronsfield MJ, Pociot F, et al: Susceptibility to human type 1 diabetes at IDDM2 is determined by tandem repeat variation at the insulin gene minisatellite locus. Nat Genet 1995;9:284–292.
89 Pugliese A, Zeller M, Fernandez A Jr, Zalcberg LJ, Bartlett RJ, Ricordi C, Pietropaolo M, Eisenbarth GS, Bennett ST, Patel DD: The insulin gene is transcribed in the human thymus and transcription levels correlated with allelic variation at the INS VNTR-IDDM2 susceptibility locus for type 1 diabetes. Nat Genet 1997;15:293–297.
90 Vafiadis P, Bennett ST, Todd JA, Nadeau J, Grabs R, Goodyer CG, Wickramasinghe S, Colle E, Polychronakos C: Insulin expression in human thymus is modulated by INS VNTR alleles at the IDDM2 locus. Nat Genet 1997;15:289–292.
91 Mathis D, Benoist C: Back to central tolerance. Immunity 2004;20:509–516.

Dr. Anette-G. Ziegler, MD
Diabetes Research Institute, Koelner Platz 1
DE–80804 Munich (Germany)
Tel. +49 89 3079 3121, Fax +49 89 3081 733, E-Mail anziegler@lrz.uni-muenchen.de

Chiarelli F, Dahl-Jørgensen K, Kiess W (eds): Diabetes in Childhood and Adolescence.
Pediatr Adolesc Med. Basel, Karger, 2005, vol 10, pp 72–83

# Neonatal Diabetes mellitus

*Michel Polak*[a], *Julian Shield*[b]

[a]Paediatric Endocrinology and INSERM EMI 0363, Hôpital Necker-Enfants Malades, Paris, France; [b]Department of Child Health, Royal Hospital for Children, Bristol, UK

Neonatal diabetes mellitus (NDM) is a rare (1/400,000 newborns) but potentially devastating condition. Two main groups have been recognized that mainly differ in the duration of insulin dependence, transient NDM (TNDM) and permanent NDM (PNDM). Advances have recently been made in the understanding of the molecular mechanisms of pancreatic development that are relevant to both PNDM and TNDM. This review focuses on the clinical features, treatment and molecular biology of these varied conditions.

## 'Transient' Neonatal Diabetes mellitus

TNDM is a developmental insulin production disorder that resolves postnatally. TNDM contributes to 50–60% of the cases of neonatal diabetes [1, 2]. Intrauterine growth retardation is usually present. The high rate of IUGR is in keeping with the crucial role of insulin in fetal growth, especially during the last trimester of pregnancy. Hyperglycemia, failure to thrive and, in some cases, dehydration occur after birth. Insulin production is inadequate, requiring exogenous insulin therapy. Tests are negative for anti-islet antibodies and for HLA class II haplotypes conferring susceptibility to type 1 diabetes [2]. A defect in β-cell maturation has been suggested [3]. Interestingly, exocrine pancreatic insufficiency is present in only a few patients [4]. However, the cellular basis of TNDM remains unknown. Most patients go into remission within a year, but a few have persisting intermittent glucose intolerance whilst many relapse with diabetes in late childhood or adulthood. Although these recurrences are usually consistent with non-autoimmune type 1 diabetes, whether they are ascribable to insulin deficiency and/or insulin resistance remains unclear [1, 5]. Indeed permanent hyperglycemia requiring insulin therapy developed in 5 of the 7 TNDM patients who were older than 8 years of age in a French cohort [6]. Similarly, in another large cohort of TNDM patients, diabetes mellitus recurred in 11 of 18 patients older than 4 years of age [7a]. Thus, the 'transient' form of the disease is probably a permanent β-cell defect with variable expression during growth and development. A major factor in the onset of recurrent diabetes is probably puberty, which is associated with significant insulin resistance.

Recently, we examined derived indices of β-cell function, peripheral insulin sensitivity and the pancreatic response to intravenous glucose loading in children with a previous history of transient neonatal diabetes currently in remission repeated after a period of 2 years to try and better understand the apparent persisting β-cell defect. We used standard Intravenous glucose tolerance tests measuring the first phase insulin response cumulatively at 1 and 3 min. The insulin measurements on all the cases were centralized. In addition, fasting insulin and glucose values were used to estimate HOMA-B% and insulinogenic indices (derived indices of β-cell function) and HOMA-S and QUICKI (derived measures of insulin sensitivity). Six cases (median age initially 7.5 years) with known previous TNDM currently in remission with no exogenous insulin requirement were tested. Two cases had chromosome 6 uniparental disomy, 1 case had a 6q2.4 region methylation defect whereas in 3 cases no chromosome 6 genetic anomaly could be detected. Control data from 16 children of a similar age was available for derived fasting indices of β-cell functional capacity and insulin sensitivity. One child had a subnormal insulin secretory response to intravenous glucose that remained abnormal 2 years later. The other children had relatively normal or entirely normal responses over 2 years. Measures of β-cell function and insulin sensitivity in the fasting state showed comparable results to those obtained from normal controls. The majority of children with TNDM in remission have no evidence of β-cell dysfunction or insulin resistance in the fasting state. Measures of insulin response to intravenous glucose loading are often normal but suggestive of future recurrence if profoundly abnormal [7b].

TNDM is usually sporadic, but paternal transmission has been documented in about one-third of the reported patients, some of whom had non-diabetic fathers [1, 8]. Paternal isodisomy of chromosome 6 has been demonstrated in several unrelated patients with TNDM (fig. 1) [9, 10]. Other patients had partial duplications of the long arm of the paternal chromosome 6 [10, 11]. These unbalanced duplications are inherited within families. Only if the duplication is inherited from the father does TNDM result, suggesting a disorder of imprinting. More recently, a region in which methylation differs between the maternal and the paternal chromosome 6 has been identified [12]. Abnormal methylation patterns have been demonstrated in some TNDM

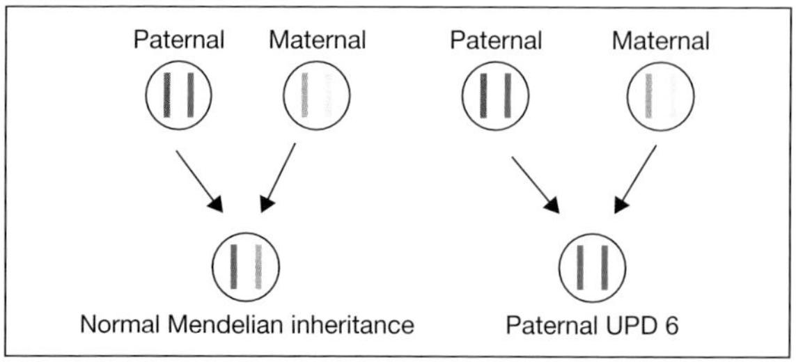


***Fig. 1.*** Schematic representation of paternal uniparental disomy of chromosome 6. Given the non-Gaussian distribution of age in the study population, the nonparametric Mann-Whitney U test was used to compare age in the two groups.

***Table 1.*** Etiologies of neonatal diabetes

| |
|---|
| *Transient neonatal diabetes mellitus* |
| Chromosome 6 anomalies detected |
| Paternal duplications |
| Paternal isodisomy |
| Methylation defect |
| No chromosome 6 anomaly detected |
| *Permanent neonatal diabetes mellitus* |
| IPEX syndrome: diffuse autoimmunity |
| Mitochondrial disease |
| Severe pancreatic hypoplasia associated with IPF1 (PDX1) mutation |
| Homozygous glucokinase mutation: insensitivity to glucose, parental MODY 2 |
| Associated with epiphyseal dysplasia: Wolcott-Rallison syndrome |
| Possibly associated with enterovirus infection |
| Association with cerebellar hypoplasia |

patients without other chromosome 6 abnormalities (table 1) [12, 13]. These observations strongly suggest that TNDM may result from overexpression of an imprinted gene located on chromosome 6q24 and displaying paternal expression. Two paternally expressed genes are located in the region and, therefore, have been considered candidate genes for the disease: one is the transcription factor *ZAC* that regulates cell cycle arrest and apoptosis and also the pituitary adenylate cyclase-activating polypeptide receptor 1 (PACAP1

*Table 2.* Comparison of several features in PNDM and TNDM cases in the French cohort (n = 50) (from Metz et al. [6], with permission)

| | PNDM (n = 21) | TNDM (n = 29) | p |
|---|---|---|---|
| Gestational age, weeks | 39.2 ± 1.6 | 38.2 ± 2.2 | 0.15 |
| Birth weight, g | 2,497 ± 690 | 1,987 ± 510 | <0.006 |
| Birth length, cm | 47.5 ± 2.4 | 44.3 ± 3.4 | <0.006 |
| Head circumference, cm | 33 ± 1.9 | 31.5 ± 1.8 | <0.02 |
| Intrauterine growth retardation | n = 7/19 36% | n = 20/27 74% | <0.03 |
| Median age at diagnosis, days (range)* | 27(1–127) | 6(1–81) | <0.01 |
| Initial insulin dose, unit/kg/day | 1.4 ± 1.2 | 0.6 ± 0.25 | <0.006 |

being a potent insulin secretagogue) and the other the *HYMAI* gene, whose function is unknown [13]. No other loci have been implicated in TNDM to date.

### Permanent Neonatal Diabetes

Permanent neonatal diabetes mellitus in our experience is less common than the transient form of the condition. By definition, diabetes develops in the neonatal period never to go into remission. There are no clinical features that can predict whether a neonate with diabetes but no other dysmorphology will eventually have permanent or transient disease although cases with the permanent form do not always have intra-uterine growth retardation as is universally seen in the transient 6q phenotype (table 2) [6, 7]. Diabetes in infancy is nearly always unrelated to classical type 1 diabetes [14]. In an Italian study conducted in all infants developing diabetes before the age of 1 year, a clear difference was demonstrated between those getting diabetes before the age of 180 days and those after. The children developing diabetes early had a very high presence of 'protective' HLA alleles to classical type 1 diabetes (76% with 0 or 1 susceptibility heterodimers) compared to only 12% in the late (>180 days) onset group [15]. In addition, autoimmune markers were far less prevalent in the early onset compared to late onset children (15 vs. 65%).

A number of discrete clinical syndromes have been identified associated with PNDM.

### *Insulin Promoter Factor-1*

The first to be described was in a child with pancreatic agenesis and marked endocrine and exocrine failure. Insulin promoter factor-1 appeared to be a good candidate for pancreatic agenesis given its role as a master control of exocrine and endocrine pancreatic development from studies of gene disruption [16] and later as a regulator of insulin and somatostatin gene expression [17].

The child was homozygous for a single nucleotide deletion within codon 63 of *IPF-1* (Pro63fsdelC) [18].

Furthermore, within the extended family there were 8 individuals in 6 generations with early-onset diabetes akin to type 2 diabetes. These were identified as heterozygotes for the same mutation with the mutant truncated isoform of *IPF-1* acting as a dominant negative inhibitor of wild-type *IPF-1* activity [19]. The illness resultant on heterozygosity was reassigned as maturity-onset diabetes of the young (MODY) 4. Additional studies have also identified that less-severe *IPF-1* mutations can cause autosomal-dominant late-onset forms of type 2 diabetes that account for around 6% of a French cohort of multiplex type 2 diabetic families [20].

### *Glucokinase*

MODY 2 is caused by mutations in the glucokinase gene and usually leads to mild hyperglycemia in affected individuals [21]. Glucokinase is a key regulator of glucose metabolism in islet cells controlling the levels of insulin secretion. However, within two families (one Norwegian, one Italian) with multiple forms of diabetes in their pedigree, 2 infants with classical PNDM (presenting on day one) have been identified who are homozygous for missense mutations within the glucokinase gene rendering them completely deficient in glycolytic activity whilst their apparently consanguineous and mild-to-moderately glucose-intolerant parents were heterozygous for the same mutations [22]. A search for further permanent neonatal diabetes cases caused by homozygosity in glucokinase mutations both in British and French cohorts (total number 18) yielded none, suggesting that this is unlikely to be a major cause of PNDM [23, 24]. However, we would recommend that if there is a history of gestational diabetes, testing for fasting glucose levels in both parents is needed. If both parents have mild glucose intolerance a screen for *glucokinase* mutations is then warranted.

### *FOXP3 (IPEX)*

A number of authors have reported an X-linked syndrome with a combination of exfoliative dermatitis, intractable diarrhea with villous atrophy, hemolytic anemia, autoimmune thyroid disease and neonatal-onset diabetes. Most children die in the first year of life of overwhelming sepsis [25]. In some of these cases, agenesis of the islets of Langerhans has been described [26]. The idea of an autoimmune basis to this disease was strengthened by the apparent success of cyclosporin A in improving the condition of 1 or 2 cases [27]. Identification of glutamic acid decarboxylase (GAD) antibodies in a patient with this condition prior to bone marrow transplantation implies that this is a form of neonatal diabetes with an autoimmune origin. Bone marrow transplantation conditioning led to a resolution of the diabetes a week before transplantation and subsequently the diarrhea resolved, as did the dermatitis. The patient remained in remission for 2 years prior to the development of hemophagocytic syndrome that proved fatal [28]. The mutation in this condition lies in the FOXP3 gene that encodes a forkhead domain-containing protein [29]. The scurfy mouse with a frame-shift mutation in Foxp3 is characterized by over-proliferation of CD4+/CD8− T lymphocytes with multiorgan infiltration. The males die 15–25 days after birth [30]. It has now been demonstrated that the protein product 'scurfin', is essential for normal immune homeostasis.

### *EIF2AK3*

Wolcott-Rallison syndrome is an autosomal-recessive disorder characterized by infancy-onset (often within the neonatal period) diabetes associated with a spondyloepiphyseal dysplasia. In addition, there is a constellation of others features such as hepatomegaly, mental retardation, renal failure and early death [31]. In 2000, Delepine et al. [32] used two consanguineous families to map the condition to the locus 2p12. Within this locus lies the gene EIF2AK3 that is highly expressed in islet cells acting as a regulator of protein synthesis. Proteins and insulin are manufactured in the endoplasmic reticulum. In response to environmental stresses, cells down-regulate protein synthesis by phosphorylation of the alpha subunit of eukaryotic translation initiation factor-2 (eif2-alpha) by eukaryotic translation initiation factor-2 kinase3 (*EIF2AK3).* Mal-folded proteins in the ER inhibit further translation initiation mediated by increased phosphorylation of eif2-alpha. A targeted mutation of the mouse Eif2ak3 gene (PERK) led to an accumulation of mal-folded proteins in the endoplasmic reticulum (ER) with resultant abnormally elevated protein synthesis and increased stress on the ER-folding machinery [33]. PERK is highly expressed in mouse pancreas. The PERK knock-out mouse demonstrates normal pancreatic endocrine and exocrine development. However, postnatally it develops endoplasmic reticulum distension accompanied by increased cell death and progressive diabetes mellitus and pancreatic exocrine failure [34]. Further analysis within the consanguineous Wolcott-Rallison families confirmed frameshift or amino acid substitution mutations occurring in EIF2AK3 segregating with the disorder in each family [32].

### *Other Permanent Neonatal Diabetes Syndromes*

In 1992, Christen et al. [35] described two boys with X-linked phosphoribosyl-ATP pyrophosphatase hyperactivity who became diabetic on day one of life. Glucose intolerance persisted throughout life although there were periods off insulin as the children grew older. Both boys had other major problems including mental retardation, ataxia and a progressive axonal neuropathy. The mother also had hyperuricemia (gout) and glucose intolerance with a history of gestational diabetes.

In 1994, Yorifuji et al. [36] described a condition of neonatal diabetes associated with severe hypoplasia of the pancreas (only head and uncus present) and congenital cyanotic heart disease (transposition of great arteries or tetralogy of Fallot) in a single family of apparent autosomal-dominant inheritance. Not all the cases developed diabetes as a neonate, and the timing is probably related to the size of the remaining pancreatic tissue.

A further severe syndrome described more recently was that of three members of a consanguineous family described with neonatal diabetes and cerebellar hypoplasia with a suggested autosomal-recessive inheritance pattern. The infants all died within a few months of birth from a combination of metabolic dysfunction, respiratory compromise and apparent sepsis [37]. Interestingly, there are a number of specific transcriptional activators which regulate gene expression shared in common by β-cells and neuronal tissues [38]: dysfunction in any of these might explain both components of this syndrome although genetic linkage analysis has so far proven unsuccessful.

A single case report has suggested that maternal enterovirus (echovirus 6) infection in pregnancy (end of first trimester) can lead to autoimmune, neonatal-onset diabetes with the presence of anti-insulin and glutamic acid decarboxylase antibodies at or very soon after birth. In this female child (ruling out IPEX), the pancreas was very hypoplastic and the authors suggested a role for maternally transmitted enterovirus either by direct influence on pancreatic organogenesis or through aggressive β-cell-targeted autoimmune attack [39].

It is worth mentioning that neonatal diabetes may exist in the context of a mitochondrial disorder [6]. It is usually associated with other organ dysfunction which may be recognized after the diagnosis of diabetes mellitus.

*Gene Knockout Studies in Mice that May Cause PNDM in Humans*

Both Pax 4 and 6 are members of the paired box gene family. These are developmental control genes that encode transcription factors expressed in distinct spatially and temporally restricted patterns during embryogenesis. Pax 4 and Pax 6 knockout mice result in severe pancreatic anomalies [40, 41]. Although no human disease has yet been identified akin to these or other mice knockouts with similar effects such as beta2/neuroD and Isl-1 they remain good candidates for further unrecognized permanent diabetes syndromes, as will other transcription genes identified to play a role in pancreatic development.

## Management of Insulin Therapy in the Neonatal Period

Insulin therapy is crucial in NDM to obtain satisfactory weight gain and growth in these infants with intra-uterine growth retardation. Sometimes glucose and caloric deprivation has been instituted in these children in the face of hyperglycemia to avoid insulin therapy. This leads to further difficulties in weight gain. In fact, high caloric intake should be maintained in these newborns and insulin therapy is given. Although pediatricians face numerous difficulties in managing insulin therapy in the newborn period, very few data are available on the methods of insulin delivery in neonatal diabetes. In infants with transient neonatal diabetes mellitus, control of the blood glucose concentration was attained with ultralente insulin treatment, without any episodes of hypoglycemia [42]. The authors recommended subcutaneous injection of ultralente insulin, rather than lente or isophane (NPH) insulin, to avoid hypoglycemia during the treatment of transient neonatal diabetes mellitus. This has not been our experience. Multiple injections of regular insulin are sometimes difficult to manage. Short-acting insulins, both human and analogue, are best avoided except when using intravenous soluble insulin infusions to initially stabilize the infant. However, in the UK, isophane insulin on a once daily basis has afforded reasonable control. Potentially, the insulin analogue (insulin glargine) with its very steady, flat pharmacokinetic profile might prove useful in this condition although there is currently no licence for children of this age.

In some centers in France, we have chosen the continuous subcutaneous insulin infusion (CSII) in all the cases of neonatal diabetes requiring subcutaneous insulin therapy for more than 15 days (Drs N. Tubiana-Rufi, G. Munz-Licha, Professors M. Polak and P. Czernichow, Department of Pediatric

Endocrinology and Diabetology, Hôpital Robert Debre and Hôpital Necker Enfants Malades, Paris). We have used this approach in 5 cases within our departments. Four of the cases were TNDM (follow-up 7 months to 10 years). The practical aspects of the treatment were as follows. During the first days, the daily dose requirement was evaluated with intravenous insulin and glucose infusions. When good glycemic control was obtained, CSII therapy was started. Insulin was diluted to 4–10 units per milliliter. Insulin strategy to start CSII depended on the feeding conditions. Under enteral continuous feeding, 100% of the total daily dose was administered at a basal rate. Under bottle feeding, the basal rate represented 30% of the total daily dose and boluses 70%, with the same insulin dose before each feed (number of feeds 8, then 7, then 6). Blood glucose was monitored every 3–4 h. Basal rate was adjusted on the night blood glucose measurements and boluses on the postprandial ones. CSII therapy was started between day 7 and 55, 1–13 days after the initiation of insulin therapy. During the first month of CSII therapy (dose at day 15 of CSII: 0.3–1 unit per kg/day), good glycemic control was achieved on a mean number of 240 blood glucose measurements (5 patients). Mean blood glucose was 1.73 g/l (9.5 mmol/l), no severe episodes of hypoglycemia were noted, and the mean number of hypoglycemia episodes (blood glucose <0.6 g/l) (3.3 mmol/l) was 4.2 per month. Similar excellent results were achieved for the rest of the CSII in both the TNDM and the PNDM cases. We did not observe any cutaneous side effects. We conclude that during the neonatal period, CSII therapy is safe, more physiological, more accurate and easier to manage than injections. CSII allows us to match the insulin requirements of a newborn. However, CSII requires management and supervision by an experienced team of physicians and nurses.

## Summary and Conclusions

Current evidence from the literature and our personal data suggest that: (1) patients with TNDM are more likely to have IUGR and less likely to develop ketoacidosis than patients with PNDM; (2) TNDM patients are younger at the diagnosis of diabetes and have lower initial insulin requirements; (3) considerable overlap occurs between the two groups, so that TNDM cannot be distinguished from PNDM based on clinical features; (4) very early onset diabetes mellitus seems to be unrelated to autoimmunity in most instances; (5) recurrent diabetes is common in patients with 'transient' neonatal diabetes mellitus and, consequently, prolonged follow-up is imperative; (6) molecular diagnosis of chromosome 6 anomalies provide a tool to identify transient from permanent neonatal diabetes mellitus in the neonatal period; (7) realizing how difficult it is to take care of a child of this age with diabetes mellitus should prompt clinicians to transfer these children to specialized centers; (8) insulin therapy and high caloric intake are the basis of the treatment; (9) insulin pump therapy may offer an interesting therapeutic tool in this age group in experienced hands.

Neonatal diabetes is a very rare condition. However, it is probably of great relevance to our understanding of the causation of type 2 diabetes within the general population. We believe these rare single gene disorders are natural models identifying new genes that might have relevance to type 2 diabetes. As already illustrated, the IPF-1 mutation is important in MODY 4 and in some familial forms of early-onset type 2 diabetes. In TNDM, Lindsay et al. [43] have demonstrated a weak linkage of diabetes in Pima Indians to paternally derived alleles at 6q24. We hope that elucidating the etiology of other forms of neonatal diabetes will give information on normal pancreatic development and the basis of the pathology underlying pancreatic dysfunction.

## Acknowledgments

We thank the non-profit organization *Aide aux Jeunes Diabétiques* (AJD) and the Diabetes UK for its generous support of some of our work on neonatal diabetes. We thank our collaborators in the network 'EURONEODIA' dedicated to neonatal diabetes: Prof. P. Czernichow pediatric endocrinology and Dr. H. Cavé genetic biochemistry, Hôpital Robert Debré, Paris, France; Dr. K. Temple, Wessex Clinical Genetics Service, Department of Human Genetics, Southampton University, Southampton, UK; Drs D. Mackay and D. Robinson, Wessex Regional Genetics Laboratory, Salisbury District Hospital, Salisbury, UK; Drs L. Journot and A. Varrault, CNRS UPR 9023 – CCIPE, Montpellier, France.

## References

1 Von Mühlendahl KE, Herkenhoff H: Long-term course of neonatal diabetes. N Engl J Med 1995;333:704–708.

2 Shield JP, Gardner RJ, Wadsworth EJ, et al: Aetiopathology and genetic basis of neonatal diabetes. Arch Dis Child 1997;76:39–42.

3 Ferguson AW, Milner RDG: Transient neonatal diabetes mellitus in sibs. Arch Dis Child 1970;45:80–81.

4 Fösel S: Transient and permanent neonatal diabetes. Eur J Pediatr 1999;154:944–948.

5 Shield JPH, Baum JD: Transient neonatal diabetes and later onset diabetes. A case of inherited insulin resistance. Arch Dis Child 1995;72:56–57.

6 Metz C, Cave H, Bertrand AM, Deffert C, Gueguen-Giroux B, Czernichow P, Polak M, NDM French Study Group: Neonatal diabetes mellitus: Chromosomal analysis in transient and permanent cases. J Pediatr 2002;141:483–489.

7a Temple IK, Gardner RJ, MacKay DJG, Barber JCK, Robinson DO, Shield JPH: Transient neonatal diabetes mellitus: Widening our understanding of the aetiopathogenesis of diabetes. Diabetes 2000;49:1359.

7b Shield JPM, H Templ IK, Sabin M, et al: An assessment of pancreatic endocrine function and insulin sensitivity in patients with transient neonatal diabetes in remission. Arch Dis Childhood 2004;89:341–343.

community [15]. Effective therapy of DKA requires attention to the pathophysiologic changes caused by insulin deficiency and the secondary consequences of such deficiencies: hyperglycemia, glycosuria and osmotic diuresis, sodium and water losses, total body potassium deficit, glycogenolysis and also protein and fat catabolism generating more hyperglycemia and ketonuria, ketonemia and eventually ketoacidosis. Prompt institution of fluid and electrolyte replacement along with appropriate insulin administration should produce slow but steady corrections of such imbalances thereby preventing or minimizing complications associated with DKA [16–24].

All stages of ketoacidosis from the earliest increases in blood glucose through increasing generation of ketone bodies to ketonemia, acidemia and eventually ketoacidosis may lead to coma and death. Despite appropriate use of insulin and fluids and continuous clinical observation, the mortality rate of DKA has not improved and has remained the same as that reported in the 1970s [25, 26]. Diabetic ketoacidosis must be distinguished from a chronic state of hyperglycemia whose diabetes is merely 'out of control'. There is no uniform definition of what constitutes DKA. Many articles and many textbook chapters use idiosyncratic definitions which may or may not be consistent with others' definitions. Diabetic ketoacidosis might be defined in reference to carbon dioxide levels (or serum bicarbonate) equal to or less than 10 mEq/l [4]. When comparing what is written in textbooks and the literature, especially concerning outcome and associated problems, it is very important to define pH, acid-base status as well as level of glycemia. The exact level of hyperglycemia or ketosis in DKA can be extremely variable. The term 'diabetic coma' in the medical literature often is misleading since most patients with severe diabetic ketoacidosis are not necessarily 'unconscious'.

Proper early recognition and treatment by the patient and/or his or her family before hospitalization is a necessity. Younger patients more often present in DKA than older youth or adults [27]. This must be followed up by identification of precipitating factors [28] and education to prevent recurrence. Physicians and nurses should be taught how diabetes presents as well as how subtle symptoms and signs might be in the very youngest babies in an effort to prevent more serious metabolic decompensation. In many places around the world, newly diagnosed diabetes in children and adolescents remains unrecognized or is diagnosed only in its most severe manifestations [25, 29–31]. In one study in New York [32], if the diagnosis of diabetes itself was missed, up to 68% of children presented in DKA compared to less than half if the diagnosis was considered and made. In underprivileged adult communities, drug or alcohol abuse is commonly associated with diabetic ketoacidosis [33] so this should be not forgotten when teenagers or young adults present to emergency facilities or clinics. DKA is slightly more likely to occur in those patients treated with subcutaneous insulin infusion pumps compared to similarly aggressive management with multidose insulin protocols [34] because interruption of the pump insulin produces fat and absolute insulin deficiency and there is no long-acting or intermediate-acting insulin depot (no NPH, lente or glargine being used, for example).

Special efforts to educate and re-educate pump treated patients is needed to sustain frequent blood glucose as well as urine or blood ketone monitoring during any unexplained instances of hyperglycemia in pump-treated patients. They should be taught, like all patients with diabetes, details of how to respond early enough to prevent most episodes of full decompensation although some catheter disconnections or insulin delivery problems (battery failure, alarm failure, clogged catheters) will always be inevitable.

### Sick Day Guidelines and at Home Management to Prevent DKA

As health care professionals, a main goal of learning about living with diabetes must remain teaching recognition of what happens with an intercurrent illness and how to make adjustments in fluid intake and insulin administration accordingly. Most illnesses can be managed at home with such adjustments and with phone consultation available. DKA does not happen very quickly and usually allows sufficient time to adjust insulin [35] – if one is aware of the possibility of DKA and metabolic decompensation as well as willing to take steps (i.e. give extra insulin, provide extra salty fluids, monitor for possible dehydration, check ketone levels) to counterbalance such metabolic needs. Education is a necessity but the ability and willingness to use such self-care education and skills is also a requirement to prevent DKA from becoming a serious and life-threatening event [36]. Studies in Germany [27] and Scotland [37] elegantly document the importance of emphasis on teaching sick day rules (table 1) and applying them satisfactorily to decrease emergency room visits and to increase family home competence to manage illnesses, adjust insulin upwards if hyperglycemia and/or ketonuria/ketosis occur and also to occasionally adjust insulin downwards with other illness. All this is based upon frequent home glucose monitoring coupled with either urine or blood ketone monitoring as well. If a patient or family does not monitor or is unable to monitor or keep records, they obviously lose the ability to detect any subtle or changing patterns of glycemia so that recognition of impending hyperglycemic crises is delayed or absent. Urine glucose monitoring serves the same purpose in situation where blood glucose testing is unavailable. The benefit of home or self blood glucose monitoring is its ability to provide prompt recognition of a changing pattern

*Table 1.* Sick day guidelines

Preventive measures include the following *sick day guidelines*. These should be taught to all families and, as age-appropriate, to children and adolescents with type 1 diabetes mellitus. Fathers and not just mothers should be taught such guidelines. Periodic (annual) review should be documented in the medical record. These sick day guidelines should be started whenever symptoms suggest the possibility of DKA, whenever blood sugars exceed 240–250 mg/dl (approximately 14 mmol/l) or with any unexplained weight loss or evidence for an intercurrent illness (i.e. cough, fever, runny nose, GI upset, rash or similar exposure):

1. Home/self blood glucose monitoring (HBGM or SBGM) – with adult supervision even in adolescents – at least every 3–4 h and occasionally every 1–2 h and with results recorded in a log book
2. A minimum of urine ketone testing – or β-hydroxybutyric acid blood testing – every 2–4 h with results recorded in a log book
3. Continued monitoring in the middle of the night (no matter how tired the patient or family)
4. Increased salty fluid (i.e. clear salty broth) to combat dehydration or sugar/salt solutions such as Gatorade®, Lytren®, Pedialyte® if eating is also decreased and some source of fast sugar is needed; decarbonated cola or ginger ale sodas may also provide some electrolytes as well as added water and sucrose under such circumstances
5. Weight obtained every 8–12 h each day at home to monitor for clinical dehydration
6. Treatment of underlying illnesses (appropriate antibiotics for bacterial infections)
7. Antipyretics (usually acetominophen) if needed
8. Antiemetics (such as Pepto Bismol®) if severe vomiting prevents adequate fluid intake
9. Continue insulin and usually *extra* insulin '*booster shots*' (10–20% extra based upon previous total day's insulin doses and repeated every 2–4 h) for as long as hyperglycemia and/or ketonuria persists
10. Recognize when insulin dose (rarely) needs to be temporarily decreased – based upon documented hypoglycemia rather than hyperglycemia during illness; most often this involves a gastrointestinal illness rather than a respiratory illness
11. Contact (telephone) with health care team if symptoms persist, worsen or resolution does not occur (especially persistent and severe abdominal pains, persistent emesis, deeper and/or more labored respirations, weight loss or change in neurologic status of any kind)

*All too frequently a physician or nurse advises omission of insulin because the patient is ill and not eating. Under no condition should this be routinely done since most episodes of DKA require more insulin despite less food intake.* There are some occasions when fast-acting or even intermediate/long-acting insulin doses should be temporarily decreased or discontinued but this should occur only when blood glucose levels are documented to be low. The health care team may be able to recognize certain patterns of community epidemics and use this information to advice patients and family members of what to expect.

especially when any illness occurs. Such monitoring can signal a changing pattern of increasing glycemia as well as provide an increasing attention to accompanying other warning signs as increasing thirst, polyuria, nocturia, enuresis, malaise, weight loss, nausea, vomiting and ketonuria. Home blood capillary β-hydroxybutyric acid testing with readily available and inexpensive blood testing strips may provide information for patients and/or their family members to act earlier or more aggressively to head metabolic decompensation and replace urinary acetone/acetoacetate test strips currently available [38–42]. Emphasis on identifying possible 'metabolic stresses' such as those occurring during intercurrent illnesses (respiratory and/or gastrointestinal) is extremely important to allow the patient and/or family members to increase blood glucose and ketone monitoring. Intercurrent infections sometimes produce changes in insulin effectiveness for 8–24 h prior to the onset of overt symptoms. Being alert to metabolic parameters changing in such a fashion often allows sufficient insulin and fluid compensation to altogether prevent further progression of the ketoacidotic state. Ketoacidosis does not occur because of overeating or other 'dietary indiscretions'.

### Recurrent Diabetic Ketoacidosis

Ketoacidosis is not a sudden complication of having diabetes takes from several hours to several days to develop in the vast majority of patients. Most cases of DKA can be recognized by well-educated patients and their families. Parents or another responsible adult should be taught and expected to directly supervise or actually perform blood glucose testing, ketone testing and insulin administration. Teens who are otherwise self-sufficient as well as adults when they are ill may want to sleep and not take the time and effort to monitoring appropriately. Other family members should be designated to follow sick day guidelines and assist under such circumstances. Those with elevated hemoglobin A1c values are, by definition, chronically decompensated and out of control so may have less reserve of water and minerals so that dehydration may occur more quickly. Telephone consultation with a member of the health care team is extremely important to help decide what is occurring at home and whether or not more detailed medical observation is necessary. A plan of action can be outlined with the family members 'serving as the eyes and ears' for the health care team. The extremely 'brittle' or 'labile' child or adolescent who presents with recurring DKA, often from a tumultuous family environment, may be the exception to this rule in approximately 2% of a general pediatric endocrinology or pediatric/adolescent diabetes practice [3, 43]. A study in Leicester, UK, suggested that 20% of pediatric patients accounted for 80% of all admissions for DKA at the Leicester Royal Infirmary [44]. Such youngsters, usually around adolescence [4, 32] but occasionally a few years younger, seems to be enmeshed with parental and family issues that often demand that they 'be sick' in order to gain attention from other family members [45, 46]. DKA in children and adolescents appears to occur 14 times more commonly in boys than in girls in one study [47] but just the opposite was found in other studies of DKA [48, 49]. Many episodes of diabetic ketoacidosis occur when insulin doses are 'forgotten' [4, 47] although stress-related crises are frequently part of the history obtained. Sexual abuse, physical abuse, mental abuse, parents or family members who are drug or alcohol abusers or those family situations in which patients are neglected and left to care for themselves often are the true underlying factors to explain recurrent DKA.

### Omitted Insulin – Usually the Explanation for Recurrent DKA

Since omitted insulin is usually suspected in such patients, prevention of recurrent DKA involves recognition and acknowledgement of the problem in those in the worst glucose control (highest hemoglobin A1c, for instance) and working out specific arrangements to have responsible adults at home actually administering insulin doses several times each day while psychological therapy is begun. Such cases are more common than is generally acknowledged, are difficult to diagnosis and often respond – in the midst of their DKA episodes – more quickly than other cases to routine fluid, electrolyte, and insulin administration because ongoing infections as a precipitant is not present. Recent pharmacy computer studies in Scotland document that omitted insulin is very common [5, 47]. Psychological intervention becomes mandatory under such circumstances [4, 41, 50]. A novel approach to missed insulin injections as a cause of recurrent diabetic ketoacidosis prescribed insulin pumps in an attempt to decrease the amount of time when inadequate insulin was available and documented reduced emergency room episodes as well as significant reductions in emergency room and hospitalization costs [51, 52] but this has not received wide clinical acceptance.

### Acute Hospital or Emergency Room DKA Management (table 2)

*Fluid and Electrolyte Management*

*Initial Sodium and Water Management.* The severity of mental status changes is likely related to serum osmolarity [53]. The weight of the patient can be used for initial estimation of replacement fluids on the assumption that dehydration is mainly reflected by acute body weight loss. Surface area estimations may be used to estimate fluid needs at all ages and are particularly

***Table 2.*** NEDEC DKA low-dose insulin infusion protocol for children and adolescents [adapted from Brink, SJ: New England Diabetes and Endocrinology Center, 2004®]

1. Maintain airway, breathing and circulation. Consider low flow nasal oxygen
2. Confirm diagnosis of diabetic ketoacidosis at bedside and consider infections, surgical emergencies and other possible precipitants
3. Start intravenous infusion with normal saline 10–20 $cm^3$/kg to run over 1–2 h
4. Lead II EKG for potassium status (full EKG in adults to rule out myocardial infarction)
5. Start flow sheet: weight, height, surface area calculations, pulse, BP, respiratory rate and effort, neurologic status including fundoscopy, baseline glucose, urine, electrolytes, calcium, phosphate, acid-base data and renal functioning
6. Determine estimated maintenance and deficit for electrolyte and fluid orders and assume correction over 36–48 h rather than 24 h in an effort to minimize cerebral edema complications
7. Attach piggyback short-acting insulin infusion system to existing intravenous line:
   a. Prepare 100 units regular insulin (1 cc) in 100 cc of normal saline
   b. Preflush intravenous tubing to allow adherence of insulin to plastic; no need for albumin
   c. Set up piggyback system into existing intravenous line using available pump or pediatric set
   d. Give 0.1–0.2 units/kg of body weight as intravenous push (bolus) of fast-acting regular insulin
   e. Start 0.1 unit/kg body weight/hr intravenously by continuous infusion
   f. F Expect initial drop from rehydration and then approximately 10% of blood sugar hourly (50–70 mg (or approximately 3–4 mmol)/dl/h)
   g. Monitor blood glucose at 1 h and then every 2–4 h to ensure expected response
   h. Monitor urine for ketone bodies at least every 3–4 h or, alternatively and if available, monitor blood β-hydroxybutyric acid sequentially every 2–4 h
   i. Double rate of infusion or switch to alternative insulin delivery protocol if no response
   j. Calculate estimated time when blood glucose will reach 250–300 mg/dl (or approximately 14–17 mmol/dl) to avoid hypoglycemia
   k. Stop insulin infusion when blood glucose reaches 250 mg/dl (or approximately 14 mmol/dl) and change intravenous solution to contain 5% dextrose with electrolytes
8. After initial 1–2 h of normal saline infusion, change intravenous solution to 40 mEq/l of potassium using 20 mEq/l KCl plus 20 mEq/l $K_2HPO_4$ to avoid iatrogenic hypokalemia in either 0.5 or 0.9 normal saline (see text)
9. Check electrolytes at 2–4 h and again as necessary according to clinical monitoring requirements, patient status, etc. to adjust type of fluids and rate of administration; evaluate abdominal pain appropriately
10. Must give subcutaneous insulin or intramuscular insulin 15 minutes before intravenous insulin is discontinued or if line no longer operational because of short half life of intravenous insulin to avoid recurrent ketoacidosis; adjust dosage according to newness of IDDM, degree of ketosis and/or acidosis, age of patient, known sensitivity or other factors which will affect amount of insulin needed (pregnancy, renal failure, infection, etc.)

*Table 2* (continued)

| | |
|---|---|
| 11. | Identify and treat any underlying problem (i.e. continue antibiotics as needed for urinary infection, streptococcal disease, etc.) |
| 12. | Keep *flow sheet* up to date and reassess frequently |
| 13. | Pay attention to vital signs, abdominal exam, neurologic status (including examination of the optic disk) and electrolyte changes; detect and treat cerebral edema; consider cerebral CT or MRI studies to rule out cerebral edema, cerebrovascular accidents and cerebral venous thrombosis if abnormal neurologic findings occur |
| 14. | Educate patient and family to prevent recurrence: identify contributing psychosocial problems |

useful in infants and children but can also be used in adolescents and adults for estimating maintenance needs. The severity of the signs and symptoms of dehydration reflect extracellular fluid loss with minimal clinically detectable evidence of dehydration approximately 3–5% loss of body weight. With 20% acute volume depletion the patient is, by definition, in profound shock and often moribund. (20% acute plus chronic weight loss is not all water loss so that patients who are newly diagnosed and give a history of significant weight loss are not necessarily 20% dehydrated since they have lost muscle and fat as well as water weight.) Because extracellular fluid loss represents the loss of sodium and water, immediate restitution of blood volume can be provided using estimated 10–20 cc/kg of body weight with normal (0.9%) saline given over the first 1–2 h of treatment. This effectively removes the patient from the immediate consequences of potential or overt shock and does not cause any delay searching for special/expensive intravenous solutions (blood, Ringers lactate, albumin, etc.). Because most young patients will not have pre-existing or serious cardiac or renal problems, there is not much danger in providing such initial hydration. In an adult or elderly patient, caution may be required vis-à-vis such pre-existing cardiovascular or renal problems because of problems with fluid overload and generalized vascular status, perfusion capability, etc. Maintenance water, sodium and potassium can be estimated according to standard pediatric guidelines based on surface area estimations: water: 2,000 (1,500–2,000 range) $cm^3/m^2/24\,h$; sodium: 40 (30–60 range) $mEq/m^2/24\,h$; and potassium: 40 (30–50 range) $mEq/m^2/24\,h$. Total body deficits can be enormous and not always readily reflected via initial laboratory measurements. The serum sodium may be high, normal or low but this is not an accurate measure of the absolute sodium requirement especially if there has been technical artifact because of concomitant hyperlipidemia. Most centers suggest the use of normal saline (0.9%) intravenously for the first 1–4 h with a switch to half-normal (0.45%) saline several hours into therapy. More recently, because of the chance that cerebral edema is more common than appreciated [54], recommendations to continue normal saline for a longer time period have been proposed to allow osmotic re-equilibration in a more leisurely time frame [50, 55–59]. If the total deficit of sodium is sufficiently excessive and if hypovolemia is great enough, glomerular filtration may decrease and the patient may present with oliguria or progress to acute tubular necrosis. Central venous catheters or dialysis are rarely needed in children and adolescents although may be extremely useful under specific circumstances.

*Potassium.* Because of the acidotic state, potassium is usually driven out of the intracellular space while a state of kaliuresis exists as the kidney attempts to save sodium (Bunge effect). Initially, serum potassium levels can be either normal, elevated or low depending upon where in the dynamic state one obtains potassium levels. With treatment as dehydration is corrected, lactic acid production decreases and some potassium begins to shift back intracellularly fostering peripheral hypokalemia. With insulin administration, ketoacid production decreases also fostering entry of potassium intracellularly. Serum potassium should be expected to decrease soon after appropriate DKA treatment begins so an early finding of hypokalemia can be worrisome if it presages further serious hypokalemia.

Sequential bedside EKG rhythm strips for T or U wave changes or cardiac monitoring allows identification of potential dangerous hypokalemia necessitating a change in potassium replacement (increasing potassium replenishment). Occasionally, metabolic decompensation has progressed to the point that hypokalemia is present initially; this has a more ominous prognosis because of the cardiac arrhythmias that can coexist at that time or shortly after the acidotic state begins to change. Potassium should be given immediately if hypokalemia is suspected or documented. Usually, potassium is added in the second to fourth hour of treatment. Early and vigorous treatment with potassium replacement may decrease mortality and morbidity. It has been suggested, therefore, that potassium be added to the initial intravenous solution as soon as a reliable history of polyuria has been obtained in a child or once the first urine is voided since young patients are not at high risk for cardiac or renal compromise from pre-existing abnormalities compared to adults or the elderly. Potassium can be replaced at a rate of 40 mEq/l of solution without danger of a rapid rise in blood levels or of irritation at the intravenous site. Half could be given as potassium chloride (20 mEq/l KCl) and the other half as potassium phosphate (20 mEq/l $K_2HPO_4$) for the first 6–12 h of replacement therapy although replacement only with KCl produces as good clinical outcomes in published literature as when half phosphate and half chloride salts are used. After several hours, only potassium chloride should be used so that iatrogenic hypocalcemia does not occur (see phosphate treatment section below). On rare

*Table 3.* Complications associated with bicarbonate administration in DKA

| |
|---|
| a. Abrupt osmotic changes |
| b. Precipitous potassium changes |
| c. Overshoot alkalosis |
| d. Potential hypoxia with shift of oxyhemoglobin dissociation curve |
| e. Cerebral edema, coma and death |

occasions, more potassium is needed and this requires closer cardiac monitoring, more frequent serum potassium determinations and even nasogastric potassium administration if intravenous access is problematic.

*Bicarbonate* (table 3). Since acetoacetate and β-hydroxybutyrate are metabolizable anions, restoration of serum bicarbonate concentration usually will follow insulin administration in the absence of treatment with alkali containing solutions. Acidosis results from a combination of (1) release of fatty acids secondary to insulin deficiency; (2) generation of 'ketone bodies'; (3) starvation from poor food intake and, in some instances (4) excessive production of lactic acid because of plasma volume depletion, poor tissue perfusion and an increase in anaerobic glycolysis in muscles. Concerns for consequences of severe metabolic acidosis have been balanced by fears of cerebral edema and respiratory arrest when bicarbonate is replaced 'too quickly' [55, 60]. Life-threatening hypokalemia (as potassium returns back into the cell) as well as worsening tissue hypoxia affinity for oxygen can be added to the list of possible bicarbonate treatment complications (table 3). Treatment with sodium bicarbonate should be restricted to patients with a severe metabolic acidosis as indicated by an arterial pH of 7.0–7.1 or less or a bicarbonate value of less than 5 mEq/l. Rapid infusions or large amounts over a short time span should not be routine and should be reserved for acute and life-threatening cardiorespiratory arrest situations. If sodium bicarbonate is given, the amount of sodium should be subtracted from that amount of sodium contained in the replacement fluids to avoid exacerbation of the (already) hyperosmolar state. *When sodium bicarbonate is used, it should be given by slow intravenous infusion over several hours* [55, 56, 61–63]. Frequent serial pH and/or bicarbonate determinations should be obtained so that the administration of bicarbonate can be discontinued when the pH reaches 7.2–7.25. If calculations of base deficit are utilized, a practical approach would suggest giving approximately 50% of the calculated deficit (0.3 × body weight in kg × base deficit) in mmol over 30 min. Favorable results are reported on low-dose insulin protocols [64] without routine bicarbonate administration. An increase in carbon dioxide (as respiratory effort decreases with an abatement of Kussmaul respirations) and the more slowly moving bicarbonate diffusion across the blood-brain barrier may explain a paradoxical cerebrospinal acidosis associated with bicarbonate administration. Cerebral vasodilatation and an increase in cerebral blood volume may contribute to an increase in cerebrospinal pressure and cerebral edema as well as account for the changes in levels of consciousness in patients receiving sodium bicarbonate.

*Calcium, Phosphate and Oxygen.* Patients with diabetic ketoacidosis sustain intracellular phosphate depletion. Serum phosphate often follows a pattern similar to that of potassium. Although initial serum phosphate values may be normal or elevated, within 4–6 h after insulin treatment has begun, these values often may fall dramatically as glycogen deposition resumes and phosphate moves intracellularly. The consequences of hypophosphatemia may be reflected in red blood cell levels of 2,3-diphosphoglycerate (2,3-DPG), an intermediary metabolite of glycolysis. The role of red cell 2,3-DPG in diabetic ketoacidosis is important because 2,3-DPG has the capacity to alter the affinity of the hemoglobin molecule for oxygen and thus the delivery of oxygen to tissues. A fall in 2,3-DPG content may cause tissue and cerebral hypoxia in patients with diabetic ketoacidosis, hence the recommendation that most patients being treated for DKA should receive oxygen at least for the first few hours of treatment. In any patient with known or suspected cardiac, renal and/or cerebrovascular compromise, there is potential benefit in ensuring adequate oxygen supply and minimal risk using nasal oxygen delivery under such circumstances.

If sodium bicarbonate is given in sufficient amounts to raise the pH of the blood too rapidly, the protective Bohr effect which allows oxygen to be released in the face of acidosis is reversed. Because of such theoretical concerns vis-à-vis oxygen delivery and the acid-base status of the patient, reservations about bicarbonate administration exist. The sudden rise in hemoglobin affinity for oxygen might lead to tissue hypoxia and account for the sudden deterioration of some patients receiving bicarbonate. This sequence of events following the administration of sodium bicarbonate might contribute to cerebral edema. This author [3] suggests replenishment of phosphate losses by providing 50% of the needed potassium replacement and maintenance as phosphate salts and 50% as chloride salts (see 'Potassium' section above). This is provided for the first 6–12 h of intravenous fluid therapy so that changes in calcium-phosphate ratios are not excessive. Therefore, oxygen is also recommended at low flow rates and usually delivered by nasal prongs.

*Insulin: Bolus, Intramuscular, Continuous Intravenous Protocols*

The best route of administration and the dose of insulin necessary for treatment of diabetic ketoacidosis are unknown. Successful results have been published with differing insulin regimes for several decades although most experts currently recommend continuous low-dose infusion insulin. All patients in ketoacidosis have an immediate need for insulin and, no matter which protocol is followed, fluid and electrolyte replacement as well as recognition of underlying precipitating events must remain high on the list of priorities to decrease morbidity and mortality. *Close and repeated clinical as well as laboratory observations are mandatory to enable the wisest and safest therapeutic approaches and to allow for their modification once therapy begins since DKA and its treatment require such vigilance to maximize safety and positive outcomes* (table 4).

The giving of 'enough' insulin (table 5) should be one's aim. This should be guided by initial and subsequent blood sugar levels as well as clinical follow-up, duration of symptomatology, severity of dehydration etc. Blood acetoacetate and acetone levels may rise initially despite a much greater fall in β-hydroxybutyric acid as a result of acid-base changes and insulin treatment involved with fat metabolic effects. Blood and urine ketone determinations (which only measure acetone and acetoacetate, and not β-hydroxybutyrate) may RISE rather than fall as therapy starts to proceed. New strips for rapid blood β-hydroxybutyric acid level determination [42] may help adjust treatment needs more physiologically. Urine ketone determinations are far less useful as an index of additional insulin requirement than is clinical response and blood glucose changes. Physicians should be wary of increasing insulin dosage solely because of worsening measures of only acetone and acetoacetate in blood and/or urine. In fact, this should be expected over the first few hours of successful treatment as β-hydroxybutyric acid is converted to acetoacetate and acetone [65]. Too vigorous insulin administration may lead to too rapid decreases in blood glucose and therefore excessive osmotic changes; the risks of cerebral edema might increase if this crucial metabolic fact is ignored. Human regular insulin, because it is less allergenic than other insulin preparations, should be the regular insulin of choice unless it is unavailable (or the patient is known to be using an alternative insulin product already). Rapid acting insulin analogs like lispro insulin (Humalog®) and insulin aspart insulin (NovoRapid®) can also be used under such circumstances intravenously, intramuscularly or subcutaneously. Both of these newer analogs (Humalog and NovoRapid) when given subcutaneously may be needed closer to every 2–3 h rather than every 4–6 h compared to human regular insulin (Humulin and Novolin) because of their absorption characteristics.

Many factors determine the amounts of insulin required as summarized in table 4. The largest doses are generally needed in older more overweight patients who have had diabetes for some time, particularly when insulin has not been administered regularly (i.e. chronically omitted) or when insulin has not been given during the initial hours of an illness. Newly diagnosed patients who are very acidotic may require very large amounts of insulin whereas others are

***Table 4.*** DKA flow sheet

| | Exam | | | | Blood work | | | | | | Urine | Fluids | | | | | | Insulin | |
|---|---|---|---|---|---|---|---|---|---|---|---|---|---|---|---|---|---|---|---|
| Time | BP | Resp | CNS<br><br>1 = alert<br>2 = lethargic (easily aroused)<br>3 = stupor (aroused with difficulty)<br>4 = coma/ unresponsive | Pupils | Glucose | $HCO_3$ | Na | K | Cl | BUN/ cr | Urine ketones | Start time | Type | $cm^3$/ h | Na | K | $HCO_3$ | Start time | U/h |
| | | | | | | | | | | | | | | | | | | | |
| | | | | | | | | | | | | | | | | | | | |
| | | | | | | | | | | | | | | | | | | | |
| | | | | | | | | | | | | | | | | | | | |

*Table 5.* When to modify insulin dose in DKA treatment [35]

A. Increase dose
   1. Very high usual insulin dose
   2. Longer duration of diabetes
   3. Severe infection
   4. Extreme obesity
   5. Insulin resistance
   6. Severe acidosis

B. Decrease dose
   1. Newly diagnosed patient
   2. Not unconscious
   3. Blood sugar below 400 mg/dl (approx. 22 mmol/l)
   4. Very thin person
   5. Young infant or child
   6. History of skipping insulin
   7. History of insulin sensitivity (i.e. very low insulin dose)
   8. Renal insufficiency
   9. Hypokalemia
   10. Extreme hyperosmolality

exquisitely sensitive. The new 'epidemic' of overweight adolescents presenting in DKA but who soon look more like type 2 Syndrome X/non-insulin-dependent diabetes mellitus [66] has presented peculiar challenges to health care providers because of the often enormous amounts of insulin required in the first few days of DKA and subsequent treatment – until suddenly insulin resistance appears to decrease and dramatic reductions of insulin are then needed with resolution of initial 'glucose toxicity'. Similarly, a recent review of deaths in African-American youth considered to have died from DKA but actually dying from hyperglycemic hyperosmolar states at the onset of type 2 diabetes poses major problems for the diagnostician as well as the treatment team [67]. Smaller children, infants and toddlers seem to be more sensitive to insulin than older children and teenagers. *At least one physician must at all times be in charge* and know the time of insulin administration, the relation of subsequent blood sugar determinations to each dosage, and the time of starting as well as the rate of flow of fluids and electrolytes. Keeping a flow sheet may be the single most important task (once the diagnosis is established and treatment begun) because of the dynamic state of affairs present in this condition and how much can change once treatment begins. There is not substitute formula to replace close hour-to-hour observation of the patient and supervision of treatment by the physician and hospital team.

*Bolus Insulin.* In the past, traditional insulin therapy has been given by a combination of bolus intravenous as well as bolus subcutaneous regular insulin.

Any possibility of decreased perfusion to a particular subcutaneous area, therefore, was eliminated because some insulin was available directly into the blood stream. Insulin was given according to a variety of guidelines which were related to body size, weight and/or habitus with numerous protocols described in textbooks around the world. Multiple decisions regarding initial and subsequent dosage amounts were required but most patients recovered without excess morbidity or mortality; in fact, with appropriate sequential blood sugar and electrolyte monitoring, mortality figures drastically decreased over the years that insulin has been available. Children were usually given less insulin empirically than adults. It was not infrequent to have the initial doses of insulin (given in this large bolus fashion) of sufficient magnitude so that no further insulin was needed for many hours after treatment. Hyperglycemia was rapidly corrected over a few hours and often there was an excess of subsequent hypoglycemia from all the insulin administered and accumulated in the body [40].

*Intramuscular Insulin.* The earliest reports advocating the use of intramuscular insulin in the treatment of diabetic ketoacidosis were published in the German literature [43]. Because intramuscular insulin may produce a faster absorption of insulin and a greater drop in blood glucose levels when compared to subcutaneous doses, several investigators started to look at the use of frequent but smaller doses of intramuscular insulin injections. British diabetologists [68] recommended hourly intramuscular insulin administration. For youngsters, a loading dose of 0.25 units of regular insulin per kilogram followed by 0.1 units per kilogram per hour intramuscularly. The benefits of intramuscular treatment over intravenous plus subcutaneous treatment with insulin consist of the following: (1) ease of protocol comprehension by staff; (2) no need for complex apparatus to deliver insulin; (3) no need for complicated calculations of insulin dose; (4) little risk of late hypoglycemia because of the near normal blood insulin levels achieved; (5) smooth fall in blood lactate; (6) no major potassium fluxes, and (7) decreased potential for cerebral edema because of the slower falls in blood glucose and slower osmotic changes. Potential problems utilizing intramuscular insulin protocols arise when rehydration and electrolyte disturbances receive inadequate attention particularly if the patient is already hypotensive at presentation. Another source of potential concern is the choice of injection site for the insulin; if the buttocks are used, the injected insulin may be deposited in the fat not the muscle tissues. In order to avoid this, the recommendation has been to utilize a muscle such as the deltoid which is readily and predictably accessible even in those patients who are overweight or obese.

*Intravenous Low-Dose Continuous Infusion.* More so than with intramuscular protocols, intravenous low-dose regular insulin infusion has become the standard method of treating diabetic ketoacidosis [14–21]. Although the original reports from Germany were in 1946 [69] and then again in 1960 [70], it was not until 1972 when interest was stirred and enthusiasm generated for low-dose insulin infusions for ketoacidosis based on studies [70] where such treatment was 'rediscovered' [71]. The slow and predictable decrease in blood glucose has been viewed as a marked improvement compared to larger bolus insulin treatments previously used. Generally, blood sugar falls by approximately 10% hourly once the initial 'dehydrated' blood glucose value is corrected (with the first few hours of hydration). Correction of acidemia and restoration of electrolyte status and lipid profiles presumably occurs at a slightly slower rate compared to earlier intravenous insulin protocols because of the smaller amounts of insulin being given; in some studies, no significant differences among the three types of insulin dosing protocols could be found [71–73]. Early fears of insulin resistance have not been confirmed nor has there been any noticeable increase in mortality [74–77].

One protocol for use of low-dose continuous insulin infusion is presented in table 1. Albumin is not needed to prevent insulin adsorption to glass and/or plastic bottles and tubing. Infusing insulin at these rates allows for adequate blood insulin levels to correct hyperglycemia, inhibit lipolysis, inhibit glycogenolysis and correct abnormalities in counter-regulatory hormone levels found in ketoacidosis. If blood sugars do not respond as expected, it should be verified that insulin was actually administered and delivered. Medical errors include unconnected catheters, non-transcribed medical orders, delivering fluids and electrolyte solutions but forgetting to administer insulin all are variations of the theme of not actually administering or delivering insulin to the patient in DKA. If insulin actually is being delivered and the blood sugars remain elevated, the dose should either be doubled or an alternative protocol utilized. As in all other treatment regimes, uncorrected severe dehydration and resulting hypovolemic shock remains a potential cause for nonresponse especially from underestimated ongoing losses. The presence of documented infection seems to slow down return of all parameters of metabolic control but is not significantly different clinically in low-dose vs. high-dose protocol comparisons [78].

When blood sugar falls to approximately 250 mg/dl (approximately 14 mmol/l), 5% dextrose is added to the intravenous fluids and subcutaneous insulin is started. Sometimes, the insulin infusion is then discontinued but no order follows to give subcutaneous insulin and a state of ongoing insulin deficiency then occurs! In order to avoid this type of error, it seems wise to specify in hospital DKA protocols that subcutaneous insulin be given one half hour *before* the continuous insulin infusion is terminated. Some authors recommend continuing intravenous insulin but at half the initial ordered dose and rate if the correction of hyperglycemia occurs more rapidly than the acidosis.

The benefits of continuous intravenous insulin treatment for diabetic ketoacidosis [15–18, 20, 64, 79] are the same as those for intramuscular treatment: (1) more gentle osmotic correction of hyperosmolar state; (2) reduced risk of hypoglycemia because the decrease is more predictable; (3) decreased severe hypokalemia; (4) decreased theoretical risk of cerebral edema; (5) elimination of guessing the dose required. Repeated intramuscular injections are obviously not necessarily – an especially important benefit when dealing with small children scared of needles anyway. The major drawback may be the need to ensure a continuous intravenous route, especially a problem in the severely dehydrated patient or in the child who is difficult to restrain and keep quiet. Because of the very small amounts of insulin being given per hour, infusion pumps are often required; searching for special apparatus should not cause undue delays in beginning fluid and electrolyte therapy or in actually starting insulin replacement. Often a pediatric infusion set can serve the same purposes and not require specially trained personnel for monitoring.

One additional advantage of the low-dose continuous insulin infusion method is that the infusion rate can be titrated against changes in the blood sugar in an almost instantaneous fashion because of the very short plasma half-life of insulin and the fact that no depot insulin is in use. This can also be a disadvantage if the infusion is inadvertently discontinued. As a precaution against this occurring, the protocol used by this author stipulates that the insulin be hung in piggyback fashion and that the rate of delivery of insulin be controlled and ordered separately from that of the replacement fluids and electrolytes. In addition, the infusion is continued for 15–30 min *after* the dose of subcutaneous insulin is finally administered – as a safeguard to prevent omitting the subcutaneous dose but still discontinuing infused insulin. As more people are using faster acting insulin analogs like lispro insulin (Humalog) and aspart insulin (NovoRapid), this preparatory time may not be as important as with synthetic human or animal insulins.

With both the intramuscular and the continuous intravenous protocols, physician and staff complacency must be avoided. The physician and ancillary personnel thus should have more time to consider precipitating factors and ongoing processes as well as to devote more attention to the fluid and electrolyte abnormalities which may be more lethal to the patient. It would be difficult to argue that low-dose treatment methods are MORE effective than others, but they appear to be simpler to use, easier to teach, and for these reasons, better treatment for diabetic ketoacidosis. A DKA treatment study in Tennessee [80] comparing fast-acting insulin analogs with more conventional therapy suggested equivalent therapeutic results. A population based study comparing bolus insulin injection versus continuous insulin infusion in the treatment of diabetic ketoacidosis suggested decreased hypoglycemia with continuous insulin infusion [73].

*Carbohydrates*

Carbohydrate is necessary as substrate for insulin action if fatty acid breakdown is to be rapidly halted [65]. Under many conditions of DKA presentation, lack of appetite or lack of food and caloric intake is part of the presenting picture so that starvation ketosis may add to the dilemma of ketoacidosis (insulin deficiency) and lactic acidosis (tissue dehydration). This author suggests that glucose be added to the intravenous fluids when the blood glucose is in the 250–300 mg/dl (approximately 14–17 mmol/l) range. For some patients whose problems of ketoacidosis are secondary to dehydration and vomiting, and who enter with blood sugars in the low 300 mg/dl (approximately 17 mmol/l) range, this means giving 5% dextrose with the initial fluid solution. For other patients, this means adding 5–10% dextrose at 5–12 h after initiating treatment with fluids, electrolytes and insulin. Deciding when to add glucose is facilitated with the more predictable decreases in glycemia (~10% blood glucose drop per hour after initial rehydration blood glucose is known) that occur using low-dose insulin infusion protocols and the availability of accurate bedside capillary blood glucose equipment.

*Subsequent Treatment*

Oral feeding should be reinstituted as soon as possible starting with clear liquids and progressing to soft solids and then more complex foods. This 'rule' must be a flexible one and changed according to clinical consideration, state of consciousness, presence or absence of bowel sounds, emesis or nausea, diarrhea, etc. Early refeeding can hasten recovery as it may allow increased potassium replenishment in a safe manner in addition to avoiding the body's need to continue to breakdown fats and continue to make excess ketones. When youngsters start complaining that they are hungry ('starving'), it's usually prudent to begin refeeding!

Subsequent insulin dosage remains a clinical guess which takes into account many factors such as age and weight of the patient, duration of diabetes, prior usual dose of insulin (unless newly diagnosed), other potential confounding factors (pregnancy, renal failure, use of other drugs, etc.). Since average daily insulin doses are approximately 0.5–0.8 units per kilogram in the prepubertal and postpubertal periods and approximately 0.8–1.2 units per kilogram per day in the midst of the pubertal growth spurt; these values can be used to arrive at an estimated insulin dosage and can then be divided into morning and suppertime insulin. Adults generally require about 0.5–0.8 units per kilogram as well although the more obese children, teens and adults may need significantly more insulin because of insulin resistance. Newly diagnosed patients may require much more insulin for several days to several weeks after diagnosis. In any individual patient, extra insulin may be needed for 24–48 h after resolution of the ketoacidotic crisis. Sequential blood sugar determinations are the best guide to insulin dose and help determine when to change to intermediate acting insulin since there are no hard and fast, dogmatic rules in such circumstances and each patient must be treatment in an individualized fashion based upon their actual blood glucose responses.

Philosophy of insulinization [81] dictates which protocols are to be considered for moving to twice, three or four times daily insulin subcutaneously and home treatment. Urinary ketones are not very helpful in making insulin dose decisions once clinical improvement is apparent but they should be expected to slowly and steadily decrease and be eliminated over the subsequent days after an episode of DKA. With availability of blood β-hydroxybutyric acid strips, such monitoring data may help with such treatment decisions. Some period of partial starvation is almost always part of the explanation for persistent mild ketonuria in addition to the fact that the largest proportion of ketoacid, β-hydroxybutyric acid, is cleared to acetone and acetoacetate and this clearance takes place at a slow process for hours or days after the actual acute ketoacidotic crisis [16, 65].

*DKA Complications*

Problems reflecting sodium, potassium, water, acid-base status, calcium/phosphate balance and glucose as well as insulin orders all occur and are often caused by errors in initial or subsequent orders compounded by lack of appropriate monitoring and attention to the fact that DKA is a dynamic state with its treatment adding to changing circumstances (table 6). Emphasis on avoidance of human errors and errors that occur systematically because of changing treatment teams helps to minimize such errors. Missing the underlying precipitating factors whether they are patient and family lack of knowledge concerning home recognition of impending DKA, psychosocial turmoil at home (or at school) or truly events such as pyelonephritis or appendicitis can certainly increase morbidity and mortality significantly. Similarly, in an adult population, attention to cardiovascular and cerebrovascular events as precipitants of DKA or co-existing conditions deserves attention of the emergency room and medical care establishment. Gastric lavage should be considered for any patient truly unconscious because of the frequent association of gastric atony with ketoacidosis especially in adults and the elderly. Used judiciously, however, nasogastric tubes can certainly help to prevent aspiration in the patient who is critically ill (i.e. unconscious or semi-conscious) at presentation. Abdominal pain can be diffuse and severe and perhaps suggest the need for surgical intervention. Amylase elevation, usually of pancreatic origin, is common and sometimes extremely high whereas serum lipase values are often not abnormal [14]. Leukocytosis also can be extreme causing worry about underlying bacterial infection when most often

***Table 6.*** Frequent errors and complications of DKA [35]

| | |
|---|---|
| 1. | Delay in diagnosis |
| 2. | Delay in instituting therapy |
| 3. | Inadequate fluid replacement |
| 4. | Unrecognized hypokalemia |
| 5. | Overemphasis on insulin |
| 6. | Overzealous bicarbonate usage |
| 7. | Hypoglycemia ('changing of the guard' syndrome) |
| 8. | Recurrent ketoacidosis ('changing of the guard' syndrome) |
| 9. | Overzealous phosphate replacement with resultant hypocalcemia |
| 10. | Aspiration |
| 11. | Unrecognized cerebral edema |
| 12. | Unrecognized acute tubular necrosis |
| 13. | Unrecognized cerebral venous thrombosis |
| 14. | Peripheral or pulmonary edema: (Insulin edema vs. fluid overload) |
| 15. | Not treating precipitating etiology of ketoacidosis |
| 16. | Neurologic sequelae |
| 17. | Death |

both the hyperamylasemia and leukocytosis resolve spontaneously with correction of the metabolic acidosis and dehydration [14]. Antibiotics use, per se, is not usually indicated in the treatment of DKA unless a specific infectious disease can be diagnosed.

*Insulin Edema*

The rapid appearance of edema, significant weight gain, abdominal bloating and blurred vision can occur shortly after treatment of DKA is begun. These clinical events are most often noted during or after aggressive treatment of patients with ketoacidosis or in patients in whom the diagnosis of diabetes has been made recently but who have had symptomatic diabetes for a longer duration. Unless underlying cardiovascular or renal disease is present, not often the case in pediatric or adolescent diabetes mellitus, these symptoms usually abate spontaneously and have been called 'insulin edema' for lack of a better explanation [57]. Occasionally the peripheral edema is severe enough that diuretic treatment is needed for several days after the acute DKA event has terminated.

*Cerebral Edema*

Unexpected or unusual neurologic abnormalities including changes in sensorium as well as abnormalities of vital signs (elevated temperature, hypertension, for example) should warrant consideration of either cerebral edema or cerebral venous thrombosis [82]. Imaging with computerized tomography

***Table 7.*** Cerebral edema symptoms and signs [35]

1. Progressive CNS deterioration despite improvement of laboratory parameters
   a. Headache
   b. Increasing lethargy
   c. Failure to regain consciousness
   d. Increased CSF pressure
   e. Abnormal reflexes
2. Eye changes
   a. Papilledema
   b. Unequal intraocular pressure
   c. Increasing intraocular pressure
   d. Decreasing pupillary light reflex
3. Hyperpyrexia
4. Hypertension
5. Diabetes insipidus
6. Abnormal electroencephalogram
7. Abnormal computerized tomography or magnetic resonance imaging consistent with cerebral edema

or magnetic resonance may be the only way to confirm these diagnoses and tell cerebral edema apart from cerebral venous thrombosis but table 7 presents some symptoms and signs that should raise the index of suspicion and warrant fundoscopy as well as closer medical attention so that appropriate treatment can be instituted.

While major treatment errors in fluid, electrolyte or insulin administration occur, most cases of cerebral edema remain unexplainable [50–56, 83]. An adult study from Malta [84] showed suggested cerebral dehydration on CT scanning in all brains of those with diabetes and DKA but did not show any evidence of cerebral edema in adults treated with isotonic vs. hypotonic fluids during the study. Clinical and laboratory parameters often cannot be correlated with the overall severity of the coma episode [85]. Cerebral edema in one Canadian study occurred in 0.2–1% of all cases of DKA in children [86]. Table 7 lists a series of clinical events which should lead one to be suspicious of the possibility of cerebral edema especially if the patient seems to be improving by laboratory parameters but worsening on clinical grounds. Rosenbloom [84] indicated that approximately one half of cases of cerebral edema during DKA, in retrospective analyses, had 'a premonitory period when development…could be suspected on the basis of…' clinical symptoms or signs. Any delay in diagnosis, error in treatment or worsening of acid-base, fluid or electrolyte status of the patient, if left unrecognized (or if treated incorrectly) could be invoked as a possible explanation for inadequate delivery of oxygen to the brain. Brain infarction can occur associated with or after cerebral edema [87]. Those errors that might cause a cardiac arrhythmia or interfere with respiration would be obvious candidates yet such findings are rarely documented as predisposing factors in the development of cerebral edema. Autopsy findings thought to be similar to those seen in the brains of victims of asphyxia and cerebral anoxia have been reported [54]. In a US multicentered study of 61 less than 18-year-old patients with DKA and cerebral edema (n = 61) over a 15-year time period, 28% died of cerebral edema or survived in a vegetative state and another 13% had mild-to-moderate neurologic disabilities as a consequence of the cerebral edema [88].

Other investigators have been able to show some contribution to these changes by hyperosmolality as well as rate of change of osmotic factors ('idiogenic osmols) [89] per se and, because of these changes, recent recommendations have been to replace the overall fluid and electrolyte deficiencies in a slightly slower fashion (i.e. 36 h to calculate replacement rather than 24 h) and with fewer drastic changes (i.e. avoiding boluses of sodium bicarbonate which might be associated with rapid pH changes, rapid movement of potassium and phosphorus; low-dose insulin protocols rather than high-dose bolus insulin to slow down the hyperglycemia-hyperosmotic changes over a somewhat more prolonged recovery period). The assumption that hypoxia is somehow the common final pathway has led to renewed interest in preventing rather than treating this problem. Studies demonstrating abnormalities of a nonspecific nature in electroencephalograms during a variety of phases of diabetic ketoacidosis treatment and more recently, documentation of cerebral edema via sensory evoked potentials [90], with the use of transcranial Doppler ultrasonography [91], computerized tomography or magnetic resonance imaging of the head [50] leads to the conclusion that cerebral edema, in admittedly milder forms, may be present in *all* patients with diabetic ketoacidosis [20]. Low flow oxygen delivery may help decrease cerebral edema associated with DKA just as early recognition via sequential neurologic examination (presence or absence of venous pulsations and sharp disk margins on fundoscopy by the primary health care professional supervising the DKA treatment is important. *Fundoscopy must be done and documented initially and at intervals during treatment to make sure that cerebral edema is recognized.* Early consultation by a neurologist, neurosurgeon and/or ophthalmologist might be indicated if early recognition will lead to better treatment outcomes or if fundoscopy cannot be accomplished by the primary treating health care team. Treatment, once cerebral edema is recognized, is supportive [91, 92] and includes measures to maintain cardiorespiratory function [93] and normal body temperature. The possible benefits of corticosteroids to reduce intracranial pressure and the use of other measures (such as mannitol usually felt to work through the induction of a therapeutic osmotic diuretic effect) have not been scientifically proven but are often added once cerebral edema occurs. If cerebral edema is diagnosed, the intravenous fluid rate should be reduced dramatically, mannitol should be considered at a dose of 1 g/kg intravenously (10–20 g/$m^2$) while hyperventilation may all be helpful in reducing intracranial pressure or its effects on the brain [14]. More recent reviews of cerebral edema in childhood diabetic ketoacidosis [94–96] suggest specific protocols which allow recognition of cerebral edema sufficiently early for intervention while acknowledging that early computed tomograms were often normal.

## Conclusions

DKA is a true pediatric and adult metabolic medical emergency but, like many other disease entities, prevention of DKA decreases morbidity and mortality as well as saves enormous hospital and emergency room costs. Teaching the patient and his/her family to recognize early symptoms and signs of impending DKA should be a high priority. Teaching health care professionals to understand the pathophysiology of DKA helps them provide better patient education and better treatment when DKA occurs.

## References


1 Fleckman AM: Diabetic ketoacidosis. Endocrinol Metab Clin North Am 1993;22:181–207.

2 Rewers A, Chase HP, Mackenzie T, Walravens P, Roback M, Rewers M, Hamman RF, Klingensmith G: Predictors of acute complications in children with type 1 diabetes. J Am Med Assoc 2002;287: 2511–2518.

3 Fishbein H, Palumbo PJ: Acute metabolic complications in diabetes; in Harris MI, Cowie CC, Stern MP (eds): Diabetes in America, ed. 2. Bethesda, NIH/NIDDK, 1995, pp 283–292.

4 American Diabetes Association: Diabetes Statistics. Diabetes Vital Statistics. Alexandria, American Diabetes Association, 1996, pp 13–20.

5 Javor KA, Kotsanos JG, McDonald RC, Baron AD, Kesterson JG, Tierney WM: Diabetic ketoacidosis charges relative to medical charges of adult patients with type 1 diabetes. Diab Care 1997; 20:349–354.

6 Harper DE, Waldrop RD: Infant diabetic ketoacidosis in the emergency department. Southern Med J 1996;89:729–731.

7 Brink SJ: Pediatric and Adolescent Diabetes mellitus. Chicago, Year Book Medical Publishers, 1987.

8 Morris AD, Greene SA, Boyle DIR, MacDonald TM, Newton RW: Direct evidence of missing insulin as a cause of poor glycemic control and diabetic ketoacidosis. J Pediatr Endocr Metab 1997;10:345.

9 Arslanian S, Becker DJ, Drash AL: Diabetes mellitus in the child and adolescent; in Kappy MS, Blizzard RM, Migeon CJ (eds): Wilkins. The Diagnosis and Treatment of Endocrine Disorders in Childhood and Adolescence. Springfield, Thomas, 1994, pp 961–1026.

10 Japan and Pittsburgh Childhood Diabetes Research Groups: Coma at the onset of young insulin dependent diabetes in Japan. Diabetes 1985;34:1214–1216.

11 Blanc N, Polak M, Czernichow P, Tubiana-Rufi N: Acidocetose severe par retard au diagnostic de diabet chez l'enfant. Quatre observations pour alerter les medecins. Arch Pediatrie 1997;4: 550–554.
12 Savova R, Popova G, Koprivarova K, Konstantinova M, Angelova B, Atanasova M, Goranova S, Christov V, Kalinov K: Clinical and laboratory characteristics of type 1 insulin dependent diabetes mellitus at presentation among Bulgarian children. Diab Res Clin Practice 1996;34:S159–S163.
13 Bell DS, Alele J: Diabetic ketoacidosis. Why early detection and aggressive treatment are crucial. Postgrad Med 1997;101:193–198.
14 Singh RK, Perros P, Frier BM: Hospital management of diabetic ketoacidosis: Are clinical guidelines implemented effectively? Diab Med 1997;14:482–486.
15 Dunger DB, Sperling MA, Acerini CL, Bohn DJ, Daneman D, Danne TP, Glaser NS, Hanas R, Hintz RL, Levitsky LL, Savage MO, Tasker RC, Wolfsdorf JI: ESPE;LWPES. ESPE/LWPES consensus statement on diabetic ketoacidosis in children and adolescents. Arch Dis Child 2004; 89:88–94.
16 Davidson MB: Diabetic ketoacidosis and hyperosmolar nonketotic syndrome; in Davidson MB (ed): Diabetes mellitus Diagnosis and Treatment, ed 4. Philadelphia, Saunders, 1997, pp 159–194.
17 Sperling MA: Diabetes mellitus; in Sperling MA (ed): Pediatric Endocrinology. Philadelphia, Saunders, 1997, pp 241–246.
18 Genuth SM: Diabetic ketoacidosis and hyperglycemia hyperosmolar coma. Curr Ther Endoocrinol Metab 1997;6:438–447.
19 Klekamp J, Churchwell KB: Diabetic ketoacidosis in children: Initial clinical assessment and treatment. Pediatr Annals 1996;25387–25393.
20 Brink SJ: Presentation and ketoacidosis; in Kelnar CJH (ed): Childhood and Adolescent Diabetes. London, Chapman & Hall Medical, 1995, pp 226–240.
21 Lifshitz F (ed): Pediatric Endocrinology, ed 3. New York, Marcel Dekker, 1996.
22 Rosenbloom AL, Hanas R: Diabetic ketoacidosis (DKA): Treatment guidelines. Clin Pediatr 1996;261–266.
23 Jackson RI, Guthrie A: The Physiological Management of Diabetes in Children. New York, Elsevier Science, 1986.
24 Travis LB, Brouhard BH, Schreiner BJ (eds): Diabetes mellitus in Children and Adolescents. Philadelphia, Saunders, 1987.
25 Curtis JR, To T, Muirhead S, Cummings E, Daneman D: Recent trends in hospitalization for diabetic ketoacidosis in Ontario children. Diab Care 2002;25:1591–1596.
26 Vanelli M, Chiarelli F: Treatment of diabetic ketoacidosis in children and adolescents. Acta Biomed Ateneo Parmense 2003;74:59–68.
27 Neu A, Willasch A, Ehehalt S, Hub R, Ranke MB: DIARY Group Baden-Wuerttemberg: Ketoacidosis at onset of type 1 diabetes mellitus in children – frequency and clinical presentation. Pediatr Diab 2003;4:77–81.
28 Komulainen J, Lounamaa R, Knip M, Kaprio EA, Akerblom HK: Ketoacidosis at the diagnosis of type 1 insulin dependent diabetes mellitus is related to poor residual beta cell function. Childhood Diabetes in Finland Study Group. Arch Dis Child 1996;75:410–415.
29 Solutes G, Gyro BJ, Levy-Marchal C: Clinical diagnosis of childhood insulin dependent diabetes mellitus. Hungarian Epidemiological Group for Childhood Diabetes. Orvosi Hetilap 1997;138:7–9.
30 Al Khawari M, Shaltout A, Qabazard M, Abdella N, Al Moeman J, Al-Mazidi Z, Mandani F, Moussa MA: Incidence and severity of ketoacidosis in childhood onset diabetes in Kuwait. Diab Res Clin Prac 1997;35:123–128.
31 Rosenbauer J, Icks A, Giani G: Clinical characteristics and predictors of severe ketoacidosis at onset of type 1 diabetes mellitus in children in a North Rhine-Westphalian region, Germany. J Pediatr Endocrin Metab 2002;15:1137–1145.
32 Mallare JT, Cordice CC, Ryan BA, Carey DE, Kreitzer PM, Frank GR: Identifying risk factors for the development of diabetic ketoacidosis in new onset type 1 diabetes mellitus. Clin Pediatr (Phila) 2003;42:591–597.
33 Umpierrez GE, Kelly JP, Navarrete JE, Casals MM, Kitabchi AE: Hyperglycemic crises in urban blacks. Arch Intern Med 1997;157:669–675.

34 DCCT Research Group: Implementation of treatment protocols in the Diabetes Control and Complications Trial. Diab Care 1995;18:361–376.
35 Brink SJ: Diabetic ketoacidosis; in Brink SJ, Serban V (eds): Pediatric and Adolescent Diabetes. Timisoara, Romania, Brumar, 2003, pp 129–160.
36 Laffel L: Sick-day management in type 1 diabetes. Endocrinol Metab Clin N Am 2000;29: 707–223.
37 Alexander V on behalf of DiabNet, Scotland UK. Reducing DKA: A practical approach. J Pediatr Endocrinol Metab 2002;15(suppl):22.
38 Laffel L, Brink S, Kaufman F, Bergenstal R, Fineberg SE, Jenkins M: Frequency of elevations in blood β-hydroxybutyrate (β-OHB) during home monitoring and association with glycemia in insulin-treated children and adults. American Diabetes Association Annual Scientific Meeting, 2000.
39 Fineberg SE, Brink S, Kaufman F, Bergenstal R, Hicks C, Rice KR, Pasquarello C: Comparison of blood beta-hydroxybutyrate and urine ketones in 4 weeks of home monitoring by insulin-requiring children and adults. American Diabetes Association Annual Scientific Meeting, 2000.
40 Brink SJ, Moltz KC, Holverson M, Carpenter S, Kaufman F, Rice K, Pasquarello C, Laffel L: Association of blood B-hydroxybutyrate with urine ketones and glycemia in children with type 1 diabetes during 4 weeks of home monitoring. ISPAD Annual Scientific Meeting, Los Angeles, 2000.
41 Laffel LMB, Loughlin CA, Tovar A, Zuehlke JB, Moltz KC, Miller M, Brink S: Sick day Management (SDM) using Blood beta hydroxybutyrate vs urine ketones significantly reduces hospital visits in youth with T1DM: A randomized clinical trial. American Diabetes Association Annual Scientific Meeting Poster Session, 2002.
42 Samuelsson U, Ludvigsson J: When should determination of ketonemia be recommended? Diabetes Technol Ther 2002;4:645–650.
43 Golden MP, Herrold AJ, Orr D: An approach to prevention of recurrent diabetic ketoacidosis in the pediatric population. J Pediatr 1985;107:195–200.
44 Skinner TC: Recurrent diabetic ketoacidosis: Causes, prevention and management. Horm Res 1992;57(S1):78–80.
45 Citrin W, Tapp JT, Wine HE: Diabetes counseling issues: The patient and the family; in Brink SJ (ed): Pediatric and Adolescent Diabetes mellitus. Chicago, Year Book Medical Publishers, 1987, pp 369–690.
46 Gill GV, Lucas S, Kent LA: Prevalence and characteristics of brittle diabetes in Britain. Q J Med 1996;89:839–843.
47 Dumont RH, Jacobson AM, Cole C, Hauser St, Wolfsdorf JI, Willet JB, Milley JE, Wertlieb D: Psychosocial predictors of acute complications of diabetic youth. Diab Med 1995;12:612–618.
48 Polonsky WH, Anderson BJ, Lohrer PA, Aponte JE, Jacobson Am, Cole CF: Insulin omission in women with IDDM. Diab Care 1994;17:1178–1185.
49 Thompson CJ, Cummings F, Chalmers J, Newton RW: Abnormal insulin treatment behavior: A major cause of ketoacidosis in the young adult. Diab Med 1995;12:429–432.
50 Fiese BH: Family context in pediatric psychology from a transactional perspective: Family rituals and stories as examples. J Pediatr Psychol 1997;22:183–196.
51 Steindel B, Kaufman F, Roe T: Continuous subcutaneous insulin infusion in poorly controlled patients with type 1 diabetes mellitus. Diabetes 1993;42(S1):A587.
52 Blacket PR: Insulin pump treatment for recurrent ketoacidosis in adolescence. Diab Care 1995;18:881–882.
53 Fulop M, Tannenbaum H, Dreyer N: Ketotic hyperosmolar coma. Lancet 1973;ii:637.
54 Krane EJ, Rockoff MD, Wollman JK, Wolfsdorf JI: Subclinical brain swelling in children during treatment of diabetic ketoacidosis. N Engl J Med 1985;312:1147–1151.
55 Fiordalisi I, Harris Wl, Novotny W, Mosovich LL, Finberg L: Minimizing symptomatic brain swelling by preventing low effective osmolality during repair of diabetic ketoacidemia. Pediatr Res 1992;31:185A.
56 Finberg L: Why do patients with diabetic ketoacidosis have cerebral swelling and why does treatment sometimes make it worse? Arch Pediatr Adol Med 1996;150:785–786.

Chiarelli F, Dahl-Jørgensen K, Kiess W (eds): Diabetes in Childhood and Adolescence.
Pediatr Adolesc Med. Basel, Karger, 2005, vol 10, pp 122–138

# Insulin Treatment

*Thomas M. Kapellen, A. Galler, W. Kiess*

Universitätsklinik und Poliklinik für Kinder und Jugendliche,
Universität Leipzig, Leipzig, Germany

People with type 1 diabetes mellitus are dependent on insulin for survival. Therefore, insulin should be available for all patients with type 1 diabetes mellitus (ISPAD guidelines). It should be pointed out to the patients and their parents that there is no alternative treatment other than insulin. On the other hand, insulin treatment regimens should always be individualized. Each child and family should be informed about the possible treatment regimens and their pros and cons. In principal, everything is allowed as long as it is convenient and offers the best quality of life in combination with good metabolic control.

## Insulin Action and Types of Insulin

Insulin is the primary medication in treatment of type 1 diabetes. For many years only regular and intermediate-acting neutral protamine Hagedorn (NPH) insulin were used. Purified porcine and bovine insulin is now rarely used since human insulin is readily available. Therefore, first-line therapy in children is preferably human insulin. Porcine insulin is used especially in Germany as zinc insulin Semilente® in adolescents with the dawn phenomenon. Other indications for porcine insulin include insulin resistance because of insulin antibodies. New insulins were created in the 1990s with alteration of the amino acid sequence in order to change absorption kinetics. Data provided by the manufacturers are available for each insulin preparation in respect to pharmacokinetics and pharmacodynamics (table 1). Despite these published data, we know that there is a wide range of inter- and intra-individual variability in insulin action [12].

*Table 1.* Insulins and their action profile after subcutaneous injection (mean of manufacturers' instructions)

| Insulin type | Start of action | Peak of action h | Duration h |
|---|---|---|---|
| *Rapid-acting insulin* | | | |
| Analogue (Lispro, Aspart) | 15–(30) min | 1–(2) | 3–4 |
| *Short-acting insulin* | | | |
| Regular (human) insulin | 30–60 min | 2–4 | 4–6–(7) |
| *Basal intermediate-/long-acting Insulin* | | | |
| NPH – insulin (human isophane) | 1–2 h | 4–6–8 | 8–12–18 |
| Amorphous zinc insulin (porcine) (Semilente®) | 1–2 h | 6–8 | 12–18 |
| Zinc insulin (human) (Monotard®) | 1–2 h | 6–8 | 12–18 |
| *Long-acting analogues* | | | |
| Glargine® | 2–4 h | none | 24 |
| Detemir® | 1–2 h | 6–12 | 20–24 |

Insulin's actions are mediated by binding to its receptor. This results in multiple effects on carbohydrate, lipid, and protein metabolism. Some of the effects are as follows:

- Utilization of glucose as an energy source
- Storage of glucose as glycogen
- Inhibition of liver enzymes for endogenous glucose release
- Inhibition of lipolysis
- Promotion of amino acid uptake and storage
- Stimulation of cell growth and multiplication

## Rapid-Acting Insulin (Insulin Analogues)

Insulin tends to aggregate into dimers or hexamers when injected subcutaneously. This aggregation retards the absorption of regular insulin. Insulin lispro and aspart have been modified from regular human insulin due to a change in amino acid structure and do not form dimers or hexamers. The rapid-acting insulin can be injected at the time of meals without an injection-meal interval. Therefore, the most important indication for rapid-acting analogues is the child or toddler with unpredictable eating habits [3]. Because of the very immediate onset of action, high blood glucose levels can be corrected faster with rapid- than with short-acting insulin. Therefore, in hyperglycemia, e.g. on sick days, analogues would be an alternative. In CSII rapid-acting insulin is now more widely used in pediatric patients because of the benefit of short action. Colquitt and coworkers report on a modest reduction of HbA1c of 0.26% in a meta-analysis of 6 randomized controlled trials in pump treatment. Some authors even report on lower risk of nocturnal hypoglycemia with the use of lispro as evening mealtime insulin [7]. Recently, the benefit of rapid-acting insulin analogues versus regular insulin was reviewed by a group of Cochrane reviewers [23]. This analysis suggests only a minor benefit of rapid-acting insulin analogues in the majority of patients. In the subgroup analysis of the pediatric studies there was a significant reduction of HbA1c. Some reviewed studies reported a reduction of the overall rate of hypoglycemic episodes. Severe hypoglycemia was not reduced in children and adolescents. The reviewers suggest a cautious response of physicians to the vigorous promotion of insulin analogues by the manufacturers until long-term safety data are available.

### Short-Acting Insulin

Short-acting insulin or regular insulin is still the major insulin treatment component; vast experience and a body of literature of its use is available. Regular insulin is sold as a clear solution. Human regular insulin can also be injected intravenously for example as medication during sick days, for ketoacidosis or before and during operations. It is widely used in combination with NPH insulin as a pre-meal bolus. For this purpose, it should be injected about 15–30 min before mealtimes. Used as mealtime insulin, the action lasts for an additional meal after about 2–3 h of injection and is used in our personal experience to cover breakfast and second breakfast (in school) or lunch and tea-time. Sometimes a late meal is required before sleep to avoid nocturnal hypoglycemia when regular insulin is used at dinner time.

### Intermediate-Acting Insulin

Besides NPH insulin, zinc-delayed insulins are available for intermediate basal insulin substitution. NPH insulin is widely used for basal bolus regimen in combination with short-acting or rapid-acting insulin. It can also be mixed in a syringe with regular insulin for a twice daily regimen. NPH insulin is a cloudy suspension. Vials therefore have to be properly mixed prior to each use and pens containing NPH need to be tipped at least 20 times to ensure adequate mixing and concentration. Porcine zinc insulin (Semilente®) injected late at night is frequently used in Europe by adolescents with dawn-phenomenon [16] because of its later peak than NPH insulin. In our opinion, human zinc insulin

(Monotard®) is only indicated if other regimens, e.g. for dawn phenomenon, did not result in good metabolic control. Anyhow, this intermediate-acting insulin tends to have a very variable peak of biological action and therefore is hard to dose.

### Long-Acting Insulin Analogues

Glargine was the first long-acting insulin analogue available for children and adolescents. The clear acidic solution of insulin glargine precipitates after injection and has a smooth, almost peakless 24-hour action profile. One should be aware that glargine cannot be mixed with any other insulin. There are several clinical trials with different end points that showed a reduction of hypoglycemic events especially at night time [2, 10, 20, 24]. However, glycemic control with glargine was similar as compared with NPH in most studies. Schober et al. [24] could show a slight but not significantly reduced number of cases of severe hypoglycemia. In other published trials, definition of hypoglycemia varied and results are therefore hard to compare. Insulin detemir is another basal insulin analogue. The amino acid threonine is removed at position B30. Due to acetylation of a 14-carbon myristol fatty acid to lysine at position B29 binding to albumin is enabled. This contributes to protracted release and action. Large clinical trials with children have not yet been published. Experience with adults shows a smoothened time action profile and reduced risk of hypoglycemic events and nocturnal hypoglycemia. Variability of fasting plasma glucose levels could also be reduced but metabolic control measured as HbA1c was similar in comparison to NPH control group [13, 25]. Danne et al. [4] recently published pharmacokinetic profiles of insulin detemir in children and adolescents. They found similar profiles across all age groups with detemir in comparison to a more age- and dose-related profile in NPH. The authors concluded that detemir could be used in all age groups with the same titration recommendations.

### Premixed Insulin Preparations

There are several premixed combinations of short- and rapid-acting insulin with NPH available in variable ratios. We only very rarely use premixed insulin and prefer dose-adjusted mixing pre-injection in a syringe. This is because it is easier to individualize insulin dosing and adapt the dose of the short-acting insulin for correction of hyperglycemia or variable meals. However, in some situations premixed combinations could be useful, especially in families where mixing insulin is difficult, e.g. for dyscalculia or other impairments or for psychosocial reasons.

### Free Mixing of Insulin

The short- or rapid-acting insulin should be drawn up in the syringe before the intermediate insulin. This prevents contamination of the short- or rapid-acting insulin vial and therefore prevents the conversion of the short-acting insulin into a longer-acting form. NPH insulin can be mixed with rapid- and short-acting insulin in the same syringe or vial without affecting the absorption profile of the rapid- or short-acting insulin [11, 19].

Glargine cannot be mixed. Intermediate and long-acting insulins should also not be mixed with each other. We do not recommend mixing with zinc-containing insulin.

### Storage

Unused insulin vials should be stored in the refrigerator (4–8°C). At room temperature insulin is stable for several weeks. Our recommendation is to use an opened vial for a maximum of 4 weeks when kept at room temperature. If the vial is exposed to higher temperatures (i.e. in the tropics or left in the car in summer) or direct sun or heat by ovens, the containing insulin may lose potency. Expiry dates of the manufacturers should be adhered to. When going on vacation, insulin should be stored in a cold bag or refrigerator in warm countries. If patients go skiing insulin should be kept warm near the body and freezing should be avoided.

### Insulin Concentrations

Insulin is available in two different concentrations depending on the country. One unit of insulin contains approximately 36 μg or 6 nmol of insulin. The most common concentration available all over the world is 100 U/ml (U100). In some European countries U40 (40 U/ml) is still available. In these countries suitable syringes for this concentration are available. Pen devices are only filled with U100 insulin all over the world.

If very low doses are needed for the treatment of toddlers or babies, dilutions of U10 can be processed by parents, caregivers or pharmacists. For this purpose, diluents are available from the different manufacturers. Special

*Table 2.* Influences on insulin absorption and action

| Influence factors | Effect on absorption |
|---|---|
| Insulin preparation | depending on the preparation longer or shorter action |
| Injection site | abdomen > thigh > buttocks |
| Depth of injection | intramuscular faster absorption than subcutaneous |
| Lipodystrophy | worse absorption at lipohypertrophic or atrophic sites |
| Insulin dose | the larger the dose the longer the absorption |
| Temperature | higher temperature at injection site may accelerate absorption |
| Exercise | higher blood flow may accelerate absorption |

care must be paid to the preparation and the use of standard syringes with such diluted insulins to ensure correct dosing.

## Insulin Absorption

Insulin absorption and action is dependent on various influences (table 2). The injection site contributes to absorption kinetics. Insulin is absorbed fastest if injected into the abdominal subcutis followed by the buttocks and slowest via the thigh. Thus, the recommendation is to inject rapid- and short-acting insulins into the abdominal wall. Long-acting insulins and evening doses of intermediate-acting insulins are recommended to be injected into the thigh to optimize the overnight profile of insulin action. Some people use the upper arm as the injection site; however, there is no general recommendation for this site because of the very thin layer of subcutaneous fat especially in younger children. This might increase the risk of an intramuscular injection with very fast absorption and a high risk of hypoglycemia. If insulin is injected into the muscle instead of the subcutaneous fat, the absorption is much faster and is not as consistent as with subcutaneous injection. This difference is less obvious with rapid-acting insulins. Therefore, a subcutaneous injection is preferred to obtain a slower and predictable absorption profile. The depth of the injection on different injection sites could contribute to the absorption due to accidental intramuscular injection. There is a significant risk for intramuscular injections in lean individuals and especially in boys. Young boys have a mean subcutis thickness of 9–10 mm in the abdomen and thighs and 19 mm in the buttocks. Girls have an abdominal and thigh subcutis thickness of 13–15 mm measured by ultrasound without compression compared to 26 mm in the buttocks [1]. Therefore, most children should use 8-mm needles, for lean boys 5 or 6 mm could be long enough especially if pen devices are used without a two-finger pitch. Intramuscular injection can be minimized by using the two-finger pitch technique.

The presence of lipohypertrophy, a common problem in diabetes treatment, also affects absorption. Lipohypertrophic sites have been found in 24% of adult patients with type 1 diabetes [18]. Raile et al. [21] found lipohypertrophy of injection sites in more than 50% of children. This can considerably affect the absorption of the injected insulin. Rotation of injection sites can avoid development of lipohypertrophic changes and is therefore recommended. Lipoatrophy is less common with the use of human insulins. Raile et al. [21] found lipoatrophic changes in 4 of 112 children. Factors associated with the development of lipodystrophy of injection sites are insulin antibodies.

Insulin absorption may be increased with higher body temperature or higher temperature of the injection site related to an increased subcutaneous blood flow. The surrounding temperature can also have an influence on body temperature (especially if a person is not used to hot weather). Exercise can also increase the subcutaneous blood flow. The thigh should therefore be avoided as an injection site prior or immediately after exercise.

Insulin has dose-dependent absorption kinetics. Small doses are absorbed faster than large doses. Very large doses (i.e. depending on age more than 20 IU) should be divided and injected at different injection sites for better resorption.

### Insulin Regimens

In addition to good metabolic control and near-normal glucose levels individual treatment goals are different from patient to patient. Insulin treatment should be individually adapted to the patients' and families' conditions. To reach physiological insulin replacement with subcutaneous injections of insulin is by definition very difficult. The more sophisticated the treatment regimen, the more closely can physiological insulin release be mimicked. With new treatment options like insulin analogues or insulin pump treatment, this goal can possibly be reached in a better way. In any case, treatment has to be accepted and carried out by the patient and the families and treatment adherence and compliance are therefore crucial. In pediatric diabetology every strategy should be allowed to get the best metabolic control with good adherence and optimal quality of life.

The selected insulin regimen for each patient is therefore dependent on a variety of factors including the following:

- Patients' and families' skills
- Age
- Duration of diabetes
- Endogenous insulin production (honeymoon period),

- Families' and patients' lifestyle
- Metabolic targets (of the diabetes team and the patient)
- Dietary management and preferences
- Psychosocial requirements (e.g. ethnical cultural beliefs)
- Physical activities
- Skills of patient and family
- Frequency of severe hypoglycemic events
- Associated conditions or complications (see chapter other complications)
- Experience of the pediatric diabetes team

Therefore, nowadays terms like conventional or intensive insulin treatment should no longer be used but the individual and flexible treatment regimen should be described for each patient under the given circumstances.

There is no doubt that intensified insulin treatment could reduce the risk of the development of complications in type 1 diabetes [5, 6]. This can be reached most easily by a basal-bolus regimen in adults. In the adolescent group in the DDCT study, an intensified diabetes management with multiple glucose measurements, insulin injections and dose adjustment also resulted in good metabolic control and reduced diabetic complications. In addition, weight gain and hypoglycemia were increased. Therefore, adolescents should preferably all be treated with a basal-bolus regimen if they can manage this at all. On the other hand, in the situation of partial remission one or two daily injections can be suitable to introduce the patient and family in diabetes management relatively easily. In summary, many individual regimens are in common use with limited data from clinical trials.

### One Injection Daily

This regimen is very rarely appropriate but may be indicated in patients with a profound remission. We have used this in only a very few patients for a short period of time.

### Two Daily Injections

Free mixed or premixed rapid- or short-acting insulin with intermediate-acting insulin is given before breakfast and before the evening meal. Dose adjustment is possible with variability of the carbohydrate content of breakfast and dinner. We use this regimen in younger children with relatively fixed carbohydrate balance and partial remission. 60–75% of the total daily insulin dose is given in the morning and 25–40% in the evening. Approximately 30% of each dose is short-acting insulin.

### Three Daily Injections

Free mixed or premixed rapid- or short-acting insulin with intermediate insulin is given before breakfast and before the evening meal. For lunch or afternoon snack, a short- or rapid-acting insulin is injected. We use this regimen when basal insulin supply is too short in the afternoon to maintain normal blood glucose levels in the evening especially in younger children and schoolchildren when a two-injection regimen was not able to lead to normoglycemia.

### Four or More Injections per Day

Short- or rapid-acting insulin given before the main meals with intermediate insulin given in the morning and evening (or bedtime) or combined with once-daily glargine. If treatment is sophisticated with dose adjustment for every mealtime and a fixed basal insulin supply, the so-called basal-bolus regimen is performed. This regimen is used in schoolchildren, adolescents and adults. To some extent, we use a basal-bolus regimen in young children for more flexibility or to adhere to a very variable daily lifestyle. 40–60% of the daily given insulin dose is for the basal insulin supply, the remainder is divided up into pre-meal boluses. Glargine may usually be injected once daily with a dose of about 40% of daily insulin requirement.

### Insulin Pump Therapy (Continuous Subcutaneous Insulin Infusion = CSII)

This treatment regimen can supply insulin via the most physiologic manner. The pump contains short- or rapid-acting insulin with a programmed basal insulin delivery. For every meal (or snack) patients have to calculate the required insulin dose and a bolus must be activated. For more details, see the chapter by Phillip et al. [pp. 150–162].

### Treatment Goals

Our diabetes clinic emphasizes the targets of glycemic control described in the consensus guidelines of the International Society for Pediatric and Adolescent Diabetes (ISPAD) like the German pediatric diabetes guidelines do (AGPD) (table 3).

***Table 3.*** Treatment goals (ISPAD Consensus Guidelines 2000)

| Biochemical level of control | Ideal (nondiabetic) | Optimal | Suboptimal | High-risk (action required) |
|---|---|---|---|---|
| Preprandial or fasting blood glucose, mmol/l | 3.6–6.1 | 4.0–7.0 | >8.0 | >9.0 |
| Postprandial blood glucose, mmol/l | 4.4–7.0 | 5.0–11.0 | 11.0–14.0 | >14.0 |
| Nocturnal blood glucose, mmol/l | 3.6–6.0 | Not <3.6 | <3.6 or >9.0 | <3.0 or >11.0 |
| HbA1c, % (DCCT standardized) | <6.05 | <7.6 | 7.6–9.0 | >9.0 |

It has to be emphasized that individual treatment goals have to be discussed and agreed upon with the patient and his/her family under any circumstances.

## Insulin Delivery Devices

*Insulin Syringes*

There are disposable plastic syringes designed for single use available for U40 (in some European countries) and U100 in different sizes (20, 25, 30, 40, 50 and 100 units) Needle lengths are 8, 12 and 12.7 mm. One should pay attention to the different concentrations and the adequate syringes. Our patients usually use the same syringe for 1 day. Disposal of syringes and needles should be managed in a safe and hygienic way (e.g. use of special, capped plastic containers).

*Insulin Pens*

All manufacturers of insulin provide pen devices for their pre-filled cartridges. Cartridges of rapid-acting, short-acting and intermediate-acting insulin as well as for premixed formulations and for glargine and detemir are available. Monotard® and Semilente® can only be injected by syringe. The pen-insulin concentration is U100. Most pens are adjustable in 1-unit steps, one pen is available that can be adjusted in 0.5-unit steps. Pen needles are available in lengths of 5, 6, 8, 12 and 12.7 mm. Some manufacturers provide disposable pens. Attention has to be paid to the injection of NPH insulin: The pen has to be tipped about 20 times before the suspension is injectable in order to secure uniform concentration of the insulin preparation. Before injection, the patient should check that the needle is filled with insulin by injecting 1–2 units into the air. The injection time should be minimal 10 s to ensure that the whole dose has reached the subcutaneous space. Injections of insulin with a pen seem to be as accurate as injections with an insulin syringe [8]. The use of pen devices is in our opinion much easier even for children of age 8–10 years than the use of syringes.

### Automatic Injection Devices

There are attachments to some pens or syringes available that automatically insert the needle into the skin. The needle is hidden in these devices until they are activated. These devices may be of help in some cases of needle phobia.

### Jet Injection Devices

Jet injectors use high pressure air to form a thin stream of injected solution that penetrates the skin. There are no long-term data available for the systems. Short-term metabolic control seems to be similar to that for needles as reported in an old study with a system that is no longer available [15]. The German working group for pediatric diabetes (AGPD) recommends avoiding the use of jet injectors because of the lack of data available on the accuracy of the systems.

### Insulin Pumps

There are several pumps available now with different features and styling. Management of insulin treatment with pumps is increasing all over the world now. Even babies and toddlers are treated with CSII. We try to carefully evaluate if a patient and the family is a candidate for pump therapy [see chapter by Phillip et al., pp. 150–162]. One has to keep in mind that this regimen is almost doubly cost intensive as a basis bolus regimen using pen/syringe injections. A meta-analysis of pump therapy mainly in adolescents showed an improvement in HbA1c of about 1.2% [27]! One randomized controlled cross-over designed trial in children and adolescents was published recently by Weintrob et al. [26]. These authors reported a similar metabolic control (HbA1c) in the CSII and basis-bolus group [26].

*Table 4.* Dose adjustment tables used in the Hospital for Children and Adolescents, University of Leipzig (examples dependent on age, daytime and other individual factors)

| Blood glucose level | Dose for young children, U | Dose for schoolchildren, U | Dose for adolescents, U |
|---|---|---|---|
| <3.0 mmol/l | −0.5 | −1.0 | −2.0 |
| 3.0–4.9 mmol/l | −0.25 | −0.5 | −1.0 |
| 5.0–7.9 mmol/l | ±0 | ±0 | ±0 |
| 8.0–9.9 mmol/l | +0.25 | +0.5 | +1.0 |
| 10.0–11.9 mmol/l | +0.5 | +1.0 | +2.0 |
| 12.0–13.9 mmol/l | +0.75 | +1.5 | +3.0 |
| >14.0 mmol/l | +1.0 | +2.0 | +4.0 |

− = Decrease of dose adjustment; + = increase of dose adjustment.

## Practical Aspects of Insulin Treatment

Independent of the regimen used, our patients and families are educated that hyperglycemia should be corrected by rapid- or short-acting insulin. Every patient gets an individual dose adjustment table fixed in their diabetes diary (table 4). Dose adjustment varies depending on age, daytime and other individual factors. An individual patient often has different daytime-dependent dose adjustments.

All our patients are educated in carbohydrate counting. Depending on the regimen when short- or rapid-acting insulin is injected, a dose adjustment for more or less eaten carbohydrates can be made. In the following section personal treatment experiences and strategies of our group are reported. Where available, evidence-based recommendations have been added from the literature.

## Treatment in the Remission Phase

Most patients will have a shorter or longer period of partial remission (in the literature defined as insulin requirement less than 0.5 units/kg body weight/day). For young and school-aged children, we usually try a two-injections regimen in this phase. This is an easy way to achieve good metabolic control and to get acquainted with diabetes management skills. However, in adolescents and children with vigorous exercise (e.g. competitive sports) or unusual eating habits, we tend to introduce a basis-bolus regimen already at this early phase if at all possible.

### Toddlers and Preschool Children

In the preschool age one of the most important treatment goals is the avoidance of severe hypoglycemic events because of the impact on psychomotor development [9, 14]. Our strategy is therefore a minimal number of injections with minimal hypoglycemia and good metabolic control. Many of these patients are on a two- to three-injection regimen. Daily insulin requirement is about 0.6–1.0 units/kg/day beyond the remission phase.

Some toddlers tend to have very different carbohydrate consumption at meals. In these cases, we recommend rapid-acting insulin and injection after the meal [3]. If nocturnal hypoglycemia is a major problem CSII should be considered. When injections in kindergarten or school are needed, a home-care nurse can be engaged to ensure this if the parents are not available.

### Schoolchildren

The older the children, the more can the diabetes management be devised independent from caretakers. However, there is no common age at which children are considered able to inject their insulin independently. We have made the experience that in diabetes camps independence from the parents can be taught easily. Most schoolchildren in our clinic are on a four-injection regimen adhering to a basal bolus principle. Dose adjustment is done at every mealtime. In the German school system, it is common to have a second breakfast. This can be covered by short-acting insulin in the morning. For lunch and dinner we frequently use rapid-acting insulin.

### Adolescents

One of the therapeutic challenges in this age group is the so-called dawn phenomenon. Due to counterregulatory hormones (i.e. growth hormone, cortisol, adrenalin) fasting glucose levels are elevated. A first treatment option is to inject more NPH insulin as late as possible at bedtime (22.00–23.00 h). If nocturnal hypoglycemic episodes occur or fasting glucose levels are still too high, the regimen must be changed. The use of Semilente as the nocturnal intermediate insulin injected at late night has been recommended [16]. Dosage is 40–60% of prior evening dose of NPH. Some patients still have unsatisfactory fasting blood glucose levels. Another option could be glargine injected in the evening. When Semilente does not lead to good metabolic control, CSII to maintain an individual basal nocturnal insulin supply is introduced. In addition, the common problem in some adolescents is noncompliance or adherence difficulties. In this case, simplification of the insulin regimen can sometimes avoid ketoacidosis and at least ensure minimal insulin supply. Insulin requirements during puberty are usually about 1.0–2.0 units/kg/day. Contra-insulinemic hormones and relative insulin resistance cause such relatively high insulin requirements in adolescents. Especially adolescent girls and obese patients tend to develop insulin resistance. Girls also seem to require more insulin during their menses. Some authors recommend metformin as an adjunct therapy in adolescents with type 1 diabetes and insulin resistance. Hamilton et al. [17] studied 27 adolescents with poor metabolic control in a randomized placebo-controlled design over 3 months. Adolescents treated with metformin twice daily up to 2,000 mg/day had a lower HbA1c (0.6%), a decreased insulin requirement and no weight gain at the end of the study. Another trial showed a decrease in HbA1c of 0.9% after 3 months of adjunct metformin treatment [22]. No long-term follow-up of these groups is available yet.

### Special Recommendations

Dose adjustment for days of physical activity and sports will be discussed in the chapter on exercise [pp. 181–189].

Another situation where insulin dose adjustment is required is sick day management. In the case of diarrhea and vomiting, the dose should be reduced. Basal insulin supply is nearly the same in the basis-bolus regimen whereas in the two-injections regimen the basal insulin in the morning should also be reduced (about 30%). In case of nausea and vomiting short-acting insulin should be injected with a longer time interval after food intake. Blood glucose levels should be measured at least every 2 h. Interpretation of ketonuria is difficult in this situation because of fasting. If insulin was already injected before recognizing the sickness, tea with sugar or coke could maintain an acceptable blood glucose level. In case of vomiting and imminent hypoglycemia glucose must be injected. Alternatively, small doses of glucagon could be repeatedly injected subcutaneously. In case of concomitant disease or surgery, we have developed a treatment scheme that is available in the emergency room and at the pediatric surgery department (table 5).

In case of infectious disease with fever most patients require 20–40% more insulin (basal and mealtime bolus). Some toddlers even have a higher insulin requirement in case of viral infection with mild symptoms. Cautious dose adjustment with correction of high blood glucose levels can be reached with regular blood glucose measurements and additional rapid- or short-acting insulin injections.

***Table 5.*** Emergency treatment for sick day, concomitant disease or surgery (Hospital for Children and Adolescents, University of Leipzig)

Infusion over two lines

(1) 2/3 electrolyte-glucose 5%
  0–6 years: 50 ml/kg/12 h (= 2.5g glucose/kg/12 h)
  >6 years: 40 ml/kg/12 h (= 2.0 g glucose/kg/12 h)

(2) Short-acting insulin bypass
  0.5 U insulin/kg/day in 50 ml NaCl 0.9%
  Regular dosage: 0.04 U/kg/h
  Insulin dose adjustment as follows:

Dose adjustment of insulin bypass after measurement of blood glucose level every hour

| Blood glucose level | Insulin dose U/kg/h | Infusion velocity ml/h |
|---|---|---|
| <4.0 mmol/l | 0 | 0 |
| 4.0–5.9 mmol/l | 0.02 | 2.0 |
| 6.0–7.9 mmol/l | 0.04 | 4.0 |
| 8.0–9.9 mmol/l | 0.06 | 6.0 |
| 10.0–12.0 mmol/l | 0.08 | 8.0 |
| >12.0 mmol/l | 0.1 | 10.0 |

## Conclusion

The aim of insulin treatment strategies is to provide near physiological insulin replacement and hence normoglycemia. Under different circumstances this can be managed by individual regimens with insulins using different devices. The basic treatment principle is an individualized treatment strategy that leads to good metabolic control with good quality of life for the patients and their families.

*'Everything should be allowed that achieves these goals.'*

## References

1 Birkebaek NH, Johansen A, Solvig J: Cutis/subcutis thickness at insulin injection sites and localization of simulated insulin boluses in children with type 1 diabetes mellitus: Need for individualization of injection technique? Diabet Med 1998;15:965–971.

2 Chase PH, Dixon B, Pearson J, Fiallo-Sharer R, Walravens P, Klingensmith G, Rewers M, Garg SK: Reduced hypoglycemic episodes and improved glycemic control in children with type 1 diabetes using insulin glargine and neutral protamin Hagedorn insulin. J Pediatr 2003;143: 737–740.

3 Danne T, Aman A, Schober E, Deiss D, Jacobsen JL, Friberg HH, Jensen LH: A comparison of postprandial and preprandial administration of insulin Aspart in children and adolescents with type 1 diabetes. Diabetes Care 2003;26:2359–2364.
4 Danne T, Lüpke K, Walte K, von Schütz W, Gall M-A: Insulin detemir is characterized by a consistent pharmacokinetic profile across age groups in children, adolescents, and adults with type 1 diabetes. Diabetes Care 2003;26:3087–3092.
5 Diabetes Control and Complications Trial Research Group: Effect of intensive diabetes treatment on the development and progression of long-term complications in adolescents with insulin-dependent diabetes mellitus: Diabetes Control and Complications Trial. J Pediatr 1994;125: 177–881.
6 The Diabetes Control and Complications Trial Research Group: The effect of intensive treatment of diabetes on the development and progression of long-term complications in insulin-dependent diabetes mellitus. N Engl J Med1993;329:977–986.
7 Ford-Adams ME, Murphy NP, Moore EJ, Edge JA, Ong KL, Watts AP, Acerini CL, Dunger DB: Insulin lispro: A potential role in preventing nocturnal hypoglycemia in young children with diabetes mellitus. Diabet Med 2003;20:656–660.
8 Gnanalingham MG, Newland P, Smith CP: Accuracy and reproducibility of low dose insulin administration using pen-injectors and syringes. Arch Dis Child 1998;79:59–62.
9 Hannonen R, Tupola S, Ahonen T, Riikonen R: Neurocognitive functioning in children with type-1 diabetes with and without episodes of severe hypoglycaemia. Dev Med Child Neurol 2003; 45:262–268.
10 Hathout EH, Fujishige L, Geach J, Ischandar M, Marou S, Mace JW: Effect of therapy with insulin glargine (Lantus) on glycemic control in toddlers, children, and adolescents with diabetes. Diabetes Technol Ther 2003;5:801–806.
11 Heine RJ, Bilo HJ, Fonk T, van der Meer J, van der Veen EA: Absorption kinetics and action profiles of mixtures of short- and intermediate-acting insulins. Diabetologie 1986;27:558–562.
12 Heinemann L: Variability of insulin absorption and insulin action. Diabetes Technol Ther 2002;4:673–682.
13 Hermansen K, Madsbad S, Perrild H, Kristensen A, Axelsen M: Comparison of the soluble basal insulin analog insulin detemir with NPH insulin: A randomized open crossover trial in type 1 diabetic subjects on basal-bolus therapy. Diabetes Care 2001;24:296–301.
14 Hershey T, Lillie R, Sadler M, White NH: The effect of severe hypoglycaemia on cognition in children and adolescents with type 1 diabetes mellitus. Diab Nutr Metab 2002;15:426–429.
15 Houtzagers CM, Visser AP, Berntzen PA, Heine RJ, van der Veen EA: The Medi-Jector2: Efficacy and acceptability in insulin dependent diabetic patients with and without needle phobia. Diab Med 1988;5:135–138.
16 Holl RW, Teller WM, Heinze E: Semilente at bedtime is superior to NPH-insulin for the suppression of the dawn-phenomenon in adolescents with type 1 diabetes. Exp Clin Endocrinol Diab 1996;104:360–364.
17 Hamilton J, Cummings E, Zdravkovic V, Finegood D, Daneman D: Metformin as an adjunct therapy in adolescents with type 1 diabetes and insulin resistance. Diabetes Care 2003;26:138–143.
18 Hauner H, Stockamp B, Haastert B: Prevalence of lipohypertrophy in insulin-treated diabetic patients and predisposing factors. Exp Clin Endocrinol Diab 1996;104:106–110.
19 Joseph SE, Korzon-Burakowska A, Woodworth JR, Evans M, Hopkins D, Janes JM, Amiel SA: The action profile of lispro is not blunted by mixing in the syringe with NPH insulin. Diabetes Care 1998;21:2098–2102.
20 Murphy NP, Keane SM, Ong KK, Ford-Adams M, Edge JA, Acerini CL, Dunger DB: Randomized cross-over trial of insulin glargine plus lispro or NPH insulin plus regular human insulin in adolescents with type 1 diabetes on intensive insulin regimens. Diabetes Care 2003;26:799–804.
21 Raile K, Noelle V, Landgraf R, Schwarz HP: Insulin antibodies are associated with lipoatrophy but also with lipohypertrophy in children and adolescents with type 1 diabetes. Exp Clin Endocrinol Diab 2001;109:393–396.
22 Sarnblad S, Kroon M, Aman J: Metformin as an additional therapy in adolescents with poorly controlled type 1 diabetes: Randomized placebo-controlled trial with aspects on insulin sensitivity. Eur J Endocrinol 2003;149:232–329.

23 Siebenhofer A, Plank J, Berghold A, Narath M, Gfrerer R, Pieber TR: Short acting insulin analogues versus regular human insulin in patients with diabetes mellitus. The Cochrane Library, Issue 2, 2004, Chichester, Wiley, 2004.
24 Schober E, Schoenle E, Van Dyk J, Wernicke-Panthen K: Comparative trial between insulin glargine and NPH insulin in children and adolescents with type 1 diabetes mellitus. J Pediatr Endocrinol Metab 2002;15:369–376.
25 Vague P, Selam J-L, Skeie S, De Leeuw I, Elte JWF, Haarh H, Kristensen A, Draeger E: Insulin detemir is associated with more predictable glycemic control and reduced risk of hypoglycaemia compared to NPH insulin in patients with type 1 diabetes on basal-bolus regimen with pre-meal insulin aspart. Diabetes Care 2003;26:590–596.
26 Weintrob N, Benzaquen H, Galatzer A, Shalatin S, Lazar L, Fayman G, Lilos P, Dickerman Z, Phillip M: Comparison of continuous subcutaneous insulin infusion and multiple daily injection regimens in children with type 1 diabetes: A randomized open crossover trial. Pediatrics 2003;112: 559–564.
27 Weissberg-Benchell J, Antisdel-Lomaglio J, Seshadri R: Insulin pump therapy: A meta-analysis. Diabetes Care 2003;26:1079–87.

Dr. Thomas M. Kapellen
Universitätsklinik und Poliklinik für Kinder und Jugendliche
Universität Leipzig, Oststrasse 21–25, DE–04317 Leipzig (Germany)
Tel. +49 341 97 972 60 00, Fax +49 341 97 972 60 09, E-Mail kapt@medizin.uni-leipzig.de

Chiarelli F, Dahl-Jørgensen K, Kiess W (eds): Diabetes in Childhood and Adolescence.
Pediatr Adolesc Med. Basel, Karger, 2005, vol 10, pp 139–149

# Medical Nutrition Therapy of Children and Adolescents with Diabetes

*Suvi M. Virtanen*

Department of Epidemiology and Health Promotion, National Institute of Public Health and Research Unit, Tampere University Hospital, and School of Public Health, Tampere, Finland

During the insulin area the diet recommended for the subjects with diabetes has gradually changed from a very high fat (up to 60% of energy intake) and low carbohydrate (from 20% of energy intake), sugar-restricted diet to a flexible, nonrestricted diet (table 1). The recommendation for the amount of fat has gone down and that of carbohydrate up finally resulting in the current situation, where large variation in the proportions of energy-yielding nutrients is allowed (table 2). The diet recommended for the subject with diabetes today is indeed nutritionally identical to the one recommended for the general population and is applicable to the whole family. This development has been firmly bound to the progress in other medical treatments of diabetes as well as to advance in the field of nutrition science. The availability of blood glucose home monitoring and the development of multiple insulin injection and insulin pump therapies during the 1980s changed the treatment in a profound way. With the more physiologic insulin therapies, the eating schedule can be more flexible. The very short-acting insulin preparations further increase flexibility. Along with the advances made in the understanding of the health effects of dietary fatty acids, emphasis has shifted from total fat to the type of dietary fatty acids in the medical nutrition therapy of diabetes.

Nutritional management is one of the cornerstones of diabetes care. Achieving good glycemic control is usually not possible without good coordination between insulin treatment, nutrition therapy and exercise by means of glucose self-monitoring. When giving dietary advice, it is important to take into account cultural, ethnic and family traditions as well as individual dietary

*Table 1.* Changes in the medical nutrition therapy of diabetes in children and adolescents by time

| Earlier | Now |
|---|---|
| Doctor prescribed treatment | Self-care with the help of multidisciplinary diabetes team |
| Rigid diet | Flexible diet |
| Some foods restricted | No forbidden foods |
| Diet according to insulin | Insulin according to diet and exercise |
| Amount of foods prescribed | Eating according to hunger and blood glucose self-monitoring taking into account exercise and growth |
| Cultural, social and psychological values of foods and eating ignored | Variety of factors affecting food choice better understood |

habits before the diagnosis of diabetes. The psychological meanings of foods and eating should not be underestimated. Although the dietary recommendations for children and adolescents with diabetes do not anymore differ from those given for the general population, they do differ from what the other children and adolescents eat.

We are facing new challenges in the treatment of diabetes: type 2 diabetes is increasing also among children and adolescents along with the increasing prevalence of overweight and obesity and sedentary life style in these age groups [5]. The increasing flexibility and alternatives in the treatment of diabetes give better possibilities to achieve good metabolic control, but this also means that more knowledge and skills are needed to successfully coordinate nutrition therapy with insulin therapy and exercise.

## Aims of Medical Nutrition Therapy

The nutritional management of children and adolescents with diabetes aims at [1]:

- providing appropriate energy and nutrient intake to ensure optimal growth, development and health
- promoting healthy lifelong eating habits while preserving social, cultural and psychological well-being
- achieving and maintaining the best possible glycemic control
- achieving and maintaining ideal body weight and taking regular physical exercise

*Table 2.* Nutritional recommendations for subjects with diabetes given by the International Society for Pediatric and Adolescent Diabetes (ISPAD), the American Diabetes Association (ADA) and the Diabetes and Nutrition Study Group (DNSG) of the European Association for the Study of Diabetes

| | ISPAD 2000 [1] | ADA 2002 [2, 3] | DNSG 2000 [4] |
|---|---|---|---|
| Carbohydrate, % energy | >50 | – | 45–60 |
| Dietary fiber, g/day | 5+ age (years)* | ↑ | ↑ |
| Sucrose, % energy | ≤10 | – | ≤10 |
| Protein, % energy | 10–15 | 15–20** | 10–20** |
| Fat, % energy | 30–35 | – | 25–35 |
| SFA and trans-unsaturated fatty acids | <10 (for SFA) | <10 (for SFA)*** | <10*** |
| MUFA | >10 | – | 10–20 |
| PUFA | <10 | 10 | <10 |
| Carbohydrate + MUFA, % energy | – | 60–70 | 60–70 |
| Dietary cholesterol, mg/day | – | <300 | ≤300 |

* For children older than 2 years.
** If renal function is normal.
***If LDL cholesterol is elevated <7 and <8% are recommended by ADA and DNSG, respectively.

- preventing and treating acute complications of diabetes such as hypoglycemia, hypoglycemic crises, hyperglycemia, illness and exercise-related problems
- preventing or delaying micro and macrovascular complications

## Dietary Advice

The complexity of nutritional issues in the lifelong management of diabetes is generally acknowledged. A registered dietitian who is experienced in childhood diabetes and in implementing nutrition therapy into diabetes management and education should belong to the multidisciplinary diabetes care team [1, 2]. Medical nutrition therapy provided by registered dietitians resulted in better glycemic control in subjects with newly diagnosed type 1 diabetes [6]. A recent workshop report revealed, however, that of the 45 pediatric clinics participating in the survey only 25 had a pediatric dietitian available for children with diabetes [7].

The giving of dietary advice should start gradually: first the emphasis is on establishing secure and supporting relationship with the family and only simple instructions are given, later more detailed education is given. Interaction in the diabetes care team is important: dietary advice given by different team members should be consistent. Dietary advice also needs to be given to the other caregivers: extended family, teachers, babysitters, etc.

Dietary advice should be based on the dietary history on the family's and child's food habits and meal pattern before the diagnosis of diabetes. Also, the child's daily activities including exercise schedules need to be interviewed. Additionally, 24-hour recalls and 3-day food diaries can be used to assess child's energy intake. Adequacy of energy intake should be evaluated by following weight gain and growth patterns on a regular basis (every 3–6 months).

## Main Dietary Recommendations

The dietary recommendations given by different diabetes expert groups are very well in line with each other (table 2) and also with recommendations given to the general population [8].

Nutrition therapy of children and adolescents with type 1 diabetes should focus on achieving blood glucose goals without excessive hypoglycemia. It is essential to provide adequate intake of energy to ensure normal growth and development and to avoid obesity. Insulin regimens need to be integrated into usual eating and physical activity habits. Varying eating and exercise patterns can be managed with adjustment of insulin doses. Self blood glucose monitoring and decision-making based on outcomes are necessary tools for achieving the best possible glycemic control. Individuals treated with insulin also need education in the management and prevention of hypoglycemia, acute illnesses, and exercise-related blood glucose problems.

Nutrition therapy of youth (or children) with type 2 diabetes includes facilitating changes in eating and physical activity habits that reduce insulin resistance and improve metabolic status. Attention should be paid to the cessation of excessive weight gain with normal linear growth and to achievement of glycemic control goals. The possible comorbidities, such as hypertension and dyslipidemia are more frequent with type 2 than type 1 diabetes and need to be addressed.

Dietary recommendations can be presented in a diagrammatic and practical way by the food pyramid: the top consists of fats, oils, sweets, and confectionary (should be use sparingly); next downward come milk, cheese, meat, fish, egg, and nuts (2–3 servings per day); then fruits and vegetables (5 servings per day), and lastly the base is formed by bread, cereals, rice, potato, and pasta (6–11 servings per day) [1].

## Sociocultural Aspects of Food and Eating

Parents and siblings have an influence on a child's food choices. The child's caretakers, teachers and friends, as well as the media, also play a role in child's food selection, their importance varying at different ages. It seems that food habits are more strongly associated within the nuclear family than between friends, even among adolescents [9]. The findings from the Framingham Children Study demonstrated that both maternal and paternal intake of saturated fatty acids was related to child's intake [10].

There are critical periods when changes in food habits take place in families. Parents seem to be more prone to change their food habits at the time the children are born [11]. The concern over the health of a family member was related to the quality of the diet of the parents [12].

Few studies have compared the diet within families with a child with diabetes. The siblings of Finnish children with diabetes changed their fat and milk choices at the time of diagnosis according to dietary guidelines and these changes persisted during the 2-year follow-up period [13]. Nondiabetic siblings of farmers' and lower socioeconomic families were less prone to change their food habits. In another Finnish subject series of very young children with diabetes, the family members (siblings, mothers, fathers) increased their consumption of skim milk, low-fat cheese, low-fat cold meat cuts, fruits, vegetables at the time of diagnosis [14].

It seems that the family members of a child with diabetes are willing to change their own food habits towards the recommended diet. Similar food choices among family members decrease the feeling of social isolation of the child with diabetes. The diet recommended to children with diabetes also promotes the health of other family members. It works well, for example, in the prevention of cardiovascular diseases and of type 2 diabetes. In the other fields of treatment of diabetes, there is evidence of the importance of family support. Parental support in blood glucose home monitoring has been shown to increase compliance, and the higher frequency of blood glucose monitoring was related to better glycemic control among adolescents with diabetes [15].

## Carbohydrates

The total amount of carbohydrates is more important for the glycemic effect than the source or type. It has been shown that there is a strong relationship between the insulin dosage before meal and the postprandial response to the carbohydrate content of the meal [16].

The insulin dose and action profile needs to be balanced to the expected intake of carbohydrates. Carbohydrates can be counted in exchanges, grams, portions/servings, as glycemic index, and in carbohydrates:insulin ratio. Some families and young people may have difficulties in counting carbohydrates in exchanges or grams and may use educational tools such as 'plate model'. There is a danger that carbohydrate counting leads to carbohydrate constraint as the child grows.

Those individuals who receive intensive insulin therapy should adjust their premeal insulin dosages according to the carbohydrate content of the meals. If fixed daily insulin dosages are given then attention should be paid to a consistent day-to-day carbohydrate intake. Twice-daily insulin regimens of short and longer-acting insulins require also frequent carbohydrate intake to prevent hypoglycemia during inevitable periods of hyperinsulinemia. Most insulin regimens require carbohydrate intake before bed to prevent nocturnal hypoglycemia. During increased exercise and sport extra carbohydrates are needed before, during and after exercise to balance the increased energy need and prevent hypoglycemia [17].

Subjects with diabetes are encouraged to choose a variety of fiber-containing foods, such as whole grains, fruits, and vegetables, because they provide vitamins, minerals, fiber, and other dietary factors important for good health. There is, however, no reason to recommend a higher intake of dietary fiber for the subjects with diabetes than for the rest of the population [3, 4]. For children with and without diabetes older than 2 years, a daily fiber intake of 5 plus age in years is recommended [1, 18].

Sucrose produces similar a glycemic response as isocaloric amounts of other carbohydrates and need not be restricted in the diet of subjects with diabetes. Sucrose should be substituted for other carbohydrate sources in the meal plan or if added to the meal plan, adequately covered with insulin. There are no health reasons for eating sucrose or sucrose-containing foods either, apart from treating hypoglycemia, so that it seems prudent for children and adolescents with diabetes to have the same recommendation as other children, which is not to receive more than 10% of their total energy from sucrose.

Fructose is a major sugar in fruits. It is somewhat sweeter than sucrose. In excess it may have adverse effects on triglyceride levels. It is not recommended as a sweetening agent, but natural sources, fruits and vegetables, are recommended.

Sugar alcohols are used in food as sweeteners and bulking agents. They are hydrogenated monosaccharides (e.g. sorbitol), disaccharides (e.g. maltitol), and mixtures of hydrogenated mono-, di- and oligosaccharides. Sugar alcohols have been designated as safe for use as food additives. They may cause diarrhea, especially in children, and are not recommended as sweeteners in children [1].

Fructose, sugar alcohols and other nutritive sweeteners, all of which are sources of energy, do not have substantial advantages over sucrose for subjects with diabetes and should not be encouraged.

### Protein

Protein intake decreases during childhood from about 2 g/kg per day in early infancy to 1 g/kg per day for a 10-year-old, and to 0.8–0.9 g/kg per day in later adolescence. Both the amount and sources of protein vary widely in different countries. There is no evidence to suggest that usual protein intake (10–15% of energy) should be modified if renal function is normal. It may be prudent to avoid higher intakes. When persistent microalbuminuria, raised blood pressure or established nephropathy occur, excessive protein intake may be harmful and therefore the intake should be at the lower end of the recommended intake. Protein restriction in adolescence requires expertise of a dietitian to ensure that it does not interfere with normal growth.

### Dietary Fat

The principal goal regarding dietary fat in subjects with diabetes is to decrease the intake of saturated and trans-unsaturated fatty acids and cholesterol. Saturated fatty acids occur mainly in animal products such as high-fat milk, cheese, butter, and red meat. Trans-unsaturated fatty acids are formed when unsaturated fats are hydrogenated and are found in manufactured confectionery products (e.g. biscuits, cakes, chocolates) and some margarines. Both saturated and trans-unsaturated fatty acids have adverse effects on lipoproteins and are associated with coronary heart disease.

Saturated fat can be replaced either with carbohydrate or (cis-)monounsaturated fat, either of which can contribute to a reduction in plasma LDL cholesterol. Monounsaturated fatty acids of cis configuration are found in olive, sesame, rapeseed, and some nut oils.

Polyunsaturated fatty acids include the essential fatty acids linoleic acid and α-linolenic acid. Polyunsaturated fatty acid intake is restricted to no more than 10% of the total energy intake because of the potential adverse consequences of increased lipid oxidation and reduced levels of HDL associated with high intakes. There is some evidence from the general population that foods containing n–3 polyunsaturated fatty acids, especially eicosapentaenoic and docosahexaenoic acid, have cardioprotective properties [19]. Fish is a good source of these fatty acids and therefore two or more servings of fish per week can be recommended.

## Vitamins and Minerals

Nutrient requirements of children and adolescents with type 1 and type 2 diabetes are apparently similar to those for same-aged nondiabetic children and adolescents [8]. Children and adolescents with diabetes should be educated how to receive the daily vitamin and mineral requirements from foods. The potential toxicity of megadoses of vitamin and mineral supplements should be stressed. In selected groups, such as strict vegetarians or in individuals with energy-restricted diets, supplementation with a multivitamin preparation can be advisable. In some countries supplementary vitamin D may be necessary to children during the winter months. There is no clear evidence of benefit from vitamin or mineral supplementation in subjects with diabetes who do not have underlying deficiencies [3].

## Salt

As in the general population, adult subjects with diabetes should be advised to restrict salt intake (sodium chloride) to 6,000 mg or sodium intake to 2,400 mg (100 mmol) per day [2]. Children aged 1–3 years have a reference intake of 500 mg of sodium, those aged 4–6 years 700 mg and 7- to 10-year-olds 1,200 mg [20]. In both normotensive and hypertensive individuals, a reduction in sodium intake lowers blood pressure.

## Non-Nutritive Sweeteners

Non-nutritive sweeteners, such as saccharin, aspartame, acesulfame potassium and sucralose are safe when consumed within the acceptable daily intake (ADI) levels and may be helpful when used in drinks.

## Dietary Compliance among Children and Adolescents with Diabetes

Dietary compliance seems to be rather good among young children with diabetes [21, 22]. In the Finnish study, for example, the consumption of roots, vegetables, and high-fiber rye products was two to three times higher among children with diabetes than among control children, and the intakes of carbohydrate, total fat and saturated fat of the children with diabetes were well within the recommended limits during the first 2 years of diabetes.

The dietary compliance of Finnish children deteriorated during adolescence, e.g. the intake of saturated fat increased and the diet changed towards that of other adolescents [23–25]. Among adolescents with diabetes, a relatively high prevalence of mismanagement has been observed: 25% had missed their insulin injection, 29% made up blood test results, 34% had taken extra insulin to cover inappropriate food, and 56% had missed meals and snacks during the previous 10 days [26].

The comparison of dietary surveys of children and adolescents with diabetes published during the last decade [21, 22, 24, 25, 27–30] revealed that the Italian children with their moderate intake of protein and saturated fatty acids and high intake of monounsaturated fatty acids and carbohydrate were closest to the recommended diet.

## Obesity and Eating Disorders

Overweight and obesity in childhood and adolescence are increasing rapidly worldwide [31, 32]. In addition, there are observations of increased overweight and obesity among adolescents with diabetes compared to other adolescents [25, 33]. Obesity seems to be related partly to multiple insulin injections [34, 35] and/or higher insulin dose [25].

Eating disorders are about two times more prevalent among adolescent girls and young women with diabetes than in the general population [36, 37]. Required dietary restraint and weight gain related to the treatment of diabetes may play a role [38]. Eating disorders are related to noncompliance with diabetes treatment, impaired glycemic control and higher frequency of microvascular complications [36].

## References

1 ISPAD (International Society for Pediatric and Adolescent Diabetes): Nutritional Management; in Swift PGF (ed): Consensus Guidelines 2000. Zeist, Publ Medforum, 2000, pp 53–62.

2 American Diabetes Association Position Statement: Evidence-based nutrition principles and recommendations for the treatment and prevention of diabetes and related complications. J Am Diet Assoc 2002;102:109–118.

3 Franz MJ, Bantle JP, Beebe CA, Brunzell JD, Chiasson J-L, et al: Evidence-based nutrition principles and recommendations for the treatment and prevention of diabetes and related complications. Diabetes Care 2002;25:148–198.

4 The Diabetes and Nutrition Study Group (DNSG) of the European Association for the Study of Diabetes (EASD): Recommendations for the nutritional management of patients with diabetes mellitus. Eur J Clin Nutr 2000;54:353–355.

5 American Diabetes Association: Type 2 diabetes in children and adolescents. Diabetes Care 2000;23:381–389.

6 Kulkarni K, Castle G, Gregory R, Holmes A, Leontos C, Powers M, Snetselaar L, Splett P, Wylie-Rosett J: Nutrition practice guidelines for type 1 diabetes mellitus positively affect dietitian practices and patient outcomes. J Am Diet Assoc 1998;98:62–70.
7 Waldron S, Hanas R, Palmvig B: How do we educate young people to balance carbohydrate intake with adjustments of insulin? Horm Res 2002;57:S62–S65.
8 US Department of Agriculture, US Department of Health and Human Services: Nutrition and Your Health: Dietary Guidelines for Americans, ed 5. Home and Garden Bulletin No 232, 2000.
9 Feunekes GIJ, de Graaf C, Meyboom S, van Staveren WA: Food choice and fat intake of adolescents and adults: Associations of intakes within social networks. Prev Med 1998;27:645–656.
10 Oliveria SA, Ellison RC, Moore LL, Gillman MV, Garrahie EJ, Singer MR: Parent-child relationships in nutrient intake: The Framingham Children's Study. Am J Clin Nutr 1992;56:593–598.
11 Laitinen S, Högström P, Räsänen L: Similarity of food choices among young Finnish couples. J Hum Nutr Diet 1997;10:353–360.
12 Schafer RB: Factors affecting food behavior and the quality of husbands' and wives' diets. J Am Diet Assoc 1978;72:138–143.
13 Virta-Autio P, Virtanen SM, Räsänen L, Aro A, Tuomilehto J, Åkerblom HK, the Childhood Diabetes in Finland Study Group: Changes in milk and fat choices of nondiabetic siblings of newly diagnosed diabetic children: A two-year prospective study. J Nutr Educ 1996;28:272–278.
14 Virtanen SM, Virta-Autio P, Räsänen L, Åkerblom HK: How the food habits change in families with a newly diagnosed child with type 1 diabetes. J Pediatr Endocrinol Metab 2001;14:627–636.
15 Anderson B, Ho J, Brackett J, Finkelstein D, Laffel L: Parental involvement in diabetes management tasks: Relationships to blood glucose monitoring adherence and metabolic control in young adolescents with insulin dependent diabetes mellitus. J Pediatr 1997;130:257–265.
16 Rabasa-Lhoret R, Garon J, Langelier H, Poisson D, Chiasson J-L: The effects of meal carbohydrate content on insulin requirements in type 1 diabetic patients treated intensively with the basal-bolus (ultralente-regular) insulin regimen. Diabetes Care 1999;22:667–673.
17 American Diabetes Association: Diabetes mellitus and exercise. Position statement. Diabetes Care 2002;25:S64–S68.
18 Williams CL, Bollella M, Wynder EL: A new recommendation for dietary fiber in childhood. Pediatrics 1995;96:S985–S988.
19 Daviglus ML, Stamler J, Orencia AJ, Dyer AR, Liu K, Greenland P, Walsh MK, Morris D, Shekelle RB: Fish consumption and the 30-year risk of fatal myocardial infarction. N Engl J Med 1997;336:1046–1053.
20 Sandström B, Aro A, Becker W, Lyhne N, Pedersen JI, Thorsdottir I: Nordiska näringsrekommendationer 1996. Nord 1996:28, Nordiska Ministerrådet, Köpenhamn, 1996.
21 Randecker GA, Smiciklas-Wright H, McKenzie JM, Shannon BM, Mitchell DC, Becker DJ, Kieselhorst K: The dietary intake of children with IDDM. Diabetes Care 1996;19:1370–1374.
22 Virtanen SM, Ylönen K, Räsänen L, Ala-Venna E, Mäenpää J, Åkerblom HK: Two year prospective dietary survey of newly diagnosed children with diabetes aged less than 6 years. Arch Dis Childh 2000;82:21–26.
23 Virtanen SM, Räsänen L, Mäenpää J, Åkerblom HK: Dietary survey of Finnish adolescent diabetics and non-diabetic controls. Acta Paediatr Scand 1987;76:801–808.
24 Virtanen SM, Räsänen L, Tumme R, Laitinen S, Mäenpää J, Virtanen M, Åkerblom HK: A follow-up study of the diet of Finnish diabetic adolescents. Acta Paediatr 1992;81:153–157.
25 Pietiläinen KH, Virtanen SM, Rissanen A, Rita H, Mäenpää J: Diet, obesity, and metabolic control in girls with insulin dependent diabetes mellitus. Arch Dis Childh 1995;73:398–402.
26 Weissberg-Benchell J, Glasgow AM, Tynan WD, Wirtz P, Turek J, Ward J: Adolescent diabetes management and mismanagement. Diabetes Care 1995;18:77–82.
27 Dorchy H, Bourguet K: Nutritional intake of Belgian diabetic children. Diabetes Care 1997,20: 1046–1047.
28 Dorchy H, Bouguert K, Pieters S, Mozin MJ: Dés équilibres alimentaires importants chez les enfants diabétiques et non-diabétiques Belges. Percentile 1996;1:45–50.
29 Pinelli L, Mormile R, Gonfiantini E, Busanto A, Kaufmann R, et al.: Recommended dietary allowances (RDA) in the dietary management of children and adolescents with IDDM: An unfeasible target or an achievable cornerstone? J Pediatr Endocrinol Metab 1998;11:335–346.

30 Schober E, Langergraber B, Rupprecht G, Rami B: Dietary intake of Austrian diabetic children 10 to 14 years of age. J Pediatr Gastr Nutr 1999;29:144–147.
31 Lazarus R, Wake M, Hesketh K, Waters E: Change in body mass index in Australian primary school children, 1985–1997. Int J Obes Relat Metab Disord 2000;24:679–684.
32 Kautiainen S, Rimpelä A, Vikat A, Virtanen SM: Secular trends in overweight, obesity and perceived weight among Finnish adolescents in 1977–1999. Int J Obes 2002;26:544–552.
33 Holl RW, Heinze E, Seifert M, Grabert M, Teller WM: Longitudinal analysis of somatic development in paediatric patients with IDDM: Genetic influences on height and weight. Diabetologia 1994;37:925–929.
34 Mortensen HB, Hougaard P: Comparison of metabolic control in a cross-sectional study of 2,873 children and adolescents with IDDM from 18 countries. Diabetes Care 1997;20:714–720.
35 Holl RW, Swift PGF, Mortensen HB, Lynggaard H, Hougaard P, Aanstoot H-J, Chiarelli F, Daneman D, Danne T, Dorchy H, Garandeau P, Greene S, Hoey HMCV, Kaprio EA, Kocova M, Martul P, Matsuura N, Robertson KJ, Schoenle EJ, Sovik O, Tsou R-M, Vanelli M, Åman J: Insulin injection regimens and metabolism control in an international survey of adolescents with type 1 diabetes over 3 years: Results from the Hvidore study group. Eur J Pediatr 2003;162:22–29.
36 Rydall AC, Rodin GM, Olmsted MP, Devenyi RG, Daneman D: Disordered eating behavior and microvascular complications in young women with insulin-dependent diabetes mellitus. N Engl J Med 1997;336:1849–1854.
37 Jones JM, Lawson ML, Daneman D, Olmsted MP, Rodin G: Eating disorders in adolescent females with and without type 1 diabetes: Cross sectional study. BMJ 2000;320:1563–1566.
38 Rodin GM, Daneman D: Eating disorders and IDDM. Diabetes Care 1992;15:1402–1412.

Suvi M. Virtanen, MD
Department of Epidemiology and Health Promotion
National Institute of Public Health
Mannerheimintie 166, FIN–00300 Helsinki (Finland)
Tel. +358 9 4744 8729 or +358 50 327 9696, Fax +358 9 4744 8591
E-Mail suvi.virtanen@ktl.fi

Chiarelli F, Dahl-Jørgensen K, Kiess W (eds): Diabetes in Childhood and Adolescence.
Pediatr Adolesc Med. Basel, Karger, 2005, vol 10, pp 150–162

# Continuous Subcutaneous Insulin Infusion in Childhood and Adolescence

*Moshe Phillip, Naomi Weintrob, Shlomit Shalitin*

Institute for Endocrinology and Diabetes, National Center for Childhood Diabetes, Schneider Children's Medical Center of Israel, Petah-Tikva, Israel

## Evolution of Insulin Pump Therapy

Since the first clinical use of insulin therapy in 1923, physicians have defined the goal of treatment of diabetes mellitus as the maintenance of the glycemic status to 'as close to normal' as possible. This notion was reinforced in 1993 by the finding of the Diabetes Control and Complications Trial (DCCT), a 9-year study of 1,441 diabetic patients [1] that improving glycemic control at an early age can help prevent the typical complications of the disease later in life. With these data, diabetic patients, along with their care-givers, faced the challenge of achieving near normal metabolic control without compromising their quality of life. It is done by tailoring the treatment personally to the patient's individual lifestyle, taking into account his or her age, pubertal status, physical activity, dietary needs, intelligence family support and socio-economic status.

The failure of conventional treatments to normalize blood glucose levels in diabetic patients prompted the development of mechanical infusion systems that try to mimic the β-cell function. The first continuous insulin delivery device was fashioned in 1960 by Kadish, but it was large, cumbersome and impractical [2]. About 15 years later, several research groups [3, 4] suggested that in patients with type 1 diabetes, the best way to improve metabolic control was to administer insulin in a manner that simulates the physiological patterns of insulin secretion, that is, continuous 24-hour 'basal' delivery with superimposed prandial-related boosts or 'boluses'. Although this could be achieved with multiple daily injections (MDI) [5], controlled insulin infusion by portable pump appeared to be more flexible and precise. Early trials in several countries, using variable rates of intravenous insulin delivery, first for several days [2, 4, 6] and then for some months [7], noted improved blood glucose control compared to traditional methods. However, the clinical application of an intravenous infusion system was limited by risks of infection, thrombosis, phlebitis, insulin precipitation and aggregation, and difficulties in maintaining arm vein patency. As a result, new efforts were invested in developing portable delivery systems for continuous subcutaneous insulin infusion (CSII). The first report was published by Pickup et al. [8] in 1978. Soon after, Tamborlane et al. [9] demonstrated that CSII, when combined with self-monitoring of blood glucose ('intensive insulin therapy'), yielded glycosylated hemoglobin values in the near-normal range. Their pump was designed to infuse small pulses of rapidly absorbed insulin every few minutes, creating a small subcutaneous reservoir from which insulin could be absorbed continuously at a predictable basal rate. The pump could also be manually activated to inject a larger bolus of insulin 15–30 min before meals, according to the blood glucose level and composition of the planned meal. The metabolic improvement in the patients using the pump was at least as good as with the intravenous route.

In view of these early successful results, different prototypes of smaller, lighter, programmable pumps were introduced, with several different types of open-loop systems. *Roller pumps* are operated by the rotary action of rollers moving over a flexible tube which transfers insulin from a reservoir to a catheter. Their major drawback is that pH changes in the relatively large reservoir or contact with the plastic materials can cause the insulin to precipitate or aggregate, thereby obstructing the catheter. *Solenoid-piston pumps* move insulin in one direction by means of inlet and outlet check valves. Although small and precise, these devices also require insulin storage in a reservoir and are thus subject to the same problems as roller pumps. Solenoid-piston pumps were recently withdrawn from the market. In *syringe pumps*, currently the most popular type, an actuator driven by a motor-powered lead depresses the plunger of a small syringe. Basal and meal-time boluses are set electronically. The reservoir holds short-acting insulin (regular insulin or insulin analogue).

Modern pump modifications that improve function and ease of use include electronic memory, multiple basal rate programming, bolus options, and suspension or temporary-rate preprogramming of insulin for set times throughout the day. In addition, pumps now come in a variety of colors, and the information screen is easier to read. The infusion sets have softened catheters which do not require that the insertion needle be left in place, and 'quick-release' options which permit the pump user to easily disconnect from the infusion tubing during activities such as showering, swimming and sexual intimacy. Some of the pumps have a safety lockout feature and a remote control, and alarms that signal the user to recharge the battery, fill the syringe, etc. Newer tapes have been developed to better secure the needle or catheter on the skin while causing less local skin irritation. The use of local anesthetics, such as EMLA cream, makes catheter insertion nearly painless.

### Implantable Pumps

Buchwald and Rohde [10] developed the first constant-rate implantable pump in the 1970s. The pumping mechanism was based on the equilibrium between the positive-pressure Freon gas stored in the pump and the insulin in the reservoir, separated by a diaphragm. The reservoir was filled by the physician with a particular insulin concentration. In the 1980s, researchers demonstrated that variable-rate, patient-controlled implantable insulin pumps were feasible for clinical use, but they were limited by the short battery life [11]. However, the programmable implantable insulin pump developed around the same time at Johns Hopkins University [12], required less power and caused less physical trauma to the implant site. Average duration of function of the pump was 3 years.

The current generation of implantable insulin pumps is variable-rate, patient-controlled devices. The pumps are implanted via an incision into a 'pocket' formed in the subcutaneous space of the abdomen; the tip of the catheter is placed in the peritoneal cavity. Changes are made in the catheter or pump by reoperation at the earlier incision. The pumps deliver insulin at a constant pre-programmed basal rate between meals and overnight, with bolus doses at meals. To make dose adjustments, the patient places a hand-held communicator over the pump and presses a keyboard. Electronic problems are detected by the pump's failure to communicate properly; a warning message is displayed or an alarm is delivered from the implant. The most common problems are catheter block and precipitation of insulin within the pump. It should be noted that the use of the implantable insulin pump has been studied only in a few selected centers and is still not a common practice.

### The Clinical Use of CSII

Insulin's secretory responses to physiologic stimuli are complex and difficult to duplicate. At present, CSII appears to offer the most physiological way of insulin delivery, by combining predetermined basal rates of insulin to meet non-prandial requirements (between meals and during sleeping hours) and bolus doses at mealtimes. The basal rate is set to the minimum insulin needed

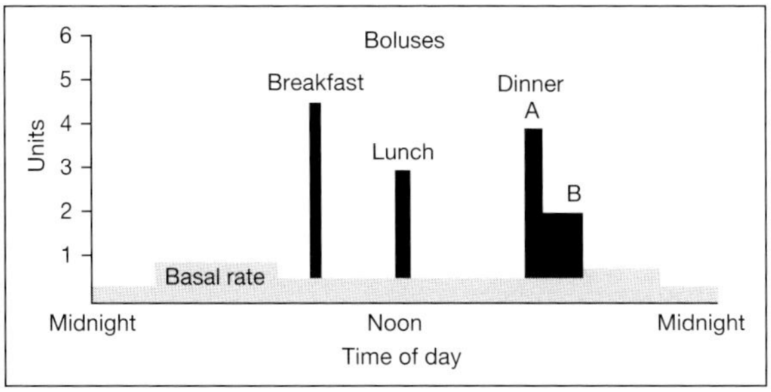


***Fig. 1.*** Changing glucose needs throughout the day. The gray band at the bottom of the figure represents the basal insulin infusion rate. It can be modified for various needs such as the dawn phenomenon or physical activity. The dark columns represent the bolus insulin injections, that is, spurts of insulin delivered quickly to bring the elevated blood glucose levels associated with meals back to normal levels. A and B represent the ability of some insulin pumps to deliver the boluses at different paces according to the carbohydrate content and composition of the meal.

to suppress gluconeogenesis and ketogenesis while keeping blood glucose levels within the normal range without inducing hypoglycemia. The mealtime boluses are calculated with the use of an algorithm and depend on the caloric and nutritive composition of the meal, the capillary glucose concentration before the meal, and the anticipated level of physical activity after the meal. For better prandial and postprandial glycemic control, according to the type of food ingested and duration of the meal, current pump technology offers several bolus options: normal, in which the programmed bolus is given immediately before the meal; square-wave bolus, in which the bolus is distributed over a chosen time; and dual-wave bolus which combines these two methods in a suitable ratio selected by the patient (fig. 1). The rate of basal insulin infusion can vary over the day to accommodate diurnal changes in insulin needs.

By using CSII, patients are spared both the need for multiple daily injections of insulin by syringe or pen and the peak-action profile that characterizes intermediate- or long-acting insulin preparations, allowing them more flexibility with meals and daily activity. In addition, the ability to set different basal profiles throughout the day – and thereby decrease or increase the insulin infusion rate – prevents the dawn phenomenon; that is, the basal rate can be increased in the early morning hours without the price of nocturnal hypoglycemia [13]. It also decreases the risk of exercise-induced hypoglycemia [13]. The multi-step adjustable basal rate is theoretically superior to the recently introduced long-acting insulin-analog glargine, which offers a fixed basal dose [14].

Studies have shown that the use of only short-acting insulin significantly decreases the variation in subcutaneous absorption of insulin compared to

Intermediate-acting insulin (~3% vs. ~30–50% difference) [15, 16]. In addition, placement of the catheter in the same area for a few days overcame the large difference in subcutaneous insulin absorption from different injection sites [17], so that blood glucose profiles are more consistent, with smaller fluctuations compared to multiple daily injections [18–20]. This has been even further improved by using insulin analogues in the CSII therapy [21].

As CSII has grown in popularity, patients and physicians have begun to recognize some of its limitations. The lack of a subcutaneous depot of intermediate- or long-acting insulin and the short half-life of serum insulin during CSII [15] increase patient susceptibility to diabetic ketoacidosis (DKA) secondary to dislodgment or occlusion of the infusion-set or pump failure [22–24]. Since the devices alarms, available today, do not warn against leakage or dislodgment, frequent self-blood glucose monitoring is needed, with rapid, appropriate action to correct high glucose levels.

Another disadvantage is the high risk of infection at the infusion-set site [22, 25, 26]. In addition, some patients show local allergic reactions to components of the infusion system [27]. These local complications can be prevented by meticulous management of the insertion sit, changing the insulin delivery catheter every 2–3 days, changing components of the infusion system and applying of local antibiotic cream to the site, as necessary.

Recent technological advances have made the pump less liable to mechanical failure and more user-friendly [28]. The pumps of the eighties were large and heavy and often had a negative impact on body image [29]. Today, pumps are pager size, easy to carry and, in our era of cellular phones, much more socially acceptable. The development of electronic memory, several basal profiles, enhanced safety alarms, a soft cannula, remote control and being waterproof have dramatically improved the day-to-day use of insulin therapy [30]. Nevertheless, the pump is still a complex, sophisticated instrument and its handling requires cognitive abilities, technical expertise, good understanding and familiarity with the device, environmental support, and careful follow-up by the health-care provider [31, 32]. Also, some patients still feel burdened by the need to carry the pump and to leave the cannula in the subcutaneous tissue 24 h a day.

The transition from one mode of insulin therapy to another is usually the result of a discussion between the child or adolescent, the parents and the medical care-givers. Choosing the CSII as the mode of intensive therapy requires an appropriate education and adjustment to the new therapeutic modality. Adolescents with type 1 diabetes often find it hard to maintain good metabolic control, possibly because of the unique emotional and hormonal changes associated with this age group. Therefore, insulin pump therapy, which provides greater lifestyle flexibility, may be better suited for this population. In a 1980 study, Tamborlane et al. [33] reported that CSII is not only a feasible tool for the management of blood glucose levels in diabetic adolescents; it actually improves their metabolic control. A few years later, Schiffrin et al. [29] demonstrated that in adolescents with type 1 diabetes, CSII was actually more effective in achieving metabolic control than intensive therapy with MDI.

The transition from MDI to CSII is usually achieved by decreasing the average total insulin dosage per day, calculated based on the dose used over the preceding 2 weeks, by about 20%. Of the total new daily dose, 50% is given as the basal insulin and 50% as pre-meal boluses. At the first days, patients are asked to perform frequent self blood glucose monitoring (before meals, after meals, and during the night). The target glycemic range for children and adolescents is 4.4–8.3 mmol/l before meals and at midnight and 6.6–10 mmol/l 2 h after meals. Different target glycemic range should be designed for infants, toddlers and young children and insulin dose should be adjusted accordingly. The use of CSII usually requires less insulin to achieve similar glycemic targets, but the initial starting insulin dose should be adjusted according to age, puberty and physical activity. Conrad et al. [34] recently showed that switching from MDI to CSII was associated with the need to decrease the insulin dose by 18% in pubertal patients, but only a small (1.7%) change was needed in prepubertal children. They therefore suggested consideration of a smaller dose change during transition from MDI to CSII in prepubertal children. They also demonstrated that the maximal basal rate in pubertal patients occurred from 3 to 9 a.m. and from 9 p.m. to 12 a.m. and in prepubertal children, from 9 p.m. to 12 a.m.

For many years pump users infused only regular insulin for both the basal needs and the pre-meal boluses. Later it was shown that the use of rapid-acting insulins results in better glycemic control [21, 35] and smoother glucose profiles [21]. Therefore, most clinicians recommend today the use of rapid-acting insulins during CSII therapy: lispro (Humalog, Eli Lilli, Indianapolis, Ind., USA) or aspart (Novorapid, Novo Nordisk, Bagsvaerd, Denmark). Nevertheless, it is noteworthy that some studies have shown similar glycemic control and blood glucose profiles with the use of regular, lispro and aspart insulins [36].

In many diabetic centers, patients are taught carbohydrate counting and insulin bolus dosing based on the insulin-to-carbohydrate ratio, before the initiation of CSII therapy. Several ways how to calculate the starting bolus insulin dose have been developed; we are using 1 U of insulin per 10–20 g of carbohydrate in the anticipated meal. According to the post-meal SBGM and food diary, additional insulin is added to the regimen to cover for elevated blood glucose levels, as necessary. In addition, elevated blood glucose levels (above 8.3 mmol/l) are corrected with additional insulin given in-between meals and snacks, using 1 U for every 2.8–5.5 above 8.3 mmol/l. This, of course, can be done without the need for additional needle pricks by the patient. Most clinicians will ask their patients to change the infusion site every 3 days in regular circumstances, but to do that earlier if blood glucose is >16.6 mmol/l and the urine is positive for ketones or when blood glucose is >16.6 mmol/l and fails to respond to corrective insulin doses as well as when any sign of infection in the insertion site is apparent.

### CSII vs. MDI

Studies comparing glycemic control and adverse events between CSII and MDI have yielded contradictory results. Most of the studies so far were lacking a control group, randomization, or crossover design, and were conducted retrospectively by paired-comparison (i.e. pre- vs. post-pump control). Furthermore, the vast majority was done in the adult population.

A recent meta-analysis of 12 randomized control trials comparing CSII with MDI in adults with type 1 diabetes found a decrease of ~1 mmol/l in mean blood glucose concentration, ~0.5% decrease in HbA1c and ~14% in insulin dose during CSII [37]. A second meta-analysis [38] of 52 studies of patients of all ages, including 41 paired studies (same individuals assessed before and after initiation of CSII) and 11 parallel studies (comparison of subjects using conventional therapy with subjects using CSII) yielded slightly better mean blood glucose levels and HbA1c with CSII. However, most of these studies enrolled self-selected patients, and their samples included patients who before CSII were treated by both 'conventional' therapy and intensive insulin therapy with MDI. The main finding of the meta-analysis was the impact of the duration of CSII therapy on the improvement in glycemic control. Specifically, a significant improvement in glycohemoglobin (mean $\pm$ SD, 8.68 $\pm$ 0.06 before vs. 7.48 $\pm$ 0.22 after, $p < 0.001$) was noted in the patients who used pump therapy for at least one year, but not in those who did so for less time (9.4 $\pm$ 0.23 vs. 9.2 $\pm$ 0.01, $p = 0.3$). Both meta-analyses failed to compare the rate of adverse events, and the descriptive data were equivocal with regard to the rates of DKA, severe hypoglycemia, catheter site infections, and psychosocial functioning.

By contrast to the adult population with type 1 diabetes, data on CSII in toddlers, children and adolescents are still sparse. The few studies already conducted were mostly small and nonrandomized, with a short duration of CSII use [39]. Those comparing conventional therapy to CSII generally showed better glycemic control with CSII [40–44], but those comparing MDI to CSII had contradictory results [28, 45–50]. Boland et al. [47], in a parallel nonrandomized study of 1 year's duration, noted significantly better glycemic control and a decreased rate of severe hypoglycemia in adolescents using CSII, similar to the results of Kaufman et al. [48] who performed a short-term randomized crossover study using pumps only during the night. However, in a paired longitudinal study, Kaufman et al. [28] reported a decreased rate of severe hypoglycemia in the CSII treated patients but, similar glycemic control, while Maniatis et al. [49] and Raile et al. [50] failed to show any significant differences between the groups.

These discrepancies, combined with the lack of randomized crossover studies comparing the two modes of intensive therapy in young patients and the growing interest of patients and their families in pump therapy, prompted our group to conduct two open, randomized, crossover studies in children [33] and adolescents [51]. We evaluated CSII and MDI for glycemic control, incidence of hypoglycemia and hyperglycemia, dose requirements, weight gain, quality of life and satisfaction. In the children, glycemic control and rate of adverse events were similar for the two modalities. However, body mass index increased during MDI and did not change during CSII, while treatment satisfaction was greater for CSII. Comparing glycemic patterns by mode of therapy using the Continuous Subcutaneous Glucose Sensor (CGMS, MiniMed, Sylmar, Calif., USA) in the same group of patients, we found a smaller nocturnal area under the curve for hypoglycemia and a longer duration of within-target glucose tracings during CSII compared to MDI, with similar glycemic control [51]. In the adolescents [52], HbA1c level decreased by 0.43% during CSII and increased by 0.1% during MDI; this difference did not reach statistical significance due to the small number of subjects. Again, treatment satisfaction was greater for CSII. The rate of severe hypoglycemia was slightly lower during CSII for similar levels of glycemic control. Despite the increased rate of ketonuric events during CSII in both studies, DKA developed in only one adolescent subject during CSII therapy. The results of our studies and previous randomized crossover studies are summarized in table 1.

Recently, a new long-acting insulin analogue glargine, reportedly as peakless insulin, was introduced as better basal insulin for MDI regimen [14]. Studies comparing MDI with glargine with CSII have yielded contradictory results. Lepore et al. [53] demonstrated in a paired study that both CSII with lispro insulin and MDI with lispro plus glargine insulin, equally improve metabolic control and reduce severe hypoglycemia in adults with type 1 diabetes compared to MDI with NPH as it's basal insulin. However, Boland et al. [54], using a randomized parallel study design, found significantly better improvement in glycemic control during CSII and rapid analogue compared to MDI with glargine and aspart in children and adolescents with type 1 diabetes.

Recently CSII was shown to be a safe and effective mode of therapy in toddlers and young children with type 1 diabetes [55] and even in infants with congenital diabetes. It is our impression, too, that infants, toddlers and very

***Table 1.*** Summary of randomized open crossover studies comparing glycemic control, adverse events and satisfaction between CSII and MDI in children and adolescents with type 1 diabetes

| Author | Age group, years (no subjects) | Arm duration | Glycemic control CSII (vs. MDI) | Severe hypoglycemia CSII vs. MDI (n events) | DKA CSII (vs. MDI) (n events) | Insulin dose CSII (vs. MDI) | Satisfaction (CSII vs. MDI) | Continued CSII (%) |
|---|---|---|---|---|---|---|---|---|
| Schiffrin et al., 1982 [45]* | 14–41/(16) | 6 months | similar | 1 vs. 0 | not reported | similar | Similar | 44 |
| Schiffrin et al., 1984 [46]* | adolescents (20) | 4 months | better HbA1c | 1 vs. 1 | not reported | decreased | Similar | 63 |
| Kaufman et al., 1999 [48]** | 7–10 (10) | 6 weeks | better fructosamine | not reported, less mild hypoglycemic events | not reported | decreased | Better adherence, diminished fear of hypoglycemia | ** |
| Weintrob et al., 2003 [32]† | 9–14 (23) | 4 months | similar | 1 vs. 3 | none | decreased | Increased satisfaction, similar impact and worry score | 70 |
| Cohen et al., 2003 [52]‡ | 14.5 –17.9 (12) | 6 months | Δ HbA1c 0.5% less (NS) | 1 vs. 4 | 1 vs. 0 | tendency to decrease | Increased satisfaction, similar impact and worry score | 75 |

*Concrete values for HbA1c were not reported.
**Pumps used during the night only.
†BMI increased with MDI but not CSII.
‡Similar BMI for both arms.

young children who have motivated and adherent parents benefit from CSII therapy: their blood glucose profiles are smoother, parental fear of hypoglycemia is decreased and management of sick days is easier.

## Cost Benefit

In most countries, the cost of the pump itself and the monthly supplies is higher than the cost of conventional or MDI therapy. Therefore, health insurance to cover pump costs is essential for most diabetic patients. In our era of budget limitations and decreased health resources, this issue must be taken up by health-care providers. Larger analyses of the long term cost-benefits of CSII compared to other modalities of intensive control of both type 1 and type 2 diabetes in different age groups are still needed.

## Closing the Loop

Current insulin pumps are based on an open-loop infusion system, wherein the rate of insulin infusion is not automatically adjusted to blood glucose levels. The patient has to decide on the basal infusion rate at different hours of the day and the amount of bolus insulin that should be given before each meal. In the future, with the development of accurate and fast-acting glucose sensors, we expect that the system will change to a closed-loop mechanism. Efforts to connect the CSII with a real-time glucose sensor have already been made in animal models and even in some human trials [56]. Operating together, the glucose sensors and insulin pumps will in effect serve as an artificial pancreas, mimicking the role of the pancreatic β-cells and freeing the patient from the need for constant daily calculations.

## References

1 The Diabetes Control and Complications Trial Research Group: The effect of intensive treatment of diabetes on the development and progression of long-term complications in insulin-dependent diabetes mellitus. N Engl J Med 1993;329:977–986.
2 Hepp KD, Renner R, Funcke HJ, Mehnert H, Haerten R, Kresse H: Glucose homeostasis under continuous intravenous insulin therapy in diabetics. Horm Metab Res 1966;7(suppl):72–76.
3 Deckert T, Lorup B: Regulation of brittle diabetes by a preplanned infusion programme. Diabetologia 1976;12:573–579.
4 Genuth S, Martin P: Control of hyperglycemia in adult diabetics by pulsed insulin delivery. Diabetes 1977;26:571–581.
5 Turner RC, Phillips MA, Ward EA: Ultralente-based insulin regimens: Clinical applications, advantages and disadvantages. Acta Med Scand 1983;671(suppl):75–86.

6 Slama G, Hautecouverture M, Assan R, Tchobroutski G: One to five days of continuous intravenous insulin infusion in seven diabetic patients. Diabetes 1974;23:732–738.
7 Irsigler K, Kritz H: Long-term continuous intravenous insulin therapy with a portable insulin dosage regulating apparatus. Diabetes 1979;28:196–203.
8 Pickup JC, Keen H, Parsons JA, Alberti KGMM: Continuous subcutaneous insulin infusion: an approach to achieving normoglycemia. Br Med J 1978;i204–207.
9 Tamborlane WV, Sherwin RS, Genel M, Felig P: Reduction to normal of plasma glucose in juvenile diabetes by subcutaneous administration of insulin with a portable infusion pump. N Engl J Med 1979;300:573–578.
10 Buchwald J, Rohde TD: Implantable Insulin Pumps. Chicago,Year Book Medical Publishers. 1984, pp 177–222.
11 Irsigler K, Kritz H, Hagmuller G, Franetzki M, Prestele K, Thurow H, Geisen K: Long-term continuous intraperitoneal insulin infusion with an implantable remote-controlled insulin infusion device. Diabetes 1981;30:1072–1075.
12 Saudek CD, Selman JL, Pitt HA, Waxman K, Rubio M, Jeandidier N, Turner D, Fischell RE, Charles MA: A preliminary trial of the programmable implantable medication system for insulin delivery. N Engl J Med 1989;321:574–579.
13 Koivisto VA, Yki-Jarvinen H, Helve E, Karonen SL, Pelkonen R: Pathogenesis and prevention of the dawn phenomenon in diabetic patients treated with CSII. Diabetes 1986;35:78–82.
14 Lepore M, Pampanelli S, Fanelli C, Porcellati F, Bartocci L, Di Vincenzo A, Cordoni C, Costa E, Brunetti P, Bolli GB: Pharmacokinetics and pharmacodynamics of subcutaneous injection of long-acting human insulin analog glargine, NPH insulin, and Ultralente human insulin and continuous subcutaneous infusion of insulin lispro. Diabetes 2000;49:2142–2148.
15 Lauritzen T, Pramming S, Deckert T, Binder C: Pharmacokinetics of continuous subcutaneous insulin infusion. Diabeteologia 1983;24:326–329.
16 Zinman B: The physiologic replacement of insulin, an elusive goal. N Engl J Med 1989;321:363–369.
17 Koivisto VA, Felig P: Alterations in insulin absorption and in blood glucose control associated with varying insulin injection sites in diabetic patients. Ann Intern Med 1980;92:59–61.
18 Wredling R, Hannerz L, Johansson UB: Variability of blood glucose levels in patients treated with continuous subcutaneous insulin infusion: a pilot study. Practical Diabetes Int 1997;14:5–8.
19 Hanaire-Broutin H, Melki V, Bessieres-Lacombe S, Tauber JP: The Study Group for the Development of Pump Therapy in Diabetes. Comparison of continuous subcutaneous insulin infusion and multiple daily injection regimens using insulin lispro in type 1 diabetes patients on intensified treatment. Diabetes Care 2000;23:1232–1235.
20 DeVries JH, Snoek FJ, Kostense PJ, Masurel N, Heine RJ: Dutch Insulin Pump Study Group. A randomized trial of continuous subcutaneous insulin infusion and intensive injection therapy in type 1 diabetes for patients with long-standing poor glycemic control. Diabetes Care 2002; 25:2074–2080.
21 Renner R, Pfutzner A, Trautmann M, Harzer O, Sauter K, Landgraf R: Use of insulin lispro in continuous subcutaneous insulin infusion treatment: Results of a multicenter trial. German Humalog-CSII Study Group. Diabetes Care 1999;22:784–788.
22 Chantelau E, Spraul M, Muhlhauser I, Gause R, Berger M: Long-term safety, efficacy and side-effects of continuous subcutaneous insulin infusion treatment for type 1 (insulin-dependent) diabetes mellitus: A one centre experience. Diabetologia 1989;32:421–426.
23 Wang PH, Lau J, Chalmers TC: Meta-analysis of effects of intensive blood-glucose control on late complications of type 1 diabetes. Lancet 1993;341:1306–1309.
24 Diabetes Control and Complications Trial Research Group. Implementation of treatment protocols in the Diabetes Control and Complications Trial. Diabetes Care 1995;18:361–376.
25 Mecklenburg RS, Benson EA, Benson JW Jr, Fredlund PN, Guinn T, Metz RJ, Nielsen RL, Sanner CA: Acute complications associated with insulin infusion pump therapy. Report of experience with 161 patients. JAMA 1984;252:3265–3269.
26 Teutsch SM, Herman WH, Dwyer DM, Lane JM: Mortality among diabetic patients using continuous subcutaneous insulin-infusion pumps, N Engl J Med 1984;310:361–368.
27 Pietri A, Raskin P: Cutaneous complications of chronic continuous subcutaneous insulin infusion therapy. Diabetes Care 1981;4:624–626.

28 Kaufman FR, Halvorson M, Fisher L, Pitukcheewanont P: Insulin pump therapy in type 1 pediatric patients. J Pediatr Endocrinol Metab 1999;12(suppl 3):759–764.
29 Schiffrin A, Desrosiers M, Moffatt M, Belmonte MM: Feasibility of strict diabetes control in insulin-dependent diabetic adolescents. J Pediatr 1983;103:522–527.
30 Bode BW, Sabbah HT, Gross TM, Fredrickson LP, Davidson PC: Diabetes management in the new millennium using insulin pump therapy. Diabetes Metab Res Rev 2002;18(suppl 1):S14–20.
31 Schade DS, Valentine V: To pump or not to pump. Diabetes Care 2002;25:2100–2102.
32 Weintrob N, Benzaquen H, Galatzer A, Shalitin S, Lazar L, Fayman G, Lilos P, Dickerman Z, Phillip M: Comparison of continuous subcutaneous insulin infusion and multiple daily injection regimens in children with type 1 diabetes: A randomized open crossover trial. Pediatrics 2003; 112:559–564.
33 Tamborlane WV, Sherwin RS, Genel M, Felig P: Outpatient treatment of juvenile-onset diabetes with a preprogrammed portable subcutaneous insulin infusion system. Am J Med 1980;68: 190–196.
34 Conrad SC, McGrath MT, Gitelman SE: Transition from multiple daily injections to continuous subcutaneous insulin infusion in type 1 diabetes mellitus. J Pediadr 2002;140:235–240.
35 Zinman B, Tildesley H, Chiasson JL, Tsui E, Strack T: Insulin lispro in CSII: Results of a double-blind crossover study. Diabetes 1997;46:440–443.
36 Bode B, Weinstein R, Bell D, McGill J, Nadeau D, Raskin P, Davidson J, Henry R, Huang WC, Reinhardt RR: Comparison of insulin aspart with buffered regular insulin and insulin lispro in continuous subcutaneous insulin infusion: A randomized study in type 1 diabetes. Diabetes Care 2002;25:439–444.
37 Pickup J, Mattock M, Kerry S: Glycaemic control with continuous subcutaneous insulin infusion compared with intensive insulin injections in patients with type 1 diabetes: meta-analysis of randomised controlled trials. Br Med J 2002;324:1–6.
38 Weissberg-Benchell J, Antisdel-Lomaglio J, Seshadri R: Insulin pump therapy: A meta-analysis. Diabetes Care 2003;26:1079–1087.
39 Lenhard MJ, Reeves GD: Continuous subcutaneous insulin infusion: A comprehensive review of insulin pump therapy. Arch Intern Med 2001;161:2293–2300.
40 Schiffrin A, Colle E, Belmonte M: Improved control in diabetes with continuous subcutaneous insulin infusion. Diabetes Care 1980;3:643–649.
41 Davies AG, Price DA, Houlton CA, Burn JL, Fielding BA, Postlethwaite RJ: Continuous subcutaneous insulin infusion in diabetes mellitus: A year's prospective trial. Arch Dis Child 1984;59: 1027–1033.
42 Brink SJ, Stewart C: Insulin pump treatment in insulin-dependent diabetes mellitus. Children, adolescents, and young adults. JAMA 1986;255:617–621.
43 de Beaufort CE, Houtzagers CM, Bruining GJ, Aarsen RS, den Boer NC, Grose WF, van Strik R, de Visser JJ: Continuous subcutaneous insulin infusion (CSII) versus conventional injection therapy in newly diagnosed diabetic children: two-year follow-up of a randomized, prospective trial. Diabet Med 1989;6:766–771.
44 Saha ME, Huuppone T, Mikael K, Juuti M, Komulainen J: Continuous subcutaneous insulin infusion in the treatment of children and adolescents with type 1 diabetes mellitus. J Pediatr Endocrinol Metab 2002;15:1005–1010.
45 Schiffrin A, Belmonte MM: Comparison between continuous subcutaneous insulin infusion and multiple injections of insulin: A one-year prospective study. Diabetes 1982;31:255–264.
46 Schiffrin AD, Desrosiers M, Aleyassine H, Belmonte MM: Intensified insulin therapy in the type I diabetic adolescent: a controlled trial. Diabetes Care. 1984;7:107–113.
47 Boland EA, Grey M, Oesterle A, Fredrickson L, Tamborlane WV: Continuous subcutaneous insulin infusion. A new way to lower risk of severe hypoglycemia, improve metabolic control, and enhance coping in adolescents with type 1 diabetes. Diabetes Care 1999;22:1779–1784.
48 Kaufman FR, Halvorson M, Kim C, Pitukcheewanont P: Use of insulin pump therapy at nighttime only for children 7–10 years of age with type 1 diabetes. Diabetes Care 2000;23:579–582.
49 Maniatis AK, Klingensmith GJ, Slover RH, Mowry CJ, Chase HP: Continuous subcutaneous insulin infusion therapy for children and adolescents: An option for routine diabetes care. Pediatrics 2001;107:351–356.

50 Raile K, Noelle V, Landgraf R, Schwarz HP: Weight in adolescents with type 1 diabetes mellitus during continuous subcutaneous insulin infusion (CSII) therapy, J Pediatr Endocrinol Metab 2002;15:607–612.
51 Weintrob N, Schechter A, Benzaquen H, Shalitin S, Lilos P, Galatzer A, Phillip M: Glycemic patterns detected by continuous subcutaneous glucose sensing in children with type 1 diabetes treated by MDI or CSII. Diabetes 2003;52(suppl 1):430.
52 Cohen D, Weintrob N, Benzaquen H, Galatzer A, Fayman G, Phillip M: Continuous subcutaneous insulin infusion (CSII) versus multiple daily injections (MDI) in adolescents with type 1 diabetes: A randomized open crossover trial. J Pediatr Endocrinol Metab 2003;16:1047–1050.
53 Lepore G, Dodesini AR, Nosari I, Trevisan R: Both continuous subcutaneous insulin infusion and a multiple daily insulin injection regimen with glargine as basal insulin are equally better than traditional multiple daily insulin injection treatment. Diabetes Care 2003;26:1321–1322.
54 Boland E, Weinzimer S, Ahern JA, Steffen A, Tamborlane W: Randomised, prospective trial of CSII vs MDI with glargine in Children: A preliminary report. Diabetes 2003;52(suppl1):192.
55 Weinzimer S, Ahern J, Boland E, Steffen A, Tamborlane W: Continuous subcutaneous insulin infusion (CSII) is safe and effective in very young children with type 1 diabetes (T1DM). Diabetes 2002;51(suppl 2):1744.
56 Renard E, Shah R, Miller M, Kolopp M, Costalat G, Bringer J: Sustained safety and accuracy of cental IV glucose sensors connected to implanted insulin pumps and short-term closed-loop trials in diabetic patients. Diabetes 2003;52(suppl 2):155.

Prof. Moshe Phillip
Schneider Children's Medical Center of Israel
Institute for Endocrinology and Diabetes
National Center for Childhood Diabetes
14 Kaplan Street, Petah Tikva 49202 (Israel)
Tel. +972 3 9253731, Fax +972 3 9253836, E-Mail mosheph@post.tau.ac.il

Chiarelli F, Dahl-Jørgensen K, Kiess W (eds): Diabetes in Childhood and Adolescence.
Pediatr Adolesc Med. Basel, Karger, 2005, vol 10, pp 163–180

# Quality Management in Pediatric Diabetology

*Reinhard W. Holl, Matthias Grabert, Ulrike Krause, Franz Schweiggert for the German Initiative on Quality Control in Paediatric Diabetology*

Computer Assisted Quality Management in Medicine,
University of Ulm, ZIMBT, Ulm, Germany

## Why Is Quality Management Important for Pediatric Diabetology?

The current therapy available for children and adolescents with diabetes is by no means ideal. Current guidelines [1] define good control at HbA1c-levels below 7.5%, and acceptable control at HbA1c levels between 7.6 and 9%. However, in real life, the actual level of control achieved in children and adolescents is considerably worse: While excellent metabolic control in the majority of children is reported from few pediatric centers only (for example, mean HbA1c in 144 children in Brussels: 6.6% [2]), multicenter studies in most countries report considerably higher average HbA1c levels: Denmark: 9.7% in 339 pediatric patients [3], Scotland: 9.1% based on 1,755 patients [4], Germany: mean 7.9% in 21,335 patients with T1-DM younger than 20 years, with 66.5% of patients >7.5 and 35.9% above 9% [5], Australia: 8.2% in 1,190 children and adolescents (1.2–15.8 years of age) [6]. This fact is confirmed by a multinational survey from 18 countries, including 2,873 children and adolescents [7]. Even as HbA1c falls considerably above recommended targets in most pediatric patients, at the same time the rate of severe hypoglycemic events is also unacceptably high, especially in the youngest age group [7, 8]. In the short run, diabetes in children and adolescents causes a major burden for affected families, psychological disturbances and financial costs for the individual and the society [9]. In the long run, insufficient metabolic control in diabetic patients is a major predictor for diabetic microvascular and macrovascular complications, with hard end-points including blindness, end-stage kidney disease, cardiovascular disease and considerable morbidity and mortality.

How can the outlook for children and adolescents with diabetes be improved? Many patients and families, but also health care professionals caring for pediatric patients hope for new technical developments (closed-loop systems, implantable insulin pumps, continuous and/or noninvasive blood glucose monitoring), for islet cell transplantation, genetically engineered cells or stem cell technology, or just for pharmacological improvements like new insulin preparations or analogs, insulin-sensitizing drugs, co-therapy to reduce glycation and subsequent organ damage, etc. However, even the most optimistic researchers will admit that such developments are not likely to provide a cure for type 1 diabetes in the next 5–10 years for the majority of patients currently affected. It is beyond the scope of this chapter to go into detail on all the chances and risks of such potential developments. While the vision of a definitive cure provides hope and spirit for the patient and family, small practical improvements are much more likely to have a significant impact on the foreseeable future for pediatric patients with diabetes.

Both health care professionals and affected patients/families will agree that the situation for children and adolescents with diabetes has improved considerably during the last 20 years. However, this improvement was not due to a major technological breakthrough: While new insulin analogues beyond doubt provide a certain advantage for some patients, and currently available blood glucose meters are faster and more convenient, the major tools for modern diabetes therapy have been available for many years: insulin preparations with different kinetics, blood-glucose self-monitoring, insulin dose adjustment, education for patients and families, psychological and social support for affected children and their families.

Therefore, the basic philosophy of quality management for childhood diabetes can be summarized in one sentence: Use the available tools for diabetes care more and more efficiently. This is an evolutionary approach, in contrast to a revolution in diabetes care based on hypothetical biotechnological breakthroughs.

An additional point has to be mentioned as a major force to justify quality management: All healthcare systems in the world are currently under considerable financial pressure. This fact has to be accepted, and even the allocation of more resources towards pediatrics, or towards diabetes care, will in itself not be able to solve this problem. Given the vast number of equally important health challenges for the future, it is very unlikely that any modern society will be able to considerably increase the financing for pediatric diabetes care. In this economic light the concept of outcome research will be necessary to convince

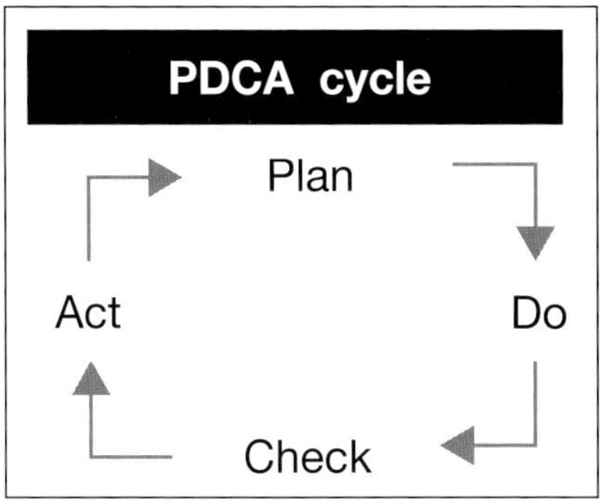


*Fig. 1.* Visualization of the PDCA-cycle. Adapted from Deming [10].

politicians and society of the long-term cost-effectiveness of pediatric diabetes care.

In view of these economic constraints, it is no surprise that modern concepts like 'evidence-based medicine', 'health technology assessment' or 'managed care' have primarily been developed in the United Kingdom in response to considerable under-financing of health care. Currently, many societies – in European and overseas – adopt similar approaches to make medicine more efficient.

## The Quality Control Cycle

Quality management is a continuous process, generally described as a cycle: With every turn, some improvement is likely to be achieved; however, the optimum, the ideal diabetes care, is probably never reaches. A common visualization of the quality control cycle is the PDCA-approach: Plan – Do – Check – Act (fig. 1), but other acronyms have been used as well.

Before quality improvement is feasible, the basic philosophy of quality control has to be accepted wholeheartedly by an institution. In other words, a health care team, a hospital or practice, or society as a whole has to be convinced that quality management is a way to improve the results achieved [11]. This decision should be based on concrete shortcomings of present care, and the step towards improvement should be as focused as possible: Improve metabolic control, or reduce the number of severe hypoglycemic events, or make the system more cost-effective.

The more precisely the problem is defined, the more efficient is the quality management likely to be. If a concrete remedy for a perceived deficit is available, the next step of course would be to implement these changes. Did these changes work? In order to get the answer, one of the basics of quality management has to be implemented: objective documentation of the results, which are then to be interpreted carefully. Further action can then be based upon the results already achieved.

A practical example for such a cycle would follow-up the current insufficient level of metabolic control achieved in many pediatric patients with diabetes: A diabetes team may decide to improve the situation by switching to intensified insulin therapy [12], by using insulin pumps [13] or by intensifying diabetes education [14]. Which approach is the most promising will depend on the current therapeutic strategy at this institution, available evidence in the literature, or personal experience reported by other diabetes teams. However, the crucial point is objective documentation of changes in metabolic control achieved in response to this intervention, and base subsequent actions on these evaluations.

### Where to Look: Structure, Process or Outcome of Care?

Based on a generally accepted suggestion by Donabedian [15], it is common in the medical area to discriminate between structural aspects of health care, the process of delivering care, and the final results or outcome. In pediatric diabetology, structure of care relates to the personnel and training/experience in a diabetes team, the availability of a 24-hour telephone hotline or continuous presence of a diabetes specialist. Availability of a pediatric psychologist, a diabetes nurse specialist, a dietician and/or a health care worker are other aspects of structural quality. It is difficult to provide high-level diabetes care without sufficient trained personnel. Consequently, in many quality initiatives, the availability of a multi-professional diabetes team which is dedicated full-time to the care of children and adolescents with diabetes is considered as perhaps the most important component.

The availability and integration of inpatient and outpatient care is also an important structural component – despite the fact that diabetes care is provided more and more on an outpatient basis. Structured teaching courses for group or individual education, the availability of teaching materials for children of different age groups, a room dedicated entirely to education or psychosocial support groups for parents and relatives are additional components. Medical aspects related to the structure of diabetes care are for example the quality of lab measurements (blood glucose readily available for the patient, precise methods for HbA1c, lipids and urine albumin), the availability of medical literature, internet, current guidelines, etc. In contrast to adult diabetology, technical devices for eye examinations, ultrasound, vascular diagnosis, etc. have a limited importance in pediatric diabetes care and are therefore not part of structural requirements in this age group.

Many services expect progress primarily from structural improvements. This view may actually be true for health services in underdeveloped areas of the world, or when new facilities are initiated. However, it has to be realized that investments into the structure and personnel alone – while invariably expensive – will not necessarily guarantee an improvement in outcome.

The process of care is probably more important: How are available resources utilized? Which standard operating procedures, guidelines, etc. are implemented and how closely are they followed during everyday work? The process of care is therefore probably the most import component of quality management, therefore many current quality initiatives focus entirely on this area:

- How is the patient's history taken?
- Does every patient get the necessary control exams?
- Is diabetes education focussed on the problems of the patient?
- Is insulin therapy tailored to the needs of the family?
- How often are patients seen by the doctor or a diabetes nurse?
- Are patients screened for hypertension?
- Do patients with hypertension receive adequate treatment?
- Are there follow-up exams?
- How are patients and private physicians informed about the care provided by the specialist diabetes team?

These are just some examples for questions relevant for the process of diabetes care.

The philosophy to focus primarily on the process of diabetes care is based on the assumption that optimization of patient care will invariably lead to better long-term results. Is this true? Unfortunately, little data are available for the pediatric age group: No studies comparable to the DCCT or the UKPDS are currently available for pediatric patients. This becomes even more relevant when outcome indicators are considered, as few long-term, multicenter, population-based studies with children or adolescents are available. This lack of data has to be considered when pediatric quality initiatives are initiated.

### What to Record: Standardized, Objective Documentation

To get an objective picture of the process and outcome of medical care at an institution is an integral part of quality management. Questionnaires for patients on their subjective view regarding the quality of care they received are definitely an important approach reflecting the 'consumer satisfaction' aspect of diabetes care: Topics like accessibility of the diabetes team, time spent with individual team members, the understandable advice given, etc. are best recorded asking patients themselves. However, other areas of medical care, especially long-term aspects, are not readily reflected by patient questionnaires: Prevention of late complications by reduction of risk factors, or prevention of rare events like DKA episodes, etc. are probably not accessible by patient questionnaire. For these aspects, a standardized medical documentation is required, focussing on process of care, as well as long-term outcome. One possibility of a standardized dataset adopted for pediatric patients with diabetes from the IDF Europe/St. Vincent basic information sheet (BIS) is given in figure 2.

It is an inherent challenge for this approach that hard, medical facts and endpoints (lab-values, examinations, complications, etc.) are relatively easy to document in an objective way, while other, equally important areas, like psychosocial adjustment or quality of life are much more difficult to record in a valid and reproducible way in a multi-center, standard-care environment.

When initiatives for the initiation of quality management are started, the discussion on the number of parameters to document, the exact definition of these parameters (what is a severe hypoglycemia in a young child?) and the way to analyze these data (subgroups? adjustment for differences in case-mix) is a crucial, by very time-consuming step. Unfortunately, little standardization has been reached so far, both in adult as well as in pediatric diabetology.

### Paper or PC: How to Document?

On an agreement on quality indicators and parameters to document has been reached, the next step is to set up a documentation system. The easiest way is to design a paper form, where data are entered manually by the diabetes team (fig. 2). This approach has undoubtedly the advantage that it is easy, that no technology is required at the participating institutions, and that not only doctors but also nurses and other members of a health-care team feel secure with this approach. Paper documentation is probably the way to go when quality management for a rare disease is initiated. However, major disadvantages of this approach have to be kept in mind, which become more and more relevant with increasing numbers of patients included, which is equivalent to a higher frequency of the disease: When documentation covers only a fragment of patients, the risk for bias is high. Using the paper approach, a double documentation is necessary (patient chart plus quality sheet), which increases the workload for the team. For analysis, including feedback and benchmarking, data have to be available in electronic form. If this data entry is performed in a central institution, additional workforce is required, increasing the overall cost

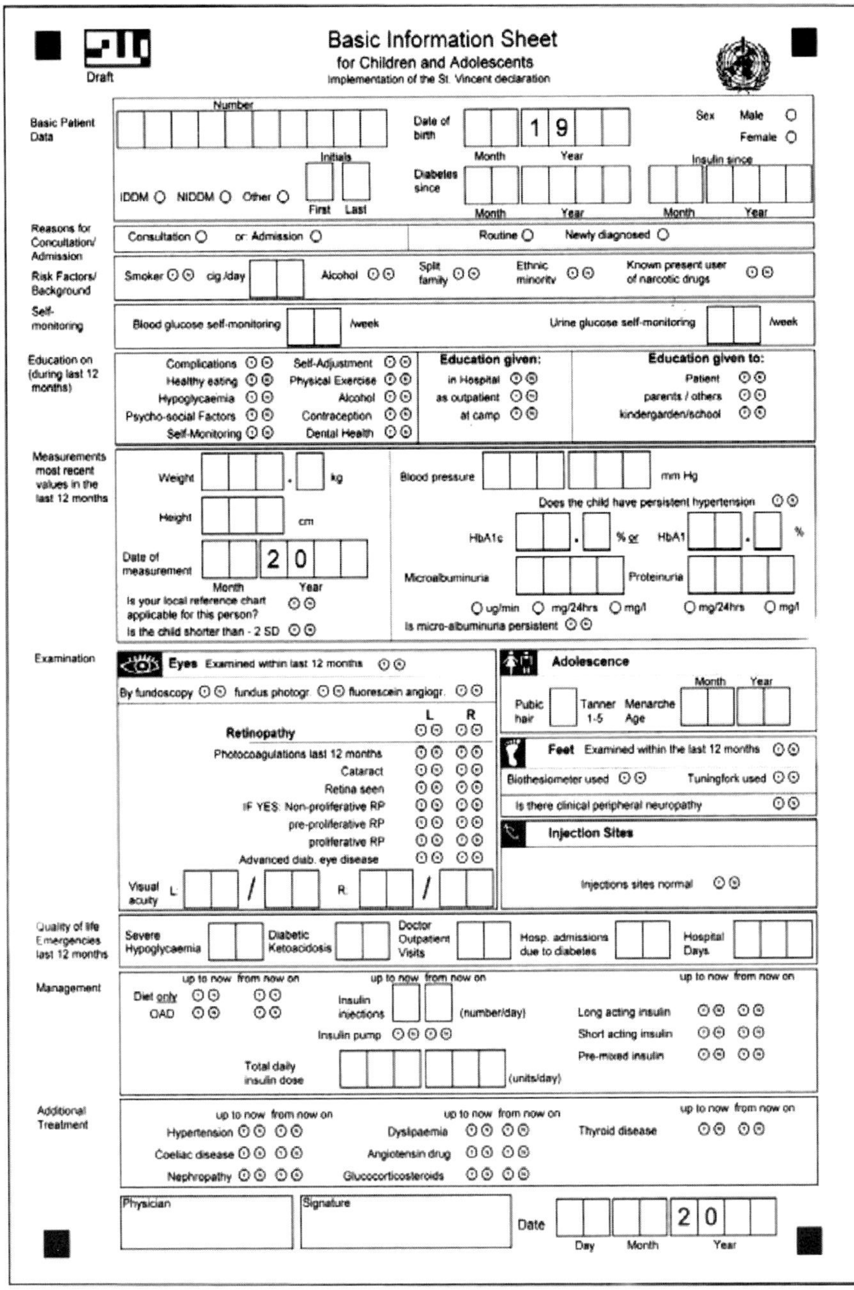

Draft

**Basic Information Sheet**
for Children and Adolescents
Implementation of the St. Vincent declaration

Basic Patient Data
Number
Date of birth: Month / Year 1 9
Sex: Male ○ Female ○
Initials: First / Last
IDDM ○ NIDDM ○ Other ○
Diabetes since: Month / Year
Insulin since: Month / Year

Reasons for Concultation/ Admission
Consultation ○ or: Admission ○ | Routine ○ Newly diagnosed ○

Risk Factors/ Background
Smoker ⊙⊙ cig./day | Alcohol ⊙⊙ | Split family ⊙⊙ | Ethnic minority ⊙⊙ | Known present user of narcotic drugs ⊙⊙

Self-monitoring
Blood glucose self-monitoring /week | Urine glucose self-monitoring /week

Education on (during last 12 months)
Complications ⊙⊙ | Self-Adjustment ⊙⊙
Healthy eating ⊙⊙ | Physical Exercise ⊙⊙
Hypoglycaemia ⊙⊙ | Alcohol ⊙⊙
Psycho-social Factors ⊙⊙ | Contraception ⊙⊙
Self-Monitoring ⊙⊙ | Dental Health ⊙⊙

**Education given:**
in Hospital ⊙⊙
as outpatient ⊙⊙
at camp ⊙⊙

**Education given to:**
Patient ⊙⊙
parents / others ⊙⊙
kindergarden/school ⊙⊙

Measurements most recent values in the last 12 months
Weight . kg
Height cm
Date of measurement: Month / Year 2 0
Is your local reference chart applicable for this person? ⊙⊙
Is the child shorter than - 2 SD ⊙⊙
Blood pressure mm Hg
Does the child have persistent hypertension ⊙⊙
HbA1c . % or HbA1 . %
Microalbuminuria | Proteinuria
○ ug/min ○ mg/24hrs ○ mg/l | ○ mg/24hrs ○ mg/l
Is micro-albuminuria persistent ⊙⊙

Examination
**Eyes** Examined within last 12 months ⊙⊙
By fundoscopy ⊙⊙ fundus photogr. ⊙⊙ fluorescein angiogr. ⊙⊙

| | L | R |
|---|---|---|
| **Retinopathy** | ⊙⊙ | ⊙⊙ |
| Photocoagulations last 12 months | ⊙⊙ | ⊙⊙ |
| Cataract | ⊙⊙ | ⊙⊙ |
| Retina seen | ⊙⊙ | ⊙⊙ |
| IF YES: Non-proliferative RP | ⊙⊙ | ⊙⊙ |
| pre-proliferative RP | ⊙⊙ | ⊙⊙ |
| proliferative RP | ⊙⊙ | ⊙⊙ |
| Advanced diab. eye disease | ⊙⊙ | ⊙⊙ |

Visual acuity L: / R: /

**Adolescence**
Pubic hair | Tanner 1-5 | Menarche Age: Month / Year

**Feet** Examined within the last 12 months ⊙⊙
Biothesiometer used ⊙⊙ | Tuningfork used ⊙⊙
Is there clinical peripheral neuropathy ⊙⊙

**Injection Sites**
Injections sites normal ⊙⊙

Quality of life Emergencies last 12 months
Severe Hypoglycaemia | Diabetic Ketoacidosis | Doctor Outpatient Visits | Hosp. admissions due to diabetes | Hospital Days

Management
| | up to now | from now on |
|---|---|---|
| Diet only | ⊙⊙ | ⊙⊙ |
| OAD | ⊙⊙ | ⊙⊙ |

Insulin injections (number/day)
Insulin pump: up to now ⊙⊙ from now on ⊙⊙
Total daily insulin dose (units/day)

| | up to now | from now on |
|---|---|---|
| Long acting insulin | ⊙⊙ | ⊙⊙ |
| Short acting insulin | ⊙⊙ | ⊙⊙ |
| Pre-mixed insulin | ⊙⊙ | ⊙⊙ |

Additional Treatment
| | up to now | from now on |
|---|---|---|
| Hypertension | ⊙⊙ | ⊙⊙ |
| Coeliac disease | ⊙⊙ | ⊙⊙ |
| Nephropathy | ⊙⊙ | ⊙⊙ |
| Dyslipaemia | ⊙⊙ | ⊙⊙ |
| Angiotensin drug | ⊙⊙ | ⊙⊙ |
| Glucocorticosteroids | ⊙⊙ | ⊙⊙ |
| Thyroid disease | ⊙⊙ | ⊙⊙ |

Physician | Signature | Date: Day / Month / Year 2 0

***Fig. 2.*** The St. Vincent basic information sheet (DiabCare BIS) for a standardized documentation of relevant items in pediatric diabetes care.

for documentation. And probably the most important point: If data are not readily available at the institution, important functions like accounting, patient summaries, research projects, etc. need separate data entry, thereby increasing the overall workload and subsequently the costs. It is therefore no surprise that all quality initiatives based on separate paper documentation (quality sheet approach) suffer from the fact that health care teams do not participate in the initiative continuously over several years, that the quality of documentation (completeness of data and internal validity) is low, and that members of the diabetes team often display a negative attitude towards quality management, as they primarily see it as an additional work-load.

Therefore, several approaches on the documentation for quality management use computer-based technology, integrating electronic patient records and the quality indicators required [16]. Due to the IT hardware required, the necessary training of personnel, but also the difficulties with data integration in heterogeneous IT environments is still present in many hospital settings as the initial investment necessary to implement such a system is considerably higher [17]. However, once the system works satisfactorily, relevant data are documented once and then made available for various tasks, many of them providing a direct advantage for the health care team. Therefore, the long-term acceptance is much better compared to the data-sheet approach [18]. In figure 3, this basic concept is illustrated by the functionality of the DPV Software, an electronic patient record developed in Germany primarily for pediatric patients with diabetes, and subsequently adopted for adult diabetes care. 150 pediatric centers, 250 adult clinics and 500 diabetes specialists in private practice currently use this system.

## Quantifying Success: Quality Indicators

How can we measure the effect of medical care? With acute diseases, quantifying the percentage of patients successfully cured from their disease, together with the rate of patients suffering from complications, seems quite easy. It is somewhat more difficult with chronic disorders, where no cure is available so far. One group of indicators assesses the process of care. We all agree that patient education is a prerequisite for long-term success and we also agree that certain control exams (HbA1c, blood pressure, BMI, lipid levels, eye exams, urine albumin excretion) have to be performed at regular intervals. The performance of a diabetes center in both areas can easily be quantified. The idea behind this approach is that optimal therapy (education, insulin therapy, control exams, psychosocial counselling, etc.) will invariably lead to optimal results. In the age of evidence-based medicine, this should be based on randomized intervention studies.

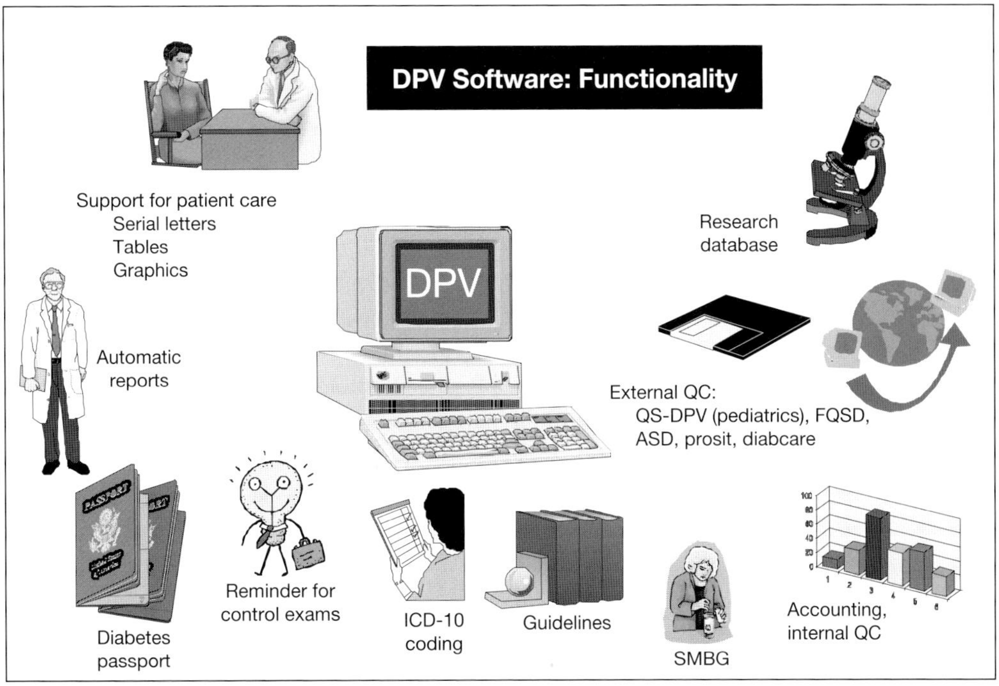


*Fig. 3.* One example of an electronic patient management system, including direct support for the diabetes team, internal and external quality control, as well as anonymous accumulation of data for research purposes. This system was originally developed in Germany for pediatric diabetes patients only, it is now widely used both for pediatric and adult diabetology [8, 22, 24].

Outcome indicators, or hard endpoints, like survival, myocardial infarct, blindness or end-stage kidney disease are the gold-standard to determine the success of medical therapy. For pediatric patients, the interval until such endpoints can be evaluated is well beyond 20 or 30 years. This is certainly one reason why practically no intervention studies with hard endpoints are available for children: For adults, the DCCT has unequivocally shown that intensive insulin therapy results in lower HbA1c levels and lower rates of microvascular complications [19]. However, in pediatric diabetology, no simple relationship seems to exist between the intensity of insulin therapy and metabolic control achieved [20]. While numerous observational studies indicate that early metabolic control is important for subsequent micro- and macrovascular complications, so far no definitive intervention studies are available relating the mode of insulin therapy – or any other aspect of long-term patient care – to such hard endpoints in young patients. However, intermediate indicators as well as some outcome indicators could be evaluated for pediatric patients: final height achieved, presence of microvascular changes (microaneurysms, miroalbuminuria) after a certain duration of diabetes, or long-term metabolic control, as Hba1c correlates with nearly all hard endpoints in diabetology.

A difficult area, which has not been solved convincingly, is the objective reflection of the psychosocial burden for patient and family, or in wider terms, their 'quality of life' (QOL). While there is no doubt that QOL aspects should be part of a quality management systems, psychosocial aspects are difficult of document objectively during routine care. However, recent research has demonstrated that QOL is positively related to HbA1c – indicating that this metabolic parameter will reflect psychosocial adjustment as well [21, 22].

Which indicators should be chosen as a basis for quality control management? The answer depends on the regional/national context, the preferences of the group, but also on the financing of the health care system. Even if pediatricians would like to be guided only by medical, psychological or social directives, one has to admit that all health care systems are currently under financial pressure, and the question of cost-effectiveness has to be an integral part of all quality management systems.

When a new quality initiative is initiated it is wise to start with a limited number of relevant quality indicators, and step by step add new, additional indicators. In table 1 some potential quality indicators relevant for pediatric diabetology are listed together with the treatment goal they reflect. This list is not comprehensive.

## How to Compare: Benchmarking

Internal quality management alone will not be sufficient to achieve optimal results in all areas. Every critical physician will ask the question how his work compares to that of his colleagues in the same area. Usually, the results from external comparisons are compiled as histograms for each quality indicator (example in fig. 4), but other graphical forms for data visualization have also been proposed.

Who should receive benchmarking reports? While some competition is healthy to stimulate one's potential, it is difficult to decide whether such external comparisons should be discussed openly or anonymously, and who should have access to the results (participating physicians only? insurance companies? government agencies? individual patients and patient organizations?). Many institutions are reluctant to publicize their results. Fears are based on insufficient results at an institution, on perceived disadvantages in the comparison

***Table 1.*** Examples for quality indicators reflecting the process and outcome of diabetes care, relevant for paediatric services

| Treatment goal | Quality indicator |
|---|---|
| Normal growth | percentage of patients with height <3rd percentile |
| Normal physical development | average BMI in diabetic children compared to nondiabetic children |
| | percentage of patients with BMI >97th percentile |
| Normal pubertal development | mean age at menarche in girls with diabetes |
| Low rate of acute complications | frequency of severe hypoglycaemia (definition!) in all patients |
| | frequency of severe hypoglycaemia (definition!) in patients younger than 5 years of age |
| | frequency of admission due to DKA after onset of diabetes |
| Prevention of microvascular complications | percentage of patients with eye exams during the last year |
| | percentage of patients with urine albumin excretion rate determined during last year |
| | mean HbA1c achieved in all patients |
| | mean HbA1c achieved in adolescent patients |
| | percentage of patients beyond 5 years of diabetes with diabetic retinopathy |
| | percentage of patients beyond 5 years of diabetes with diabetic nephropathy |
| | percentage of patients with persistent microalbuminuria not receiving ACE-inhibitors (or other interventions for microalbuminuria) |
| Prevention of cardiovascular complications | percentage of patients with lipid levels available during the last year |
| | percentage of patients with blood pressure recordings available during the last year |
| | percentage of patients with hypertension |
| | percentage of patients with hyperlipidemia |
| | percentage of patients with hypertension not receiving antihypertensive therapy |
| | percentage of patients with hyperlipidemia not receiving lipid-lowering therapy |
| | mean HbA1c achieved in all patients |
| | mean HbA1c achieved in adolescent patients |
| | percentage of patients beyond 5 years of diabetes with diabetic |

*Table 1* (continued)

| Treatment goal | Quality indicator |
|---|---|
| Optimal social adjustment | average number of days spent in hospital<br>average number of days where school was missed due to diabetes<br>percentage of patients on flexible insulin regimen (beyond remission)<br>QOL in patients with diabetes<br>QOL in parents from patients with diabetes<br>percentage of patients missing appointments |

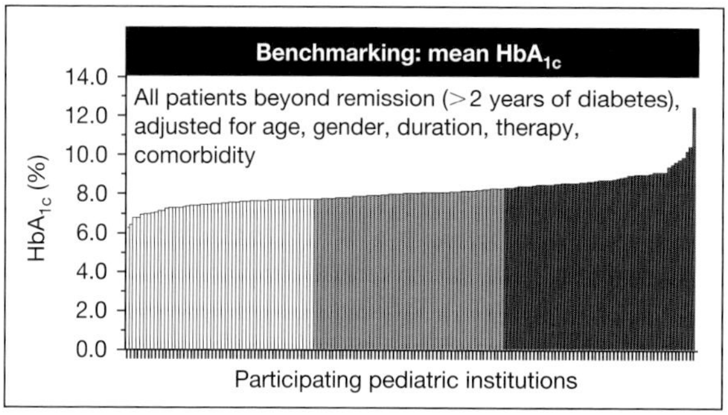


***Fig. 4.*** Benchmarking for metabolic control achieved beyond the remission phase, adjusted for various influencing factors, for 159 pediatric institutions participating in the German external quality control initiative. Color-coding (white = good, gray = acceptable, dark gray = improvement urgently recommended) is used to render results more visible.

based on the patient population (more adolescent patients, more patients referred due to insufficient metabolic control, more patients from ethnic minorities, etc.) or on the fear that future reimbursement might depend on the presentation of 'excellent' results. While some inequalities in the case-mix can be mathematically corrected (e.g. fig. 4), it has to be admitted that such corrections may not be absolutely perfect for all quality indicators.

External comparisons require critical discussions among participating centers in order to identify strengths and weaknesses, and give practical clues, how improvements might be achieved [23].

Quality of care invariably has financial implications: health care officials, insurance companies/managed care providers as well as patient organizations have a legitimate interest in benchmarking results and will more and more force institutions to implement components of quality management. Therefore, institutions who engage themselves early in this area will have considerable advantages.

### Repeating the Cycle: The Longitudinal Aspect

Quality of care is not static, both structural components and the process of care change over time. Therefore, repeated analyses of relevant quality indicators at quarterly, half-yearly or yearly intervals are necessary to document improvements but also potential deteriorations over time [24]. Repeated benchmarking also provides an overall picture of the current level of diabetes care within the quality initiative. In figure 5, changes of 3 relevant indicators over 8 years are presented from the German pediatric quality control initiative [25, 26].

### Quality Circles: How to Discuss Strengths and Weaknesses

Benchmarking alone will most likely not improve the outcome of medical services. The whole diabetes team has to critically discuss the feedback from both internal quality control (for an example, compared the outcome achieved last year to results from this year) as well as external comparisons (benchmarking). The following questions have to be discussed: Why do other centers achieve better results? Where are our weaknesses, where are our strengths? How do patient characteristics (case-mix, referral practices, etc.) affect our results?

A quality circle will only be successful if all members are motivated, open to change and accept the methodology of quality assessment as a way to improve results achieved. Due to the hierarchic structure, this is often difficult in a university setting, where excellence is defined by academic achievements or impact factors of publications, rather than outcome of patient care. As in many other areas, the concept that every member of a diabetes team can learn from their peers will gain ground and is currently supported by most medical and professional associations. Specialized training for quality-circle moderators is now offered by many medical associations or by external consultants. Regular participation in quality circles is often a prerequisite for board-certification of health-care professionals, or for accreditation of an institution.

A quality circle provides a bottom-up approach: Members of a diabetes treatment team, who are in everyday contact with the patients, generate the

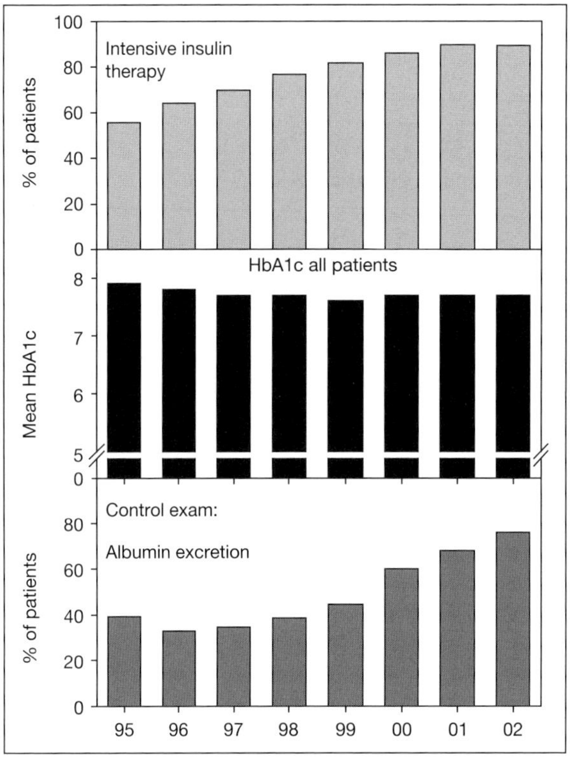


*Fig. 5.* Assessing quality indicators longitudinally (German pediatric diabetes quality initiative, 1995 until 2002) top panel: percentage of pediatric patients (age <18 years) on intensive insulin therapy (3 or more injections per day or insulin pump therapy) over the years 1995 to 2002. Middle panel: average HbA1c achieved in all pediatric patients. Bottom panel: percentage of pediatric patients (age >11 years or diabetes' duration >5 years) with a documented urine check for albumin excretion during the last year.

information, and a non-hierarchical quality control circle allows them to draw meaningful conclusions, leading to procedural changes, which will improve the quality of care they provide. Thus, a quality circle differs fundamentally from traditional, top-down, continuing medical education, where specialists pass on knowledge to a predominantly passive audience, with often minimal effects on patient outcome.

The exchange possible in quality circles can be further augmented by extended visits (hospitalizations) at other centers providing a similar level of care: individual members of a diabetes team passively observe and/or actively participate for example in education courses at the hospital where the visit takes place. A joint discussion of the observations of the visiting team member, and sometimes also a written report, provide the basis of intensive exchange. Such visits become more and more part of center certification and/or continuous education for team members.

### Quality Reports and Audits

Based on the EFQM (European Foundation for Quality Monitoring) quality model, an institution aiming to improve the quality of products or services starts by compiling a quality report: During this self-assessment step, all relevant information, based on consumer (patient) interviews, internal quality assessment, benchmarking etc is compiled. During this process, the institution is forced to identify strengths as well as deficits of the present quality level achieved.

The next step is often an external audit, either by peers from different institution, or by specially trained auditors, who objectively confirm the facts in the quality report. Based on their findings, if certain requirements are fulfilled, the institution can apply for certification. Different institutions offer such certification for medical institutions (in Germany for example DIN ISO 2000, KTQ, ProCumcert, medical communities, etc.). Primarily structural requirements and process quality (guidelines, SOP = standard operational procedures) are evaluated during external audits as a basis for subsequent certification. Following the example from industry, more and more medical institutions seek such certifications, in part for marketing reasons, in part as a prerequisite for financial reimbursement. It has to be critically acknowledged that so far – in the medical area – it has not been shown that outcome is better in certified institutions, and the certification process implies considerable costs – both internally for the preparation of a quality report and for the reimbursement of external audits.

### The Future: Chances and Limitations

Is quality management just a passing trend or will it become an integral part of all areas of health care? There are many facts supporting the latter assumption: In industry, both production and consumer services, quality management is accepted as a valuable tool to improve competitiveness and to reduce costs. As health care adopts more and more management components from business and industry, it is likely that quality management will become even more important for health care providers. Insurance companies follow the concepts of 'controlling' and 'cost-effectiveness' and will pay only for those medical services that can prove their quality. But the most important driving force will be the patient in his/her new role as 'health care consumer', demanding proofs for the quality of care provided [27]. While traditionally patients judge the quality of care by aspects like hotel quality (food, rooms, friendliness of staff) or the empathy of their doctor, more and more objective results of an institution will become the basis of patient-doctor relationship: As some cardiac patients in the US choose their surgeon based on operation frequency and rates of bypass patency and complications [28], diabetes patients in the near future will ask questions like 'average metabolic control achieved', hospitalization rate or amputation frequency [29]. In order to guide the individual patient in their search for the 'best diabetes care available', the impact of patient organizations will dramatically increase during the next years. This may sound unfamiliar or even frightening for some doctors and nurses, who are personally convinced to provide the best advice available. However, we will all realize that being personally convinced of our quality may not be enough, and quality control methodology will help us to improve further, step by step [30]. Therefore, we should not be afraid and defensive against quality control, but accept this approach as one way towards a better future for our children with diabetes.

## References


1 Swift PGF (ed): ISPAD Consensus Guidelines. Zeist, Publ. Medforum, 2000.

2 Dorchy H, Roggemans MP, Willems D: Glycated hemoglobin and related factors in diabetic children and adolescents under 18 years of age: A Belgian experience. Diabetes Care 1997; 209:2–6.

3 Olsen BS, Johannesen J, Sjolie AK, Borch-Jonsen K, Hougaard P, Thorsteinsson B, Prammig S, Marinelli K, Mortensen HB: Metabolic control and prevalence of microvascular complications in young Danish patients with type 1 diabetes mellitus. Diab Med 1999;16:79–85.

4 Scottish Study Group for the Care of the Young Diabetic: Factors influencing glycemic control in young people with type 1 diabetes in Scotland. Diabetes Care 2001;24:239–244.

5 Holl RW, Schwab O, Wiemann D, Rami B, Dost AG, Klinkert C, Grabert M for the DPV-Wiss Group: Cardiovascular risk factors in patients with type-1 diabetes mellitus during the first two decades of life. 29th Annual Meeting of ISPAD, Saint-Malo, 2003. J Pediatr Endocrinol Metab 2003;16(suppl 4):919.

6 Craig ME, Handelsman P, Donaghue KC, Chan A, Blades B, Laina R, Bradford D, Middlehurst A, Ambler G, Verge CF, Crock P, Moore P, Silink M: Predictors of glycemic control and hypoglycemia in children and adolescents with type 1 diabetes from NSW and the ACT. Med J Aust 2002;177:235–238.

7 Mortensen HB, Hougaard P, Aanstoot HJ, Atchison JA, Chiarelli F, Daneman D, Danne T, Dinesen B, Dorchy H, Garandeau P, Greene S, Hoey H, Holl RW, Kaprio EA, Kocova M, Martul P, Matsuura N, Robertson KJ, Schoenle EJ, Sovik O, Swift P, Tsou RM, Vanelli M, Aman J: Comparison of metabolic control in a cross-sectional study of 2873 children and adolescents with insulin-dependent diabetes from 18 nations. Diabetes Care 1997;20:714–720.

8 Holl RW, Grabert M, Schwab O, Schweiggert F, for the German Prospective Documentation Initiative in Pediatric Diabetology: Severe hypoglycemia in 7940 children and adolescents with type-1 diabetes mellitus treated at 74 German pediatric diabetes centers. 17th International Congress, IDF, Mexico City, 2000. Diab Res Clin Pract 2000;50:S226(P963).
9 Icks A, Rosenbauer J, Haastert B, Rathmann W, Grabert M, Grandjour A, Giani G, Holl RW: Direct costs of pediatric diabetes care in Germany and their predictors. Exp Clin Endocrinol Diab 2004;112:302–309.
10 Deming WE: Out of the crisis – Quality, productivity and competitive position. Cambridge, Cambridge University Press, 1991.
11 Holl RW, Grabert M: The Quality Circle: How to improve the outcome of pediatric diabetes care. Horm Res 2002;57(suppl 1):105–109.
12 Holl RW, Swift PGF, Mortensen HB, Lynggaard H, Hougaard P, Aanstoot HJ, Chiarelli F, Daneman D, Danne T, Dorchy H, Garandeau P, Greene S, Hoey HMCV, Kaprio EA, Kocova M, Martul P, Matsuura N, Robertson KJ, Schoenle EJ, Sovik O, Tsou RM, Vanelli M, Åman J: Insulin injection regimens and metabolic control in an international survey of adolescents with type-1-diabetes over 3 years: Results from the Hvidore Study Group. Eur J Pediatr 2003; 162:22–29.
13 Tamborlane WV, Bonfig W, Boland E: Recent advances in treatment of youth with type 1 diabets: Better care through technology. Diab Med 2001;18:864–870.
14 Glasgow RE, Osteen VL: Evaluating diabetes education: Are we measuring the most important outcomes? Diabetes Care 1992;15:1423–1432.
15 Donabedien A: Criteria and standards for quality assessment and monitoring. Q Rev Bull 1986;12:99–108.
16 Bates DW, Gawande AA: Improving safety with information technology. N Engl J Med 2003;348:2526–2534.
17 Hippisley-Cox J, Pringle R, Wynn A, Hammersley V, Coupland C, Hapgood R, Horsfiled P, Teasdale S, Johnson C: The electronic patient record in primary care – Regression or progression? BMJ 2003;326:1439–1443.
18 O'Connor PJ: Electronic medical records and diabetes care improvement. Diabetes Care 2003;26:942–943.
19 The DCCT Research Group: Effect of intensive diabetes treatment on the development and progression of long-term complications in adolescents with insulin-dependent diabetes mellitus: Diabetes Control and Complications Trial. J Pediatr 1994;125:177–188.
20 Holl RW, Swift PGF, Mortensen HB, Lynggaard H, Hougaard P, Aanstoot HJ, Chiarelli F, Daneman D, Danne T, Dorchy H, Garandeau P, Greene S, Hoey HMCV, Kaprio EA, Kocova M, Martul P, Matsuura N, Robertson KJ, Schoenle EJ, Sovik O, Tsou RM, Vanelli M, Åman J: Insulin injection regimens and metabolic control in an international survey of adolescents with type-1-diabetes over 3 years: Results from the Hvidore Study Group. Eur J Pediatr 2003;162:22–29.
21 Hesketh KD, Wake MA, Cameron FJ: Health-related quality of life and metabolic control in children with type 1 diabetes. Diabetes Care 2004;27:415–420.
22 Hoey H, Aanstoot HJ, Chiarelli F, Daneman D, Danne T, Dinesen B, Dorchy H, Fitzgerald M, Garandeau P, Greene S, Holl RW, Hougaard P, Kaprio EA, Kocova M, Lynggaard H, Martul S, Matsuura N, McGee H, Mortensen HB, Robertson KJ, Schoenle EJ, Sovik O, Swift P, Tsou RM, Vanelli M, Aman J: Good metabolic control is associated with better quality of life in 2101 adolescents with type-1-diabetes. Diabetes Care 1923–1928,2001;24(11).
23 Hecker W, Holl RW for the German Pediatric Diabetology Group: Quality of paediatric IDDM care in Germany: A multicenter analysis. J Pediatr Endocrinol Metab 1999;12:31–38.
24 Grabert M, Holl RW, Krause U, Melzer I, Schweiggert F: Predicting the level of metabolic control using collaborative filtering; in Crespo J, Maojo V, Martins F (eds): Medical Data Analysis. Lecture Notes in Computer Science, 2001, vol 2199, pp 108–112.
25 Grabert M, Schweiggert F, Holl RW: A framework for diabetes documentation and quality management in Germany: 10 years of experience with DPV. Comput Methods Programs Biomed 2002;69:115–121.
26 McClain MR, Steinmann WC, Wennberg DE, Rice JC, Sherwin RW: Trends in the diabetes quality improvement project measures in Maine from 1994 to 1999. Diabetes Care 2003;26:597–601.

Chiarelli F, Dahl-Jørgensen K, Kiess W (eds): Diabetes in Childhood and Adolescence.
Pediatr Adolesc Med. Basel, Karger, 2005, vol 10, pp 190–201

# Invasive and Noninvasive Means of Diabetes Self-Management

*Dorothee Deiss, Reinhard Hartmann, Olga Kordonouri*

Clinic of General Pediatrics, Otto-Heubner-Centrum,
Charité, Campus Virchow-Klinikum, Humboldt University,
Berlin, Germany

## Historical Background

*'If one wants to dose the insulin exactly, one must determine the blood sugar level.'*

Already in 1926, Richard Wagner of the University Hospital in Vienna observed that the most important goal of every rational diabetes treatment to achieve normal blood glucose levels is not easy to be obtained in everyday life, due to the need for permanent blood glucose determination. At the same time, the pediatrician Karl Stolte developed an 'intensive insulin therapy', which was checked by means of metabolic self-control 'three times per day via a urine test which was performed directly prior to the insulin injection'. However, in the following decades, this liberal viewpoint was suppressed by strict and conventional principles of therapy and nutrition, caused, in part, by minimal possibilities of metabolic self-control.

Up to the 1970s, one had to be satisfied with the indirect estimation of blood glucose concentration by means of semiquantitative testing of urine glucose. With the introduction of high specific and economic enzymatic methods utilizing glucose dehydrogenase, hexokinase, or glucokinase in conjunction with colormetric, photometric or electrochemical detection devices, the urine glucose determination was gradually replaced by blood glucose measurements [1]. Through small inexpensive hand-held meters, the era of home glucose monitoring based on capillary blood had begun and 'the path towards intensive forms of insulin therapy was open' [2].

## Means of Diabetes Self-Management

*Urine Glucose Testing*

Semiquantitative test-strip methods using specific reactions for glucose are recommended for the limited application of urine glucose determination. Most commercial strips are based on glucose oxidase reaction [3] and use a color chart with which the test strip color is compared. The measurement of urine glucose has become less important due to very different renal thresholds for glucosuria and because the correlation between urinary and blood glucose is subjected to considerable inter- and intraindividual fluctuations [4]. Furthermore, it is not possible to assess glucose concentration in the normo- or hypoglycemic range by urine testing of glucose. Since the urine measurements are not invasive and provide an overview of a certain time interval, they still play a role in the self-monitoring of pediatric patients with non-insulin dependent diabetes like dietary-treated type 2 diabetes or MODY [3, 5].

*Blood Glucose Testing*

Routine monitoring by blood glucose measurements firstly became possible since 1975 by using strips impregnated with glucose oxidase to estimate the blood glucose concentration by comparison with a color scale [6]. The disadvantages of this method are sources of error in improper application, changes in hematocrit and possible interfering with drugs. In the meantime, these methods have been almost completely replaced by electrochemical methods of blood glucose measurements based on electrical signals generated by glucose oxidase reaction. The advantages of these meter devices are small sample volume requirements (minimal 0.3 μl), rapid measurements even within 5s, and the ability to store up to several hundred results that can be downloaded for analysis.

An additional simplification of diabetes self-management is being initiated with the development of a blood glucose monitor, which automatically sends test results wireless by radio frequency to an insulin pump [7].

*Ketone Testing*

Due to the importance of testing ketone during hyperglycemia, urine tests are still used. The principal ketone bodies, β-hydroxybutyrate and acetoacetate are usually present in approximately equimolar amounts; however, in diabetic ketoacidosis β-hydroxybutyrate increases more than 6-fold than acetoacetate. The semiquantitative test of urine ketone bodies is basically a reaction with acetoacetate, none of the tests detect β-hydroxybutyrate. Urine testing is very unpopular in children and adolescents and is not performed even in impending ketoacidosis. Recently, inexpensive quantitative tests for β-hydroxybutyrate (β-OHB) concentration have become available for use with small blood samples in a hand-held meter which is also able to measure blood glucose (MediSense Xtra®). The diagnosis of ketosis can be obtained with fingerstick determinations of β-OHB levels more than 60 min earlier than with urine testing [8]. In this way, patients would have an earlier warning mechanism for detecting the development of metabolic deterioration, for example by interruption of insulin infusion in pump therapy. Thus, they immediately can take self-measures for adjustment in time in their home setting to prevent ketoacidosis and hospital admission. On the other side, during recovery from ketoacidosis, ketone bodies in urine may be persisting long after blood concentrations have been normalized [8] leading to overdosed and prolonged insulin therapy.

*Hemoglobin A1c Testing*

Glycated hemoglobin (GHb) describes a series of stable minor hemoglobin components formed slowly and nonenzymatically from hemoglobin and glucose. In the late 1970s, it became clear that the minor hemoglobin fraction HbA1c resulted from a posttranslational modification of HbA and that there was a linear correlation with average glycemia of the proceeding 6–12 weeks [9]. The different HbA1c assays can be divided into two major categories: methods based on charge differences between GHb and non-GHb like cation-exchange chromatography, electrophoresis, and isoelectric focusing and methods based on structural characteristics of glycogroups of hemoglobin like affinity chromatography and immunoassay [10, 11]. The widely used method for HbA1c determination is the high-performance liquid chromatography (HPLC) method, which has been used since 1985 in important long-term studies like the Diabetes Control and Complications Trial (DCCT) [12] and in routine patient care. The analysis is bound to a clinical laboratory and offers only a delayed overview of glycemic control to patient and physician. With the introduction of the DCA2000 Analyzer (Bayer Diagnostics, Germany), the HbA1c value is available within 6 min during the patient's visit at the outpatient clinic. Thus, therapy adjustments can be discussed directly and realized faster. The most recent development is a potentially home self-monitoring method with a single-use test for HbA1c (A1cNow®, Metrika, Sunnyvale, Calif., USA) [13].

Up to now, there are many different commercial methods available for measuring HbA1c, but without international standardization. However, national initiatives for the harmonization of HbA1c results did important steps toward improvement of methods comparability and the future basis for international standardization may be a reference system developed by the IFCC Working Group on HbA1c Standardization [14].

## Clinical Relevance of Means for Diabetes Self-Management

*Capillary Blood Glucose Measurements*

In the past years, it became increasingly apparent that glycemic control before and during puberty is of great importance concerning the development of microvascular complications in young patients with type 1 diabetes [15–17]. To achieve near-normoglycemia is considerably more difficult in children than in adults. In addition to intensified insulin management, frequent blood glucose self-measurements are required to improve metabolic control [12]. The frequency of self-monitoring blood glucose (SMBG) has been shown to be predictive for HbA1c concentration. Increased frequency of SMBG testing corresponded with lower HbA1c [18, 19]. Performing capillary finger sticks is for many children and adolescents much more cumbersome than insulin injections. Moreover, despite of frequent capillary blood glucose monitoring, a high number and even prolonged hypo- and hyperglycemic episodes may remain undetected, because information on blood glucose concentration between the single-pointed self-measurements is lacking. Therefore, already in the 1970s and 1980s, two parameters for the estimation of 24-hour glucose profiles by means of repeated capillary self-measurements were proposed:

- MAGE (mean amplitude glycemic excursions) to determine within-day blood glucose swings [20].
- MODD (mean of daily differences) to determine day-to-day variation as a measure of diabetic instability [21].

*HbA1c*

Up to now, HbA1c has been the primary measure of diabetes treatment efficacy and the best parameter to extrapolate the individual's risk for the development of late complications [22]. The relationship of glycemic exposure (HbA1c) to the risk of development and progression of retinopathy and nephropathy was clearly demonstrated in the DCCT [23]. In the Berlin Retinopathy Study, the risk of background retinopathy has been shown to be mainly influenced by long-term HbA1c in pediatric patients. However, it remained unclear why, in individual cases, HbA1c was a poor predictor [24].

During the past years, the limitations of HbA1c as the golden standard for measuring glycemic control and diabetes treatment success became more and more apparent. High and low glucose fluctuations are masked in a mean value of HbA1c. Low HbA1c values can be achieved with frequent hypoglycemic episodes despite of glycemic excursions.

## Means of Continuous Glucose Monitoring

The need of more sophisticated methods and parameters for the evaluation of metabolic control was increasing. The concept of continuous glucose monitoring was already developed in the mid-1970s [25]. However, even the mobile version of the Biostator device (artificial pancreas) could hardly be regarded as a glucose home-monitor.

In recent years, significant efforts have been directed toward the development of technologies providing minimal invasive approaches for continuous glucose monitoring which should allow ambulatory monitoring of patients.

The glucose sensors must fulfill the accuracy and safety conditions required for any clinically usable device and the specific requirements of long-term stability and high reactivity in glucose measurement [26]. Although various approaches in glucose sensing have been and are still being investigated, only a limited number can presently fulfill the requirements for clinical use.

*Minimally Invasive Enzymatic Glucose Sensors*

Enzymatic sensors using glucose oxidase still remain the most clinically usable approach for glucose sensing. The generated electrical signal is proportional to the glucose concentration in the sensor environment [26]. However, altered stability of signal can impair sensor accuracy. Efforts to improve accuracy and stability of enzymatic sensors continue.

The Continuous Glucose Monitoring System (CGMS®, MedtronicMinimed, Northridge, Calif., USA), is a needle-type sensor, implanted in the subcutaneous tissue, which has been approved by FDA for clinical use in 1999 and received a CE marking in 2000. The sensor provides measurement of interstitial glucose concentration between 40 and 400 mg/dl. It is connected by a cable to a portable pager-size monitor that records the sensor signals every 5 min for at least 3 days. Real-time data are not given, but downloaded to a computer for retrospective analysis, presented as a continuous glucose curve and statistical data. The sensor signal must be calibrated against capillary blood glucose at least four times a day [27]. The delay between the blood glucose level and sensor signal, which corresponds to glucose concentration in interstitial fluid, is around 4 min, indicating a good reactivity [28]. There is some literature to suggest that CGMS suffers from accuracy problems in the hypoglycemic range [29]. In recent studies, it could be demonstrated that subcutaneous sensor glucose values are closely parallel to blood glucose during insulin-induced hypoglycemia [30, 31]. In clinical practice, the quality of generated data depends on the comprehensiveness of instructions given to the patient on handling the CGMS [32].

The Guardian®RT (MedtronicMinimed, Northridge, Calif., USA) representing a cableless version of the CGMS with real-time display and hyper-/ hypoglycemic alerts needs two capillary blood glucose measurements per day for calibration. The device is CE marked since 2004.

The GlucoWatch G2 biographer® (Cygnus, Redwood City, Calif., USA) is based upon the principle of reverse iontophoresis for glucose recovery. An electric current of low intensity applied on intact skin extracts interstitial fluid, in which glucose is measured by glucose oxidase reaction [33]. Several limitations of the technique such as a warm-up phase for several hours, an average time lag of sensor data behind blood glucose of 10 minutes [34], local skin irritations at the site of electrodes, and false low glucose readings have been reported. The GlucoWatch is CE marked and FDA approved for children since 2002.

The GlucoDay® (A. Menarini Diagnostics, Basel, Switzerland) uses a microdialysis system with a subcutaneous probe. Calibration of sensor data is performed against one capillary blood glucose measurement once the dialysis system is in steady state [36]. However, sufficient data presented in real-time are lacking so far, especially in children, for whom the system may be to large and uncomfortable to use. The device is CE marked, but not yet FDA approved for children.

*Minimally-Invasive Non-Enzymatic Glucose Sensors*

GlucOnline® (Roche Diagnostics, Basel, Switzerland) is also using microdialysis with a viscometric method [37]. Reported clinical data are few and a possible long-term side effect of the concanavalin A used in the glucose sensor has still to be proven (pending FDA submission).

*Noninvasive Nonenzymatic Glucose Sensors*

Pendra® (Pendragon Medical, Florence, Italy) with an attractive appearance of a wristwatch uses impedance spectroscopy and electrolytic changes related to glucose fluctuations measured through the skin [38]. There are not yet sufficient studies about data accuracy and reliability under usual life conditions (CE marked, not yet FDA approved).

## Clinical Relevance of Continuous Glucose Monitoring

Since CGMS and GlucoWatch G2 biographer were the first devices of continuous glucose monitoring approved for children, most experiences about feasibility and applicability of continuous glucose monitoring in children are based on studies with these devices.

*Detection of Hypoglycemic Episodes*

Asymptomatic and nocturnal hypoglycemia is a common problem in pediatric patients with type 1 diabetes. Prevalence rates up to 70% in children and 50% in adolescents are reported [39, 40]. Failure to recognize hypoglycemia may cause defective counter-regulatory responses resulting in hypoglycemia unawareness [40], which could then increase the risk of subsequent prolonged and severe hypoglycemia. The results of the DCCT show that a history of one or more episodes of severe hypoglycemia may predict further hypoglycemic episodes [12]. Nocturnal hypoglycemia has been suggested to contribute to fasting and post-meal hyperglycemia during the morning due to long-lasting post-hypoglycemic insulin resistance [41].

The detection of hypoglycemic episodes may be difficult. Particularly in children, asymptomatic and nocturnal hypoglycemia may often remain undetected in spite of frequent blood glucose monitoring by finger pricks [35, 39, 42–44]. Moreover, the treatment of type 1 diabetes is often complicated by the presence of the dawn phenomenon, i.e. early morning hyperglycemia, particularly in children and adolescents during puberty [45]. Continuous glucose monitoring is a useful tool to diagnose asymptomatic hypoglycemia, which often remain undetected although lasting up to eight hours [39, 46]. With CGMS, hypoglycemic events were diagnosed in more than 70% of toddlers and preschool children with type 1 diabetes, but less than 30% were detected by finger pricks [39]. Many children and adolescents are not aware of hypoglycemia and cannot react by adequate supply of carbohydrates – the consequence of which is uncontrolled glucose fluctuations. Thus, continuous glucose monitoring is a great help for patients with reduced awareness of hypoglycemia which mostly can be improved by appropriate education. Furthermore, without performing finger pricks, continuous glucose monitoring allows glucose measurements and, thereby, changes in attitude and therapy adjustment in patients with an increased risk of hypoglycemia under daily life conditions like during sport.

*Monitoring of Postprandial Hyperglycemia*

Rapid and marked glycemic excursions after the meals often remain undetected. Despite excellent HbA1c and target preprandial glucose levels, profound postprandial hyperglycemia could be detected in children using continuous glucose monitoring [46]. Therefore, there are controversial discussions whether fasting or postprandial glucose values have more impact on metabolic control [47]. In a small number of children changing to insulin pump therapy (continuous subcutaneous insulin infusion, CSII), an improvement of HbA1c could be demonstrated as a result of reduced postprandial glycemic excursions according to the evaluation of CGMS data [48]. Similarly, in 50 pediatric patients starting with CSII in our center, the improvement of HbA1c was mainly related to an overall hyperglycemic decrease [49]. Not only bolus but also correction insulin dose is assumed to be fitted more exactly and individually by the diagnostic possibilities of continuous glucose monitoring. Moreover, usage of continuous glucose monitoring may provide more insight into different glycemic effects of meals and kind of food in patients with type 1 diabetes.

*Monitoring of Therapy Changes*

Changing insulin therapy, it seems very helpful to evaluate a continuous glucose curve over some days. Before changing from multiple daily injections (MDI) to CSII, the primary bolus and basal doses can be individually determined and tailored for CSII by means of CGMS measurements. During pump therapy, CGMS facilitates to optimize the basal rate. Conventional basal tests are often unpopular in adolescents and parents of younger children, whereas the application of CGMS could be superior for realizing this monitoring. After change to CSII, glycemic control improves for a short time period in most patients, but HbA1c values increase up to previous levels after a few months. Possible causes such as poor compliance concerning the performance of recommended blood glucose measurements and omission of meal related insulin boluses could be identified by using read-out memory from pumps and information of CGMS [50]. Information from CGMS can be used to identify underlying problems and may be helpful for the patient's consulting and compliance.

*Correlation between CGMS Data and HbA1c*

HbA1c reflects the average glycemic control over a period up to 3 months, while the current methods of continuous glucose monitoring provide information about metabolic conditions over 12 h (GlucoWatch G2 biographer) or 3 days (CGMS). With continuous glucose monitoring, the association between HbA1c and several new metabolic parameters, as measured by CGMS, can be assessed. The area under the glucose curve (AUC) is a measure for hypo- and hyperglycemic amount offering more extensive information than the number of hypo- and hyperglycemic events documented by SMBG. In pediatric patients with CSII, we found a strong correlation of HbA1c with AUC $>$180 mg/dl and AUC/24 h, particularly at day [49]. In another cohort of 145 children and adolescents treated with MDI or CSII, the glucose AUC$>$180 mg/dl was the most predictive independent factor of HbA1c (fig. 1).

## Conclusion

Intensive diabetes self-management, particularly by means of frequent SMBG, is the condition to achieve good metabolic control in patients with type 1

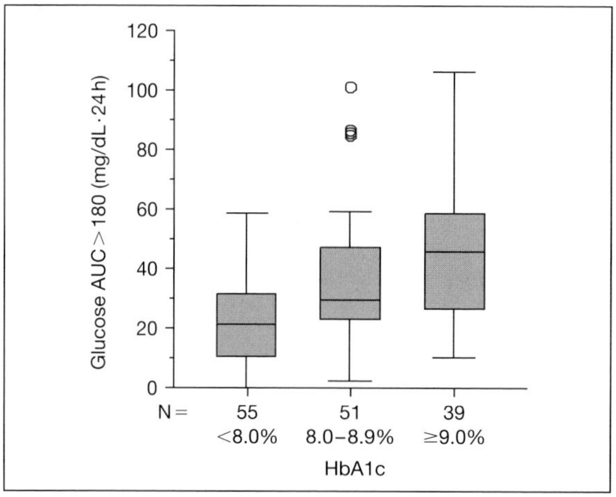


***Fig. 1.*** Relationship between glycemic control (HbA1c) and area under the curve (AUC) of glucose values above 180 mg/dl·24 h as measured by CGMS (continuous glucose monitoring system) in 145 children with type 1 diabetes. AUC values are represented by box-and-whisker plots with median (line in the box), interquartile range (box), 95th percentile range (whisker), and outlier (circle).

diabetes. For this purpose, glucose meter devices offering rapid measurements and using very small amounts of capillary blood are available. However, frequent SMBG is a painful procedure leading to a poor compliance, particularly in young patients with diabetes. New systems enabling accurate continuous measurement of interstitial glucose concentrations with good correlation to blood glucose levels have been developed recently offering new possibilities for diabetes management both in patients and diabetes specialists. Patients are faced with devices which are able to continuously measure glucose levels, to detect and assess rapid fluctuations and unmask otherwise undetected glycemic situations. Furthermore, waiting for new systems with real-time display, they are hoping to get better diabetes self-management with fewer invasive and painful procedures like conventional finger sticks. On the other hand, diabetes health care providers are getting the opportunity to better assess metabolic control of their patients analyzing a variety of data retrospectively or even prospectively with real-time devices. To our opinion, a great challenge will be the use of continuous real-time glucose monitoring in clinical application of new insulin preparations and treatment. These are all steps striking the goal that the external and internal closed-loop system of continuous glucose monitoring and insulin delivery systems will be available for daily use in diabetes patients in the near future.

## References


1 Tattersall RB: Home blood glucose monitoring. Diabetologia 1979;16:71–74.
2 Hürter P: Diabetes bei Kindern und Jugendlichen, ed 5. Berlin, Springer, 1997.
3 Sacks DB, Bruns DE, Goldstein DE, Maclaren NK, McDonald JM, Parrott M: Guidelines and recommendations for laboratory analysis in the diagnosis and management of diabetes mellitus. Clin Chem 2002;48:436–472.
4 Tattersall R, Walford S, Peacock I, Gale E, Allison S: A critical evaluation of methods of monitoring diabetic control. Diabetes Care 1980;3:150–154.
5 American Diabetes Association: Standards of medical care in diabetes (position statement). Diabetes Care 2004;27(suppl 1):S15–S35.
6 Christensen SE, Jorgensen OL, Moller N, Andersen KJ, Moller J, Orskov H: A test strip method for visual and reflectometric reading of blood glucose. Diabet Med 1985;2:272–273.
7 Halvorson MJ KF, Carpenter SD, Cooper K, Kolopp M, Mueller J: The Medtronic Minimed Paradigm 522 continuous glucose monitoring system for patient use: Real-time sensor glucose values. Diabetes 2004;53(suppl 2):3-LB.
8 Guerci B, Drouin P, Grange V, Bougneres P, Fontaine P, Kerlan V, et al: Self-monitoring of blood glucose significantly improves metabolic control in patients with type 2 diabetes mellitus: The Auto-Surveillance Intervention Active (ASIA) study. Diabetes Metab 2003;29:587–594.
9 Koenig RJ, Peterson CM, Jones RL, Saudek C, Lehrman M, Cerami A: Correlation of glucose regulation and hemoglobin AIc in diabetes mellitus. N Engl J Med 1976;295:417–420.
10 Benjamin RJ, Sacks DB: Glycated protein update: Implications of recent studies, including the diabetes control and complications trial. Clin Chem 1994;40:683–687.
11 Goldstein DE, Little RR, Lorenz RA, Malone JI, Nathan D, Peterson CM, et al: Tests of glycemia in diabetes. Diabetes Care 2004;27:1761–1773.
12 Diabetes Control and Complications Trial Research Group: Effect of intensive diabetes treatment on the development and progression of long-term complications in adolescents with insulin-dependent diabetes mellitus: Diabetes Control and Complications Trial. J Pediatr 1994; 125:177–188.
13 Stivers CR, Baddam SR, Clark AL, Ammirati EB, Irvin BR, Blatt JM: A miniaturized self-contained single-use disposable quantitative test for hemoglobin A1c in blood at the point of care. Diabetes Technol Ther 2000;2:517–526.
14 Hoelzel W WC, Jeppsson JO, Miedema K, Barr JR, Goodall I, Hoshino T, John WG, Kobold U, Little R, Mosca A, Mauri P, Paroni R, Susanto F, Takei I, Thienpont L, Umemoto M, Wiedmeyer HM, IFCC Working Group on HbA1c Standardization: IFCC reference system for measurement of hemoglobin A1c in human blood and the national standardization schemes in the United States, Japan, and Sweden: A method-comparison study. Clin Chem 2004;50:166–174.
15 Donaghue KC, Fung AT, Hing S, Fairchild J, King J, Chan A, et al: The effect of prepubertal diabetes duration on diabetes. Microvascular complications in early and late adolescence. Diabetes Care 1997;20:77–80.
16 Svensson M, Eriksson JW, Dahlquist G: Early glycemic control, age at onset, and development of microvascular complications in childhood-onset type 1 diabetes: A population-based study in northern Sweden. Diabetes Care 2004;27:955–962.
17 Kordonouri O, Danne T, Enders I, Weber B: Does the long-term clinical course of type 1 diabetes mellitus differ in patients with prepubertal and pubertal onset? Results of the Berlin Retinopathy Study. Eur J Pediatr 1998;157:202–207.
18 Haller MJ SM, Silverstein JH: Predictors of control of diabetes: Monitoring may be the key. J Pediatr 2004;144:660–661.
19 Levine BS, Anderson BJ, Butler DA, Antisdel JE, Brackett J, Laffel LM: Predictors of glycemic control and short-term adverse outcomes in youth with type 1 diabetes. J Pediatr 2001;139:197–203.
20 Service FJ, Molnar GD, Rosevear JW, Ackerman E, Gatewood LC, Taylor WF: Mean amplitude of glycemic excursions, a measure of diabetic instability. Diabetes 1970;19:644–655.
21 Molnar GD, Taylor WF, Langworthy AL: Plasma immunoreactive insulin patterns in insulin-treated diabetics. Studies during continuous blood glucose monitoring. Mayo Clin Proc 1972;47:709–719.

22 Diabetes Control and Complications Trial Research Group: The effect of intensive treatment of diabetes on the development and progression of long-term complications in insulin-dependent diabetes mellitus. N Engl J Med 1993;329:977–986.
23 The relationship of glycemic exposure (HbA1c) to the risk of development and progression of retinopathy in the diabetes control and complications trial. Diabetes 1995;44:968–983.
24 Danne T, Weber B, Hartmann R, Enders I, Burger W, Hovener G: Long-term glycemic control has a nonlinear association to the frequency of background retinopathy in adolescents with diabetes. Follow-up of the Berlin Retinopathy Study. Diabetes Care 1994;17:1390–1396.
25 Pfeiffer EF: On the way to the automated (blood) glucose regulation in diabetes: The dark past, the gray present and the rosy future. XII Congress of the International Diabetes Federation, Madrid, 22–28 September 1985. Diabetologia 1987;30:51–65.
26 Gough DA, Armour JC: Development of the implantable glucose sensor. What are the prospects and why is it taking so long? Diabetes 1995;44:1005–1009.
27 Mastrototaro J: The MiniMed Continuous Glucose Monitoring System (CGMS). J Pediatr Endocrinol Metab 1999;12(suppl 3):751–758.
28 Rebrin K, Steil GM, van Antwerp WP, Mastrototaro JJ: Subcutaneous glucose predicts plasma glucose independent of insulin: Implications for continuous monitoring. Am J Physiol 1999;277: E561–E571.
29 The accuracy of the CGMS in children with type 1 diabetes: Results of the diabetes research in children network (DirecNet) accuracy study. Diabetes Technol Ther 2003;5:781–789.
30 Caplin NJ, O'Leary P, Bulsara M, Davis EA, Jones TW: Subcutaneous glucose sensor values closely parallel blood glucose during insulin-induced hypoglycemia. Diabet Med 2003;20: 238–241.
31 Monsod TP, Flanagan DE, Rife F, Saenz R, Caprio S, Sherwin RS, et al: Do sensor glucose levels accurately predict plasma glucose concentrations during hypoglycemia and hyperinsulinemia? Diabetes Care 2002;25:889–893.
32 Melki V, Hanaire-Broutin H: Indication of CGMS (Continuous Glucose Monitoring System) in the functional investigations of adult type 1 diabetic patients. Diabetes Metab 2001;27:618–623.
33 Garg SK, Potts RO, Ackerman NR, Fermi SJ, Tamada JA, Chase HP: Correlation of fingerstick blood glucose measurements with GlucoWatch biographer glucose results in young subjects with type 1 diabetes. Diabetes Care 1999;22:1708–1714.
34 Tamada JA, Garg S, Jovanovic L, Pitzer KR, Fermi S, Potts RO: Noninvasive glucose monitoring: Comprehensive clinical results. Cygnus Research Team. JAMA 1999;282:1839–1844.
35 Chase HP, Roberts MD, Wightman C, Klingensmith G, Garg SK, Van Wyhe M, et al: Use of the GlucoWatch biographer in children with type 1 diabetes. Pediatrics 2003;111:90–94.
36 Maran A, Crepaldi C, Tiengo A, Grassi G, Vitali E, Pagano G, et al: Continuous subcutaneous glucose monitoring in diabetic patients: A multicenter analysis. Diabetes Care 2002;25:347–352.
37 Beyer U, Schafer D, Thomas A, Aulich H, Haueter U, Reihl B, et al: Recording of subcutaneous glucose dynamics by a viscometric affinity sensor. Diabetologia 2001;44:416–423.
38 Caduff A, Hirt E, Feldman Y, Ali Z, Heinemann L: First human experiments with a novel non-invasive, non-optical continuous glucose monitoring system. Biosens Bioelectron 2003;19:209–217.
39 Deiss D, Kordonouri O, Meyer K, Danne T: Long hypoglycaemic periods detected by subcutaneous continuous glucose monitoring in toddlers and pre-school children with diabetes mellitus. Diabet Med 2001;18:337–338.
40 Matyka KA, Wigg L, Pramming S, Stores G, Dunger DB: Cognitive function and mood after profound nocturnal hypoglycaemia in prepubertal children with conventional insulin treatment for diabetes. Arch Dis Child 1999;81:138–142.
41 Fowelin J, Attvall S, von Schenck H, Smith U, Lager I: Postprandial hyperglycaemia following a morning hypoglycaemia in type 1 diabetes mellitus. Diabet Med 1990;7:156–161.
42 Schiaffini R, Ciampalini P, Fierabracci A, Spera S, Borrelli P, Bottazzo GF, et al: The Continuous Glucose Monitoring System (CGMS) in type 1 diabetic children is the way to reduce hypoglycemic risk. Diabetes Metab Res Rev 2002;18:324–329.
43 Amin R, Ross K, Acerini CL, Edge JA, Warner J, Dunger DB: Hypoglycemia prevalence in prepubertal children with type 1 diabetes on standard insulin regimen: Use of continuous glucose monitoring system. Diabetes Care 2003;26:662–667.

44 Kaufman FR, Austin J, Neinstein A, Jeng L, Halvorson M, Devoe DJ, et al: Nocturnal hypoglycemia detected with the Continuous Glucose Monitoring System in pediatric patients with type 1 diabetes. J Pediatr 2002;141:625–630.
45 Danne T, Deiss D, Hopfenmuller W, von Schutz W, Kordonouri O: Experience with insulin analogues in children. Horm Res 2002;57(suppl 1):46–53.
46 Boland E, Monsod T, Delucia M, Brandt CA, Fernando S, Tamborlane WV: Limitations of conventional methods of self-monitoring of blood glucose: Lessons learned from 3 days of continuous glucose sensing in pediatric patients with type 1 diabetes. Diabetes Care 2001;24:1858–1862.
47 Bastyr EJ 3rd, Stuart CA, Brodows RG, Schwartz S, Graf CJ, Zagar A, et al: Therapy focused on lowering postprandial glucose, not fasting glucose, may be superior for lowering HbA1c. IOEZ Study Group. Diabetes Care 2000;23:1236–1241.
48 Heptulla RA, Allen HF, Gross TM, Reiter EO: Continuous glucose monitoring in children with type 1 diabetes: Before and after insulin pump therapy. Pediatr Diabetes 2004;5:10–15.
49 Deiss D, Hartmann R, Hoeffe J, Kordonouri O: Assessment of glycemic control by continuous glucose monitoring system (CGMS) in 50 children with type 1 diabetes starting on insulin pump therapy. Pediatr Diabetes 2004;5:117–121.
50 Burdick J, Chase HP, Slover RH, Knievel K, Scrimgeour L, Maniatis AK, et al: Missed insulin meal boluses and elevated hemoglobin A1c levels in children receiving insulin pump therapy. Pediatrics 2004;113:e221–e224.

Olga Kordonouri, MD
Klinik für Allgemeine Pädiatrie
Otto-Heubner-Zentrum für Kinder- und Jugendmedizin
Charité Universitätsmedizin Berlin, Campus Virchow-Klinikum
Augustenburger Platz 1, DE–13353 Berlin (Germany)
Tel. +49 30 450 566181, Fax +49 30 450 566916, E-Mail olga.kordonouri@charite.de

Chiarelli F, Dahl-Jørgensen K, Kiess W (eds): Diabetes in Childhood and Adolescence.
Pediatr Adolesc Med. Basel, Karger, 2005, vol 10, pp 202–224

# Adolescence

*David B. Dunger, Carlo L. Acerini, Marion L. Ahmed*

Department of Paediatrics, University of Cambridge,
Addenbrooke's Hospital, Cambridge, UK

Adolescence is a period of transition from physical immaturity to maturity and from parental dependency to independence. It is a period of rapid change, and for the young person with type 1 diabetes mellitus (T1DM) striving for independence, the daily ritual of injections, blood testing and awareness of diet represent additional burdens. Thus, although it may be frustrating for those trying to care for these young people, their occasional disinterest and poor compliance are predictable. However, whereas the focus is often on behaviour and issues of compliance, the transition through puberty also poses considerable challenges in providing appropriate insulin replacement, and improving glycaemic control whilst avoiding hypoglycaemia and excess weight gain. These problems were highlighted by the Diabetes Care and Complications Trial (DCCT), where for the intensively treated adolescents, glycated haemoglobin indices (HbA1c) were on average 1% higher than those in adults, and achieving similar benefits from blood glucose control in terms of complications outcome came at the expense of an increased frequency of hypoglycaemia and obesity [1]. It is unlikely that these differences were related to poor compliance but rather reflect the inherent difficulties in diabetes management during adolescence (table 1).

## Pubertal Growth and Development

The age at onset of puberty is rarely delayed in subjects with T1DM and the sequence of events is identical to that observed in normal children [2]. Some investigators have reported a degree of disassociation between adrenarche and gonadarche with reduced levels of adrenal androgens during early puberty in boys [3]. In contrast, features of both ovarian hyperandrogenism and polycystic ovarian syndrome may be evident during late puberty in girls [4].

***Table 1.*** Comparison of efficacy and safety of intensive treatment between adolescents and adults

| | Adults | Adolescents | p |
|---|---|---|---|
| Mean HbA1c, % | | | |
| Intensive | 8.06 ± 0.13 | 7.12 ± 0.03 | <0.001 |
| Conventional | 9.76 ± 0.12 | 9.02 ± 0.05 | <0.001 |
| Decreased risk, % | | | |
| Retinopathy | 61 | 63 | 0.802 |
| Microalbuminuria | 35 | 45 | 0.886 |
| All severe hypoglycaemia | | | |
| Rate/100 PYR | 85.7 | 56.9 | 0.004 |
| Coma/seizure | | | |
| Rate/100 PYR | 26.7 | 14.4 | 0.001 |



During puberty there is a rapid increase in statural growth and marked changes in body composition. An adolescent will gain around 16% of their mature height, around 45% of their adult weight and experience a near doubling of lean body mass as they pass through puberty. Predictably, insulin requirements increase during this time, but in addition, pubertal development is characterised by increasing insulin resistance.

*Insulin Resistance*

In young people without diabetes, although plasma glucose levels are maintained within a very narrow range through puberty, fasting insulin levels increase, returning to pre-pubertal levels only in early adult life [5, 6]. Maximal fasting plasma insulin levels are observed around Tanner Stage 3–4 and a consistent finding has been that the fasting insulin levels tend to be slightly higher in females than in males [6, 7]. There is a strong relationship between fasting plasma insulin concentrations and height velocity in normal children [8] and the higher levels in girls may reflect their earlier maturation and pubertal growth, although similar findings have been reported in prepubertal subjects. Stimulated insulin concentrations following oral or intravenous glucose are also greater during puberty and are accompanied by parallel changes in C-peptide levels [9, 10]. Stephanie Amiel and colleagues were the first to demonstrate that puberty was associated with alterations in insulin stimulated glucose metabolism that could be reduced by 34 to 40% during mid-puberty [11]. These changes largely relate to reduced peripheral glucose uptake

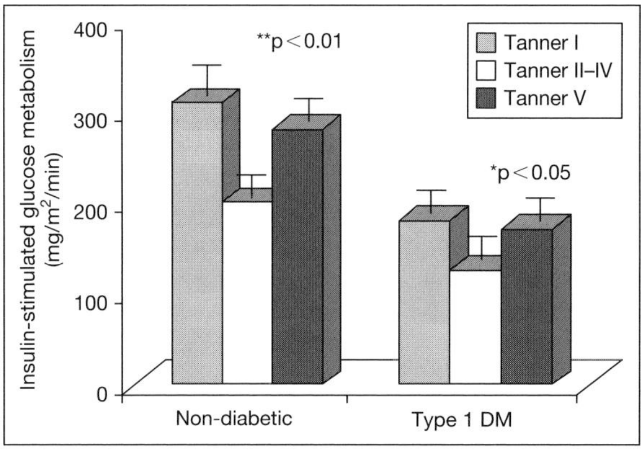


***Fig. 1.*** The impact of puberty on insulin stimulated peripheral glucose uptake. Comparison between healthy controls and subjects with type 1 diabetes. Puberty according to Tanner Stage [Copyright 1986 Massachusetts Medical Society. All rights reserved. Reproduced with permission from [15]].

rather than changes in hepatic glucose production [12]. Insulin resistance is associated with compensatory hyperinsulinaemia that leads to progressive falls in fasting free fatty acids and branch chain amino acids levels, suggesting an inhibition of lipid and protein breakdown [13]. Furthermore, hyperinsulinaemia also leads to consistent falls in levels of the inhibitory insulin-like growth factor (IGF) binding protein-1 (IGFBP-1) through puberty suggesting that the insulin resistance of puberty may play a physiological role in pubertal growth and development [14]. Adolescents with T1DM show the same pattern of change in insulin sensitivity during puberty, but at all stages they are more insulin resistant than control subjects without diabetes [15] (fig. 1).

*The Growth Hormone/IGF-I Axis*

Amiel et al. [15] identified a correlation between insulin sensitivity during puberty and mean 24-hour plasma growth hormone (GH) levels. The insulin antagonistic effects of GH have been well characterised and have been shown to be due to reductions in peripheral glucose metabolism and, to a lesser extent, to enhancements in hepatic glucose production [12, 16, 17]. GH may be acting directly through its own receptor (interacting with post receptor insulin signalling), but may also be acting indirectly through mobilisation of non-esterified free fatty acids (NEFAs) from adipose tissue. NEFAs have suppressive effects on peripheral glucose metabolism [18, 19] and have been implicated in regulating hepatic glucose metabolism [20, 21]. The characteristics of the GH pulses produced overnight are thought to be important determinants of the metabolic actions of GH, and increases in GH pulse amplitude lead to sustained changes in insulin sensitivity [12]. There is compelling evidence to suggest that the accentuated insulin resistance in T1DM results from GH hypersecretion; the overnight pattern of GH secretion leading to the 'Dawn Phenomenon' of increasing insulin requirements during the early hours of the morning [22].

Abnormalities of the GH/ IGF-I axis have been consistently reported in adolescents with T1DM. Compared to healthy controls they have increased nocturnal GH concentrations and GH pulses are characterised by increases in both pulse amplitude and baseline concentrations [23]; there is some evidence that GH clearance may also be delayed [24] and deconvolution analysis suggest that there may be decreases in GH pulse periodicity and increases in overall GH secretion rate [25].

The GH hypersecretion seen in T1DM results from an increased feedback drive at the level of hypothalamus/pituitary secondary to the presence of paradoxically low circulating IGF-I levels. Circulating IGF-I levels are frequently observed to be low, or in the low-normal range, as are those of the principal IGF-binding protein, IGFBP-3 [26, 27]. These abnormalities are thought to arise because of partial insensitivity to GH at the level of the hepatic GH receptor and are largely explained by the central role of insulin in the regulation of the GH/ IGF-I axis. Insulin enhances IGF-I production either by direct regulation of the hepatic GH receptor, or by way of permissive effects on post-GH receptor signalling [28].

Insulin also has an important role in regulating IGF bioavailability and bioactivity through regulation of circulating concentrations of IGFBP-1. IGFBP-1 is a potent inhibitor of IGF-I action and its production by the liver is inversely regulated by insulin [29]. Raised serum IGFBP-1 levels may, by mopping up 'free' or 'unbound' IGF-I within the circulation, be directly implicated in the development of the 'Dawn Phenomenon' [30]. Reduced IGF-I levels and bioavailability may also have direct effects on insulin sensitivity. IGF-I exhibits a high degree of structural homology (42–50%) with both proinsulin and insulin and has been shown to exert metabolic effects through its own receptor that are distinct from those of insulin [31].

Therefore, insulin, or rather portal insulin, concentrations play a pivotal role in the regulation of GH/IGF-I axis, and the low IGF-I levels in T1DM reflect the peripheral rather than portal route of insulin delivery [32]. In T1DM, the GH hypersecretion, reduced IGF-I bioactivity and increased IGFBP-1 levels are linked to deteriorating glycaemic control [33].

*Height and Weight Gain*

Historically, T1DM was associated with quite considerable growth impairment as exemplified by the case reports from Mauriac [34] in the 1930s.

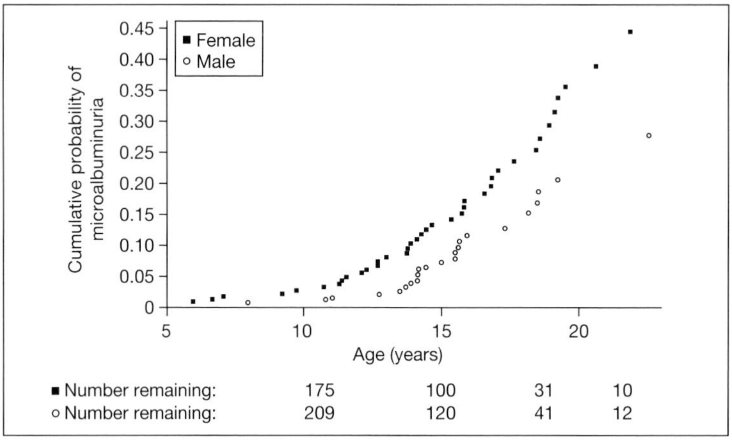


***Fig. 3.*** Cumulative probability for the development of microalbuminuria with age. [Copyright 1999 American Association. From [58]. Reprinted with permission from the American Diabetes Association].

seemed to be at increased risk of MA during puberty, compared to boys, suggesting that the hormonal changes of puberty may be an important for the development of microvascular complications [59, 60] (fig. 3).

Although some early studies have suggested that increased circulating IGF-1 levels might be associated with the development of proliferative retinopathy [61], the majority of clinical studies to date have indicated that microvascular complications develop in the presence of low circulating IGF-1 levels [62–64]. That is not to say that 'free' or easily dissociable IGF-1 may not be playing a role in the development of these complications, as suggested by clinical trials where administration of high, supraphysiological doses of recombinant human IGF-1 (rhIGF-I) to adult patients with T1DM was associated with a worsening of retinopathy scores [65, 66].

GH hypersecretion has been consistently linked with the development of microvascular complications [67] ever since the early studies showing that pituitary ablation could retard the development of proliferative retinopathy [68]. The role of GH, particularly in the pathogenesis of diabetic nephropathy, has also been highlighted by recent studies in the NOD mouse where, as in humans, low circulating IGF-1 levels are accompanied by GH hypersecretion [69]. As resistance to the effects of GH are specific to the hepatic GH receptor and not to the GH receptor in other tissues, high circulating GH levels have been shown to have direct effects in mediating both renal hypertrophy and hyperfiltration [70]. Furthermore, these changes are reversible with the use of specific GH receptor antagonists [71]. Recent data indicate that similar mechanisms may be important in the development of MA during puberty. Subjects developing MA have lower circulating IGF-1 levels and increased GH secretion compared to control T1DM subjects without MA [60, 72].

The gender differences in the risk for developing either severe retinopathy or MA are harder to explain. Whereas the lifetime risk for the development of MA is greatest in males [73], during puberty females show a 2-fold increased risk compared with males for developing MA [58]. Two studies have demonstrated that in females with T1DM low levels of the sex hormone binding globulin (SHBG) and a raised free androgen index are associated with the development of MA [59, 60]. This has raised speculation that a degree of ovarian hyperandrogenism secondary to high GH and insulin levels may also be contributing to complications risk in girls during puberty.

## Psychological Problems

It has to be remembered that for many young people adolescence can be a psychologically stressful time and the prevalence of psychological and psychiatric disorders is remarkably high. However, psychiatric disorders have been shown to be more common in both adolescents and young adults with T1DM than in non-diabetic populations [74, 75] and psychological problems may have an important impact on outcome with respect of glycaemic control and risk of complications [76, 77].

*General Psychological Morbidity*

A great number of cross-sectional studies have demonstrated increased psychological problems during adolescents in children with diabetes [74, 75], but there have been few longitudinal studies looking at the outcome with respect to glycaemic control and complications [76–78]. In a recent longitudinal study from Oxford, female adolescents tended to have more emotional symptoms than male patients and this may be associated with lower self esteem [79]. Anxiety and depression tend to be associated with slightly better glycaemic control and it has been suggested by some authors that anxious children may be more diligent in monitoring and may take more effective action in response to poor glucose levels [80]. In contrast, adolescent behavioural problems of aggression and anti-social conduct have been associated with poor outcome with respect of HbA1c [79]. Overall, studies show high levels of psychological morbidity and, with long term follow up, around 10% of males and 23% of females require some degree of psychiatric support [81] (table 2).

***Table 2.*** Multiple regression analysis with mean HbA1c as dependent variable

| | β | SE(β) | t | p | 95% CI |
|---|---|---|---|---|---|
| Sex | 0.81 | 0.53 | 1.53 | | (−0.25, 1.87) |
| Baseline behavioural state | 0.15 | 0.04 | 3.61 | <0.001 | (0.07, 0.24) |
| Baseline emotional state | 0.06 | 0.03 | 1.96 | <0.06 | (−0.002, 0.13) |
| Baseline self-esteem | 0.004 | 0.02 | 0.17 | | (−0.04, 0.05) |



*Eating Disorders*

Several studies have highlighted the importance of eating disorders as a risk factor for later complications [75, 82–84]. In the study of Rydall et al. [78], out of the 91 young women who had eating disorders at baseline, HbA1c levels and rates of retinopathy were higher on follow-up compared to a non-eating disorder group. However, studies reporting an increased frequency of eating disorders in adolescents with T1DM have reported conflicting results, largely because of the instruments used to detect eating disorders are difficult to apply in populations with diabetes [83]. The prevalence of frank eating disorders is probably relatively low and not much greater or different from that in the normal population. However, anxiety about weight gain is common (and probably justified) and may be associated with less overt evidence of eating disorder. In a recent long-term follow-up study from Oxford, 30% of young women interviewed in their twenties admitted to insulin misuse during the adolescent years [84]. The likelihood of insulin misuse increased with baseline anxiety about weight gain and was present in 69% of those who developed a frank eating disorder. Overall, covert eating disorder and insulin misuse could have a considerable impact on the risk of complications and may explain some of the increased risk observed in adolescent girls.

*Brittle Diabetes*

The term 'brittle diabetes' was first applied to subjects with the problem of recurrent admissions with diabetic ketoacidosis (DKA). Although rare cases have been described, with the apparent problems in insulin absorption from subcutaneous depots or the development of severe neutralising antibodies to insulin, it is now generally accepted that the majority of cases of DKA result from insulin omission [85, 86]. However, adolescence is a relatively high risk period for the development of other conditions such as Crohn's disease, autoimmune hypothyroidism and Addison's disease and these too can lead to unstable diabetes. Overall, recurrent admissions with DKA are more common in females than in males and usually reflect serious psychological problems or family dysfunction [87]. The degree to which eating disorders and insulin misuse contributes to these problems is unclear, but it may be more common than previously suspected. Many of these subjects with recurrent DKA become profoundly insulin resistant as a consequence of recurrent chronic poor glycaemic control, and the vicious cycle may prove difficult to break without intensive monitoring and psychological support.

### Management of Diabetes during Adolescence

The management of diabetes during adolescence is complex; reflecting the rapid physiological changes and the emotional issues of puberty. It is a period when the young person is trying to gain independence from the family; but the demand for greater independence may not be equalled by the desire to take greater responsibility for the diabetes. Often, considerable effort is required to broker deals whereby families can reach appropriate compromise. Motivation may also be difficult to engender as 'risk taking' is part of normal adolescent development. Treatment goals may need to be continually reviewed and revised so that if adolescents are motivated to change, the outcome in terms of improved control can be tangible.

*Insulin Therapy and Diet*

The increasing insulin requirements of puberty are considerable and insulin doses may need to be increased from the typical 0.25 to 0.5 units/kg/day required in the pre-pubertal period, to 1 or 1.5 units/kg/day during puberty. Equally important, insulin requirements decline after the peak height velocity of puberty is achieved and will gradually fall back to prepubertal levels in the early to mid-twenties. The major increase in insulin requirement during puberty is in the background or basal insulin component and this can only be successfully achieved with either basal-bolus or continuous subcutaneous insulin infusion (CSII) pump therapy regimens. Many teenagers may need up to four or five subcutaneous bolus injections of fast acting insulin a day as part of their basal bolus or CSII insulin regimen, reflecting the variable and flexible eating habits commonly seen in this age group. The use of short or rapid acting insulin analogues such as insulin lispro or insulin aspart in this situation may provide some advantage by offering a more physiological control of the post-prandial glucose excursions. The relatively recently introduced long acting insulin analogue preparations, such as insulin glargine and insulin detemir, also provide better and more stable background basal insulin delivery [88, 89].

The short- and long-acting insulin analogue preparations given in combination may therefore be more advantageous to the teenager with T1DM, although and this may predispose to hyperglycaemia and poor long-term glycaemic control.

Adolescents are sexually aware and active at an increasingly younger age. Sex education is now part of the school curriculum in early teenage years. Contraception and advice should be routinely discussed; given the potential deleterious effects of poor glycaemic control on fetal development. Appropriate contraceptive advice for the young female with diabetes is also important given the wide choice of methods and agents available, and the potential for increased cardiovascular disease risk associated with the use of some of the combined oestrogen/progesterone oral contraceptive preparations. It is recommended that patients starting oral contraceptive treatment should be prescribed a so-called 3rd-generation pill, preferably a preparation with the lowest dose of oestrogen which is sufficient to control break-through bleeding. Caution should be taken in prescribing these agents however, particularly when there is evidence of obesity, hypertension or a positive family history of venous thromboembolism or early (age <50 years) cardiovascular disease and premenopausal breast cancer. In this situation, alternative means of contraception should be considered, such as the progesterone-only pill or barrier methods.

Adolescence is also a period of life in which there is often an increasing interest in sporting activities and in the taking of regular exercise, although secular trends suggest that young people in general are becoming less active. There are very few sports in which patients with diabetes are either prohibited or restricted from participation, and given the potential benefits in terms of insulin sensitivity [124] and cardiovascular health all patients with diabetes should be encouraged to participate in some form of regular activity.

*Transition of Care*

Adolescence inevitably involves the transfer of responsibility for the care of the diabetes from the parents to the child. However, for many adolescents, accepting such responsibility at a time in their life when they still feel vulnerable and insecure and where the diabetes is considered low in their priorities due to other interests may prove difficult. The years when young people first move away from home may be equally difficult and some studies indicate that the worst HbA1c levels are seen around the age of 18–19 years [79]. Sadly, in some countries a significant cause of morbidity and death is neglect of diabetes and untreated DKA occurring at home, often in young men [125, 126] (fig. 4).

It has been increasingly realised that many young adults with T1DM share a lot of the psychological problems seen in the adolescent. The prognosis and psychological morbidity continues to be poor well into the young adult years [79]. For the adolescent with T1DM, transition from the paediatric to the adult clinic represents a major obstacle to future health care. Transitional health care

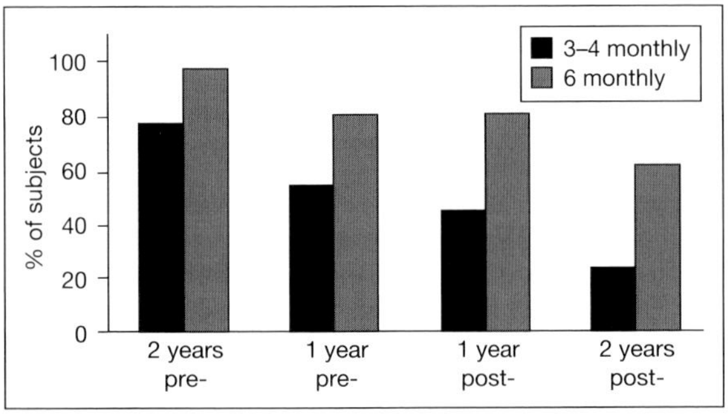


*Fig. 4.* Hospital clinic attendance during the 2 years before and after transfer, in a cohort of 96 subjects with type 1 diabetes [Copyright © 2002, Blackwell Publishing Ltd. Adapted from [127]].

is therefore important and has been 'ideally' defined as the 'planned purposeful movement of the adolescent from child-centered to adult-orientated care'. The process of transition should ideally; be uninterrupted, well coordinated, and comprehensive, yet sufficiently flexible to take into account the psychological and social development of the adolescent; the complexity of the health problems for the family, and their readiness for change. The fact that in many countries, young people with diabetes are arbitrarily transferred from the paediatric to the adult service in the middle of this period of high risk is unfortunate. Adolescents clearly do not want to go on being part of the paediatric diabetes clinic indefinitely, yet the optimal methods of transfer remain to be determined and evaluated. Whatever the age of transfer from the paediatric clinic, patients often have concerns over potential differences in approach to diabetes care. Furthermore, while the change from the family-based paediatric clinic to the larger-size adult clinic may promote independence, it can also lead to anxiety and reduced attendance. In one study, as many as 30% of the young people have dropped out the clinic system 2 years after transfer to the adult diabetes clinic [127]. Many innovative methods of transfer are being proposed and several strategies have been devised to address these problems. These include the establishment of 'joint clinics' staffed by both paediatric and adult physicians, or 'young adult clinics' staffed by adult physicians, but run separately from the main adult clinic. Although some data suggest that the provision of young adult clinics improves attendance [128], there has been little systematic evaluation of the various methods of transitional care and the perceptions of the patients themselves have not been determined. The success of any of these interventions often depends on the individual commitment of the physicians or paediatricians, to the overall aim of promoting good diabetes care during adolescence.

42 Holl RW, Heinze E, Seifert M, Grabert M, Teller WM: Longitudinal analysis of somatic development in paediatric patients with IDDM: Genetic influences on height and weight. Diabetologia 1994;37:925–929.
43 Pitukcheewanont P, Alemzadeh R, Jacobs WR, Jones BH, Eberle AJ: Does glycemic control affect growth velocity in children with insulin-dependent diabetes mellitus. Acta Diabetol 1995;32: 148–152.
44 Mortensen HB, Hougaard P: Comparison of metabolic control in a cross-sectional study of 2,873 children and adolescents with IDDM from 18 countries. The Hvidore Study Group on Childhood Diabetes. Diabetes Care 1997;20:714–720.
45 Holl RW, Grabert M, Sorgo W, Heinze E, Debatin KM: Contributions of age, gender and insulin administration to weight gain in subjects with IDDM. Diabetologia 1998;41:542–547.
46 Gregory JW, Wilson AC, Greene SA: Body fat and overweight among children and adolescents with diabetes mellitus. Diab Med 1992;9:344–348.
47 Domargard A, Sarnblad S, Kroon M, Karlsson I, Skeppner G, Aman J: Increased prevalence of overweight in adolescent girls with type 1 diabetes mellitus. Acta Paediatr 1999;88:1223–1228.
48 Ahmed ML, Ong KK, Watts AP, Morrell DJ, Preece MA, Dunger DB: Elevated leptin levels are associated with excess gains in fat mass in girls, but not boys, with type 1 diabetes: Longitudinal study during adolescence. J Clin Endocrinol Metab 2001;86:1188–1193.
49 Kiess W, Anil M, Blum WF, Englaro P, Juul A, Attanasio A, Dotsch J, Rascher W: Serum leptin levels in children and adolescents with insulin-dependent diabetes mellitus in relation to metabolic control and body mass index. Eur J Endocrinol 1998;138:501–509.
50 Mortensen HB, Robertson KJ, Aanstoot HJ, Danne T, Holl RW, Hougaard P, Atchison JA, Chiarelli F, Daneman D, Dinesen B, Dorchy H, Garandeau P, Greene S, Hoey H, Kaprio EA, Kocova M, Martul P, Matsuura N, Schoenle EJ, Sovik O, Swift PG, Tsou RM, Vanelli M, Aman J: Insulin management and metabolic control of type 1 diabetes mellitus in childhood and adolescence in 18 countries. Hvidore Study Group on Childhood Diabetes. Diab Med 1998;15: 752–759.
51 Escobar-Morreale HF, Roldán B, Barrio R, Alonso M, Sancho J, Hermenegildo De La Calle, García-Robles R: High prevalence of the polycystic ovary syndrome and hirsutism in women with type 1 diabetes mellitus. J Clin Endocrinol Metab 2000;85:4182–4187.
52 Trzeciak B: Effect of diabetes mellitus on the incidence of abnormal genital bleedings in women. Ginekol Pol 1978;49:119–123.
53 Djursing H, Nyholm HC, Hagen C, Carstensen L, Pedersen LM: Clinical and hormonal characteristics in women with anovulation and insulin-treated diabetes mellitus. Am J Obstet Gynecol 1982;143:876–882.
54 Strotmeyer ES, Steenkiste AR, Foley TP, Berga SL, Dorman JS: Menstrual cycle differences between women with type 1 diabetes and women without diabetes. Diabetes Care 2003;26: 1016–1021.
55 Burger W, Hovener G, Dusterhus R, Hartmann R, Weber B: Prevalence and development of retinopathy in children and adolescents with type 1 (insulin-dependent) diabetes mellitus. A longitudinal study. Diabetologia 1986;29:17–22.
56 Danne T, Weber B, Hartmann R, Enders I, Burger W, Hovener G: Long-term glycemic control has a nonlinear association to the frequency of background retinopathy in adolescents with diabetes. Follow-up of the Berlin Retinopathy Study. Diabetes Care 1994;17:1390–1396.
57 Barkai L, Vamosi I, Lukacs K: Enhanced progression of urinary albumin excretion in IDDM during puberty. Diabetes Care 1998;21:1019–1023.
58 Schultz CJ, Konopelska-Bahu T, Dalton RN, Carroll TA, Stratton I, Gale EA, Neil A, Dunger DB: Microalbuminuria prevalence varies with age, sex, and puberty in children with type 1 diabetes followed from diagnosis in a longitudinal study. Oxford Regional Prospective Study Group. Diabetes Care 1999;22:495–502.
59 Rudberg S, Persson B: Indications of low sex hormone binding globulin (SHBG) in young females with type 1 diabetes, and an independent association to microalbuminuria. Diab Med 1995;12: 816–822.
60 Amin R, Schultz C, Ong K, Frystyk J, Dalton RN, Perry L, Orskov H, Dunger DB, Oxford Regional Prospective Study: Low IGF-I and elevated testosterone during puberty in subjects with

type 1 diabetes developing microalbuminuria in comparison to normoalbuminuric control subjects: The Oxford Regional Prospective Study. Diabetes Care 2003;26:1456–1461.
61 Merimee TJ: A follow-up study of vascular disease in growth-hormone-deficient dwarfs with diabetes. N Engl J Med 1978;298:1217–1222.
62 Hyer SL, Sharp PS, Brooks RA, Burrin JM, Kohner EM: Serum IGF-1 concentration in diabetic retinopathy. Diab Med 1988;5:356–360.
63 Dills DG, Moss SE, Klein R, Klein BE, Davis M: Is insulinlike growth factor I associated with diabetic retinopathy? Diabetes 1990;39:191–195.
64 Dills DG, Moss SE, Klein R, Klein BE: Association of elevated IGF-I levels with increased retinopathy in late-onset diabetes. Diabetes 1991;40:1725–1730.
65 Moller N, Orskov H: Does IGF-I therapy in insulin-dependent diabetes mellitus limit complications? Lancet 1997;350:1188–1189.
66 Thrailkill KM, Quattrin T, Baker L, Kuntze JE, Compton PG, Martha PM Jr: Cotherapy with recombinant human insulin-like growth factor I and insulin improves glycemic control in type 1 diabetes. RhIGF-I in IDDM Study Group. Diabetes Care 1999;22:585–592.
67 Alzaid AA, Dinneen SF, Melton LJ 3rd, Rizza RA: The role of growth hormone in the development of diabetic retinopathy. Diabetes Care 1994;17:531–534.
68 Lundbaek K, Christensen NJ, Jensen VA, Johansen K, Olsen TS, Hansen AP, Orskov H, Osterby R: Diabetes, diabetic angiopathy, and growth hormone. Lancet 1970;ii:131–133.
69 Landau D, Domene H, Flyvbjerg A, Gronbaek H, Roberts CT Jr, Argov S, LeRoith D: Differential expression of renal growth hormone receptor and its binding protein in experimental diabetes mellitus. Growth Horm IGF Res 1998;8:39–45.
70 Flyvbjerg A, Bennett WF, Rasch R, Kopchick JJ, Scarlett JA: Inhibitory effect of a growth hormone receptor antagonist (G120K-PEG) on renal enlargement, glomerular hypertrophy, and urinary albumin excretion in experimental diabetes in mice. Diabetes 1999;48:377–382.
71 van Neck JW, Dits NF, Cingel V, Hoppenbrouwers IA, Drop SL, Flyvbjerg A: Dose-response effects of a new growth hormone receptor antagonist (B2036-PEG) on circulating, hepatic and renal expression of the growth hormone/insulin-like growth factor system in adult mice. J Endocrinol 2000;167:295–303.
72 Amin R, Williams RW, Frystyk J, Dalton N, Orskov H, Matthews D, Dunger D: Abnormalities in the growth hormone-IGF-I axis in association with microalbuminuria in young adults with T1DM: The Oxford Regional Prospective Study. Diabetes 2003;52:S1, abstr 208–OR.
73 Hovind P, Tarnow L, Rossing P, Jensen BR, Graae M, Torp I, Binder C, Parving HH: Predictors for the development of microalbuminuria and macroalbuminuria in patients with type 1 diabetes: Inception cohort study. Br Med J 2004;328:1105.
74 Mayou R, Peveler R, Davies B, Mann J, Fairburn C: Psychiatric morbidity in young adults with insulin-dependent diabetes mellitus. Psychol Med 1991;21:639–645.
75 Blanz BJ, Rensch-Riemann BS, Fritz-Sigmund DI, Schmidt MH: IDDM is a risk factor for adolescent psychiatric disorders. Diabetes Care 1993;16:1579–1587.
76 Kovacs M, Goldston D, Obrosky DS, Iyengar S: Prevalence and predictors of pervasive noncompliance with medical treatment among youths with insulin-dependent diabetes mellitus. J Am Acad Child Adolesc Psychiatry 1992;31:1112–1119.
77 Dumont RH, Jacobson AM, Cole C, Hauser ST, Wolfsdorf JI, Willett JB, Milley JE, Wertlieb D: Psychosocial predictors of acute complications of diabetes in youth. Diabet Med 1995;12: 612–618.
78 Rydall AC, Rodin GM, Olmsted MP, Devenyi RG, Daneman D: Disordered eating behavior and microvascular complications in young women with insulin-dependent diabetes mellitus. N Engl J Med 1997;336:1849–1854.
79 Bryden KS, Peveler RC, Stein A, Neil A, Mayou RA, Dunger DB: Clinical and psychological course of diabetes from adolescence to young adulthood: A longitudinal cohort study. Diabetes Care 2001;24:1536–1540.
80 Fonagy P, Moran GS, Lindsay MK, Kurtz AB, Brown R: Psychological adjustment and diabetic control. Arch Dis Child 1987;62:1009–1013.
81 Bryden KS, Dunger DB, Mayou RA, Peveler RC, Neil HA: Poor prognosis of young adults with type 1 diabetes: A longitudinal study. Diabetes Care 2003;26:1052–1057.

82 Steel JM, Young RJ, Lloyd GG, Clarke BF: Clinically apparent eating disorders in young diabetic women: Associations with painful neuropathy and other complications. Br Med J (Clin Res Ed) 1987;294:859–862.
83 Peveler RC, Fairburn CG, Boller I, Dunger D: Eating disorders in adolescents with IDDM. A controlled study. Diabetes Care 1992;15:1356–1360.
84 Bryden KS, Neil A, Mayou RA, Peveler RC, Fairburn CG, Dunger DB: Eating habits, body weight, and insulin misuse. A longitudinal study of teenagers and young adults with type 1 diabetes. Diabetes Care 1999;22:1956–1960.
85 Malone JI, Root AW: Plasma free insulin concentrations: Keystone to effective management of diabetes mellitus in children. J Pediatr 1981;99:862–867.
86 Morris AD, Boyle DI, McMahon AD, Greene SA, MacDonald TM, Newton RW: Adherence to insulin treatment, glycaemic control, and ketoacidosis in insulin-dependent diabetes mellitus. The DARTS/MEMO Collaboration. Diabetes Audit and Research in Tayside Scotland. Medicines Monitoring Unit. Lancet 1997;350:1505–1510.
87 Rewers A, Chase HP, Mackenzie T, Walravens P, Roback M, Rewers M, Hamman RF, Klingensmith G: Predictors of acute complications in children with type 1 diabetes. JAMA 2002; 287:2511–2518.
88 Lepore M, Pampanelli S, Fanelli C, Porcellati F, Bartocci L, Di Vincenzo A, Cordoni C, Costa E, Brunetti P, Bolli GB: Pharmacokinetics and pharmacodynamics of subcutaneous injection of long-acting human insulin analog glargine, NPH insulin, and ultralente human insulin and continuous subcutaneous infusion of insulin lispro. Diabetes 2000;49:2142–2148.
89 Danne T, Lupke K, Walte K, Von Schuetz W, Gall MA: Insulin detemir is characterized by a consistent pharmacokinetic profile across age-groups in children, adolescents, and adults with type 1 diabetes. Diabetes Care 2003;26:3087–3092.
90 Schober E, Schoenle E, Van Dyk J, Wernicke-Panten K; Pediatric Study Group of Insulin Glargine: Comparative trial between insulin glargine and NPH insulin in children and adolescents with type 1 diabetes mellitus. J Pediatr Endocrinol Metab 2002;15:369–376.
91 Murphy NP, Keane SM, Ong KK, Ford-Adams M, Edge JA, Acerini CL, Dunger DB: Randomized cross-over trial of insulin glargine plus lispro or NPH insulin plus regular human insulin in adolescents with type 1 diabetes on intensive insulin regimens. Diabetes Care 2003;26:799–804.
92 Vague P, Selam JL, Skeie S, De Leeuw I, Elte JW, Haahr H, Kristensen A, Draeger E: Insulin detemir is associated with more predictable glycemic control and reduced risk of hypoglycemia than NPH insulin in patients with type 1 diabetes on a basal-bolus regimen with premeal insulin aspart. Diabetes Care 2003;26:590–596.
93 Maniatis AK, Klingensmith GJ, Slover RH, Mowry CJ, Chase HP: Continuous subcutaneous insulin infusion therapy for children and adolescents: An option for routine diabetes care. Pediatrics 2001;107:351–356.
94 Doyle EA, Weinzimer SA, Steffen AT, Ahern JA, Vincent M, Tamborlane WV: A randomized, prospective trial comparing the efficacy of continuous subcutaneous insulin infusion with multiple daily injections using insulin glargine. Diabetes Care 2004;27:1554–1558.
95 DAFNE Study Group: Training in flexible, intensive insulin management to enable dietary freedom in people with type 1 diabetes: Dose adjustment for normal eating (DAFNE) randomised controlled trial. Br Med J 2002;325:746.
96 Acerini CL, Patton CM, Savage MO, Kernell A, Westphal O, Dunger DB: Randomised placebo-controlled trial of human recombinant insulin-like growth factor I plus intensive insulin therapy in adolescents with insulin-dependent diabetes mellitus. Lancet 1997;350:1199–1204.
97 Sarnblad S, Kroon M, Aman J: Metformin as additional therapy in adolescents with poorly controlled type 1 diabetes: Randomised placebo-controlled trial with aspects on insulin sensitivity. Eur J Endocrinol 2003;149:323–329.
98 Hamilton J, Cummings E, Zdravkovic V, Finegood D, Daneman D: Metformin as an adjunct therapy in adolescents with type 1 diabetes and insulin resistance: A randomized controlled trial. Diabetes Care 2003;26:138–143.
99 Diabetes Control and Complications Trial Research Group: Effect of intensive diabetes treatment on the development and progression of long-term complications in adolescents with insulin-dependent diabetes mellitus: Diabetes Control and Complications Trial. J Pediatr 1994;125: 177–188.

100 Ahern JA, Boland EA, Doane R, Ahern JJ, Rose P, Vincent M, Tamborlane WV: Insulin pump therapy in pediatrics: A therapeutic alternative to safely lower HbA1c levels across all age groups. Pediatr Diabetes 2002;3:10–15.
101 Whincup G, Milner RD: Prediction and management of nocturnal hypoglycaemia in diabetes. Arch Dis Child 1987;62:333–337.
102 Porter PA, Byrne G, Stick S, Jones TW: Nocturnal hypoglycaemia and sleep disturbances in young teenagers with insulin dependent diabetes mellitus. Arch Dis Child 1996;75:120–123.
103 Beregszaszi M, Tubiana-Rufi N, Benali K, Noel M, Bloch J, Czernichow P: Nocturnal hypoglycemia in children and adolescents with insulin-dependent diabetes mellitus: Prevalence and risk factors. J Pediatr 1997;131:27–33.
104 Lopez MJ, Oyarzabal M, Barrio R, Hermoso F, Lopez JP, Rodriguez M, Blasco L, Gastaldo E: Nocturnal hypoglycaemia in IDDM patients younger than 18 years. Diab Med 1997;14:772–777.
105 Porter PA, Keating B, Byrne G, Jones TW: Incidence and predictive criteria of nocturnal hypoglycemia in young children with insulin-dependent diabetes mellitus. J Pediatr 1997;130: 366–372.
106 Matyka KA: Sweet dreams?–nocturnal hypoglycemia in children with type 1 diabetes. Pediatr Diab 2002;3:74–81.
107 Edge JA, Matthews DR, Dunger DB: Failure of current insulin regimes to meet the overnight insulin requirements of adolescent diabetics. Diab Res 1990;15:109–102.
108 Mohn A, Strang S, Wernicke-Panten K, Lang AM, Edge JA, Dunger DB: Nocturnal glucose control and free insulin levels in children with type 1 diabetes by use of the long-acting insulin HOE 901 as part of a three-injection regimen. Diabetes Care 2000;23:557–559.
109 Mohn A, Matyka KA, Harris DA, Ross KM, Edge JA, Dunger DB: Lispro or regular insulin for multiple injection therapy in adolescence. Differences in free insulin and glucose levels overnight. Diabetes Care 1999;22:27–32.
110 Jones TW, Porter P, Sherwin RS, Davis EA, O'Leary P, Frazer F, Byrne G, Stick S, Tamborlane WV: Decreased epinephrine responses to hypoglycemia during sleep N Engl J Med 1998;338:1657–1662.
111 Matyka KA, Wigg L, Pramming S, Stores G, Dunger DB: Cognitive function and mood after profound nocturnal hypoglycaemia in prepubertal children with conventional insulin treatment for diabetes. Arch Dis Child 1999;81:138–142.
112 Thompson CJ, Cummings JF, Chalmers J, Gould C, Newton RW: How have patients reacted to the implications of the DCCT? Diabetes Care 1996;19:876–879.
113 Tattersall RB, Gill GV: Unexplained deaths of type 1 diabetic patients. Diab Med 1991;8:49–58.
114 Robinson RT, Harris ND, Ireland RH, Macdonald IA, Heller SR: Changes in cardiac repolarization during clinical episodes of nocturnal hypoglycaemia in adults with Type 1 diabetes. Diabetologia 2004;47:312–315.
115 Murphy NP, Ford-Adams ME, Ong KK, Harris ND, Keane SM, Davies C, Ireland RH, MacDonald IA, Knight EJ, Edge JA, Heller SR, Dunger DB: Prolonged cardiac repolarisation during spontaneous nocturnal hypoglycaemia in children and adolescents with type 1 diabetes. Diabetologia 2004;in press.
116 Daneman D, Olmsted M, Rydall A, Maharaj S, Rodin G: Eating disorders in young women with type 1 diabetes. Prevalence, problems and prevention. Horm Res 1998;50:79–86.
117 Schultz CJ, Neil HAW, Dalton RN, Dunger DB on behalf of the Oxford Regional Prospective Study group: Risk of nephropathy can be detected before the onset of microalbuminuria during the early years from diagnosis of type 1 diabetes. Diabetes Care 2000;23:1811–1815.
118 Cook J, Daneman D, Spino M, Sochett E, Perlman K, Balfe JW: Angiotensin converting enzyme inhibitor therapy to decrease microalbuminuria in normotensive children with insulin-dependent diabetes mellitus. J Pediatr 1990;117:39–45.
119 Rudberg S, Osterby R, Bangstad HJ, Dahlquist G, Persson B: Effect of angiotensin converting enzyme inhibitor or beta blocker on glomerular structural changes in young microalbuminuric patients with type I (insulin-dependent) diabetes mellitus. Diabetologia 1999;42:589–595.
120 O'Hare P, Bilbous R, Mitchell T, O' Callaghan CJ, Viberti GC: ACE-Inhibitor Trial to Lower Albuminuria in Normotensive Insulin-Dependent Subjects Study Group: Low-dose ramipril reduces microalbuminuria in type 1 diabetic patients without hypertension: results of a randomized controlled trial. Diabetes Care 2000;23:1823–1829.

121 Dahlquist G, Stattin EL, Rudberg S: Urinary albumin excretion rate and glomerular filtration rate in the prediction of diabetic nephropathy: A long-term follow-up study of childhood onset type-1 diabetic patients. Nephrol Dial Transplant 2001;16:1382–1386.
122 Glasgow AM, Tynan D, Schwartz R, Hicks JM, Turek J, Driscol C, O'Donnell RM, Getson PR: Alcohol and drug use in teenagers with diabetes mellitus. J Adolesc Health 1991;12:11–14.
123 Ng RS, Darko DA, Hillson RM: Street drug use among young patients with type 1 diabetes in the UK. Diabet Med 2004;21:295–296.
124 Yki-Jarvinen H, DeFronzo RA, Koivisto VA: Normalization of insulin sensitivity in type I diabetic subjects by physical training during insulin pump therapy. Diabetes Care 1984;7:520–527.
125 Edge JA, Ford-Adams ME, Dunger DB: Causes of death in children with insulin dependent diabetes 1990–96. Arch Dis Child 1999;81:318–323.
126 Laing SP, Swerdlow AJ, Slater SD, Botha JL, Burden AC, Waugh NR, Smith AW, Hill RD, Bingley PJ, Patterson CC, Qiao Z, Keen H: The British Diabetic Association Cohort Study. I. All-cause mortality in patients with insulin-treated diabetes mellitus. Diab Med 1999;16: 459–465.
127 Kipps S, Bahu T, Ong K, Ackland FM, Brown RS, Fox CT, Griffin NK, Knight AH, Mann NP, Neil HA, Simpson H, Edge JA, Dunger DB: Current methods of transfer of young people with type 1 diabetes to adult services. Diab Med 2002;19:649–654.
128 Kinmonth AL, Donovan C: The approach of general practice; in Kurtz Z, Hopkins A (ed): Services for Young People with Chronic Disorders in Their Transition from Childhood to Adult Life. London, Royal College of Physicians, 1996.

D. Dunger, MD
Department of Paediatrics, University of Cambridge
Box 116, Addenbrooke's Hospital, Hills Road, Cambridge, CB2 2QQ (UK)
Tel. +44 0 1223 336886, Fax +44 0 1223 336996, E-Mail dbd25@cam.ac.uk

Chiarelli F, Dahl-Jørgensen K, Kiess W (eds): Diabetes in Childhood and Adolescence.
Pediatr Adolesc Med. Basel, Karger, 2005, vol 10, pp 225–258

# Diabetic Nephropathy in Children and Adolescents

*Francesco Chiarelli, Francesca Santilli*

Department of Pediatrics, University of Chieti, Chieti, Italy

Overt diabetes-related microvascular and macrovascular complications, with particular reference to nephropathy, are almost unknown in younger children and are extremely uncommon even in adolescents with fairly long disease duration [1–4]. Nonetheless, their onset can be presumed to start very early in the course of diabetes, perhaps at the disease onset, and the earliest stages can be often detected as soon as 2 to 5 years after diagnosis [5–7]. Health care professionals involved in the management of type 1 diabetes (T1DM) in children and adolescents should be aware of these complications and must provide appropriate education and surveillance.

## Natural History of Nephropathy

The cumulative risk for diabetic nephropathy is approximately 30–40% after 40 years of disease although the risk seems considerably greater in patients in whom T1DM develops during childhood [8]; in recent studies, however, a declining incidence of diabetic nephropathy has been observed [9, 10]. Nephropathy is associated with a major portion of the excess morbidity and mortality in patients with T1DM [11]. Overt nephropathy, which rarely occurs in childhood or adolescence, accounts for the highest proportion of new patients entering renal dialysis and transplantation programs in developed countries [12].

Children and adolescents with T1DM might manifest microalbuminuria, the first clinically identifiable sign of diabetic nephropathy, but the real incidence, prevalence and prognostic significance are still unknown. In fact, most of the studies performed so far have a cross-sectional design, and only limited data are

*Table 1.* Cross-sectional studies on microalbuminuria prevalence

| Author | Screening procedure (methods and timing) | Population | Microalbuminuria % | Mean duration of diabetes years |
|---|---|---|---|---|
| Mathiesen et al. [7] | AER, overnight | 97 | 20 | 10 |
| Dahlquist and Rudberg [14] | AER, overnight | 129 | 20 | 10 |
| Mortensen et al. [16] | AER, overnight | 957 | 4 | 6 |
| Joner et al. [15] | AER, overnight | 371 | 12 | 10.5 |
| Moore and Shield (MIDAC study) [13] | AER, overnight | 1007 | 9.7 | >1 |

AER = Albumin excretion rate.

available from longitudinal studies based on small clinical samples. In contrast, the determination of microalbuminuria prevalence in relation to risk factors requires a large prospective population-based study. From cross-sectional studies, the microalbuminuria prevalence rate has been estimated to be between 12 and 20% in patients between 15 and 20 years (table 1) [13–16]. In Italy, a lower prevalence of 5.9% has been observed in a cross-sectional study recruiting 977 children and adolescents with a mean age of 12.7 ± 4.6 years and with a mean diabetes duration of 5.1 years [17]. On the other hand, the prevalence of microalbuminuria in longitudinal studies varies from 4.8 to 21% (table 2) [18–21], and this large variation in prevalence rate for microalbuminuria might be explained by differences in glycemic control in the various studies.

The Oxford Regional Prospective Study (ORPS) of childhood diabetes is the only study providing accurate data concerning prevalence of microalbuminuria in a community cohort with patients recruited at diagnosis of T1DM [21]. Of a total of 514 children followed longitudinally for more than 4.5 years, 12.8% developed microalbuminuria, which became persistent in 4.8%. The cumulative risk for developing microalbuminuria in this cohort was around 40% after 11 years' duration of T1DM. However, subjects diagnosed with diabetes before puberty showed a silent period followed by a more rapid development of microalbuminuria during puberty, whereas the rate of development of microalbuminuria in subjects diagnosed at puberty was relatively constant, indicating that differences in pubertal stages have a profound effect on the prevalence of microalbuminuria.

*Table 2.* Longitudinal studies on MA prevalence

| Author | Screening procedure (methods and timing) | Population | Follow-up years | Microalbuminuria |
|---|---|---|---|---|
| Norgaard et al. [18] | AER, 24-hour urine | 113 | 2 | 15% |
| Jones et al., 1998 | AER, morning spot urine | 233 | 8 | intermittent: 9%<br>permanent: 14% |
| Janner et al. | AER, 12-hour urine; 3-monthly | 164 (83F, 81M) | 8 | 20 |
| Barkai et al. [19] | AER, 24-hour urine, 6-month intervals | 74 (20 prepubertal, 28 pubertal, 26 postpubertal) | 3 | 6/28 pubertal subjects<br>2/26 postpubertal subjects |
| Rudberg et al. [20] | AER, 3-month intervals | 156 | 3–9 | 4.8% |
| Danne et al. [2] | AER, overnight | 249 | 9 | intermittent: 3%<br>permanent: 5% |
| Schultz et al. [21] | AER, overnight or morning | 514 | 10 (>4.5 years in 287 children) | permanent: 4.8% |

AER = Albumin excretion rate.

Diabetic nephropathy evolves through five stages as follows [22, 23]:

1. In the first stage, often at the time of diagnosis of diabetes, kidney size is increased, and the glomerular filtration rate (GFR) is elevated. These abnormalities are usually reversible with the establishment of good metabolic control. Nevertheless, in some instances, nephromegaly and raised GFR persist, whereas in others these findings may return after a few years.
2. The second stage develops in virtually all persons with T1DM in the 2nd to 5th years after diagnosis. Although no functional impairment is detectable other than the possibility of a raised GFR, pathologic features can be found on biopsy and include mesangial matrix expansion and glomerular basement membrane thickening. Progression to the later stages of nephropathy can be prevented or delayed by the maintenance of excellent metabolic control [6].
3. The third stage is determined by the presence of microalbuminuria, defined by an albumin excretion rate (AER) in at least two to three timed (either 24-hour or overnight) urine collections of greater than

diabetic patients compared with that of patients without family history for cardiovascular disease and enhances the likelihood of cardiovascular disease in diabetic patients who have nephropathy [98]. This observation has been confirmed by studies that have revealed that first-degree nondiabetic relatives of type 1 diabetic patients with albuminuria have reduced insulin sensitivity and abnormal lipid profiles [99]. This familial aggregation of renal and cardiovascular disease and their risk factors has led to the suggestion that these disorders may share a common pathogenetic basis.

Family studies of blood pressure have provided further insights [44, 59]. Higher arterial pressure was measured in parents of diabetic patients with proteinuria than in parents of patients without proteinuria. A higher prevalence of arterial hypertension among the parents of type 1 diabetic patients with nephropathy was also found by subsequent studies. A relative risk for development of overt nephropathy of approximately 3.3 was found if at least one of the parents had hypertension. All these studies suggest that hypertension or a predisposition to it may be important components in determining the susceptibility to renal disease in diabetes [44, 59].

*Hyperlipidemia*

There is a close correlation between metabolic control and disturbances in lipid metabolism.

Despite experimental data implicating lipids in the pathogenesis of early diabetic nephropathy, no association has been noted between abnormal lipids and the development of microalbuminuria [2]. Although increased lipid levels may contribute to the progression of microalbuminuria to overt nephropathy, intervention studies are needed to evaluate the impact of lipid-lowering agents on the progression of DN.

*Smoking*

Available data suggest that persons with diabetes are as likely as persons without diabetes to start smoking [100]. Furthermore, people who choose to smoke are at greater risk for the onset and progression of complications than are persons who do not smoke or who quit smoking. Although most of the studies to date address outcomes in older age groups, it is generally believed in the teen years that smoking begins and when prevention programs may be most likely to succeed. In the EURODIAB IDDM Complications Study of 3,250 men and women between 15 and 60 years of age, current smokers were more likely to have poorer metabolic control and to get microalbuminuria and retinopathy [101]. Ex-smokers had findings similar to nonsmokers, except for the presence of more advanced complications. In a study of 241 patients with T1DM and 5,876 controls, it has been found that smokers with diabetes reported morbidity three to ten times more frequently than nonsmoking controls and two to three times more often than nonsmokers with diabetes [102]. The smoking versus diabetes interaction was more than multiplicative for all morbidity measures.

Smoking seems to enhance the progression of microalbuminuria to overt nephropathy [103]. The frequency of smoking in adolescents with type 1 diabetes is unclear, although one study has suggested that it may be lower when compared with smoking among nondiabetic peers [104].

### Puberty

Early manifestations of microvascular complications are rarely found in prepubertal children with T1DM [2–4]. In contrast, both nephropathy and retinopathy show an increasing prevalence during the pubertal and postpubertal years [2–4, 105]. Investigators have sought to answer two important questions arising from these observations: (a) the contribution made by puberty to the expression of these complications, and (b) the significance of the prepubertal years to their development. Support for the idea that puberty accelerates the development of DN comes from several sources. A significant relationship has been found between pubertal duration and the prevalence of both microalbuminuria and nephromegaly (early markers of diabetic nephropathy) in a cohort of prepubertal, pubertal, and postpubertal children and adolescents with similar durations of T1DM [105]. Thus, robust evidence suggests that puberty enhances the development of microvascular disease. The mediators of this effect have not been clearly delineated, but growth factors such as growth hormone/IGF-1, TGF-β, and other hormonal factors such as androgens have been implicated [52, 106].

The evidence is much less clear with regard to the contribution of the prepubertal years to the onset of microvascular disease [107, 108]. However, as previously stated, it seems likely that poor glycemic control may accelerate DN also during prepubertal years and contributes to the long-term prognosis of childhood diabetes, although the risk may only become evident at puberty [16, 19]. In a study of prepubertal, pubertal, and postpubertal subjects, all having a similar diabetes duration (5–10 years), nephromegaly (an early indicator of diabetic nephropathy) was observed in 14% of prepubertal subjects [105]. Similar observations have been made in the ORPS of T1DM, where children with an early onset of diabetes were at risk of developing microalbuminuria before puberty [21]. Recently, an increasing delay in onset of complications was found in adolescents with longer prepubertal diabetes duration [109]. These findings imply some effect of the prepubertal diabetic milieu on the nephropathic process.

In conclusion, through much of the natural history of DN, renal disease develops without detectable clinical expression, with normal AER and blood pressure, and with GFR normal to elevated. Therefore, methods for early identification of diabetic patients at risk for development of DN are needed. Recently, to investigate the contribution of several variables such as age, diabetes duration, sex, puberty, glycemia, systemic blood pressure, hyperfiltration, lipids, genetic susceptibility, on the development of the early lesions of DN, a longitudinal study has been carried out by the International Diabetic Nephropathy Study Group in a cohort of 243 almost entirely normoalbuminuric type 1 diabetic patients (age 10–40 years, 50% 10–18 years) [110]. Using two renal biopsies performed over 5 years, changes in renal structure have been assessed with regard to the above mentioned variables. The main findings of this study are that DN lesions occurring in young normoalbuminuric type 1 diabetic patients are significantly related to disease duration, but are less closely related to glycemia or renal hemodynamics than previously reported; and that systemic blood pressure within the normal range may be a more important determinant of early DN lesions than previously appreciated [111]. A succeeding report from the International Diabetic Nephropathy Study examined the effects of disease duration and age at onset of T1DM on glomerular morphometry obtained from kidney biopsy in 243 normoalbuminuric young diabetic subjects, with prepubertal, pubertal or postpuberty onset. Glomerular abnormalities progressed slowly in the first 14 or 15 years after disease onset but more rapidly thereafter, with no statistically significant differences in the effect of duration among the three age-at-onset subgroups, even with multivariate adjustment for sex, center, baseline HbA1c, diastolic blood pressure, height and BMI [112].

## Screening for Complications in Adolescents

Surveillance for complications requires that the basic components of a screening program be met. A sensitive and specific method must be used to detect the disorder before it becomes irreversible or causes serious morbidity, the screening procedure should be cost-effective, and there should be effective management of the disorder detected. Surveillance for nephropathy and hypertension all meet these criteria because effective intervention can slow or stop the progress of these conditions.

Table 3 details the specific screening processes recommended for adolescents with diabetes. Regular measurement of HbA1c is an indispensable part of routine diabetes care because it is the best surrogate marker of the risk for microvascular, and probably also macrovascular, complications. HbA1c is the best available marker of long-term diabetes control. Because excellent

*Table 3.* Screening for diabetic nephropathy

| |
|---|
| *Hemoglobin A1c:* Every 3–4 months to assess and track degree of metabolic control and to make changes to achieve and maintain the best possible control from the very beginning of diabetes |
| *Blood pressure:* Every 3–6 months to assess presence of hypertension; no data available to determine when this should be started; it seems reasonable to recommend measurement at all clinic assessments |
| *Nephropathy:* Annual timed urine collections for albumin excretion rate (AER) beginning at onset of puberty and 3–5 years' diabetes duration; if positive, confirmation of microalbuminuria requires repeat testing at three monthly intervals over 6 months |

metabolic control is known to prevent or delay the onset and progression of complications, this measurement also provides information about the effectiveness of interventions aimed at improving metabolic control. Similarly, blood pressure measurement on a twice-yearly basis is sufficient for detecting early hypertension, the presence of which should signal the need for more frequent assessments and appropriate intervention.

### Microalbuminuria

The focus of screening for diabetic nephropathy needs to be on its prevention or early detection and intervention. Microalbuminuria provides a sufficiently reliable screening method for early nephropathy in children and adolescents with type 1 diabetes [83, 113]. Prospective studies have clearly demonstrated that microalbuminuria is highly predictive of subsequent proteinuria and overt nephropathy in type 1 diabetes. Many different approaches have been used to screen adolescents for microalbuminuria: the one yielding the most pathophysiologic information is the AER measured in a 24-hour urine collection, although this method is often inconvenient for the patients and is susceptible to the influences of posture and exercise [114, 115]. An acceptable and easier way is the use of a timed overnight collection. Shorter timed specimens and determinations of albumin to creatinine ratio in a spot urine sample are other possibilities but are less sensitive and specific than longer timed specimens. The high day-to-day variability in AER (up to 40%) makes it essential that more than one specimen is collected at any time before a diagnosis of microalbuminuria is made [116]. The most accepted definition of persistent microalbuminuria is an albumin excretion rate <20 μg/min in timed overnight urine collections in two out of three consecutive urine specimens in 6 months. The cutoffs for AER of 15, 20, or 30 μg/min are all somewhat arbitrary because the upper limit of AER is 7.2 μg/min as determined in nondiabetic adolescents [117]. Clearly, the predictive value of a positive test increases as the cutoff increases.

In accordance with the guidelines proposed by the American Diabetes Association (ADA) and the International Society for Pediatric and Adolescent Diabetes (ISPAD) [118, 119], in patients with prebubertal onset of diabetes, screening for microalbuminuria should be performed 5 years after onset, at age 11 years or at puberty (whichever is earlier), and annually thereafter; in patients with pubertal onset of diabetes, microalbuminuria screening should be performed 2 years after onset, and annually thereafter.

In patients in whom initial screening tests are negative for microalbuminuria, it is safe to presume that the development of renal changes will take place relatively slowly, and that annual screening will be sufficient. This presumption is supported by the relatively slow accretion of new cases of microalbuminuria seen in DCCT [6, 86]. In patients who are positive for microalbuminuria, repeat testing over a 3- to 6-month period should be performed to determine the presence of persistent microalbuminuria. If the microalbuminuria is persistent, appropriate intervention should be instituted. In patients in whom the microalbuminuria is intermittent, three monthly checks should continue because these patients may be at risk for accelerated progression of nephropathy [117].

It has also been suggested that subjects at risk for diabetic nephropathy can be identified during the first few years after diagnosis by sequential annual measurements of the AER. In fact, the development of microalbuminuria seems associated with AER levels lying within the second half of the normoalbuminuric range, which can already be observed between 1 and 2.5 years after diagnosis [120].

Recently, the rate of change of albuminuria over 1 year has been shown to independently predict mortality and cardiovascular disease in both type 1 and type 2 diabetic patients with DN [121] and may have clinical utility as a risk marker in identifying a subgroup of patients at greater risk.

### Primary Prevention and Secondary Intervention

Over the past 35 years, there has apparently been a highly significant decrease in the prevalence of DN in T1DM [10]. Improved glycemic control, lower blood pressure (in part due to early aggressive antihypertensive treatment), and reduced prevalence of smoking rates were associated with improved prognosis [10].

Interventions can be divided into those that prevent onset of the complication (primary prevention) and those that slow or halt its progression (secondary intervention). The major interventions include intensive diabetes management to achieve and maintain excellent metabolic control and antihypertensive therapy. Data are available to support the use of antihypertensives in general, and ACE inhibitors in particular, in slowing the progression of both early (microalbuminuria) and advanced (macroalbuminuria) DN [122]. Other less well-studied interventions may also hold the promise of decreasing complication onset or progression [123].

### Intensive Diabetes Management

The DCCT and other studies demonstrated the effectiveness of improved metabolic control as both a primary prevention and secondary intervention for all the three main microvascular complications [86, 87]. The level of HbA1c that must be achieved to prevent the onset or slow the progression of complications remains uncertain. In the DCCT, there was a linear relationship between HbA1c and the relative risk of complications, with decreasing risk into the nondiabetic range. In contrast, in a recent study [124] it has been reported a threshold effect for microalbuminuria at an HbA1c level of about 8.1%. The risk for the development of DN has been quantitated in a recent prospective 4-year study [125]. Although it is not commonly believed that the weight of evidence supports a threshold effect, it is nevertheless a reasonable first step to target HbA1c levels below 8% when managing adolescents [126, 127]. This practice would provide a level of metabolic control somewhat tighter than that achieved by the adolescents in the intensive treatment group in the DCCT and significantly more so than the average metabolic control achieved by children and adolescents with diabetes throughout the world [128, 129]. A European study group documented that such a level of good control is not easily obtained in children with T1DM. In fact, only 34% of 2,227 patients were able to achieve the recommended HbA1c level below 8% [128]. The ability to achieve and maintain this level of control is dependent on the allocation of sufficient resources to provide experienced multidisciplinary health care team support to these adolescents and their families. It is highly unlikely that such resources will be made available on a worldwide basis.

In the DCCT, despite a significant reduction in the occurrence of microalbuminuria and albuminuria, 16% in the primary prevention cohort and 26% in the secondary prevention cohort developed microalbuminuria during the nine years of intensified treatment. This clearly documents that additional treatment modalities are needed to reduce or avoid the increasing burden of DN.

### Reduction in the Dietary Protein Content

As mentioned earlier, arterial hypertension, albuminuria, and poor glycaemic control are the most important risk factors for a progressive decline in GFR in DN, while dietary protein intake generally has been found to play a minor or no role. However, a meta-analysis based on five studies in patients with T1DM and microalbuminuria or proteinuria showed that a low-protein diet (<0.8 g/kg/day) significantly slowed the increase in urinary AER or the decline in GFR or creatinine clearance (relative risk 0.56; 95% CI 0.40–0.77) [130]. Flaws in design (short-term, nonrandomized cross-over study and self-control studies), methods (creatinine clearance), and insufficient adjustment for other progression promoters, including antihypertensive treatment with ACE inhibitors, have weakened the strength of that conclusion [131]. Given the individual variability in the response of GFR following the introduction of a low protein diet [132], it should be reserved only to 'responders'.

### Angiotensin-Converting Enzyme Inhibition/ Antihypertensive Therapy

ACE inhibition and angiotensin receptor blockade have been shown to reduce the progression of both microalbuminuria and overt proteinuria in adults with T1DM. Many studies have confirmed the effectiveness of these agents in slowing the progression of DN at any stage after its onset (secondary intervention) [25, 133].

A randomized placebo-controlled trial in normotensive type 1 diabetic patients with normoalbuminuria has suggested a beneficial effect of ACE-inhibitors on the development of microalbuminuria [134]. In a placebo-controlled study performed in 12 normotensive adolescents with diabetes, a 3-month treatment with ACE inhibitors was able to reduce microalbuminuria in 10 of the 12 patients [135].

ACE inhibitors should be considered the agents of first choice in the management of both microalbuminuria and hypertension in patients with diabetes [133]. Few studies of ACE inhibitor therapy have been reported in adolescents with microalbuminuria: a significant decrease in AER has been obtained in a 3-month crossover trial with the ACE inhibitor captopril when compared with a placebo [136, 137].

A meta-analysis of 12 trials in 698 type 1 diabetic patients with microalbuminuria who were followed for at least one year has revealed that ACE inhibitors reduced the risk of progression to macroalbuminuria by 62% compared to that of the placebo group [odds ratio 0.38 (95% CI 0.25–0.57)] [138]. Regression to normoalbuminuria was three times greater than in patients receiving a placebo. At 2 years, the urinary AER was 50% lower in the patients taking ACE inhibitors than in those receiving placebo. Moreover, it has been shown that the beneficial effect of ACE inhibitors on preventing progression from microalbuminuria to overt nephropathy is long lasting (8 years) and, more importantly, it is associated with preservation of normal GFR [139]. Furthermore, the Captopril Collaborative Study Group demonstrated a significant risk reduction for doubling of serum creatinine concentrations in patients with T1DM and nephropathy who received captopril (48%; 95% CI 16–69%). The placebo-treated patients received conventional antihypertensive treatment excluding calcium channel blockers. It has been recently reported that long-term treatment (4 years) with an ACE inhibitor and long-acting dihydropyridine calcium antagonist has similar beneficial effects on progression of diabetic nephropathy in hypertensive patients with T1DM [140].

There are no obvious contraindications to ACE inhibitor use in the pediatric population, although there is concern that noncompliance or intermittent compliance with therapy may provide a misguided sense of security. The teratogenic effects of ACE inhibitors must be kept in mind when using these drugs in adolescent girls.

### Angiotensin II Receptor Antagonists

The recently introduced angiotensin II (ATII) receptor antagonists seem to have further advantages in patients with early diabetic nephropathy [141].

A double-blind, randomized, cross-over study has been performed, comparing an ATII T1DM antagonist, losartan, with enalapril in patients with type 1 diabetes and nephropathy [142]: this study showed that losartan's ability to reduce albuminuria and blood pressure is similar to the effect of ACE inhibitors, indicating that the reduction in albuminuria and blood pressure induced by ACE inhibition is primarily caused by interference with the renin-angiotensin system and that losartan represents a valuable new drug in the treatment of hypertension and proteinuria in patients with T1DM and nephropathy.

Recently, an 8-week randomized double-blind placebo-controlled crossover trial was performed to test the hypothesis that dual blockade of the RAS with both an ACE inhibitor (benazepril) and an angiotensin receptor antagonist (valsartan) is superior to either drug alone in type 1 diabetic patients with DN [143]. Dual blockade induced an additional reduction in albuminuria (43%) and systolic blood pressure (6–7 mm Hg) compared to both monotherapies.

### Other Interventions

Other strategies have not been tested in adolescents with T1DM. Any new interventions that become available should be rigorously tested in this age group. The use of aldose reductase inhibitors has not proved effective in complications intervention [66].

As previously stated, especially in children and adolescents, the natural history of microalbuminuria is not necessary the progression to frank proteinuria and overt nephropathy. In fact, there is increasing evidence that microalbuminuria can be non-progressive or even transient [27]. Some longitudinal studies suggest that as many as 50% of subjects might revert to normoalbuminuria at the end of the pubertal year [4, 21, 144]. However, these longitudinal data are not sufficient to answer the question as to whether this observed regression will be permanent or whether microalbuminuria during puberty might represent the first sign of progressive nephropathy.

To investigate the reversibility of early renal abnormalities, a recent study was aimed to determine the frequency of a significant reduction in urinary AER and factors affecting such reduction in 386 patients with T1DM and microalbuminuria. Regression of microalbuminuria was frequent, with a six-year cumulative incidence of 58 percent. The use of ACE-inhibitors was not associated with the regression of microalbuminuria, whereas microalbuminuria of short duration, levels of HbA1c less than 8%, low systolic blood pressure (less than 115 mm Hg), and low levels of both cholesterol and triglycerides were independently associated with the regression of microalbuminuria (table 4) [145].

In conclusion, the decision to start a pharmacological treatment of microalbuminuria in adolescents should always be made individually [146]. Until now, a general consensus within the pediatric population on who should receive treatment with renoprotective drugs and when has not been achieved. This may be due mainly to the lack of enough longitudinal data on the natural history of microalbuminuria in children and adolescents with T1DM. On the basis of available information on the risk factors, it may be possible to establish some rules (fig. 2) in order to avoid unnecessary treatment or delay of potential beneficial therapy. It seems obvious that type 1 diabetic patients with persistent microalbuminuria and hypertension should receive treatment with

***Table 4.*** Clinical characteristics of patients with T1DM according to the presence or absence of regression of microalbuminuria during follow-up

| Characteristic | Regression (n = 196) | No regression (n = 190) | p value |
|---|---|---|---|
| Female sex, % | 55 | 47 | 0.16 |
| Age, years | 29 ± 8 | 31 ± 8 | 0.02 |
| Duration of diabetes, years | 17 ± 9 | 18 ± 9 | 0.41 |
| Albumin excretion rate, μg/min | | | |
| Initial | | | |
| Median | 59 | 57 | |
| Interquartile range | 41 – 122 | 37 – 110 | |
| At the end of the study | | | |
| Median | 17 | 87 | |
| Interquartile range | 11 – 34 | 38 – 262 | |
| Microalbuminuria of short duration (incidence cohort), % | 26 | 25 | 0.86 |
| Use of non-ACE inhibitor antihypertensive drugs | | | |
| Initial | 8 | 10 | 0.52 |
| At the end of the study | 15 | 16 | 0.68 |
| Use of ACE inhibitors, % | | | |
| Initial | 23 | 28 | 0.22 |
| At the end of the study | 41 | 53 | 0.02 |
| Systolic blood pressure, mm Hg | 121 ± 16 | 124 ± 14 | 0.07 |
| Diastolic blood pressure, mm Hg | 74 ± 9 | 76 ± 8 | 0.11 |
| Glycosylated hemoglobin, % | 8.8 ± 1.5 | 9.3 ± 1.6 | 0.001 |
| Total cholesterol, mg/dl | 193 ± 40 | 203 ± 40 | 0.01 |
| HDL cholesterol, mg/dl | 53 ± 13 | 53 ± 16 | 0.59 |
| Triglycerides, mg/dl | 109 ± 57 | 146 ±134 | <0.001 |
| Current smoking, % | 33 | 34 | 0.25 |
| Mean follow-up time, years | 4.3 ± 1.7 | 4.6 ± 1.5 | 0.12 |

Data are means ± SD or %.

antihypertensive drugs. Patients with persistent microalbuminuria and other signs of long-term complications, such as retinopathy, should be started with ACE-inhibitors or ATII receptor antagonists especially if raising GFR is detected or if the AER exceeds 50 μg/min. This cut-off point is justified by previous longitudinal studies where patients with an AER >70 μg/min at the start of the study developed persistent microalbuminuria or even an AER >200 μg/min [147]. However, the presence of retinopathy might be a robust

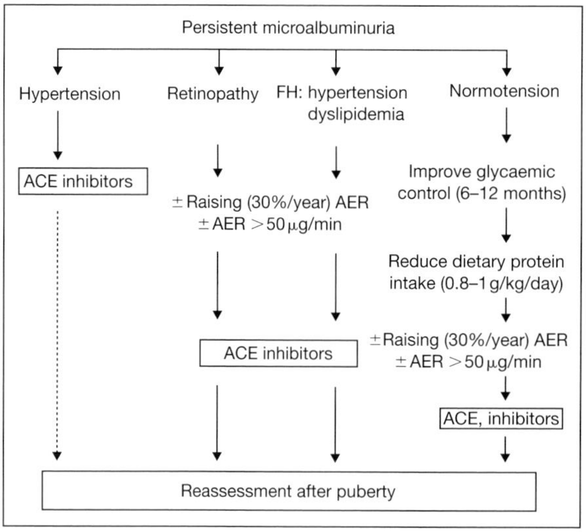


*Fig. 2.* Flow-chart of treatment intervention in diabetic patients with persistent microalbuminuria.

indication of treatment, especially if the independent effect of ACE inhibitors on retinopathy is confirmed in other studies.

Patients with microalbuminuria and family history of hypertension and/or family dyslipidemia constitute a special group, as both might be an inheritable trait, and both are well-known risk factors for progressive renal and cardiovascular damage: in these patients treatment with renoprotective drugs may be indicated, especially during puberty and in the case of worsening microalbuminuria.

In normotensive patients with persistent microalbuminuria, it might be reasonable to first try to optimize glycemic control, to reduce dietary protein intake and discourage smoking. In case of persistent microalbuminuria or rising AER despite these measurements, it can be worthwhile to start treatment in order to avoid further injury.

As previously stated, microalbuminuria might be transient and only strictly related to puberty. Therefore, treatment should be stopped in all those patients at the end of puberty that never presented hypertension and reverted microalbuminuria. During this period, repeated AER and blood pressure measurements will help to detect promptly the reappearance of raising AER.

In the few prepubertal children with persistent microalbuminuria as the only risk factor, it seems reasonable to wait until puberty to start treatment unless during a careful follow-up rising AER or blood pressure occur.

## Conclusion

Although children and adolescents with T1DM are faced with the treatment of the acute complications of hypoglycemia and ketoacidosis on a day-to-day basis, in the long-term, the microvascular complications of the disease with particular reference to nephropathy place them at greatest risk for serious morbidity and earlier than expected mortality. The families of children with diabetes should be provided with information about the complications of diabetes beginning at the time of diagnosis, and this information needs to be reinforced throughout the follow-up period. Appropriate surveillance for the earliest evidence of nephropathy should be performed following the recommendations of the ISPAD. Therapeutic interventions, particularly excellent metabolic control and timely blood pressure control may be exceedingly effective in preventing nephropathy onset or significantly retarding the rate of progression.

## References


1 Cook J, Daneman D: Microalbuminuria in adolescents with insulin-dependent diabetes: Prevalence and associated characteristics. Am J Dis Child 1990;144:234–237.

2 Danne T, Kordonouri O, Hovener G, Weber B: Diabetic angiopathy in children. Diabet Med 1997;14:1012–1025.

3 Donaghue KC, Fung AT, Hung S, Fairchild J, King J, Chan A, Howard NJ, Silink M: The effect of prepubertal diabetes duration on diabetes microvascular complications in early and late adolescence. Diabetes Care 1997;20:77–80.

4 Rudberg S, Dalhlquist G: Determinants of progression of microalbuminuria in adolescents with IDDM. Diabetes Care 1996;19:369–371.

5 Silverstein JH, Fenell R, Donelly W: Correlates of biopsy-studied nephropathy in young patients with insulin-dependent diabetes mellitus. J Pediatr 1985;106:196–201.

6 DCCT Research Group: The effect of intensive therapy on the development and progression of diabetic nephropathy in the Diabetes Control and Complications Trial. Kidney Int 1995;47: 1703–1720.

7 Mathiesen ER, Saurbrey N, Hommel E, Parving HH: Prevalence of microalbuminuria in children with type 1 (insulin-dependent) diabetes mellitus. Diabetologia 1986;29:640–643.

8 Lapuz MHS: Diabetic nephropathy. Med Clin North Am 1997;81:679–688.

9 Bojestig M, Arnqvist HJ, Hermansson G, Karlberg B, Ludvigsson J: Declining incidence of nephropathy in insulin-dependent diabetes mellitus. N Engl J Med 1994;330:15–18.

10 Hovind P, Tarnow L, Rossing K, Eising S, Larsen N, Binder C, Parving HH: Decreasing incidence of severe diabetic microangiopathy in type 1 diabetes. Diabetes Care 2003;26:1258–1264.

11 Wang SL, Head J, Stevens L, Fuller JH: Excess mortality and its relation to hypertension and proteinuria in diabetic patients: The WHO multinational study of vascular disease in diabetes. Diabetes Care 1996;19:305–312.

12 Casani A, Bangstad HJ, Chiarelli F: Detection and management of diabetic glomerulopathy in children and adolescents with insulin-dependent diabetes mellitus: Need for improved knowledge and better care. J Pediatr Endocrinol Metab 2000;13:467–474.

13 Moore THM, Shield JPH, on behalf of the Microalbuminuria in Diabetic Adolescents and Children (MIDAC) Research Group: Prevalence of abnormal urinary albumin excretion in adolescents and children with insulin dependent diabetes: The MIDAC study. Arch Dis Child 2000;83:239–243.

14 Dahlquist G, Rudberg S: The prevalence of microalbuminuria in diabetic children and adolescents and its relation to puberty. Acta Pediatr Scand 1987;76:795–800.
15 Joner G, Brinchman-Hansen O, Torres CG, Hanssen KF: A nationwide cross-sectional study of retinopathy and microalbuminuria in young Norwegian type 1 (insulin-dependent) diabetic patients. Diabetologia 1992;35:1049–1054.
16 Mortensen HB, Marinelli K, Norgaard K, et al: A nation-wide cross-sectional study of urinary albumin excretion rate, arterial blood pressure and blood glucose control in Danish children with type 1 diabetes mellitus. Danish Study Group of Diabetes in Childhood. Diab Med 1990;7: 887–897.
17 Tumini S: Prevalenza di ipertensione in bambini e adolescenti con T1DM normo e microalbuminurici. Abstract Book XIII SIEDP Congress, Firenze, 2001, p 4.
18 Norgaard K, Storm B, Graae M, Feldt-Rasmussen B: Elevated albumin excretion and retinal changes in children with type 1 diabetes are related to long-term poor blood glucose control. Diab Med 1989;6:325–328.
19 Barkai L, Vamosi I, Lukacs K: Enhanced progression of urinary albumin excretion in IDDM during puberty. Diabetes Care 1998;21:1019–1023.
20 Rudberg S, Ullman E, Dahlquist G: Relationship between early metabolic control and the development of microalbuminuria: A longitudinal study in children with type 1 (insulin-dependent) diabetes mellitus. Diabetologia 1993;36:1309–1314.
21 Schultz CJ, Konopelska-Bahu T, Dalton RN, et al: Microalbuminuria prevalence varies with age, sex, and puberty ion children with type 1 diabetes followed from diagnosis in a longitudinal study. Oxford Regional Prospective Study Group. Diabetes Care 1999;22:495–502.
22 Mathiesen ER, Ronn B, Strom B, Foght V, Deckert T: The natural course of microalbuminuria in insulin-dependent diabetes mellitus. A 10 year prospective study. Diabet Med 1995;12: 482–487.
23 Mogensen CE: How to protect the kidney in diabetic patients: With special reference to IDDM. Diabetes 1997;46(suppl 2):104–111.
24 Mogensen CE, Christensen CK: Predicting diabetic nephropathy in insulin-dependent patients. N Engl J Med 1984;311:89–93.
25 The Microalbuminuria Captopril Study Group: Captopril reduces risk of nephropathy in IDDM patients with microalbuminuria. Diabetologia 1996;39:587–593.
26 Caramori ML, Fioretto P, Mauer M: Low glomerular filtration rate in normoalbuminuric type 1 diabetic patients: An indicator of more advanced glomerular lesions. Diabetes 2003;52: 1036–1040.
27 Gorman D, Sochett E, Daneman D: The natural history of microalbuminuria in adolescents with type I diabetes. J Pediatr 1999;134:333–337.
28 Chiarelli F, Mohn A, Tumini S, Trotta D, Verrotti A: Screening for microvascular complications in children with diabetes. Horm Res 2002;57(suppl 1):113–116.
29 Mogensen CE, Hansen KW, Osterby R, Damsgaard EM: Blood pressure elevation versus abnormal albuminuria in the genesis and prediction of renal disease in diabetes. Diabetes Care 1992;15:1192–1204.
30 Chiarelli F, Casani A, Verrotti A, Morgese G, Pinelli L: Diabetic nephropathy in children and adolescents: A critical review with particular reference to angiotensin-converting enzyme inhibitors. Acta Paediatr 1998;425:42–45.
31 DeFronzo R: Diabetic nephropathy; in Porte D, Sherwin RS (eds): Diabetes mellitus. Stamford, Appleton & Lange, 1997, pp 971–1008.
32 UK Prospective Diabetes Study Group: Intensive blood glucose control with sulphonylureas or insulin compared with conventional treatment and risk of complications in patients with type 2 diabetes. Lancet 1998;352:837–853.
33 Trevisan R, Viberti GC: Pathophysiology of diabetic nephropathy; in LeRoith D, Taylor SI, Olefsky JM (eds): Diabetes mellitus. A Fundamental and Clinical Text. Philadelphia, Lippincott Williams & Wilkins, 2000, pp 898–910.
34 Singh R, Barden A, Mori T, Beilin L: Advanced glycation end-products: A review. Diabetologia 2001;44:129–146.

35 Chiarelli F, de Martino M, Mezzetti A, Catino M, Morgese G, Cuccurullo F, Verrotti A: Advanced glycation end-products in children and adolescents with diabetes: Relation to glycemic control and early microvascular complications. J Pediatr 1999;134:486–491.
36 Chiarelli F, Spagnoli A, Basciani F, Tumini S, Mezzetti A, Cipollone F, Cuccurullo F, Morgese G, Verrotti A: Vascular endothelial growth factor (VEGF) in children, adolescents and young adults with type 1 diabetes mellitus: Relation to glycaemic control and microvascular complications. Diab Med 2000;17:650–656.
37 Santilli F, Spagnoli A, Mohn A, Tumini S, Verrotti A, Cipollone F, Mezzetti A, Chiarelli F: Increased VEGF serum concentrations may help to identify patients with onset of type diabetes during childhood at risk for developing persistent microalbuminuria. J Clin Endocrinol Metab 2001;86:3871–3876.
38 Lorenzi M: Glucose toxicity in the vascular complications of diabetes: The cellular perspective. Diab Metab Rev 1992;8:85–103.
39 Koya D, King GL: Protein kinase C activation and the development of diabetic complications. Diabetes 1998;47:859–866.
40 Idris I, Gray S, Donnelly R: Protein kinase C activation: Isoenzyme-specific effects on metabolism and cardiovascular complications in diabetes. Diabetologia 2001;44:659–673.
41 Iori E, Marescotti MC, Vedovato M, Ceolotto G, Avogaro A, Tiengo A, Del Prato S, Trevisan R: In situ protein Kinase C activity is increased in cultured fibroblasts from type 1 diabetic patients with nephropathy. Diabetologia 2003;46:524–530.
42 Wilmer WA, Dixon CL, Hebert C: Chronic exposure of human mesangial cells to high glucose enviroments activates the p38 MAPK pathway. Kidney Int 2001;60:858–871.
43 Igarashi M, Wakasaki H, Takahara N, Ishii H, Jiang ZY, Yamauchi T, Kuboki K, Meier M, Rhodes CJ, King GL: Glucose or diabetes activates p38 mitogen-activated protein kinase via different pathways. J Clin Invest 1999;103:185–195.
44 Estacio RO, Schrier RW: Diabetic nephropathy: Pathogenesis, diagnosis, and prevention of progression. Adv Intern Med 2001;46:359–408.
45 Lee LK, Meyer TW, Pollock AS, Lovett DH: Endothelial cell injury initiates glomerular sclerosis in the rat remnant kidney. J Clin Invest 1995;96:953–964.
46 Gruden G, Thomas S, Burt D, Lane S, Chusney G, Sacks S, Viberti GC: Mechanical stretch induces vascular permeability factor in human mesangial cells: Mechanisms of signal transduction. Proc Natl Acad Sci USA 1997;94:12112–12116.
47 Lopes de Faria GB, Friedman R, Tariq T, Viberti GC: Prevalence of raised sodium-lithium countertransport activity in type 1 diabetic patients. Kidney Int 1992;41:877–882.
48 Chiarelli F, Catino M, Tumini S, de Martino M, Mezzetti A, Verrotti A, Vanelli M: Increased $Na^+/Li^+$ countertransport activity may help to identify type 1 diabetic adolescents and young adults at risk for developing persistent microalbuminuria. Diabetes Care 1999;22:1158–1164.
49 Lurbe A, Fioretto P, Barbosa J, Mauer M, LaPointe MS, Battle D: Growth phenotype of cultured skin fibroblasts from IDDM patients with and without nephropathy and overactivity of the Na/H antiporter. Kidney Int 1996;50:1684–1693.
50 Trevisan R, Fioretto P, Barbosa J, Mauer M: Insulin-dependent diabetic sibling pairs are concordant for sodium-hydrogen antiport activity. Kidney Int 1999;55:2383–2389.
51 Koren W, Koldanov R, Pronin VS, Postnov IY, Peleg E, Rosenthal T, Berezin M, Postnov YV: Enhanced erythrocyte Na/H exchange predicts diabetic nephropathy in patients with IDDM. Diabetologia 1998;41:201–205.
52 Chiarelli F, Santilli F, Mohn A: Role of growth factors in the development of diabetic complications. Horm Res 2000;53:53–67.
53 Flybjerg A: Putative pathophysiological role of growth factors and cytokines in experimental diabetic kidney disease. Diabetologia 2000;43:1205–1223.
54 Landau D, Chin E, Bondy C, Domene H, Roberts CT, Gronbaek H, Flybjerg A, Leroith D: Expression of insulin-like growth factor binding proteins in the rat kidney: Effects of long-term diabetes. Endocrinology 1995;136:1835–1842.
55 Ziyadeh FN, Sharma K: Role of transforming growth factor beta in diabetic glomerulosclerosis and renal hypertrophy. Kidney Int 1995;48(suppl 51):34–36.

93 Young LA, Kimball TR, Daniels SR, Standiford DA, Khoury PR, Eichelberger SM, Dolan LM: Nocturnal blood pressure in young patients with insulin-dependent diabetes mellitus: Correlation with cardiac function. J Pediatr 1998;133:46–50.
94 Sochett EB, Poon I, Balfe W, Daneman D: Ambulatory blood pressure monitoring in insulin-dependent diabetes mellitus adolescents with and without microalbuminuria. J Diab Compl 1998;12:18–23.
95 Verdecchia P, Schillaci G, Guerrieri M, Gatteschi C, Benemio G, Boldrini F, Porcellati C: Circadian blood pressure changes and left ventricular hypertrophy in essential hypertension. Circulation 1991;81:528–536.
96 Borch-Johnsen K, Norgaard K, Hommel E, Mathiesen ER, Jensen JS, Deckert T, Parving HH: Is diabetic nephropathy an inherited complication? Kidney Int 1992;41:719–722.
97 Quinn M, Angelico MC, Warram JH, Krolewski AS: Familial factors determine the development of diabetic nephropathy in patients with IDDM. Diabetologia 1996;39:940–945.
98 Earle K, Walker J, Hill C, Viberti GC: Familial clustering of cardiovascular disease in patients with insulin-dependent diabetes and nephropathy. N Engl J Med 1992;326:673–677.
99 De Cosmo S, Bacci S, Piras GP, Cignarelli M, Placentino G, Margaglione M, Colazzo D, Di Minno G, Giorgino R, Liuzzi A, Viberti GC: High prevalence of risk factors for cardiovascular disease in parents of IDDM patients with albuminuria. Diabetologia 1997;40:1191–1196.
100 Ford ES, Malarcher AM, Herman WH, Aubert RE: Diabetes mellitus and cigarette smoking. Findings of the 1989 National Health Interview Survey. Diabetes Care 1994;17:688–692.
101 Chaturvedi N, Stephenson JM, Fuller JH: The relationship between smoking and microvascular complications in the EURODIAB Complications Study. Diabetes Care 1995;18:785–792.
102 Gay EC, Cai Y, Gale SM, Baron A, Cruickshanks KJ, Kostraba JN, Hamman RF: Smokers with IDDM experience excess morbidity: The Colorado IDDM Registry. Diabetes Care 1992;15:947–952.
103 Sawicki PT, Didjurgeit U, Muhlhauser I, Bender R, Heinemann L, Berger M: Smoking is associated with progression of diabetic nephropathy. Diabetes Care 1994;17:1216–1231.
104 Scott LJ, Warram JH, Hanna LS, Laffel LM, Ryan L, Krolewski AS: A nonlinear effect of hyperglycemia and current cigarette smoking as major determinants of the onset of microalbuminuria in type 1 diabetes. Diabetes 2001;50:2842–2849.
105 Lawson M, Sochett EB, Chait PG, Balfe JW, Daneman D: Effect of puberty on markers of glomerular hypertrophy and hypertension in diabetes. Diabetes 1996;45:51–55.
106 Cummings EA, Sochett EB, Dekker M, Lawson ML, Daneman D: Contribution of growth hormone and IGF-I to early diabetic nephropathy in type 1 diabetes. Diabet Med 1997;14:766–771.
107 Kostraba JN, Dorman JS, Orchard TJ, Becker DJ, Ohki Y, Ellis D, Doft BH, Lobes LA, LaPorte RE, Drash AL: Contribution of diabetes duration before puberty to development of microvascular complications in IDDM subjects. Diabetes Care 1989;12:686–693.
108 Krolewski AS, Warram JH, Christlieb AR, Busick EJ, Kahn CR: The changing natural history of nephropathy in type 1 diabetes. Am J Med 1985;78:785–794.
109 Donaghue KC, Fairchild JM, Craig ME, Chan AK, Hing S, Cut Howard NJ, Silink M: Do all prepubertal years of diabetes duration contribute equally to diabetes complications? Diabetes Care 2003;26:1224–1229.
110 Mauer M, Drummond K, for the International Diabetic Nephropathy Study Group: The early natural history of nephropathy in type 1 diabetes. I. Study design and baseline characteristics of the study participants. Diabetes 2002;51:1572–1579.
111 Drummond K, Mauer M, for the International Diabetic Nephropathy Study Group: The early natural history of nephropathy in type 1 diabetes. II. Early renal structural changes in type 1 diabetes. Diabetes 2002;51:1580–1587.
112 Drummond KM, Kramer MS, Suissa S, Levy-Marchal C, Dell'Aniello S, Mauer M: Effects of duration and age at onset of type 1 diabetes on preclinical manifestations of nephropathy. Diabetes 2003;52:1818–1824.
113 Chiarelli F, Casani A, Tumini S, Kordonouri O, Danne T: Diabetic nephropathy in children and adolescents. Diab Nutr Metab 1999;12:144–152.
114 Shield JP, Hunt LP, Karachliou F, Karavanaki K, Baum JD: Is microalbuminuria progressive? Arch Dis Child 1995;73:512–514.

115 Sochett E, Daneman D: Microalbuminuria in children with insulin-dependent diabetes mellitus. J Pediatr 1988;112:744–748.
116 Krolewski AS, Warram JH: Natural history of nephropathy: How can it be changed? Diab Rev 1995;3:446–459.
117 Couper JJ, Clarke CF, Byrne GC, Jones TW, Donaghue KC, Nairn J, Boyce D, Russell M, Stephens M, Raymond J, Bates DJ, McCaul K: Progression of borderline increase in albuminuria in adolescents with insulin-dependent diabetes. Diab Med 1997;14:766–771.
118 American Diabetes Association: Clinical practice recommendations 2003. Diabetes Care 2003;26:S94–S98.
119 ISPAD Guidelines for the Management of Type 1 Diabetes mellitus in Children and Adolescents, 2000.
120 Schultz CJ, Neil HA, Dalton RN, Dunger DB: Risk of nephropathy can be detected before the onset of microalbuminuria during the early years after diagnosis of type 1 diabetes. Diabetes Care 2000;23:1811–1815.
121 Yuyun MF, Dinneen SF, Edwards OM, Wood E, Wareham NJ: Absolute level and rate of change of albuminuria over 1 year independently predict mortality and cardiovascular events in patients with diabetic nephropathy. Diabet Med 2003;20:277–282.
122 Mogensen CE, Keane WF, Bennett PH, Jerums G, Parving HH, Passa P, Steffes MW, Striker GE, Viberti GC: Prevention of diabetic renal disease with special reference to microalbuminuria. Lancet 1995;346:1080–1084.
123 Seaquest ER: Microvascular complications of diabetes: Strategies for managing retinopathy, nephropathy and neuropathy. Postgrad Med 1998;103:61–63.
124 Krolewski AS, Laffel LM, Krolewski M, Quinn M, Warram JH: Glycosylated hemoglobin and the risk of microalbuminuria in patients with insulin-dependent diabetes mellitus. N Engl J Med 1995;332:1251–1255.
125 Warram JH, Scott LJ, Hanna LS: Progression of microalbuminuria to proteinuria in type 1 diabetes: Nonlinear relationship with hyperglycemia. Diabetes 2000;49:94–100.
126 Skyler JS: Microvascular complications. Retinopathy and nephropathy. Endocrinol Metab Clin N Am 2001;30:833–856.
127 Parving HH: Diabetic nephropathy: Prevention and treatment. Kidney Int 2001;60:2041–2055.
128 Mortensen HB, Robertson KJ, Aanstoot H-J, Danne T, Holl RW, Hougaard P, Atchinson JA, Chiarelli F, et al: Insulin management and metabolic control in type 1 diabetes in childhood and adolescence in 18 countries. Diabet Med 1998;15:752–759.
129 Danne T, Mortensen HB, Hougaard P, Lyngaard H, Aanstoot H-J, Chiarelli F, et al: Persistent center differences over 3 years in glycemic control and hypoglycemia in a study of 3,805 children and adolescents with type 1 diabetes from the Hvidøre Study Group. Diabetes Care 2001;24:1342–1347.
130 Pedrini MT, Levey AS, Lau J, Chalmers TC, Wang PH: The effect of dietary protein restriction on the progression of diabetic and nondiabetic renal diseases: A meta-analysis. Ann Intern Med 1996;124:627–632.
131 Parving HH: Effects of dietary protein on renal disease. Ann Intern Med 1997;126:330–331.
132 Mogensen CE: Microalbuminuria predicts clinical proteinuria and early mortality in maturity-onset diabetes. N Engl J Med 1984;310:365–370.
133 Bohlen L, Schneider M, De Courten M: Comparative study of the effect of ACE inhibitors and other antihypertensive agents on proteinuria in diabetic patients; in Mogensen CE (ed): The Kidney and Hypertension in Diabetes mellitus, ed 3. Boston, Kluwer Academic Publishers, 1996, pp 361–374.
134 The EUCLID Study Group: Randomised placebo-controlled trial of lisinopril in normotensive patients with insulin-dependent diabetes and normoalbuminuria or microalbuminuria. Lancet 1997;349:1787–1792.
135 Cook J, Daneman D, Spino M: Angiotensin converting enzyme inhibitor therapy to decrease microalbuminuria in normotensive children with diabetes mellitus. J Pediatr 1990;117:39–45.
136 Hansen HP, Lund SS, Rossing P, Tarnow L, Nielsen FS, Jensen T, Parving HH: Preventing diabetic nephropathy: An audit. Scand J Clin Lab Invest 2001;61:471–477.

*Thermal threshold discrimination* can be tested with automated machines using the 'forced choice' principle, whereby the individual must fulfil an algorithm of correct responses at a given level in order to progress to the next (lower) level. Loss of heat detection can cause burns if the individual walks on hot surfaces without wearing shoes. Heat pain thresholds can also be measured.

### Studies of Clinical Neuropathy in Adults

The Rochester Diabetic Neuropathy Study studied a population-based sample in which the minimal criteria for polyneuropathy were two abnormalities from among neuropathic symptoms, nerve conduction, quantitative sensory examination (vibration or heat discrimination) or quantitative autonomic examination, with at least one being from nerve conduction or autonomic testing [59]. In the group aged 20–39 years, 42% had subclinical polyneuropathy and 2% mild symptomatic neuropathy. A further 6% of patients had motor involvement displayed by weakness of ankle dorsiflexion so that they could not walk on their heels.

The EURODIAB IDDM study examined prevalence of diabetic neuropathy in 3,250 randomly selected patients from 16 countries [8]. Neuropathy was defined as two of four abnormal measures on physical examination, symptoms, autonomic tests or vibration perception. In the age group 15–29 years, 19% had neuropathy and in the age group 30–44 years, 28% had neuropathy.

In the Pittsburgh Epidemiology of Diabetes Complications Study, poor vibration discrimination increased the risk fivefold for developing clinical neuropathy at two-year follow-up, but nerve conduction and thermal threshold abnormalities were not predictive [60]. Regression of abnormalities occurred in 16% for thermal threshold, 9% for vibration threshold and 9% for peroneal motor nerve conduction.

Even at a later stage of neurological involvement, 'confirmed clinical neuropathy', there can be resolution. In the Feasibility Phase of the DCCT, 39% had clinical neuropathy diagnosed by abnormalities of at least two of the following: physical symptoms, peripheral sensation, or decreased or absent reflexes [61]. The DCCT defined this category as abnormal physical examination and or history with abnormal neurophysiological tests. Only 43 of 84 with this diagnosis were still confirmed as such 5 years later: 54% in IT and 76% in CT. This lack of persistence was due to resolution of symptoms and neurological signs rather than improvement in nerve conduction or autonomic nerve testing.

Peripheral neuropathy predisposes to foot ulceration. Poor vibration discrimination has been found a predictor for foot ulceration 4 years later [62]; and for ulceration and amputation over a 12-year period in patients without a previous history of ulceration [63]. The sensitivity of vibration discrimination was 70% compared with 50% for clinical testing, with both modalities having a specificity of 72–79%.

However not all patients with neuropathy develop plantar ulceration. Other contributors are limited joint mobility, callus formation and high plantar pressure. High plantar pressure is a major determinant of ulceration [64]. High plantar pressure in patients with neuropathy is uncommon in the absence of limited joint mobility [65]. At CHW, we found that 35% of adolescents had reduced range of motion at the subtalar joint [66]. In a later study using pedar analysis of gait, 10% of adolescents were found to have elevated plantar pressure [67], which was associated with limited foot joint mobility, confirming the association reported in adults.

### Studies of Peripheral Nerve Function in Children and Adolescents

Even adolescents in very good metabolic control were found to have abnormal nerve conduction: 19% with a single abnormal parameter, 23% with 2 abnormal, 29 with 3–5 abnormal parameters (a total of 7 parameters were measured) [68]. The most common abnormality was motor nerve conduction, especially in the peroneal nerve. The diabetic group had lower motor (median and peroneal nerves) and sensory nerve conduction and lower sensory action potential (median and sural nerves) compared to healthy age-matched controls.

A recent study has linked abnormal nerve conduction (motor NCV H-reflex and sensory nerve action potential) to higher pubertal staging and worse metabolic control [69]. On neurophysiological criterion 10 of 138 had distal diabetic polyneuropathy, three of whom had signs or symptoms.

Other studies have utilized the quantitative sensory tests in children and adolescents (table 3). Some have found their diabetic adolescent group to have poorer vibration discrimination than controls [58, 70] but not universally [56, 71]. Abnormal biothesiometry in diabetic children has been found to have high specificity (75%) and sensitivity (82%) for nerve conduction abnormalities [58].

Heimans et al. [71] found diabetic children had significantly worse thermal discrimination than controls, and they had more thermal than vibratory discrimination abnormalities. Thermal abnormalities were also more frequent in a group of 60 diabetic men with subclinical neuropathy, (98% for cold discrimination and 58% for heat) than vibration abnormalities (33%) [72]. However others, using different techniques, have not found this to be so (44% vibratory vs. 35% thermal abnormalities) [73].

More recently, cold and warm thresholds were found significantly higher as a group in children and adolescents with diabetes (aged 8–16 years)

*Table 3.* Summary of recent studies of peripheral neuropathy and subclinical neuropathy

| Authors, year | n | Age years | Duration years | HbA1c % | % | Method abnormal |
|---|---|---|---|---|---|---|
| Heimans et al., 1987 [71] | 55 | 11.3 ± 3.9 | 5.1 ± 3.8 | | 2<br>15 | biothesiometry<br>thermal threshold |
| DCCT, 1988 [61] | 278 | 13–39 | 1–15 | 9.0 ± 2 | 39 | clinical neuropathy |
| Maser et al., 1989 [9] | 400 | 28.4 ± 7.8 | 19.9 ± 7.4 | 10.1* | 34 | clinical neuropathy |
| Donaghue et al., 1993 [56] | 181 | 15.0 ± 1.9 | 7.5 (5–10.3) | 8.2 (5.7–12.3) | 20<br>7 | biothesiometry<br>thermal threshold >95th PC |
| Dyck et al., 1993 [59] | 50 | 41 ± 15.4 | 14.5 (1.7–64) | | 54<br>15 | polyneuropathy<br>symptomatic |
| Olsen et al., 1994 [70] | 61 | 15.5 (10–21) | 6.9 (1–19) | | 20 | biothesiometry >95th PC |
| Hyllienmark et al., 1995 [68] | 75 | 15.4 ± 3.6 | 8.2 ± 3.5 | 7.0 ± 1.1 | 57 | nerve conduction >95th PC |
| EURODIAB, 1996 [8] | 1,348 | 15–29 | | | 19 | 'neuropathy' |
| Davis et al., 1997 [58] | 307 | 13.3 ± 4.6 | 5.1 ± 4.9 | 10.7 ± 3.5 | 9 | biothesiometry >97th PC |
| Riihimaa et al., 2001 [69] | 100 | 13.7 ± 2.0 | 7.0 ± 3.5 | 8.5 ± 1.7 | 10 | nerve conduction <1st >99th PC |
| Abad et al., 2002 [74] | 35 | 8–16 | 5.8 ± 3.2 | 8.7 ± 1.6 | 43 | thermal threshold |

*$HbA_1$: Normal range: 4.9–7.3%, range in parentheses.

compared to controls [74]. Heat-induced pain thresholds were not different from controls. However, 43% showed abnormality on one of 5 thresholds.

In our institution, after establishing normal ranges we found heat discrimination was more frequently abnormal than vibration in the foot (12 vs. 5%) [56]. However, our coefficient of variation was higher for heat discrimination in the foot compared with vibration (40–60 vs. 19–20%). When we subsequently followed a subgroup of our adolescents for up to 10 years, heat discrimination in the foot was the most consistently abnormal test which increased significantly over time [38] (GEE, $p = 0.005$, from 4% to 20%) (fig. 2). Vibration perception abnormalities did not increase.

More longitudinal studies are required in adolescents and young adults to determine the significance of abnormalities and the natural history of neuropathy.

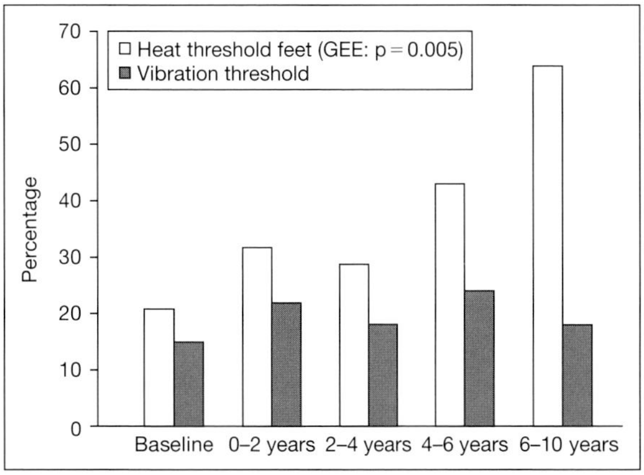


*Fig. 2.* Longitudinal study of peripheral nerve tests in 150 adolescents studied at The Children's Hospital at Westmead (1990–2001): comparison of percentage with abnormal heat threshold and abnormal vibration perception. ι = Heat threshold feet (GEE: p = 0.005); Ξ = vibration threshold.

## Acute Painful Neuropathy

Diabetic patients are at risk of acute and disabling pain at any stage of their diabetes [75]. It can occur in a stocking distribution, in the thighs (femoral neuropathy) or in the trunk as a radiculopathy. Correlation with physical examination and electrophysiological abnormalities may be poor. The pain is protracted and unremitting lasting on average 10 months till complete recovery, when return of lost tendon reflexes may occur. Exquisite contact discomfort is characteristic. It is unrelated to other complications of diabetes and can be precipitated by a period of improved glycemic control. It has been associated with eating disorders in young women [76].

Symptomatic improvement has been shown for tricyclic antidepressants, serotonin reuptake inhibitors, carbamazepine and topical capsaicin. Mexiletine, the oral analogue of lignocaine, has more recently been shown effective in reducing pain and dysesthesia, presumably due to its capacity to block sodium channels.

## Treatment of Neuropathy

Aldose reductase inhibitors have been successful in rodents as primary prevention of neuropathy. In type 2 diabetic patients with subclinical or mild peripheral neuropathy, three pupillary light reflex parameters improved, as did one CVS 'instantaneous' test and minimum latencies of F wave in median and tibial motor nerves during a 12 month trial of placebo-controlled trial of aldose reductase inhibitors [77].

## Conclusions

For the adolescent with diabetes in reasonable glycemic control, there appears to be a low rate of progression or persistence of abnormal nerve tests. Power spectral analysis of the 24-hour heart rate, 24-hour blood pressure and pupillary tests have promise for detecting autonomic neuropathy but have not yet been shown to have prognostic significance for the young person without renal disease. Nerve conduction is the most sensitive for detecting abnormalities of the peripheral nerves but only vibration discrimination has been shown to predict foot ulceration. Young adults with childhood onset of diabetes are at risk of disability due to diabetic neuropathy. Primary prevention of neuropathy during childhood is not yet a consideration.

## References


1 White NH, Waltman SR, Krupin T, Santiago JV: Reversal of neuropathic and gastrointestinal complications related to diabetes mellitus in adolescents with improved metabolic control. J Pediatr 1981;99:41–45.

2 Watkins PJ: Clinical observations and experiments in diabetic neuropathy. Diabetologia 1992; 35:2–11.

3 Ewing DJ, Campbell IW, Clarke BF: The natural history of diabetic autonomic neuropathy. Q J Med 1980;49:95–108.

4 Pirart J: Diabetes mellitus and its degenerative complications: A prospective study of 4,400 patients observed between 1947 and 1973. Diab Metabol 1977;3:173–182.

5 DCCT Research Group: The effect of intensive treatment of diabetes on the development and progression of long-term complications in insulin-dependent diabetes mellitus. N Engl J Med 1993;329:977–986.

6 DCCT Research Group: Effect of intensive diabetes treatment on the development and progression of long-term complications in adolescents with insulin-dependent diabetes mellitus: Diabetes Control and Complications Trial. J Pediatr 1994;125:177–188.

7 Dejgaard A: Pathophysiology and treatment of diabetic neuropathy. Diab Med 1998;15:97–112.

8 Tesfaye S, Stevens LK, Stephenson JM, Fuller JH, Plater M, Ionescu-Tirgoviste C, Nuber A, Pozza G, Ward JD: Prevalence of diabetic peripheral neuropathy and its relation to glycaemic control and potential risk factors: The EURODIAB IDDM Complications Study. Diabetologia 1996;39:1377–1384.

9 Maser RE, Steenkiste AR, Dorman JS, Nielsen VK, Bass EB, Manjoo Q, Drash AL, Becker DJ, Kuller LH, Greene DA: Epidemiological correlates of diabetic neuropathy. Report from Pittsburgh Epidemiology of Diabetes Complications Study. Diabetes 1989;38:1456–1461.

10 Rabinowe SL, Brown FM, Watts M, Smith AM: Complement-fixing antibodies to sympathetic and parasympathetic tissues in IDDM. Autonomic brake index and heart-rate variation. Diabetes Care 1990;13:1084–1088.

11 Hoeldtke RD, Bryner KD, Hobbs GR, Horvath GG, Riggs JE, Christie I, Ganser G, Marcovina SM, Lernmark A: Antibodies to glutamic acid decarboxylase and peripheral nerve function in type 1 diabetes. J Clin Endocrinol Metab 2000;85:3297–3308.
12 Hepburn DA, Patrick AW, Eadington DW, Ewing DJ, Frier BM: Unawareness of hypoglycaemia in insulin-treated diabetic patients: Prevalence and relationship to autonomic neuropathy. Diab Med 1990;7:711–717.
13 Ewing DJ, Campbell IW, Clarke BF: The natural history of diabetic autonomic neuropathy. Q J Med 1980;49:95–108.
14 Moss AJ, Schwartz PJ, Crampton RS, Locati E, Carleen E: The long QT syndrome: A prospective international study. Circulation 1985;71:17–21.
15 Smith SA, Dewhirst RR: A simple diagnostic test for pupillary abnormality in diabetic autonomic neuropathy. Diabet Med 1986;3:38–41.
16 Schwingshandl J, Simpson JM, Donaghue K, Bonney MA, Howard NJ, Silink M: Pupillary abnormalities in type I diabetes occurring during adolescence. Comparisons with cardiovascular reflexes. Diabetes Care 1993;16:630–633.
17 Rathmann W, Ziegler D, Jahnke M, Haastert B, Gries FA: Mortality in diabetic patients with cardiovascular autonomic neuropathy. Diab Med 1993;10:820–824.
18 Sampson MJ, Wilson S, Karagiannis P, Edmonds M, Watkins PJ: Progression of diabetic autonomic neuropathy over a decade in insulin-dependent diabetics. Q J Med 1990;75:635–646.
19 Orchard TJ, Lloyd CE, Maser RE, Kuller LH: Why does diabetic autonomic neuropathy predict IDDM mortality? An analysis from the Pittsburgh Epidemiology of Diabetes Complications Study. Diab Res Clin Prac 1996;S165–S171.
20 Maser RE, Pfeifer MA, Dorman JS, Kuller LH, Becker DJ, Orchard TJ: Diabetic autonomic neuropathy and cardiovascular risk. Pittsburgh Epidemiology of Diabetes Complications Study III. Arch Intern Med 1990;150:1218–1222.
21 Stella P, Ellis D, Maser RE, Orchard TJ: Cardiovascular autonomic neuropathy (expiration and inspiration ratio) in type 1 diabetes. Incidence and predictors. J Diab Compl 2000;14:1–6.
22 Ziegler D, Dannehl K, Muhlen H, Spuler M, Gries FA: Prevalence of cardiovascular autonomic dysfunction assessed by spectral analysis, vector analysis, and standard tests of heart rate variation and blood pressure responses at various stages of diabetic neuropathy. Diabet Med 1992;9:806–814.
23 Burger AJ, Charlamb M, Weinrauch LA, D'Elia JA: Short- and long-term reproducibility of heart rate variability in patients with long-standing type I diabetes mellitus. Am J Cardiol 1997;80: 1198–1202.
24 Burger AJ, D'Elia JA, Weinrauch LA, Lerman I, Gaur A: Marked abnormalities in heart rate variability are associated with progressive deterioration of renal function in type I diabetic patients with overt nephropathy. Int J Cardiol 2002;86:281–287.
25 Kleiger RE, Miller JP, Bigger JT Jr, Moss AJ: Decreased heart rate variability and its association with increased mortality after acute myocardial infarction. Am J Cardiol 1987;59:256–262.
26 Ewing DJ, Boland O, Neilson JM, Cho CG, Clarke BF: Autonomic neuropathy, QT interval lengthening, and unexpected deaths in male diabetic patients. Diabetologia 1991;34:182–185.
27 Veglio M, Sivieri R, Chinaglia A, Scaglione L, Cavallo-Perin P: QT interval prolongation and mortality in type 1 diabetic patients: A 5-year cohort prospective study. Neuropathy Study Group of the Italian Society of the Study of Diabetes, Piemonte Affiliate. Diabetes Care 2000;23: 1381–1383.
28 DCCT Research Group: Effect of intensive diabetes treatment on nerve conduction in the Diabetes Control and Complications Trial. Ann Neurol 1995;38:869–880.
29 DCCT Research Group: The effect of intensive diabetes therapy on the development and progression of neuropathy. The Diabetes Control and Complications Trial Research Group. Ann Intern Med 1995;122:561–568.
30 DCCT Research Group: The effect of intensive diabetes therapy on measures of autonomic nervous system function in the Diabetes Control and Complications Trial (DCCT). Diabetologia 1998;41:416–423.
31 Kennedy WR, Navarro X, Goetz FC, Sutherland DE, Najarian JS: Effects of pancreatic transplantation on diabetic neuropathy. N Engl J Med 1990;322:1031–1037.

32 Burger AJ, Weinrauch LA, D'Elia JA, Aronson D: Effect of glycemic control on heart rate variability in type I diabetic patients with cardiac autonomic neuropathy. Am J Cardiol 1999;84: 687–691.
33 Young RJ, Ewing DJ, Clarke BF: Nerve function and metabolic control in teenage diabetics. Diabetes 1983;32:142–147.
34 Young RJ, Macintyre CC, Martyn CN, Prescott RJ, Ewing DJ, Smith AF, Viberti G, Clarke BF: Progression of subclinical polyneuropathy in young patients with type 1 (insulin-dependent) diabetes: Associations with glycaemic control and microangiopathy (microvascular complications). Diabetologia 1986;29:156–161.
35 Solders G, Thalme B, Aguirre-Aquino M, Brandt L, Berg U, Persson A: Nerve conduction and autonomic nerve function in diabetic children. A 10-year follow-up study. Acta Paediatr 1997;86: 361–366.
36 Donaghue KC, Fung AT, Fairchild JM, Howard NJ, Silink M: Prospective assessment of autonomic and peripheral nerve function in adolescents with diabetes. Diabet Med 1996;13:65–71.
37 Donaghue KC: Autonomic neuropathy: Diagnosis and impact on health in adolescents with diabetes. Horm Res 1998;50(suppl 1):33–37.
38 Donaghue KC, Fairchild JM, Chan A, Silink M: Ten year results of diabetes complications screening: Superiority of pupillometry (abstract). J Pediatr Endocrinol Metabol 2001;14(suppl 3):1065.
39 Khan N, Couper JJ: Diurnal variation of blood pressure in adolescents with type 1 diabetes: Dippers and non-dippers. Diab Med 1996;13:531–535.
40 Lafferty AR, Werther GA, Clarke CF: Ambulatory blood pressure, microalbuminuria, and autonomic neuropathy in adolescents with type 1 diabetes. Diabetes Care 2000;23:533–538.
41 Poulsen PL, Hansen KW, Mogensen CE: Ambulatory blood pressure in the transition from normo- to microalbuminuria. A longitudinal study in IDDM patients. Diabetes 1994;43:1248–1253.
42 Wawryk AM, Bates DJ, Couper JJ: Power spectral analysis of heart rate variability in children and adolescents with IDDM. Diabetes Care 1997;20:1416–1421.
43 Tanaka H, Hyllienmark L, Thulesius O, Brismar T, Ludvigsson J, Ericson MO, Lindblad LE, Tamai H: Autonomic function in children with type 1 diabetes mellitus. Diab Med 1998;15: 402–411.
44 Massin MM, Derkenne B, Tallsund M, Rocour-Brumioul D, Ernould C, Lebrethon MC, Bourguignon JP: Cardiac autonomic dysfunction in diabetic children. Diabetes Care 1999;22: 1845–1850.
45 Suys BE, Huybrechts SJ, De Wolf D, Op DB, Matthys D, Van Overmeire B, Du Caju MV, Rooman RP: QTc interval prolongation and QTc dispersion in children and adolescents with type 1 diabetes. J Pediatr 2002;141:59–63.
46 Pittasch D, Lobmann R, Behrens-Baumann W, Lehnert H: Pupil signs of sympathetic autonomic neuropathy in patients with type 1 diabetes. Diabetes Care 2002;25:1545–1550.
47 Ziegler D, Mayer P, Muhlen H, Gries FA: The natural history of somatosensory and autonomic nerve dysfunction in relation to glycemic control during the first 5 years after diagnosis of type 1 (insulin-dependent) diabetes mellitus. Diabetologia 1991;34:822–829.
48 Clarke CF, Piesowicz AT, Spathis GS: Pupillary size in children and adolescents with type 1 diabetes. Diab Med 1989;6:780–783.
49 Karavanaki K, Davies AG, Hunt LP, Morgan MH, Baum JD: Pupil size in diabetes. Arch Dis Child 1994;71:511–515.
50 Karachaliou F, Karavanaki K, Greenwood R, Baum JD: Consistency of pupillary abnormality in children and adolescents with diabetes. Diabet Med 1997;14:849–853.
51 Pena MM, Donaghue KC, Fung AT, Bonney M, Schwingshandl J, Howard NJ, Silink M: The prospective assessment of autonomic nerve function by pupillometry in adolescents with type 1 diabetes mellitus. Diabet Med 1995;12:868–873.
52 Report and Recommendations of the San Antonio Conference on Diabetic Neuropathy: Consensus statement. Diabetes 1988;37:1000–1004.
53 Proceedings of a Consensus Development Conference on Standardized Measures in Diabetic Neuropathy: Summary and recommendations. Diabetes Care 1992;15:1104–1107.
54 Sindrup SH, Ejlertsen B, Gjessing H, Froland A, Sindrup EH: Peripheral nerve function during hyperglycemic clamping in healthy subjects. Acta Neurol Scand 1988;78:141–145.

55 Morley GK, Mooradian AD, Levine AS, Morley JE: Mechanism of pain in diabetic peripheral neuropathy. Effect of glucose on pain perception in humans. Am J Med 1984;77:79–82.
56 Donaghue KC, Bonney M, Simpson JM, Schwingshandl J, Fung AT, Howard NJ, Silink M: Autonomic and peripheral nerve function in adolescents with and without diabetes. Diab Med 1993;10:664–671.
57 Wiles PG, Pearce SM, Rice PJ, Mitchell JM: Vibration perception threshold: Influence of age, height, sex, and smoking, and calculation of accurate centile values. Diab Med 1991;8:157–161.
58 Davis EA, Jones TW, Walsh P, Byrne GC: The use of biothesiometry to detect neuropathy in children and adolescents with IDDM. Diabetes Care 1997;20:1448–1453.
59 Dyck PJ, Kratz KM, Karnes JL, Litchy WJ, Klein R, Pach JM, Wilson DM, O'Brien PC, Melton LJ 3rd, Service FJ: The prevalence by staged severity of various types of diabetic neuropathy, retinopathy, and nephropathy in a population-based cohort: The Rochester Diabetic Neuropathy Study. Neurology 1993;43:817–824.
60 Forrest KY, Maser RE, Pambianco G, Becker DJ, Orchard TJ: Hypertension as a risk factor for diabetic neuropathy: A prospective study. Diabetes 1997;46:665–670.
61 DCCT Research Group: Factors in development of diabetic neuropathy. Baseline analysis of neuropathy in feasibility phase of Diabetes Control and Complications Trial (DCCT). Diabetes 1988;37:476–481.
62 Coppini DV, Young PJ, Weng C, Macleod AF, Sonksen PH: Outcome on diabetic foot complications in relation to clinical examination and quantitative sensory testing: A case-control study. Diab Med 1998;15:765–771.
63 Young MJ, Breddy JL, Veves A, Boulton AJ: The prediction of diabetic neuropathic foot ulceration using vibration perception thresholds. A prospective study. Diabetes Care 1994;17:557–560.
64 Veves A, Murray HJ, Young MJ, Boulton AJ: The risk of foot ulceration in diabetic patients with high foot pressure: A prospective study. Diabetologia 1992;35:660–663.
65 Masson E: What causes high foot pressures in diabetes: How can they be relieved? Foot 1992;2:212–217.
66 Duffin AC, Donaghue KC, Potter M, McInnes A, Chan AK, King J, Howard NJ, Silink M: Limited joint mobility in the hands and feet of adolescents with type 1 diabetes mellitus. Diab Med 1999;16:125–130.
67 Duffin AC, Kidd R, Chan A, Donaghue K: Plantar pressure and callus in diabetic and nondiabetic adolescents and the efficacy of three pressure reducing interventions in diabetic adolescents. Am J Pediatr Med 2003;in press.
68 Hyllienmark L, Brismar T, Ludvigsson J: Subclinical nerve dysfunction in children and adolescents with IDDM. Diabetologia 1995;38:685–692.
69 Riihimaa PH, Suominen K, Tolonen U, Jantti V, Knip M, Tapanainen P: Peripheral nerve function is increasingly impaired during puberty in adolescents with type 1 diabetes. Diabetes Care 2001;24:1087–1092.
70 Olsen BS, Nir M, Kjaer I, Volund A, Mortensen HB: Elevated vibration perception threshold in young patients with type 1 diabetes in comparison to non-diabetic children and adolescents. Diab Med 1994;11:888–892.
71 Heimans JJ, Bertelsmann FW, de Beaufort CE, de Beaufort AJ, Faber YA, Bruining GJ: Quantitative sensory examination in diabetic children: Assessment of thermal discrimination. Diab Med 1987;4:251–253.
72 Hendriksen PH, Oey PL, Wieneke GH, Bravenboer B, van Huffelen AC: Subclinical diabetic polyneuropathy: Early detection of involvement of different nerve fibre types. J Neurol Neurosurg Psychiatry 1993;56:509–516.
73 Dyck PJ, Bushek W, Spring EM, Karnes JL, Litchy WJ, O'Brien PC, Service FJ: Vibratory and cooling detection thresholds compared with other tests in diagnosing and staging diabetic neuropathy. Diabetes Care 1987;10:432–440.
74 Abad F, Diaz-Gomez NM, Rodriguez I, Perez R, Delgado JA: Subclinical pain and thermal sensory dysfunction in children and adolescents with type 1 diabetes mellitus. Diab Med 2002;19:827–831.
75 Watkins PJ: Clinical observations and experiments in diabetic neuropathy. Diabetologia 1992; 35:2–11.

76 Steel JM, Young RJ, Lloyd GG, Clarke BF: Clinically apparent eating disorders in young diabetic women: Associations with painful neuropathy and other complications. Br Med J Clin Res Ed 1987;294:859–862.
77 Nakayama M, Nakamura J, Hamada Y, Chaya S, Mizubayashi R, Yasuda Y, Kamiya H, Koh N, Hotta N: Aldose reductase inhibition ameliorates pupillary light reflex and F-wave latency in patients with mild diabetic neuropathy. Diabetes Care 2001;24:1093–1098.
78 Barkai L, Madacsy L: Cardiovascular autonomic dysfunction in diabetes mellitus. Arch Dis Child 1995;73:515–518.
79 Holder M, Holl RW, Bartz J, Hecker W, Heinze E, Leichter HE, Teller W: Influence of long-term glycemic control on the development of cardiac autonomic neuropathy in pediatric patients with type I diabetes. Diabetes Care 1997;20:1042–1043.

Assoc. Prof. Kim C. Donaghue
Institute of Endocrinology and Diabetes
The Children's Hospital at Westmead
Locked Bag 4001, Sydney, NSW 2145 (Australia)
Tel. +61 2 9845 3167, Fax +61 9845 3170, E-Mail KimD@chw.edu.au

Chiarelli F, Dahl-Jørgensen K, Kiess W (eds): Diabetes in Childhood and Adolescence.
Pediatr Adolesc Med. Basel, Karger, 2005, vol 10, pp 279–298

# Macrovascular Disease

*K. Dahl-Jørgensen, J.R. Larsen*

Diabetes Research Centre, Pediatric Department,
Ullevål University Hospital, Oslo, Norway

## Epidemiology

Several studies have shown that mortality and morbidity is increased 2- to 4-fold compared to nondiabetics in type 1 diabetes [1, 2]. A Finnish study showed a 3.8-fold increased mortality in men and 4.5 in women who did not have diabetic nephropathy. This increased to 58-fold in men and 126-fold in women who had diabetic nephropathy. [3]. The British Diabetic Association Cohort Study reported a standardized mortality ratio of 2.7 in men and 4.0 in women [4]. For comparison, a standardized mortality ratio of 3.3 was reported in familial hypercholesterolemia [5]. Also in that disease the relative risk is increased especially in young patients.

In 16 European countries, the prevalence of cardiovascular disease in cross-sectional studies varied from 3 to 19% [6, 7]. Similar rates were reported in the USA [2, 8]. The Diabetes UK Cohort of 23,000 insulin-treated patients diagnosed before 30 years of age between 1972 and 1993 has been followed until 2000 [9]. 34 men and 34 females died of ischemic heart disease before the age of 40 years. The comparable number in the general population was 10 males and 2 females. The death rate in males per 100,000 person-years compared to the general population was 12 vs. 1 between 20 and 29 years and 69 vs. 9 between 30 and 39 years, and in females 14 vs. 0 and 84 vs. 2, respectively. Thus, the risk of mortality from ischemic heart disease is exceptionally high in young women with type 1 diabetes, with rates similar to those in men with diabetes. They have lost the cardioprotection enjoyed by young women without diabetes. This agrees with the similar incidence of new coronary events before 40 years of age in men and women with type 1 diabetes in Pittsburgh, Pa., USA [10].

Also, the prognosis of myocardial infarction is clearly impaired in diabetics; however, most studies do not distinguish between type 1 and type 2 diabetes [11].

### Atherosclerosis Starts in Childhood and Adolescence

The epidemiological studies are based on evidence of clinical disease with specific symptoms. The symptoms of coronary vascular disease is seldom before the age of 40 years in nondiabetic individuals, but necropsy studies have demonstrated that atherosclerotic changes in the vessel wall begin early in life [12–14].

The Pathobiological Determinants of Atherosclerosis in Youth Research Group (PDAY) has reported the prevalence and extent of atherosclerosis from autopsies of 2,876 adolescents and young adults who died of external causes from 1987 to 1994 [15]. The first intimal lesions (fatty streaks) appeared in all the aortas and in half of the right coronary arteries of the youngest age group (15–19 years) and increased in prevalence and extent with age through the oldest age group (30–34 years). Fibrous plaques evolving more than 5% of the vessel surface area were found in 13% of the aortas and 23% of the right coronaries in the youngest age group. They concluded that primary prevention of atherosclerosis must begin in childhood and adolescence. The PDAY investigators have shown that very-low-density lipoproteins (VLDL) and low-density lipoprotein (LDL) cholesterol concentrations were positively and high-density lipoprotein (HDL) cholesterol were negatively associated with both fatty streaks and raised intimal lesions [16, 17]. Smoking was associated with both fatty streaks and raised lesions [16]. Elevated glycohemoglobin values were associated with a substantial excess of fatty streaks and raised lesions in the right coronary artery and a lesser excess of raised lesions in the aorta [18]. Associations with hypertension and body mass index were also described [19]. Thus, not only does atherosclerosis begin in childhood, the risk factors for adult coronary heart disease and the other clinical syndromes resulting from atherosclerosis determine to a large degree its rate of progression.

Such necropsy studies have some limitations, particularly the presence of non-physiological conditions (arteries are not distended by blood pressure) and fixation artifacts, which may overestimate lesions. New development of very small high-frequency transducers has made it possible to perform direct intravascular ultrasound imaging (IVUS) of the vessel wall in living humans. Due to ethical reasons it is not possible to collect normal reference values by cardiac catheterization of young healthy subjects. However, healthy hearts that have been used for heart transplantations have to be examined for vessel function some weeks after the transplantation. In a recent IVUS study of 262 heart transplant recipients, the prevalence of atherosclerosis was 17% in hearts from individuals below 20 years of age [20].

Long-term prospective studies of more than 20 years' follow-up have demonstrated the association of traditional cardiovascular risk factors in healthy children and carotid vascular changes in adulthood [21, 22]. This calls for intensive efforts at coronary disease prevention at an early age, also in nondiabetics.

## Pathophysiology of Atherosclerosis

The fatty streaks are local accumulation of foam cells, i.e. macrophages loaded with lipids. The causal relationship between blood cholesterol and atherosclerosis is no longer in doubt [22, 24], but inflammation in the vessel wall is of major importance [25, 26]. The sequence of events leading to the formation of fatty streaks seems to be [27, 28]: (1) Circulating monocytes attach to endothelial cells by cell adhesion molecules that are induced in response to inflammatory signals. Plasma and endothelial-derived selectin mediate low-affinity binding, and integrins (VCAM-1 and ICAM-1) mediate firm attachment of the monocytes. (2) The monocytes migrate through the endothelial layer into the intima, where they differentiate further into macrophages in response to locally produced factors such as monocyte colony-stimulating factor (M-CSF). This differentiation includes upregulation of scavenger receptor A, CD36 and other receptors for oxidized LDL. (3) Serum LDL penetrates through the artery wall where it can adhere to matrix proteoglycans. These interactions are thought to trap the LDL particles and increase their susceptibility to oxidation. Enzymes contributing to LDL oxidation include lipoxygenases, myeloperoxidase and nitric oxide synthetase (iNOS) and NADPH oxidases. VLDL particles are subject to modification by lipoprotein lipase. The resulting remnant particles are also subject to trapping by proteoglycans, oxidative modification and uptake by the macrophages. The digested lipids are due to modifications, but decreased cholesterol efflux results in lipid accumulation and formation of foam cells. (4) Stimulated by inflammation and several growth factors, smooth muscle cells migrate into the area from underlying cell layers. (5) Platelets adhere to the endothelial cells. Specific adhesive substrates (as von Willebrand factor and P-selectin) exposed on the abnormal endothelial cell promote the adhesion of platelets. Adherent platelets facilitate further adhesion of leukocytes. They also release mitogenic factors such as platelet-derived growth factor (PDGF) that stimulates plaque growth. Thus, platelets may also be important in the early phase of atherogenesis, although it is of major importance later in the process by thrombus formation. (6) By further accumulation of foam cells, smooth muscle cells, leukocyte infiltration and collagen formation, the plaques increase in size. (7) By further growth, the plaque core becomes necrotic due to cell apoptosis and necrosis, increased lipolytic activity and lipid accumulation. (8) A fibrous cap, still with an endothelium cell layer, covers the plaque. (9) The fibrous cap may rupture, and expose the plaque core to the coagulation system, forming a thrombus. Plaques at risk for future thrombotic events are characterized by a large lipid core of more than 50% of the plaque volume, a thin fibrous cap, a low density of smooth muscle cells and high density of macrophages that produce metalloproteinases which destruct connective tissue and collagen [29]. (10) Many plaques disrupt without producing a thrombus that totally occludes the vessel. Fibrinolysis, either spontaneous or due to treatment, may effectively prevent that. Series of angiographies or intravascular ultrasound in the same patients have shown that this is a rather dynamic process and that remodeling of vessels occurs. However, a large acute thrombus may be catastrophic.

### Influence of Diabetes on Atherosclerosis

The most important metabolic abnormality in type 1 diabetes is hyperglycemia, but also dyslipidemia and a variable degree of insulin resistance is present, although to a lesser degree than in type 2 diabetes. King et al. [30, 31] have proposed theoretical mechanisms by which hyperglycemia and insulin resistance could cause cardiovascular diseases in diabetes. They propose that hyperglycemia, directly and via oxidants and glycated proteins, activates intracellular signal transduction systems, such as diacylglycerol (DAG) and protein kinase C levels (PKC). The activation of the PKC pathway can in vascular cells regulate permeability, contractility, extracellular matrix, cell growth, angiogenesis, cytokine actions, and leukocyte adhesions, all of which are abnormal in diabetes.

Formation of advanced glycation end-products (AGEs) may be one of the mechanisms by which hyperglycemia may induce cardiovascular disease [30]. AGE, as well as AGE receptors, has been demonstrated in atherosclerotic plaques and myocardium in patients with diabetes [33, 34]. The cross-linking abilities of AGEs may contribute to the increased stiffening of collagen and possibly to vascular hypertrophy [35, 36]. AGEs are also, through interaction with receptors, able to increase the level of nuclear factor (NF)-κB, a transcription factor suggested to be involved in the development of atherosclerosis and in apoptosis [35]. AGEs can quench nitric oxide (NO) and may impair endothelial function [38, 39]. Modifications of LDL as a result of glycation (glucoxidation) may contribute to foam cell formation [40]. Serum levels of AGEs are increased in type 2 diabetes patients with coronary heart disease [41]. Increased levels of serum AGEs has also been demonstrated in children with type 1 diabetes [42, 43].

Diabetes alters function of many different cell types, including endothelial cells, smooth muscle cells, blood cells and platelets. The single layer of endothelial cells lines the inner surface of all blood vessels, providing a metabolically active interface between blood and tissue that modulates nutrient delivery, blood flow, leukocyte migration, coagulation and fibrinolysis [44]. It synthesizes important bioactive substances, including NO and other reactive oxygen species, prostaglandins, endothelin and angiotensin II, which regulate blood vessel function and structure. NO is most importantly a potent vasodilator, but also inhibits platelet activation, limits inflammation by reducing leukocyte adhesion to the endothelium and migration into the vessel wall, and diminishes vascular smooth muscle cell proliferation and migration [45, 46]. Diabetes impairs NO-mediated endothelium-dependent vasodilation before the formation of atheromas [47]. A number of mechanisms, including hyperglycemia, contribute to the decreased bioavailability of endothelium-derived NO in diabetes, which at the same time increases the formation of reactive oxygen species (increased oxidative stress) [48]. Diabetes not only impairs vasodilation capacity, but increases the production of vasoconstrictors as endothelin-1 and angiotensin II [49]. The vasoconstriction may lead to hypertension and vascular smooth muscle cell growth.

Migration of monocytes and T lymphocytes into the intima is an important step in atherogenesis. T cells secrete cytokines that modulate lesion formation [50]. When monocytes reach the subendothelial space, they ingest oxidized LDL via specific scavenger receptors and become ‘foam cells’. Accumulation of foam cells leads to fatty streaks. Diabetes augments these processes. Hyperglycemia via decreased NO, increased oxidative stress and activation of receptor for advanced glycation end-products (RAGE) increases the activation of transcription factors (NF-κB and activator protein 1). These transcription factors regulate the expression of genes encoding a number of mediators of atherogenesis, for example leukocyte adhesion molecules on the endothelial cell surface, leukocyte-attracting chemokines, such as monocyte chemoatractant proteins that recruit lymphocytes into the vascular wall, and proinflammatory mediators including interleukin 1 and tumor necrosis factor. All these factors are important for the initiation of atheromatosis [51, 52].

Diabetes is important later in the process as well. It promotes *plaque instability*. The diabetic endothelial cells produce cytokines that decrease the synthesis of collagen by vascular smooth muscle cells [53]. Diabetes also increases the production of metalloproteinases that destruct collagen [54]. Decreased production and increased destruction of collagen may lead to disruption of the fibrous cap of the plaque.

Platelet function is also impaired in diabetes. This may both exacerbate the progression of atherosclerosis and the consequences of plaque rupture. In the platelets as in the endothelial cells, elevated glucose levels lead to activation of proteinkinase C, decreased production of platelet derived NO, and increased formation of reactive oxygen species [55]. Platelets have disturbed calcium homeostasis in diabetes [56]. This may significantly contribute to abnormal activity, since intracellular Ca regulates platelets shape change, secretion, and aggregation. Diabetes both influences intrinsic platelet activation and decreases endogenous inhibitors of platelet activity. These mechanisms may in part explain the enhanced thrombotic potential in diabetics.

Following plaque rupture, the *extent of thrombus formation* is important for the prognosis. Increased blood viscosity and disturbed blood rheology in diabetes favors thrombosis. Increased levels of fibrinogen and increased levels of plasma coagulation factors such as factor VII are described [57, 58]. Decreased levels of endogenous anticoagulants such as antithrombin III and protein C have been found in diabetic patients [59, 60]. In diabetes, endothelial cells increase the production of tissue factor, the major procoagulant found in atherosclerotic plaques [61]. Increased levels of plasminogen activator inhibitor 1 (PAI-1) is also described [62]. Many of these abnormalities correlate to hyperglycemia [63], and are preventable. In total, increased coagulation and impaired fibrinolysis [62, 63] that favor formation and persistence of thrombi are demonstrated in diabetes.

## Early and More Severe Atherosclerosis in Type 1 Diabetes

In a recent study, we demonstrated a high prevalence of *silent coronary atheromatosis* in young patients [64]. The patients were mean 43 years of age and had type 1 diabetes for a mean of 30 years and no clinical symptoms or signs of coronary heart disease. 90% of the patients had diabetes from childhood and adolescence. By IVUS examination of the coronaries all patients had significant atheromatosis. In an age-matched control group of newly transplanted hearts the expected prevalence in nondiabetics would be 65% [20]. By coronary angiography 34% had more than 50% vessel stenosis, but only 15% had pathological exercise ECG. In the same patients, a significant increased intima-media thickness of the carotid arteries was demonstrated [65]. Intima-media thickness was similar to that in nondiabetic persons who where 20–30 years older.

Increased intima-media thickness has also been shown in diabetic children. In patients with mean age 11 years and mean diabetes duration of only 4 years, a significantly increased intima-media thickness of the carotids and aorta was demonstrated compared to age-matched healthy controls [66]. The thickness was similar to that in children with hypercholesterolemia, and was more prominent in aorta than in the carotids. They concluded that aortic intima-media thickness was the best noninvasive marker of preclinical atherosclerosis in children.

Several studies have documented the increased prevalence of *symptomatic* clinical cardiovascular disease in type 1 diabetes patients [67]. The more severe coronary atherosclerosis was demonstrated in an angiography study of young type 1 diabetic patients and age- and sex-matched nondiabetic controls [68]. The diabetic patients were more likely to have severe narrowings, to have them in all three major coronary arteries, and to have them in distal segments. Involvement of distal segments makes the patients less suitable for bypass surgery.

## Risk Factors

*Impaired Blood Glucose Control*

We have clearly demonstrated that long-term blood glucose control predicts coronary atherosclerosis [65]. Coronary artery plaque formation, as judged by IVUS, was significantly associated to mean HbA1c obtained prospectively during 18 years' follow-up, after adjustment for total cholesterol and age. Regression analysis showed that a 1% increase in mean HbA1c over 18 years implied a 6.4% rise in vessel area stenosis on IVUS. A 1-mmol increase in total cholesterol implied a 10% rise in mean area stenosis. For comparison, a 10-years increase in age implied a 16.2% rise in vessel area stenosis. The increase in intima-media thickness of the carotid artery was correlated to 18 years mean HbA1c in women, but not in men [66]. In another study, the development of atherosclerosis, as judged indirectly by endothelial function and carotid artery stiffness, has been related to HbA1c, and a positive effect of tight blood glucose control over 10 years has been shown [69].

In the Diabetes Control and Complication Trial, the number of macrovascular events was fewer in the intensively treated group, but the difference between the intensively and conventionally treated group was not statistically significant. However, the patients were rather young, and the follow-up period only 6 years [70]. In the EDIC Study, a 6-years nonrandomized follow-up of the DCCT, increased intima-media thickness of the carotid artery was reported in the diabetic patients compared to controls, and it was related to HbA1c levels obtained during the DCCT. The patients that had been intensively insulin treated 6 years earlier had less progression of intima-media thickness than the conventionally treated patients [71].

In a prospective study of 177 type 1 diabetic patients diagnosed after 30 years of age, the incidence of coronary events in a 7-year follow-up was significantly related to HbA1c at the time of inclusion in the study [67]. All these findings underline the relation between glycemia and atherosclerosis, and the potential of tighter blood glucose control in slowing down the development and progression of atherosclerosis.

Also, the survival of myocardial infarction is impaired in diabetic patients [72]. In the DIGAMI study intensive insulin treatment during the acute phase and the following years improved 1 and 3 years survival [73], indicating the importance of good blood glucose control also in the late stages of atherosclerosis.

*Family History*

A family history for early cardiovascular disease (usually before age 55 years) is considered a risk factor for atherosclerosis in the general population [74]. In the literature not much attention has been given to this parameter in diabetes. In prospective studies of childhood-onset type 1 diabetics, the most important factor for cardiovascular disease was a family history of type 2 diabetes [75, 76] and hypertension [76]. In diabetic children with type 1 diabetes, the insulin requirement was higher in patients who had a family history of type 2 diabetes [77], indicating inherited insulin resistance in these patients, which is considered an independent risk factor for cardiovascular disease.

In addition to the family history of type 2 diabetes, special attention to other CVD risk factors should be made in patients with (1) parents or grandparents with signs of CVD at ≤55 years of age; (2) parents with elevated total cholesterol above 240 mg/dl or treated for dyslipidemia; (3) parents or grandparents treated for hypertension [78].

*Hypertension and Increased Urinary Albumin Excretion*

In type 1 diabetes hypertension can be essential or related to diabetes kidney disease. Both are major risk factors for atherosclerosis, and may be difficult to differ in risk calculations in clinical trials. Risk for CVD increases significantly when hypertension coexists with diabetes [79]. Moreover, hypertension has a greater impact on CVD in diabetics compared with nondiabetics [80]. Diabetic patients have a higher incidence of coronary artery disease, congestive heart failure, left ventricular hypertrophy, stroke and peripheral vascular disease when hypertension is present. Moreover, hypertension accelerates the risk for nephropathy [81], retinopathy [82] and neuropathy [83].

Several factors are involved in the pathogenesis of hypertension in diabetes. Genetic factors are important. Patients with diabetes and hypertension are reported to have a high frequency of family history of hypertension [84, 85]. Alterations in the renin-angiotensin-aldosterone system may contribute to sodium retention and hypertension in diabetes [86].

However, the most important cause of hypertension is secondary to the progression of diabetes kidney disease, which is preventable by optimal blood glucose control [87, 88]. Microalbuminuria itself is a well-established marker of increased risk for CVD [89]. If microalbuminuria develops, even without hypertension, the progression of diabetes nephropathy is much retarded by optimal blood pressure treatment [90], and the first choice of drug is ACE inhibitors, followed by angiotensin-receptor blockers, eventually in combination. ACE inhibitors have been shown to reduce CVD (i.e. myocardial infarction, stroke, death), thus further supporting the use of these agents in patients with microalbuminuria [91].

But hypertension is important to treat even if microalbuminuria is not present. Control of blood pressure (less than 140/80 mm Hg in adults) is shown in randomized trials to be effective in decreasing cardiovascular morbidity and mortality in diabetes [92, 93]. Epidemiological analyses show that blood pressures >120/80 mm Hg are associated with increased cardiovascular event rates and mortality in persons with diabetes [94]. The American Diabetes Association recommends a target blood pressure goal of <130/80 mm Hg in adult patients if it can be achieved safely [95]. Some drug classes are recommended as first choice: ACE inhibitors, beta-blockers and diuretics. If ACE inhibitors are not well tolerated angiotensin-receptor blockers are recommended [95].

The issue may be more complex in diabetic children and adolescents. Yearly screening for microalbuminuria in children that got diabetes before puberty should start 5 years after onset of the disease or at age 11 years of age (whichever is earlier). In children with pubertal onset screening should start 2 years after onset of disease [96]. Blood pressure measurement should be performed by auscultation [97]. Automated devices by oscillometric methods are less reliable, and should be used only in newborns and young infants in whom auscultation is difficult [97]. BP should be measured at every visit (or at least annually), in a relaxed setting after at least 3–5 min rest, and in a seated position with the cubital fossa supported at heart level. A technique to establish an appropriate cuff size is to choose a cuff having a bladder width that is approximately 40% of the arm circumference midway between the olecranon and the acromion. This will usually be a cuff bladder that will cover 80–100%

of the circumference of the arm. Systolic blood pressure is determined by the onset of the 'tapping' Korotkoff sound (1st phase) and diastolic BP is determined by the disappearance of the sound (5th Korotkoff phase). Some controversy existed whether to use the 4th Korotkoff phase in children, but the 5th phase is now standard [97]. BP should be recorded at least twice on each occasion, and the average of each of the systolic and diastolic BP measurement should be used to estimate the BP level. This level should be compared with reference values by age, gender and height [97]. If blood pressure is above the 90th percentile, recheck on at least two other occasions separated by at least 1 week. Hypertension is defined as BP levels at or above the 95th percentile. Blood pressure in diabetic children should be kept below the 90th percentile for kidney protection [97, 98]. This level corresponds approximately to 130/80 mm Hg in adults.

ACE inhibitors are recommended for use in children with hypertension [97]. Persistent and progressive microalbuminuria has been found to be improved by the use of ACE inhibitors. Progression to overt nephropathy may be delayed but their place in protecting long-term renal function in young people has not yet been established. There is early evidence that, even without hypertension, ACE inhibitors should be considered when persistent microalbuminuria has been confirmed [96]. Considering the lifelong glycemic exposure in childhood-onset diabetes and the early development of atherosclerosis, it seems reasonable to have an aggressive attitude, if treatment can be performed safely. ACE inhibitors have been effective and safe in children in short-term studies [99, 100]. Care has to be taken to prevent pregnancy in adolescent female patients when using ACE inhibitors.

*Lipid Disturbances*

Well-controlled type 1 diabetes is not associated with gross blood lipid disturbances when examined by conventional fasting blood sampling and analysis. However, these patients have the same variety of lipid values as non-diabetics based on genetic and diet differences, putting many of these patients at increased risk for CVD. In the DCCT patients poor glycemic control was associated with a potentially more atherogenic lipoprotein profile as measured by nuclear magnetic resonance [101]. The increased glycosylation and oxidation of LDL cholesterol may increase binding to scavenger macrophage receptors in the endothelium, giving increased foam cell formation [25]. This may be important at only moderately increased HbA1c levels. Poorly controlled type 1 diabetes is associated with abnormalities in postprandial lipid metabolism [102].

There are several studies showing the importance of cholesterol for the initiation and progression of atheromatosis [27]. Statements of the American

Academy of Pediatrics and American Heart Association recommend that in healthy children the acceptable level of LDL-cholesterol levels is 110 mg/dl, borderline 110–129 mg/dl and high risk ≥130 mg/dl [103, 104]. By higher levels repeated screening are recommended and by levels higher than 130 mg/dl (3.3 mmol/l) dietary intervention is highly recommended. The diet should have saturated fatty acids <10% of total calories, total fat over several days no more than 30% of total calories and no less than 20% of total calories, and dietary cholesterol <300 mg per day. A 'step 2' diet is recommended if the above diet is unsuccessful. Then the saturated fat should be less then 7%, polyunsaturated fat less then 10% of total calories and dietary cholesterol <200 mg per day.

The American Diabetes Association's recommendations for children and adolescents with both type 1 and type 2 diabetes [105] are similar to the established pediatric guidelines [103, 104] with modifications in response to the higher cardiovascular risk status. The goals are LDL <100 mg/dl (2.6 mmol/l), HDL >35 mg/dl (1.0 mmol/l), and triglycerides <150 mg/dl (1.7 mmol/l). Medication should be considered in children above ten years of age with LDL ≥160 mg/dl. If a high cardiovascular risk factor was present this limit was lowered to 130 mg/dl (3.3 mmol/l).The goal for treatment should be LDL <100 mg/dl (2.6 mmol/l). Resins (bile acid sequestrants) or statins (HMG CoA reductase inhibitors) may be used, but resins are associated with low compliance. Short-term trials show that the use of of statins in children and adolescents seems effective and safe [106, 107].

Screening for fasting blood lipids should be made at diagnosis after glycemic control is achieved, and then if normal every 5 years in type 1 diabetes, every 2nd year in type 2 diabetes. Screening should begin at the latest at 12 years of age, earlier (>2 years of age) if a positive family history of CVD is present. Suggestions are made that screening with other lipoproteins may be more suitable. The ratio of apolipoprotein B/apolipoprotein A1 may be a better predictor of CVD, and practically fasting values are not necessary [108]. However, better standardization of the assays and better reference values are needed before the recommendations for screening can be changed from LDL cholesterol to apolipoprotein ratio, especially in children.

Statins are effective in the primary prevention of major cardiovascular events in diabetics. The Heart Protection Study (HPS) included 5,963 patients with diabetes, of whom 10% had type 1 diabetes [109]. In this 5-years randomized, double-blind, controlled trial there was a risk reduction of one quarter of first events of myocardial infarction, stroke and limb revascularization. The effect was similar for type 1 and type 2 diabetes, and also independent of glycemic control and cholesterol levels. Mean LDL cholesterol was 2.3 mmol/l in the simvastatin group and 3.3 mmol/l in the placebo group.

ADA recommends that adult type 1 diabetics exceeding the acceptable lipid levels should be aggressively treated to prevent cardiovascular events [110]. Whether all diabetic patients, independent of type of diabetes, age and cholesterol levels, based on the results of the HPS, should be treated with statins needs to be settled. Primary prevention in diabetic children and what age to start needs to be studied. In this review several arguments for early preventive measures have been given.

*Disturbances of Platelet Function, Coagulation and Fibrinolysis*

Increased coagulation and impaired fibrinolysis [*62, 63*] favor formation and persistence of thrombi in diabetes. Primary prevention of cardiovascular events by the use of aspirin is well studied in the general population. In a meta-analysis of 55,580 randomized participants (11,466 women) aspirin treatment was associated with a statistically significant 32% reduction in the risk of a first myocardial infarction and a 15% reduction in all important vascular events, but had no significant effects on nonfatal stroke or vascular death [111]. In a position statement of the American Diabetes Association [112] aspirin therapy is recommended for primary prevention in diabetic subjects with the following risk factors: a family history of CHD, smoking, hypertension, obesity, microalbuminuria, and dyslipidemia. Use of aspirin has not been studied in diabetic individuals under the age of 30 years, and should not be recommended for patients under the age of 21 years because of the increased risk of Reye's syndrome [112].

*Lack of Exercise*

Physical exercise may improve the prognosis of type 1 diabetes patients. Prevalence of complications and mortality were followed in a large prospective study over 7 years [113]. The occurrence of microvascular complications varied inversely with the activity level. Sedentary males were three times more likely to die than the active ones. A similar although not statistically significant relationship was seen in females. The inverse association between mortality and physical activity in men remained significant when allowance was made for other mortality risk factors, such as age, BMI, smoking and diabetic complications. The study was not randomized and did not exclude a possibility of natural selection. However, the data indicate that type 1 diabetes patients actively involved in physical exercise live longer and have a better prognosis than their sedentary counterparts. Like healthy subjects, type 1 diabetes patients show a fall in total cholesterol and a rise in HDL cholesterol during physical training [114], as well as increased insulin sensitivity. These metabolic changes, and perhaps the psychological benefits of regular exercise [115], may contribute to the improved prognosis.

*Obesity and Insulin Resistance*

Obesity is a risk factor for CVD in the general population. In the Bogalusa Cohort of nearly 10,000 children between 5 and 17 years of age, the presence of cardiovascular risk factors were compared in the obese children (weight >95th percentile) and the normal weight children (<85th percentile) with significantly higher risk ratios in the obese children [116]. In the EURODIAB IDDM Complication Study, a cross-sectional study of 3,250 type 1 diabetes patients, waist-to-hip ratio in men, and BMI in women was associated with increased prevalence of CVD [7]. Also, in the Pittsburgh Epidemiology of Diabetes Complications Study waist-hip ratio correlated to CVD both in men and women [10]. Thus, the prevention of obesity in children and adolescents with diabetes is important to prevent atherosclerosis.

Obesity may result from the treatment of type 1 diabetes. It is well known that intensive insulin treatment and improved blood glucose control may induce a weight gain as a result of reduced glycosuria and increased food intake. Thus, special care has to be taken to minimize this effect, usually by decreasing caloric intake, when multiple injection or insulin pump treatment is initiated.

*Smoking*

Smoking is one of the main independent risk factors for atherosclerosis. Type 1 diabetes and smoking interact to produce excess morbidity and mortality of CVD [117, 118]. The age-adjusted prevalence of smoking was similar amongst people with or without diabetes in large surveys in the US [119] and in UK [120]. This is a big problem in teenagers with diabetes, and it is difficult to handle [121, 122]. Many teenagers use smoking as a tool to prevent weight gain. Better strategies for prevention of smoking in children with diabetes must be developed, as well as more effective smoking cessation programs in adolescents.

## Conclusion

There is increasing evidence from epidemiological, autopsy and clinical studies that atherosclerosis starts in childhood, and it is advocated to start earlier prevention of heart disease in the general population [123]. There is strong evidence that the development of atherosclerosis starts even earlier and that the progression of cardiovascular disease is much more aggressive in type 1 diabetes. The atherosclerotic process is a 'circulus vitiosus' and early intervention would be most effective. The development and progression of atherosclerosis is associated with poor glycemic control. Treatment of type 1 diabetes in childhood and adolescence is complex and a substantial part of the patients still do not reach the recommended targets of blood glucose control. It is a major challenge to improve the management of childhood diabetes by individualized intensified insulin treatment, preserving the physical and psychological well-being of the patient and the family, and ensure compliance into adulthood. Better strategies to both improve mean blood glucose and reduce the frequency of severe hypoglycemia are needed. As the development of cardiovascular disease starts in childhood, pediatric diabetologists need to focus earlier on preventive measures. Physical activity and healthy diet should actively be encouraged, and smoking abandoned. Hypercholesterolemia and hypertension should be actively screened and treated. More information is needed to decide the optimal age to start such pharmaceutical interventions in children and adolescents with diabetes.

## References


1 Pyörälä K, Laakso M, Uusitupa M: Diabetes and atherosclerosis epidemiologic view. Diabetes Metab Rev 1987;3:463–524.

2 Krolewski AS, Kosinski EJ, Warram JH, Leland OS, Busick EJ, Asmal AC, Rand LI, Christlieb AR, Bradley RF, Kahn CR: Magnitude and determinants of coronary artery disease in juvenile-onset, insulin-dependent diabetes mellitus. Am J Cardiol 1987;59:750–755.

3 Lounamaa R: Mortality in Finnish patients with insulin-dependent diabetes mellitus; thesis, Social Insurance Institution, Helsinki, 1993.

4 Laing SP, Swerdlow AJ, Slater SD, et al: The British Diabetic Association Cohort Study. I. All-cause mortality in patients with insulin-treated diabetes mellitus. Diab Med 1999;16:459–465.

5 Sijbrands EJG, Westendorp RGJ, Defesche JC, de Meier PHEM, Smelt AHM, Kastelein JPJ: Mortality over two centuries in large pedigree with familial hypercholesterolaemia: Family tree mortality study. BMJ 2001;322:1019–1022.

6 Tuomiletho J, Borch-Johnsen K, Molarius A, Forsén T, Rastenyte D, Sarti C, Reunanen A: Incidence of cardiovascular disease in type 1 (insulin-dependent) diabetic subjects with and without diabetic nephropathy in Finland. Diabetologia 1998;41:784–790.

7 Koivisto VA, Stevens LK, Mattock M, Ebeling P, Muggeo M, Stephenson J, Idzior-Walus B: The EURODIAB IDDM Complications. Study Group. Cardiovascular disease and its risk factors in IDDM in Europe. Diabetes Care 1996;19:689–697.

8 Orchard TJ, Stevens LK, Forrest KY-Z, Fuller JH: Cardiovascular disease in insulin dependent diabetes mellitus: Similar rates but different risk factors in the US compared with Europe. Int J Epidemiol 1998;27:976–983.

9 Laing SP, Swerdlow AJ, Slater SD, et al: Mortality from heart disease in a cohort of 23,000 patients with insulin-treated diabetes. Diabetologia 2003;46:760–765.

10 Lloyd CE, Kuller LH, Ellis D, Becker DJ, Wing RR, Orchard TJ: Coronary artery disease in IDDM. Gender differences in risk factors but not risk. Arterioscler Thromb Vasc Biol 1996;16:720–726.

11 Boden WE: Management of patients with diabetes and coronary artery disease; in Sobel BE, Schneider DJ (eds): Medical Management of Diabetes and Heart Disease. New York, Marcel Dekker, 2002, pp 185–209.

12 Enos WF, Holmes RH, Beyer J: Coronary disease among United States soldiers killed in action in Korea: Preliminary report. JAMA 1953;152:1090–1093.
13 McNamara JJ, Molot MA, Stremple JF, et al: Coronary artery disease in combat casualties in Vietnam. JAMA 1971;216:1185–1187.
14 Berenson GS, Wattigney WA, Tracy RE, et al: Atherosclerosis of the aorta and coronary arteries and cardiovascular risk factors in persons aged 6 to 30 years and studied at necropsy (the Bogalusa Heart Study). Am J Cardiol 1992;70:851–858.
15 Strong JP, Malcom GT, McMahan CA, Tracy RE, Newman WP, Herderick EE, Cornhill JF: Prevalence and extent of atherosclerosis in adolescents and young adults. Implications for prevention from the Pathobiological Determinants of Atherosclerosis in Youth Study. JAMA 1999;281:727–735.
16 McGill HC Jr, McMahan CA, Malcom GT: Effects of serum lipoproteins and smoking on atherosclerosis in young men and women. Arterioscler Thromb Vasc Biol 1997;17:95–106.
17 McGill HC Jr, McMahan CA, Tracy RE, et al: Relation of a postmortem renal index of hypertension to atherosclerosis and coronary artery size in young men and women. Arterioscler Thromb Vasc Biol 1998;18:1108–1118.
18 McGill HC Jr, McMahan CA, Malcom GT, et al: Relation of glycohemoglobin and adiposity to atherosclerosis youth. Arterioscler Thromb Vasc Biol 1995;15:431–440.
19 McGill HC Jr, Strong JP, Tracy RE, et al: Relation of a postmortem renal index of hypertension to atherosclerosis in youth. Arterioscler Thromb Vasc Biol 1995;15:2222–2228.
20 Tuzcu EM, Kapadia SR, Tutar E, Ziada KM, Hobbs RE, McCarthy PM, Young JB, Nissen SE: high prevalence of coronary atherosclerosis in asymptomatic teenagers and young adults. Evidence from intravascular ultrasound. Circulation 2001;103:2705–2710.
21 Li S, Chen W, Srinivasan SR, Bond MG, Tang R, Urbina EM, Berenson GS: Childhood cardiovascular risk factors and carotid vascular changes in adulthood. The Bogalusa Heart Study. JAMA 2003;290:2271–2276.
22 Raitakari OT, Juonala M, Kähönen M, Taittonen L, Laitinen T, Mäki-Torkko N, Jävisalo MJ, Uhari M, Jokinen E, Rönnamaa T, Åkerblom HK, Viikari JSA: Cardiovascular risk factors in childhood and carotid artery intima-media thickness in adulthood. The Cardiovascular Risk in Young Finns Study. JAMA 2003;290:2277–2283.
23 Steinberg D: The cholesterol controversy is over. Why did it take so long? Circulation 1989;80: 1070–1078.
24 Ross R: The pathogenesis of atherosclerosis: A perspective for the 1990s. Nature 1993;362: 801–809.
25 Libby P, Ridker PM, Maseri A: Inflammation and atherosclerosis. Circulation 2002;105: 1135–1143.
26 Ross R: Atheroslcerosis – an inflammatory disease. N Engl J Med 1999;340:115–126.
27 Steinberg D: Atherogenesis in perspective: Hypercholesterolemia and inflammation as partners in crime. Nature Medicine 2002;8:1211–1217.
28 Li AC, Glass CK: The macrophage foam cell as a target for therapeutic intervention. Nat Med 2002;8:1235–1242.
29 Davies MJ: The pathophysiology of acute coronary syndromes. Heart 2000;83:361–366.
30 King G, Wakasaki H: Theoretical mechanisms by which hyperglycemia and insulin resistance could cause cardiovascular diseases in diabetes. Diabetes 1999;22 (suppl 3):C31–C36.
31 Sheetz MJ, King L: Molecular understanding of hyperglycemia's adverse effects for diabetic complications. JAMA 2002;288:2579–2588.
32 Brownlee M, Cerami A, Vlassara H: Advanced glycation end products in tissue and the biochemical basis of diabetic complications. N Engl J Med 1988;318:1315.
33 Cipollone F, Iezzi A, Fazia M, Zuccheli M, Pini B, Cuccurullo C, Cesare DD, Blasi GD, Muraro R, Bei R, Chiarelli F, Achmidt AM, Cuccurullo F, Mezzetti A: The Receptor RAGE as a progression factor amplifying arachidonate-dependent inflammatory and proteolytic response in human atherosclerotic plaques. Role of glycemic control. Circulation 2003;106:1321.
34 Nakamuru Y, Horii Y, Nishino T, Shiiki H, Sakaguchi Y, KagoshimaT, Dhoi K, Makita Z, Vlassara H, Buccala R: Immunohistochemical localization of advanced glycosylation endproducts in coronary atheroma and cardiac tissue in diabetes mellitus. Am J Pathol 1993;143:1649–1656.

35 Sims TJ, Rasmussen LM, Oxlund H, Bailey AJ: The role of glycation cross-links in diabetic vascular stiffening. Diabetologia 1996:39; 964–951.
36 Rumble JR, Cooper ME, Soulis T, Cox A, Youssef S, Jasik M, Jerums G, Gilbert RE: Vascular hypertrophy in experimental diabetes: Role of advanced glycation endproducts. J Clin Invest 1997;99:1016–1027.
37 Bierhaus A, Chevion S, Chevion M, Hoffmann M, Quehenberger P, Illmer T, Luther T, Berenstein E, Tritschler H, Müller M, Wahl P, Ziegler R, Nawroth PP: Advanced glycation endproduct-induced activation of NF-kappa-B is suppressed by a alfa-lipoic acid in cultured endothelial cells. Diabetes 1997;46:1481–1490.
38 Bucala R, Tracey KJ, Cerami A: Advanced glycosylation products quench nitric oxide and mediate defective endothelium-dependent vasodilatation in experimental diabetes. J Clin Invest 1991;87: 432–438.
39 Hogan M, Cerami A, Bucala R: Advanced glycosylation endproducts block the antiproliferative effects of nitric oxide. J Clin Invest 1992;90:1110–1115.
40 Bucala R, Makita Z, Vega G, Grundy S, Koschinsky T, Cerami A, Vlassara H: Modification of low density lipoprotein by advanced glycation endproducts contributes to the dyslipidemia of diabetes and renal insufficiency. Proc Natl Acad Sci USA 1994;91:9441–9445.
41 Kilhovd BK, Berg TJ, Birkeland KI, Thorsby P, Hanssen KF: Serum levels of advanced glycation end products are increased in patients with type-2 diabetes and coronary heart disease. Diabetes Care 1999;22:1543–1548.
42 Berg TJ, Torjesen PA, Dahl-Jørgensen K, Hanssen KF: Increased serum levels of advanced glycation endproducts (AGEs) in children and adolescents with IDDM. Diabetes Care 1997;20:1006–1008.
43 Chiarelli F, de Martino M, Mezzetti A, Catino M, Morgese G, Cuccurullo F, Verrotti A: Advanced glycation end products in children and adolescents with diabetes: Relation to glycemic control and early microvascular complications. J Pediatr 1999;134:486–491.
44 Cines DB, Pollak ES, Buck CA, et al: Endothelial cells in physiology and in the pathophysiology of vascular disorders. Blood 1998;91:3527–3561.
45 Verma S, Anderson TJ: The most commonly asked questions about endothelial function in cardiology. Cardiol Rev 2001;9:250–252.
46 Kubes P, Suzuki M, Granger DN: Nitric oxide: An endogenous modulator of leukocyte adhesion. Proc Natl Acad Sci USA 1991;88:4651–4655.
47 Johnstone MT, Creager SJ, Scales KM, et al: Impaired endothelium-dependent vasodilation in patients with insulin-dependent diabetes mellitus. Circulation 1993;88:2510–2516.
48 De Vries AS, Verbeuren TJ, Van de Voorde J, et al: Endothelial dysfunction in diabetes. Br J Pharmacol 2000;130:963–974.
49 Hopfner RL, Gopalakrishnan V: Endothelin: Emerging role in diabetic vascular complications. Diabetologia 1999;42:1383–1394.
50 Binder CJ, Chang M-K, Shaw PX, Miller YI, Hartvigsen K, Dewan A, Witztum JL: Innate and acquired immunity in atherogenesis. Nat Med 2002;8:1218–1226.
51 Schmidt AM, Stern D: Atherosclerosis and diabetes. Curr Atheroscler Rep 2000;2:430–436.
52 Rosen P, Nawroth PP, King G, et al: The role of oxidative stress in the onset and progression of diabetes and its complications. Diabetes Metab Res Rev 2001;17:189–212.
53 Hussain MJ, Peakman M, Gallati H, et al: Elevated serum levels of macrophage-derived cytokines precede and accompany the onset of IDDM. Diabetologia 1996;39:60–69.
54 Uemura S, Matsushita H, Li W, et al: Diabetes mellitus enhances vascular matrix metalloproteinase activity. Circ Res 2001;88:1291–1298.
55 Assert R, Scherk G, Bumbure A, et al: Regulation of protein kinase C by short term hyperglycaemia in human platelets in vivo and in vitro. Diabetologia 2001;44:188–195.
56 Li Y, Woo V, Bose R: Platelet hyperactivity and abnormal Ca(2+) homeostasis in diabetes mellitus. Am J Physiol 2001;280:H1480–H1489.
57 Schneider DJ, Sobel BE: The coagulation and fibrinolytic systems, diabetes and the heart; in Sobel BE, Schneider DJ (eds): Medical Management of Diabetes and Heart Disease. New York, Marcel Dekker, 2002, pp 105–115.
58 Ceriello A, Giugliano D, Quatraro A, et al: Blood glucose may condition factor VII levels in diabetic and normal subjects. Diabetologia 1988;31:889–891.

59 Ceriello A, Giugliano D, Quatraro A, et al: Evidence for a hyperglycaemia-dependent decrease of antithrombin III-thrombin complex formation in humans. Diabetologia 1990;33:163–167.
60 Ceriello A, Giacomello R, Stel G, et al: Hyperglycemia-induced thrombin formation in diabetes. Diabetes 1995;44:924–928.
61 Kario K, Matsuo T, Kobayashi H, et al: Activation of tissue factor-induced coagulation and endothelial cell dysfunction in non-insulin-dependent diabetic patients with microalbuminuria. Arterioscler Thromb Vasc Biol 1995;15:1114–1120.
62 Carr ME: Diabetes mellitus: A hyperocoagulable state. J Diab Compl 2001;15:44–54.
63 Nordt TK, Bode C: Impaired endogenous fibrinolysis in diabetes mellitus. Semin Thromb Hemost 2000;26:495–501.
64 Larsen J, Brekke M, Sandvik L, Arnesen H, Hanssen KF, Dahl-Jørgensen K: Silent coronary atheromatosis in type 1 diabetic patients and its relation to long-term glycemic control. Diabetes 2002;51:2637–2641.
65 Larsen J, Bergengen L, Sandvik L, Arnesen H, Hanssen KF, Dahl-Jorgensen K: Mean HbA1c during 18 years predicts common carotid artery intima-media thickness in women with diabetes type 1. Diabetes 2003;52(suppl 1):A160.
66 Järvisalo MJ, Jarrti L, Näntö-Salonen K, Irjala K, Rönnema T, Hartiala JJ, Celermajer DS, Raitakari OT: Increased aortic intima-media thickness. A marker of preclinical atherosclerosis in high-risk children. Circulation 2001;104:2943–2947.
67 Lehto S, Ronnemaa T, Pyorala K, Laakso M: Poor glycemic control predicts coronary heart disease events in patient with type 1 diabetes without nephropathy. Arterioscler Thromb Vasc Biol 1999;19:1014–1019.
68 Valsania P, Zarich SW, Kowalchuk GJ, Kosinski E, Warram JH, Krolewski AS: Severity of coronary artery disease in young patients with insulin-dependent diabetes mellitus. Am Heart J 1991;122:695–700.
69 Jensen-Urstad KJ, Reichard PG, Rosfors JS, Lindblad LE, Jensen-Urstad MT. Early atherosclerosis is retarded by improved long-term blood glucose control in patients with IDDM. Diabetes 1996;45:1253–1258.
70 The Diabetes Control and Complications Trial Research Group: Effect of intensive diabetes management on macrovascular events and risk factors in the Diabetes Control and Complications Trial. Am J Cardiol 1995;75:894–903.
71 The Diabetes Control and Complications Trial/Epidemiology of Diabetes Interventions and Complications Research Group: Intensive diabetes therapy and carotid intima-media thickness in type 1 diabetes mellitus. N Engl J Med 2003;348:2294–2303.
72 Miettinen H, Lehto S, Salomaa V, Mahonen M, Niemela M, Haffner E, Pyorala K, Tuomilehto J: Impact of diabetes on mortality after the first myocardial infarction. The FINMONICA Myocardial Infarction Register Study Group. Diabetes Care 1998;21:69–75.
73 Malmberg K, for the DIGAMI Study Group: Prospective randomized study of intensive insulin treatment on long-term survival after myocardial infarction in patients with diabetes mellitus. BMJ 1997;314:1512–1515.
74 Grundy SM, Balady GJ, Criqui MH, Fletcher G, Greenland P, Hiratzka LF, et al: Primary prevention of coronary heart disease: Guidance from Framingham. Circulation 1998;97:1876–87.
75 Erbey JR, Kuller LH, Becker DJ, Orchard DJ: The association between a family history of type-2 diabetes and coronary artery disease in a type-1 diabetes population. Diabetes Care 1998;21: 610–614.
76 Mäkimattila S, Ylitalo K, Schlenzka A, Taskinen M-R, Summanen P, Syvänne M, Yki-Järvinen H: Family history of type-2 diabetes and hypertension predict intima-media thickness in patients with type-1 diabetes. Diabetologia 2002;45:711–718.
77 Dahl-Jørgensen K, Margeirsdòttir HD, Larsen JR, Lande K, Torsby P, Sandvik L: Heredity of type 2 diabetes is an important predictor for insulin requirement in children and adolescents with type 1 diabetes mellitus. Horm Res 2002;58(suppl 2):21.
78 American Academy of Pediatrics, Committee on Nutrition: Cholesterol in children. Pediatrics 1998;101:141–147.
79 Rossing P, Hougaard P, Borch-Johnsen K, Parving HH: Predictors of mortality in insulin dependent diabetes: 10-year observational follow up study. Br Med J 1996;313:779–784.

80 Stamler J, Vaccaro O, Neaton JD, Wenworth D: Diabetes, other risk factors, and 12-year cardiovascular mortality for men screened in the Multiple Risk Intervention Trial. Diabetes Care 1993;16:434–444.
81 Christensen CK, Mogensen CE: The course of incipient diabetic nephropathy: Studies of albumin excretion and blood pressure. Diab Med 1985;2:97–102.
82 Klein R, Klein BE, Moss SE, Davis MD, de Mets DL: Is blood pressure a predictor of the incidence or progression of diabetic retinopathy? Arch Intern Med 1989;149:2427–2432.
83 Maser RE, Steenkiste AR, Dorman JS, Nielsen VK, Bass EB, Manjoo Q, Drash AL, Becker DJ, Kuller LH, Green DA, et al: Epidemiological correlates of diabetic neuropathy. Report form Pittsburgh Epidemiology of Diabetes Complications Study. Diabetes 1989;38:1456–1461.
84 Barzilay J, Warram JH, Bak M, Laffel LMB, Canessa M, Krolewski AS: Predisposition to hypertension: Risk factor for nephropathy and hypertension in IDDM. Kidney Int 1992;41:723–730.
85 Krolewski AS, Canessa M, Warram JH, Laffel LM, Christliev AR, Knowler WC, Rand LI: Predisposition to hypertension and susceptibility to renal disease in insulin-dependent diabetes mellitus. N Engl J Med 1998;318:140–145.
86 Christlieb AR, Kaldany A, D'Elia JA: Plasma rennin activity and hypertension in diabetes mellitus. Diabetes 1976;25:969–974.
87 Dahl-Jørgensen K, Bjoro T, Kierulf P, Sandvik L, Bangstad HJ, Hanssen KF: Long-term glycemic control and kidney function in insulin-dependent diabetes mellitus. Kidney Int 1992;41:920–923.
88 The Diabetes Control and Complications Trial Research Group: The effect of intensive treatment of diabetes on the development and progression of long-term complications in insulin-dependent diabetes mellitus. N Engl J Med 1993;329:977–986.
89 Gall MA, Hougaard P, Borch-Johnsen K, Parving HH: Risk factors for development of incipient and overt diabetic nephropathy in patients with non-insulin dependent diabetes mellitus: Prospective, observational study. BMJ 1997;314:783–788.
90 Mogensen CE, Keane WF, Bennet PH, Jerums G, Parving HH, Passa P, Steffes MW, Striker GE, Viberti GC: Prevention of diabetic renal disease with special reference to microalbuminuria. Lancet 1995;346:1080–1084.
91 Heart Outcomes Prevention Evaluation (HOPE) Study Investigators: Effects of ramipril on cardiovascular and microvascular outcomes in people with diabetes mellitus: Results of the HOPE study and MICRO-HOPE study. Lancet 2000;355:253–259.
92 Joint National Committee on Prevention, Detection, Evaluation and Treatment of High Blood Pressure: The sixth report of the Joint National Committee on Prevention, Detection, Evaluation and Treatment of High Blood Pressure (JNC VI). Arch Intern Med 1997;157:2413–2446.
93 UK Prospective Diabetes Study Group: Tight blood pressure control and risk of macrovascular and microvascular complications in type 2 diabetes: UKPDS 38. BMJ 1998;317:703–713.
94 Hansson L, Zanchetti A, Carruthers SG, Dahlof B, Elmfeldt D, Julius S, Menard J, Rahn KH, Wedel H, Westerling S: Effects of intensive blood-pressure lowering and low-dose aspirin on patients with hypertension: Principal results of the Hypertension Optimal Treatment (HOT) randomized trial: HOT Study Group. Lancet 1998;351:1755–1762.
95 American Diabetes Association: Position Statement. Treatment of hypertension in adults with diabetes. Diabetes Care 2003;26(suppl 1):S80–S82.
96 ISPAD (International Society for Pediatric and Adolescent Diabetes) Consensus Guidelines for the Management of Children and Adolescents with Diabetes 2000. Internet access www.ispad.org.
97 National High Blood Pressure Education Program Working Group on Hypertension Control in Children and Adolescents: Update on the 1987 Task Force Report on high blood pressure in children and adolescents. Pediatrics 1996;98:649–658.
98 National High Blood Pressure Education Program Working Group report on hypertension in diabetes. Hypertension 1994;23:145–158.
99 Wells T, Frame V, Soffer B, Shaw W, Zhang Z, Herrera P, Shahinfar S: A double-blind, placebo-controlled, dose-response study of the effectiveness and safety of enalapril for children with hypertension. J Clin Pharmacol 2002;42:870–880.
100 Soffer B, Zhang Z, Miller K, Vogt BA, Shahinfar S: A double-blind, placebo-controlled, dose-response study of the effectiveness and safety of lisinopril for children with hypertension. Am J Hypertension 2003;16:795–800.

101 Jenkins AJ, Lyons TJ, Zheng D, Otvos JD, Lackland DT, McGee D, Garvey WT, Klein RL, The DCCT/EDIC Research Group: Serum lipoproteins in the Diabetes Control and Complications Trial/Epidemiology of Diabetes Intervention and Complication cohort. Diabetes Care 2003;26: 810–818.
102 Ginsberg HN: Hyperlipidemia, diabetes and the heart; in Sobel BE, Schneider DJ (eds): Medical Management of Diabetes and Heart Disease. New York, Marcel Dekker, 2002, pp 85–104.
103 American Academy of Pediatrics Committee of Nutrition: Cholesterol in childhood. Pediatrics 1998;101:141–147.
104 Williams C, Hayman L, Daniels S, Robinson T, Steinberger J, Paridon S: Cardiovascular health in childhood: A statement for health professionals from the Committee on Atherosclerosis, Hypertension and Obesity in the Young (AHOY) of the Council on Cardiovascular Disease in the Young: American Heart Association. Circulation 2002;106:143–160.
105 American Diabetes Association: Position statement: Treatment of hypertension in children and adolescents with diabetes. Diabetes Care 2003;26; 2194–2197.
106 De Jongh, Ose L, Szamosi T, Gagne C, Lambert L, Scott R, Perron P, Dobbelaere D, Saborio M, Tuohy MB,Stepanavage M, Sapre A, Gumbiner B, Mercuri M, van Trotsenburg AS, Bakker HD, Kastelein JJ: Simvastatin in Children Study Group: Efficacy and safety of statin therapy in children with familial hypercholesterolemia: A randomized, double-blind, placebo-controlled trial with simvastatin. Circulation 2002;106:2231–2237.
107 Stein EA, Illingworth DR, Kwiterovich PO Jr, Liacouras CA, Siimes MA, Jacobson MS, Brewster TG, Hopkins P, Davidson M, Graham K, Arensman F, Knopp RH, DuJovne C, Williams CL, Isaacsohn JL, Jacobsen CA, Laskarzewski PM, Ames S, Gormley GJ: Efficacy and safety of lovastatin in adolescent male with heterozygous familial hypercholesterolemia: A randomized controlled trial. JAMA 1999;281:137–144.
108 Walldius G, Jungner I, Holme I, Aastveit AH, Kolar W, Steiner E: High apolipoprotein B, low apolipoprotein A-1, and improvement in the prediction of fatal myocardial infarction (AMORIS study): A prospective study. Lancet 2001;358:2026–2033.
109 Heart protection Study Collaboratory Group: MRC/BHF Heart Protection Study of cholesterol-lowering with simvastatin in 5963 people with diabetes: A randomized placebo-controlled trial. Lancet 2003;361:2005–2016.
110 American Diabetes Association: Position statement: Management of dyslipidemia in adults with diabetes. Diabetes Care 2003;26(suppl 1):S83–S86.
111 Eidelman RS, Hebert PR, Weisman SM, Henneckens CH: An update on aspirin in the primary prevention of cardiovascular disease. Arch Intern Med 2003;163:2006–2010.
112 American Diabetes Association: Position statement. Aspirin therapy in diabetes. Diabetes Care 2003;26(suppl 1):S87–S88.
113 Moy CS, Songer TJ, LaPorte R, et al: Insulin-dependent diabetes mellitus, physical activity, and death. Am J Epidemiol 1993;137:74–81.
114 Wallberg-Henriksson H, Gunnarson R, Henriksson J, et al: Increased peripheral insulin sensitivity and muscle mitochondrial enzymes but unchanged blood glucose control in type-1 diabetics after physical training. Diabetes 1982;31:1044–1050.
115 Rowland T, Swadba LA, Biggs DE, Burke EJ, Reiter EO: Glycemic control with physical training in insulin-dependent diabetes mellitus. Sports Med 1985;139:307–310.
116 Freedman DS, William H, Dietz WH, Sathanur R, Srinivasan SR, Berenson GS: The relation of overweight to cardiovascular risk factors among children and adolescents: The Bogalusa Heart Study. Pediatrics 1999;103:1175–1182.
117 Gay EC, Cai Y, Gale SM, et al: Smokers with IDDM experience excess morbidity. The Colorado IDDM registry. Diabetes Care 1992;15:947–952.
118 Suarez L, Barret-Connor E: Interaction between cigarette smoking and a diabetes mellitus in the prediction of death attributed to cardiovascular disease. Am J Epidemiol 1984;120: 670–675.
119 Ford ES, Malarcher AM, Herman WH, Aubert RE: Diabetes mellitus and cigarette smoking. Findings from the 1989 National Health Interview Survey. Diabetes Care 1994;17:688–692.
120 Jones RB, Hedley AJ: Prevalence of smoking in a diabetic population: The need for action. Diabet Med 1987;4:233–236.

121 Masson EA, MacFarlane IA, Priestly CJ, Wallymahmed ME, Flavell HJ: Failure to prevent nicotine addiction in young people with diabetes. Arch Dis Child 1992;67:100–102.
122 Shaw NJ, McClure RJ, Kerr S, Lawton K, Smith CS: Smoking in diabetic teenagers. Diabetes Med 1993;10:255–257.
123 McGill HC, McMahan CA: Starting earlier to prevent heart disease. JAMA 2003;290:2320–2322.

Prof. Knut Dahl-Jørgensen
Diabetes Research Centre, Pediatric Department
Ullevål University Hospital, NO–0407 Oslo (Norway)
Tel. +47 23 01 5577, Fax +47 23 01 5580, E-Mail knut.dahl-jorgensen@medisin.uio.no

Chiarelli F, Dahl-Jørgensen K, Kiess W (eds): Diabetes in Childhood and Adolescence.
Pediatr Adolesc Med. Basel, Karger, 2005, vol 10, pp 299–313

# Hypoglycemia in Children and Adolescents with Type 1 Diabetes

*A. Blasetti, A. Verrotti, G. de Michele, F. Chiarelli*

Department of Pediatrics, Ospedale Policlinico, Chieti, Italy

## Definition and Epidemiology

Hypoglycemia is the most common acute complication of type 1 diabetes mellitus [1]. The severity of an episode of hypoglycemia is defined by the individual's ability to self-treat a low blood glucose level: in fact, mild episodes are generally self-treated whereas severe hypoglycemia is defined as requiring external help for recovery. Severity is not determined by the intensity or nature of the symptomatic response, the resulting conscious level of the individual during hypoglycemia or by the nature of the treatment required. Thus, a severe episode does not imply the development of coma or parenteral treatment and it can include a conscious individual who can be treated effectively with oral glucose, but who has developed neuroglycopenia of such a magnitude that self-treatment has been impossible.

The Diabetes Control and Complications Trial (DCCT) demonstrated that long-term improved metabolic control avoided the occurrence of diabetic microvascular complications or their progression, which has made intensive insulin treatment widespread in the last decade [2]. As lower HbA1c and glucose levels are targeted, increased hypoglycemia frequency and severity have become major problems particularly in pediatric and adolescent patients. The results of DCCT indicated a three times higher hypoglycemia incidence in adolescents when compared to adults [3]. A common finding in incidence studies is the fact that the lower the child's age is, the more frequent and severe are the episodes of hypoglycemia [4, 5].

A large number of papers have addressed the epidemiology of hypoglycemia in both children and adults with diabetes [6–8]. The prevalence of severe hypoglycemia in an unselected population of people with type 1 diabetes

*Table 1.* Principal risk factors for severe hypoglycemia in patients with type 1 diabetes mellitus

| |
|---|
| Strict glycemic control |
| Impaired awareness of hypoglycemia |
| History of previous severe hypoglycemia |
| Sleep |
| Duration of diabetes mellitus |
| Adolescence |
| C-peptide negativity |
| Low social class |
| Diabetic neuropathy |

From Frier [9], modified.

mellitus (T1DM) is consistently around 30% per annum; this means that approximately 1 of 3 patients with diabetes people experiences one or more episodes of severe hypoglycemia each year. This prevalence has been reported in several studies [9–11]. In a recent study, the prevalence of hypoglycemia in prepubertal children has been evaluated using the continuous glucose monitoring system: the authors have demonstrated a high frequency of nocturnal hypoglycemia (18%), mainly asymptomatic (91% of episodes).

Nocturnal hypoglycemia was associated with decreasing age, increased insulin dose, insulin regimen, and increased weight standard deviation score [12].

Moreover, in diabetic populations in Northen Europe the estimated incidence of severe hypoglycemia ranged from 1.1 to 1.7 episodes/patient/year [10, 11, 13, 14]. In a recent paper, the overall incidence of severe events was 4.8/100 patient-years and of moderate hypoglycemia was 13.1/100 patient-years [6]; in particular, significant hypoglycemia was rare in the first 12 months after the diagnosis and rates of hypoglycemia were increased in children younger than 6 years of age when compared to these older than 6 years. This and other epidemiological studies are very useful to detect the risk of hypoglycemia; a summary of the main risk factors for hypoglycemia in type 1 diabetic patients is reported in table 1.

It is relevant that in the DCCT study a low incidence of severe hypoglycemia was reported (strict control group 0.62; conventional control group 0.19 episodes per patient year [15, 16]. The participants in the DCCT were highly selected and excluded people who had experienced hypoglycemic coma without symptoms. This almost certainly excluded most people who had impaired hypoglycemia awareness. The DCCT studied young patients with short duration of T1DM, who had a relatively high level of motivation, above average intelligence and who had the benefit of extensive clinical resources to support their management. They are therefore not representative of the typical population of people with T1DM who attend the average diabetic clinic.

Restriction of the definition of severe hypoglycemia to coma requiring parental therapy with i.v. dextrose or i.m. glucagon reduced the prevalence to about 10% per annum with an incidence of 0.4 episodes/patient/year [17] and records about one third of the episodes of severe hypoglycemia that are determined using the wider definition of inability to self-treat. This may partly explain the much lower frequencies of severe hypoglycemia recorded in Düsseldorf and 9 other hospitals in Germany [18, 19] in which the definition of severe hypoglycemia used was the ‘assistance of another person and injection of glucose and glucagon [19] implying that coma or severe incapacity had developed to require this level of resuscitation.

The experience was reported of 697 patients with T1DM, aged 15–40 years with no diabetic complications, who participated in a structured 5-day inpatient training programme prior to intensification of insulin therapy. This was a prospective study performed over 6 years, during which the mean HbA1c declined from 8.3 to 7.6% (n = 636) and the incidence of severe hypoglycemia was reduced from 0.28 to 0.17 episodes/patient/year (n = 538), based on the above definition. It would appear that the patients’ education programme had provided a significant benefit in substantially reducing the overall frequency of severe hypoglycemia. However, if it is assumed that these rates represent approximately one third of episodes that are defined by inability to self-treat, the adjusted incidence of severe hypoglycemia would be approximately equivalent to that observed in the intensively treated group in the DCCT [15]. While the benefits of intensive patient education to avoid hypoglycemia are not disputed, the claim that this can almost eradicate severe hypoglycemia may be exaggerated by the use of a much stricter definition of what constitutes severe hypoglycemia, and may possibly be compounded by a degree of selection bias in the recruitment of patients for these studies [9].

## Physiopathology

It is clearly established that the counterregulatory response to hypoglycemia is based on glucagon and epinephrine secretion [19]. Other anti-insulin hormones, such as cortisol and growth hormone, do not play a role in defense against acute, insulin-induced hypoglycemia [20]. In healthy overnight fasted volunteers, the only sources for glucose release are liver and kidney (which accounts for 18–25% of all glucose release) [21, 22]. Hepatic and renal glucose release are inhibited by insulin [23] and are stimulated in the liver essentially by glucagon [24], while in the kidney mainly by catecholamines [25]. In animal studies acidosis stimulates renal glucose release and inhibits hepatic glucose release [26, 27]. The gluconeogenetic substrates utilized by liver and kidney are lactate, glycerol (in both), alanine (liver), and glutamine (kidney) [28, 29]. The primary structures involved in hypoglycemia detection and initiation of symptomatic and counterregulatory response are posed in the brain, ventromedial [30] and lateral [31–33] hypothalamus. There is growing evidence of the existence of neurones expressing the β-cell glucose transporter GLUT 2 [34] and the same glucose sensor seems to be expressed in the cells of the hepatic portal vein [35]. The lateral hypothalamus, in animal models, contains neurones that are stimulated by falling glucose and inhibited by rising glucose in the portal circulation [31–33]: it is possible to hypothesize that the portal signal may influence the hypothalamic function during hypoglycemia [36]. After activation of the aforementioned glucose sensor, the counterregulatory response began: (1) suppression of insulin secretion; (2) release of counterregulatory hormones, and (3) generation of autonomic symptoms [37].

In the response to insulin-induced hypoglycemia, glucagon plays the major counterregulatory role, the catecholamine response being not critical, but becoming important only when the secretion of glucagon is suppressed [20, 38].

The modality of glucagon response to hypoglycemia is still debated: effect of low glucose as direct stimulus on the α-cell [39], disinhibition of the α-cell, secondary to the suppression of endogenous insulin [40], or activation of autonomic nervous system which in turn stimulates the α-cell [41, 42]. As previously reported, the role of adrenergic mechanism in counterregulatory response to hypoglycemia is not critical when the glucagon response is intact: pharmacological blockade do not influence plasma glucose recovery from hypoglycemia [20, 43, 44]. In the prolonged, not acute, hypoglycemia model, the role of catecholamines becomes more important: when the catecholamines are blocked pharmacologically, plasma glucose decreases more than in control experiment despite larger response of glucagon [45]. Thus, in prolonged hypoglycemia, glucagon and catecholamines are essential; in addition, the response of both cortisol and GH also plays an important counterregulatory role [46, 47].

The counterregulation in T1DM is constantly, to various degrees, impaired. First of all, the glucagon response to hypoglycemia is lost in the early stages of the disease [42,48], amplifying the importance of epinephrine in the counterregulatory response. Unfortunately, many T1DM patients also have a blunted epinephrine response [49]. The response of epinephrine may be normal or reduced in the short term [50], but becomes defective in long-term diabetes [51]. The pathogenesis of loss of adrenaline response to hypoglycemia in T1DM remains largely unknown, but it is demonstrated that the glycemic threshold for epinephrine secretion is often shifted to lower plasma glucose levels [51]. These characteristics contribute to cause the syndrome of defective counterregulation. The hypoglycemia-associated autonomic failure (HAAF) is related to a defective counterregulatory response [52, 53], and consists of a shift in glycemic thresholds for the autonomic response to lower plama glucose concentrations [52]. Some authors have hypothesized the involvement of cortisol due to the experimental evidences of reduced adrenomedullary and sympathetic response to hypoglycemia after cortisol infusion [54].

These reports are confirmed by an interesting study that shows a reduced response to hypoglycemia after physical exercise, a condition that releases endogenous cortisol [55]. Sleep also seems to impair the plasma epinephrine response to hypoglycemia: an interesting study [56] shows a decrease of counterregulatory response in T1DM subjects, as well as in normal controls; this impaired response affects epinephrine, cortisol and GH. The catecholamine response seems to be impaired mainly in stages 3 and 4 of non-REM sleep that predominates in the first third of the nighttime-sleep cycle, the time when patients with diabetes are most prone to severe hypoglycemia. The defective response of adrenaline to hypoglycemia in T1DM is further reduced in the presence of clinically overt autonomic neuropathy, also in the stage of predominant parasympathetic involvement [57].

Thus, counterregulation in diabetes is also defective in T1DM of short duration, but mainly in patients with long-term diabetes.

## Hypoglycemia Unawareness

Failure to respond to early hypoglycemia can be an important problem for diabetic patients, increasing the risk of severe hypoglycemia with cognitive impairment [58], and leading to hypoglycemia unawareness. Hypoglycemia unawareness occurs when appropriate autonomic warning symptoms (anxiety, palpitations, hunger, sweating tremor and irritability) do not prevent neuroglycopenia (confusion, dizziness, blurred vision, weakness). Risk factors for developing unawareness are the following: diabetes duration [59], autonomic neuropathy [60], decreased β-adrenergic sensitivity [61], degree of glycemic control [62, 63], and hypoglycemia itself [64]. A reduction of β-adrenergic sensitivity without a reduction of catecholamine response has been postulated; furthermore, a restored β-adrenergic sensitivity after the avoidance of hypoglycemic episodes has been demonstrated [65]. These authors studied the response to hypoglycemia comparing 10 T1DM patients without unawareness and 10 healthy controls, demonstrating a reduction of β-adrenergic sensitivity in diabetic patients, while in nondiabetic controls an increase of β-adrenergic sensitivity after a single hypoglycemic episode was shown [66]. This hypothesis was also tested by other authors [67], who studied the catecholamine response to hypoglycemia and β-adrenergic sensitivity with isoproterenol testing, in unaware and aware diabetic subjects and in normal controls: in the unaware group they showed a reduced β-adrenergic sensitivity during an isoproterenol stimulation test, together with a decrease in counterregulatory hormone response that may contribute to reduced warning symptoms during hypoglycemia. These findings were also supported by experimental animal studies: a decreased number of cardiac β-adrenergic receptors was demonstrated in streptozotocin-diabetic rats, suggesting a downregulation of catecholamine receptors as a consequence of diabetes [68]. A reversibility of impaired β-adrenergic sensitivity (by avoiding hypoglycemic episodes), but not of the counterregulatory response has also been demonstrated [53]. It is assumed that the decreased β-adrenergic sensitivity contributes to unawareness, but it is not the only determinant of this situation. In fact, while the response to hypoglycemia may be normal or reduced in T1DM of short duration [69, 50], it becomes blunted in long-term T1DM [31].

Diabetic autonomic neuropathy plays an important role in determining this blunted response. An interesting study [70] has demonstrated that in the presence of autonomic neuropathy, the response of adrenaline to hypoglycemia is further reduced despite the meticulous prevention of recent antecedent hypoglycemia, and that this defect seems to be nonselective. It has also been demonstrated that avoiding or retarding the onset of autonomic neuropathy by obtaining a tight metabolic control, makes it possible to avoid loss of adrenaline response to hypoglycemia [69].

Unawareness represents a problem especially for the brain, and for brain functions, as well as the pathogenesis of unawareness depends also from the brain, since the central nervous system seems to act as a hypoglycemia sensor and coordinator of the counterregulatory response. Some experimental animal studies [71, 72] demonstrated an activation of neuronal networks by de-oxyglucose-induced glucoprivation in the brain of rats with connections to centers in the hypothalamus and medulla. Other authors describe a population of neurones using glucose as a signalling molecule rather than a metabolic substrate, altering their firing rate in response to changes in ambient glucose supply [73]; these populations of neurones seem to respond to decreasing blood glucose concentrations (glucose-sensitive neurones), or to increasing blood glucose concentrations (glucose-responsive neurones). Changes in glucose concentration have been shown to influence the release of several neurotransmitters, dopamine, GABA [74, 75], neuropeptide Y and catecholamines [72] in studies in animals.

These studies have also shown that severe prolonged hypoglycemia can enhance glucose uptake into the brain, and the expression of both GLUT-1 and GLUT-3 are increased in response to glucose deprivation [76, 77]. The studies in humans performed with the arteriovenous difference technique have shown enhanced brain glucose uptake during hypoglycemia in healthy volunteers, and in hypoglycemia-unaware subjects with counterregulatory failure [78, 79]. On the other hand, PET studies failed to demonstrate any change of brain glucose uptake and metabolism in different groups of diabetic subjects with different counterregulatory response [80]. Regarding the sensitivity of the brain to hypoglycemia, it is possible that brain areas can have different sensitivity to hypoglycemia: different part of cortex shows detectable evidence of dysfunction at different glucose concentrations during progressive hypoglycemia [78, 79], and have a different ability to alter their sensitivity to hypoglycemia in the hypoglycemia unaware state. Finally, it is possible to conclude that hypoglycemia unawareness is a problem of the brain and for the brain, so it is demonstrated that the brain, and especially the hypothalamus, plays an important role in initiating the protective counterregulatory response [81] to hypoglycemia.

## Prevention

Although substantial progress has been made in understanding the pathophysiology and the mechanisms of hypoglycemic signs and symptoms, hypoglycemia must be prevented in order to really improve the quality of life of children with diabetes. An interesting cost-of-illness study regarding short-term effects of severe hypoglycemia in children and adolescents with T1DM has shown an average cost at EUR 239 per event of severe hypoglycemia with unconsciousness and EUR 63 per event of severe hypoglycemia without unconsciousness, but needing assistance from another person. Moreover, of all events, 20–30% had effects on school absence, parents' absence at work, increased worry for parents and poor sleep. Patients with severe hypoglycemia indicated a lower global quality of life [82].

The predictors of severe hypoglycemia have been also evaluated: in younger children the risk increased with disease duration and underinsurance; in older children the risk increased with duration, underinsurance, lower HbA1c levels, and psychiatric disorder, with 80% of episodes occurring among the 20% of children who had recurrent episodes [83].

The hypothesis of a genetic determinant for severe hypoglycemia has been also postulated by some authors that studied serum ACE levels in children and adolescents; the results of the study shown a positive correlation between serum ACE levels, and number of severe hypoglycemia levels. This study suggests that, among other factors, a genetic determinant for severe hypoglycemia exists [84].

In the last years, many authors have suggested different measures to prevent hypoglycemia with different results [85–87]. From these studies, it is clear that adequate insulin regimen, motivation among the children and their parents to follow recommendations combined with knowledge how to adjust insulin therapy in different situations are crucial components of a successful prevention; also a correct injection technique and a precise self-monitoring of blood glucose are important to avoid mistakes in the insulin therapy. About self-monitoring of blood glucose, it is essential that the patient learns the importance of these determinations, in particular in the evening and at bedtime. In fact, hypoglycemia during the night is probably more common than we thought and, of course, nocturnal hypoglycemia can profoundly affect brain function [88]. A correct adjustment of insulin doses on the basis of actual blood glucose is essential for prevention of hypoglycemia, particularly during the night.

However, the cornerstone of hypoglycemia prevention is education: without knowledge of how to use insulin and self-monitoring of blood glucose, no insulin regimen will be successful [82]. Of course, learning becomes effective when it gives answers to relevant questions which are experienced as real problems for the one who is learning. A recent study has analyzed the reasons for severe hypoglycemia [89]. Although mistakes seem to be the most common cause of hypoglycemic episodes, there are certain steps that can be taken:

- Different pens for different types of insulin to prevent mixing;
- No pen on the night table;
- Adequate individual interval between insulin injection and the following meal;
- Late spring-early summer is accompanied by increased physical activity, and risk for hypoglycemia;
- When school starts after the summer holidays the risk of hypoglycemia is increased;
- Unusually heavy exercise may need not only a reduction of insulin dose just before the exercise, but sometimes also reduction the following night;
- Alcohol can cause dangerous hypoglycemia.

Beside the regular information and education on these matters, the authors have produced a pamphlet on hypoglycemia which was sent to all patients and families and also 2 video films on how to prevent hypoglycemia and how to use the tools (mainly self-monitoring of blood glucose and adjustment of insulin doses) to get a stable blood glucose. All patients get these video films for free 3 months after diagnosis and the other 9 months after diagnosis, in connection with a special education day at the hospital. A positive effect of these films has been found in a controlled study [90].

The main practical measures to prevent hypoglycemia are reported in table 2. Moreover, it has been shown that continuous subcutaneous insulin infusion (CSII) may significantly reduce the risk for severe hypoglycemia, especially at night, when hypoglycemia is common and insidious, and decrease the Hb1c levels [91, 92]. An interesting study performed on 100 children and adolescents treated with CSII showed a reduction of hypoglycemic episodes [93]. Several

*Table 2.* Main measures to prevent hypoglycemia

| |
|---|
| Near-physiological insulin regimen, with adaptation of insulin doses to meals, meals plans and exercise |
| Enlightening of the patients on good injection technique, including adequate time interval between injection and meal |
| Self-monitoring of blood glucose, including regular blood glucose determinations during the night |
| Adjustments of treatment based on blood glucose patterns/profiles and what is going to happen, but not based on the actual blood glucose value |
| Strive for near-normal blood glucose with less wide fluctuations, which gives better counterregulation |
| Education to make the patients and people in their surroundings aware of symptoms/signs |
| Information about the influence of seasonal variation effect of holidays and sport days psychological support to increase confidence. |
| Psychological support to increase confidence. |
| Increase general awareness of hypoglycemia through education. |

From Ludvigsson and Nordfeldt [90], modified.

reports in children underline the safety of the CSII, and the reduction of hypoglycemia despite improved glycemic control [94, 95]. Treatment with CSII of course requires at least the same knowledge and motivation as the use of multiple insulin therapy.

Evidence is now accumulating on the effect of insulin analogues on hypoglycemia. The impact of DCCT and lispro insulin on glycemic control and severe hypoglycemia was studied: the number of severe hypoglycemic episodes did not increase after the introduction of lispro, despite a further decrease in HbA1c levels [96]. A recent study on insulin lispro in children focused attention on nocturnal hypoglycemia, demonstrating the efficacy of lispro given before the evening meal in reducing early nocturnal hypoglycemia without compromising HbA1c [97]. The long-acting analog insulin glargine may also reduce nocturnal hypoglycemia [98].

Diabetic patients more often have EEG changes which have usually been contributed to previous hypoglycemic episodes [92], but it has been shown that there is a correlation between primary changes of EEG already at the diagnosis of diabetes and later severe hypoglycemia [99]. Thus, a low threshold for seizures may sometimes be a cause of convulsions rather than a consequence of them. Patients with epilepsy or abnormal EEG should be treated with adequate drugs. The interactions between hypoglycemia and sleep architecture were recently reported by Pillar el al. [100], demonstrating that profound nocturnal hypoglycemia increased slow wave sleep and delta power in spectral analysis of the EEG.

Finally, the incidence of moderate and severe hypoglycemia can and should be reduced parallel to near-normal HbA1c by active education and psychosocial support in combination with insulin treatment as physiological as possible. It has been suggested that, in adults, meticulous attention to the prevention of hypoglycemia can abolish the hypoglycemia unawareness syndrome. Hypoglycemia in children, with their erratic activity and eating behavior, is much more difficult to predict and therefore prevent. Yet the consequences of hypoglycemia are the greatest in this youngest age group, where these problems are paramount. In order to obtain an improving glucose control and to identify asymptomatic hypoglycemia, the continuous subcutaneous glucose monitoring (CSGM) seems to be very useful. In fact, some recent studies [101, 102] demonstrate that CSGM might be helpful in detecting unrecognized nocturnal hypoglycemia and in lowering HbA1c values in children with type 1 diabetes and poor glucose control, obtaining a drop in insulin requirement as well. This monitoring method will be useful to reduce the frequency of hypoglycemic episodes in children with diabetes.

In conclusion, hypoglycemia remains one of the most important problems in the management of insulin therapy in children and adolescents with diabetes; however, the advances in knowledge on the risk factors for hypoglycemia, and the new therapeutic and diagnostic approach, will be useful to prevent hypoglycemia and its consequences and to allow patients to achieve better metabolic control without increasing the risk of hypoglycemia.

## References


1 Allen C, Le Caire T, Mari Palta MS, Daniels K, Meredith, D'Alessio DJ: Risk factor for frequent and severe hypoglycaemia in type 1 diabetes. Diabetes Care 2001;24:1878–1881.

2 Cryer PE, Binder C, Bolli GB, Cherrigton AD, Gale JE, Sherwin RS: Conference summary: Hypoglycaemia in IDDM. Diabetes 1989;38:1193–1199.

3 Wredling R, Levander S, Adamson UL, Wredling R, Levander S, Admoson U, Lins PE: Permanent neuropsychological impairment after recurrent episodes of severe hypoglycaemia in man. Diabetologia 1990;33:152–157.

4 Cryer PE, Gerich JE: Hypoglycaemia in insulin dependent diabetes mellitus: Insulin excess and defective glucose counterregulation. Diabetes mellitus Theory Pract 1990:526–527.

5 Bell DSH, Cutter G: Characteristics of severe hypoglycaemia in the patients with insulin-dependent diabetes mellitus. N Engl J Med 1993;329:977–986.

6 Davis EA, Keating B, Byrne GC, Russel M, Jones TW: Hypoglycaemia: Incidence and clinical predictors in a large population-based sample of children and adolescence with IDDM. Diabetes Care 1997;20:22–24.

7 Goldstein D, Englan JD, Hess R, Rawling SS, Walker B: A prospective study of symptomatic hypoglycemia in young diabetic patients. Diabetes Care 1981;4:601–605.
8 The DCCT Research Group: Epidemiology of severe hypoglycemia in the Diabetes Control and Complication Trials. Am J Med 1991;90:450–459.
9 Frier BM: Epidemiology, short and long-term consequences of hypoglycaemia. Diab Nutr Metab 2002;15:378–385.
10 MacLeod KM, Hepburn DA, Frier BM: Frequency and morbidity of severe hypoglycemia in insulin-treated diabetic patients. Diabet Med 1993:10:238–245.
11 Ter Braak EWMT, Appelman AMMF, Van de Laak MF, Stolk RP, Van Haeften TW, Erkelens DW: Clinical characteristics of type 1 diabetic patients with and without severe hypoglycaemia. Diabetes Care 2000;20:1467–1471.
12 Amin R, Ross K, Acerini CL, Edge JA, Warner J, Dunger DB: Hypoglycaemia prevalence in prepubertal children with type 1 diabetes on standard insulin regimen: Use of continuous glucose monitoring system. Diabetes Care 2003;26:662–667.
13 Reichard P, Britz A, Rosenqvist U: Intensified conventional insulin treatment and neuropsychological impairment. Br Med J 1991;303:1439–1442.
14 Diabetes Control and Complications Trial Research Group: Hypoglycaemia in the Diabetes Control and Complications Trial. Diabetes 1997;46:271–286.
15 Diabetes Control and Complications Trial Research Group: Epidemiology of severe hypoglycemia in the Diabetes Control and Complications Trial. Am J Med 1991;303:1439–1442.
16 Pramming S, Pederson-Bjergaad U, Heller SR, Wallace T, Rasmussen AK, Jorgensen HV, Matthews DR, Thorsteinsson B: Severe hypoglycaemia in unselected patients with type 1 diabetes: A cross-sectional multicentre survey (abstract). Diabetologia 2000;43(suppl 1):A194.
17 Jorgens V, Gruber M, Bott U, Mulhauser I, Berger M: Effective and safe translation of intensified insulin therapy to general internal medical departments. Diabetologia 1993;36:99–105.
18 Bott S, Bott U, Berger M, Muhlhauser I: Intensified therapy and the risk of severe hypoglycemia. Diabetologia 1997;40:926–932.
19 Cryer P: Glucose counterregulation in man. Diabetes 1981;30:261–264.
20 Rizza R, Cryer PE, Gerich JE: Role of glucagon, catecholamines and growth hormone in human glucose counterregulation: effects of somatostatin and combined α and β-adrenergic blockade on plasma glucose recovery and glucose flux rates following insulin-induced hypoglycaemia. J Clin Invest 1979;64:62–71.
21 Cersosimo E, Garlick P, Ferretti J: Insulin regulation of renal glucose metabolism in humans. Am J Physiol 1979;276:E78–E84.
22 Moller N, Rizza R, Ford G, Nair K: Assessment of postabsorptive renal glucose metabolism in humans with multiple glucose tracers. Diabetes 2001;50:747–751.
23 Meyer C, Dostou J, Nadkarni V, Gerich J: Effects of physiological hyperinsulinemia on systemic, renal and hepatic substrate metabolism. Am J Physiol 1998;275:f905–f921.
24 Musson I, Rothman D, Gerard D, Kats L, Shulman G: Contribution of hepatic glycogenolysis to glucose production in humans in response to a physiological increase in plasma glucagon concentration. Diabetes 1995;44:185–189.
25 Stumvoll M, Chintallapudi U, Perriello G, Welle S, Gutierezz O, Gerich J: Uptake and release of glucagon by human kidney: Postabsorptive rates and response to epinephrine. J Clin Invest 1995; 96:2528–2533.
26 Schoolwerth AC, Smith BC, Culpepper RM: Renal gluconeogenesis. Miner Electrolyte Metab 1988;14:347–361.
27 Iles RA, Cohen RD, Rist AH, Baron PG: The mechanism of inhibition by acidosis of gluconeogenesis from lactate in rat liver. Biochem J 1977;164:1185–1191.
28 Stumvoll M, Meyer C, Perriello G, Kreider M, Welle S, Gerich J: Human kidney and liver gluconeogenesis: Evidence for organ substrate selectivity. Am J Physiol 1998;274:E817–E826.
29 Meyer C, Stumvoll M, Dostou J, Welle S, Haymond M, Gerich J: Renal substrate exchange and gluconeogenesis in normal postabsorptive humans. Am J Physyiol 2002;282:428–434.
30 Borg MA, Sherwin RS, Borg WP, Tamborlane WV, Shulman GI: Local ventromedial hypothalamus glucose perfusion blocks counterregulation during systemic hypoglycaemia in awake rats. J Clin Invest 1997;99:361–365.

31 Oomura Y, Onyama H, Suigimori M, Nekemura T, Yamada Y: Glucose inhibition of the glucose sensitive neurons in the rat lateral hypothalamus. Nature 1974;247:284–286.
32 Paton JFR, Li YW, Deuchars J, Kasparov S: Properties of solitary tract neurons receive inputs from the sub diaphragmatic vagus nerve. Neuroscience 1999;95:141–153.
33 Yettefi K, Orsini JC, Perrin J: Characteristics of glycaemia sensitive neurons in the nucleus tractus solitarii: Possible involvement in nutritional regulation. Physiol Behav 1997;61:93–100.
34 Leloupe C, Arluison M, Lepetit N, Cartier N, Marfaing yallat P, ferre P, Penicaud L: Glucose transporter 2 (GLUT 2): Expression in specific brain nuclei. Brain Res 1994;638:221–226.
35 Burcelin R, Dolci W, Thorens B: Glucose sensing by the hepatoportal sensor is GLUT 2 dependent. Diabetes 2000;49:1643–1648.
36 Ricardo JA, Koh ET: Anatomical evidence of direct projections from the nucleus of the solitary tract to the hypothalamus: A phaseous vegaris lectin tracing study in the rat. Brain Res 1978;154: 1–26.
37 De Feo P, Pampanelli S, Porcellati F, Rossetti P, Fanelli CG, Bolli GB: Adrenaline vs glucagone in the primacy of glucose counterregulation. Diab Nutr Metab 2002;15:232–238.
38 Cryer PE: Banting Lecture. Hypoglycaemia: The limiting factor in the management of IDDM. Diabetes 1994;43:1378–1389.
39 Gerich JE: Glucose in the control of glucagon secretion; in Lefebvre PJ (ed): Handbook of Experimental Pharmacology. Heidelberg, Springer, 1983, pp 3–18.
40 Samols E, Weir GC, Bonner-Weir S: Intra-islet insulin-glucagon-somatostatin relationship; in Lefebvre PJ (ed): Glucagon III. Berlin, Springer, 1983, pp 133–173.
41 Havel PJ, Taborsky GJ: The contribution of the autonomic nervous system to changes of glucagon and insulin secretion during hypoglycemic stress. Endocr Rev 1989;10:332–350.
42 Taborsky GJ Jr, Ahren B, Havel PJ: Autonomic mediation of glucagon secretion during hypoglycemia: Implication for impaired alpha-cell responses in type 1 diabetes. Diabetes 1998;47:995–1005.
43 Massara F, Camanni F, Molinatti G: Effect of propranol on some adrenaline and insulin induced metabolic changes in man. Acta Diabetol Lat 1985;12:41–51.
44 De Feo P, Perriello G, De Cosmo S, Ventura MM, Torlone E, Fanelli C, Santeusanio F, Bolli GB, Brunetti P: Adrenergic mechanism do not contribute to glucose counterregulation during acute insulin-induced hypoglycaemia in normal man. Diab Nutr Metab 1989;2:111–118.
45 De Feo P, Perriello G, Torlone E, Fanelli C, Ventura MM, Santeusanio F, Brunetti P, Gerich JE, Bolli GB: The contribution of adrenergic mechanism to glucose counterregulation in humans. Am J Physiol 1991;261:E725–E736.
46 De Feo P, Perriello G, Torlone E, Fanelli C, Ventura MM, Santeusanio F, Brunetti P, Gerich JE, Bolli GB: Contribution of cortisol to glucose counterregulation in man. Am J Physiol 1989:257; E35–E42.
47 De Feo P, Perriello G, Torlone E, Fanelli C, Ventura MM, Santeusanio F, Brunetti P, Gerich JE, Bolli GB: Demonstration of a role for growth hormone in glucose counterregulation. Am J Physiol 1989;E835–E843.
48 Gerich JE, Langlois M, Noacco C, Karam J, Forsham PH: Lack of a glucagon response to hypoglycaemia in diabetes: Evidence for an intrinsic pancreatic alpha-cell defect. Science 1973;182: 171–173.
49 Bolli GB: From physiology of glucose counterregulation to prevention of hypoglycaemia in type 1 diabetes mellitus. Diab Nutr Metab 1990;3:333–349.
50 Fanelli C, Epifano L, Rambotti AM, Campanelli S, Di Vincenzo A, Modarelli F, Lepore M, Annibale B, Ciofetta M, Bottini P, Porcellani F, Scionti L, Santeusiano F, Brunetti P, Bolli GB: Meticulous prevention of hypoglycaemia normalizes magnitude and glycemic thresholds of neuroendocrine responses to, symptoms of, and cognitive function during hypoglycaemia in intensively treated patients with IDDM of short duration. Diabetes 1993;42:1683–1689.
51 Bolli GB, De Feo P, Compagnucci P, Cartechini MG, Angeletti G, Santeusiano F, Brunetti P, Gerich J: Abnormal glucose counterregulation in insulin-dependent diabetes mellitus: Interaction of insulin antibodies and impaired glucagon and epinephrine secretion. Diabetes 1983;32: 134–141.
52 Dagago-Jack SE, Craft S, Cryer PE: Hypoglycaemia-associated autonomic failure in insulin dependent diabetes mellitus. J Clin Invest 1993;91:819–828.

53 Dagogo-Jack S, Rattarasarn C, Cryer PE: Reversal of hypoglycaemia unawareness, but not defective glucose counterregulation in IDDM. Diabetes 1994;43:1426–1434.
54 Davis SN, Shavers C, Costa F, Mosqeda-Garcia R: Role of cortisol in the pathogenesis of deficient counterregulation after antecedent hypoglycemia in normal humans. J Clin Invest 1996;98: 680–691.
55 Galassetti P, Mann S, Tate D, Neill RA, Costa F, Wassermann DH, Davis SN: Effects of antecedent prolonged exercise on subsequent counterregulation responses to hypoglycemia. Am J Physiol 2001;280:E908–E917.
56 Timothy W, Jones MB, et al: Decreased epinephrine responses to hypoglycemia during sleep. N Engl J Med 1998;338:1657–1662.
57 Porcellati F, Fanelli C, Bottini P, Epifano L, Rambotti AM, Lalli C, Pampanelli S, Scionti L, Santeusanio F, Brunetti P, Hilsted J, Bolli GB: Mechanism of arterial hypotension after therapeutic dose of subcutaneous insulin in diabetic subjects with and without autonomic neuropathy. Diabetes 1993;42:1055–1064.
58 Gold AE, Macleod KM, Deary IJ, Frier BM: Hypoglycemia-induced cognitive dysfunction in diabetes mellitus: Effect of hypoglycaemia unawareness. Physiol Behav 1995;58:501–511.
59 Laurence R: Insulin hypoglycaemia: Changes in nervous manifestations. Lancet 1941;ii:602.
60 Hepburn D, Patrick A, Eadington D, Ewing D, Frier B: Unawareness of hypoglycaemia in insulin-treated diabetic patients: Prevalence and relationship to autonomic neuropathy. Diabetic Med 1990;7:711–717.
61 Berlin I, Grimaldi A, Payan C, Sachon C, Bosquet F, Thervet F, Puech A: Hypoglycaemic symptoms and decreased beta-adrenergic sensitivity in insulin-dependent diabetic patients. Diabetes Care 1987;10:742–747.
62 Widom B, Simonson D: Glycemic control and neuropsychologic function during hypoglycaemia in patients with insulin-dependent diabetes. Ann Intern Med 1990;112:904–912.
63 Amiel S, Shervin R, Simonson D, Tamborlane W: Effect of intensive insulin therapy on glycemic thresholds for counterregulatory hormone release. Diabetes 1988;37:901–907.
64 Veneman T, Mitrakou A, Mokan M, Cryer P, Gerich J: Induction of hypoglycaemia unawareness by asymptomatic nocturnal hypoglycaemia. Diabetes 1993;42:1233–1237.
65 Fritsche A, Tschritter O, Haring H, Gerich J, Stumvoll M: The role of beta-adrenergic sensitivity in the pathogenesis of hypoglycaemia unawareness. Diab Nutr Metab 2002;15:354–361.
66 Fritsche A, Stumvoll M, Grub M, Sieslack S, Renn W, Schmulling RM, Haring HU, Gerich JE: Effect of hypoglycaemia on beta-adrenergic sensitivity in normal and type 1 diabetes subjects. Diabetes Care 1998;21:1505–1510.
67 Mary T, Korytkowsky MD: Reduced beta adrenergic sensitivity in patients with type 1 diabetes and hypoglycaemia unawareness. Diabetes Care 1998;11:1939–1943.
68 Savarese JJ, Berkowitz BA: Beta adrenergic receptor decrease in diabetic rat hearts. Life Sci 1979;25:2075–2078.
69 Campanelli S, Fanelli C, Lalli C, Ciofetta M, Rambotti AM, Campanelli S, Di Vincenzo A, Modarelli F, Lepore M, Annibale B, Ciofetta M, Bottini P, Porcellani F, Bartocci L, Brunetti P, Bolli GB: Long-term intensive insulin therapy: Effects of Hba1c, risk for severe and mild hypoglycaemia, status of counterregulation and unawareness of hypoglycaemia. Diabetologia 1996;39:677–686.
70 Bottini P, Boschetti E, Pampanelli S, Ciofetta M, Del Sindaco P, Scionti l, Brunetti P, Bolli GB: Contribution of autonomic neuropathy to reduced plasma adrenaline responses to hypoglycaemia in IDDM. Diabetes 1997;46:814–821.
71 Frizzell RT, Jones EM, Davis SN, et al: Counterregulation during hypoglycaemia is directed by widespread brain organs. Diabetes 1993;42:1253–1261.
72 Ritter S, Dinh TT, Llwellyn SI: Subgroups of hindbrain catecholamine neurons are selectively activated by 2-deoxy-*D*-glucose induced metabolic challenge. Brain Res 1998;805:41–45.
73 Song Z, Levin BE, McArdle JJ, Bakson N, Routh VH: Convergence of pre- and postsynaptic influences on glucosensing neurons in the ventromedial hypothalamic nucleus. Diabetes 2001;50: 2673–2681.
74 Levin BE: Glucose-regulated dopamine release from substantia nigra neurons. Brain Res 2000;874:158–164.

75 During MJ, Leone P, Davis KE, Kerr D, Sherwin RS: Glucose modulates rat substantia nigra GABA release in vivo via ATP-sensitive potassium channels. J Clin Invest 1995;95:2403–2408.
76 Takakura Y, Kuentzel SL, Raub TJ, Davies A, Baldwin SA, Borchardt RT: Hexose uptake in primary cultures of bovine brain microvessel endothelial cells. Basic characteristics and effects of *D*-glucose and insulin. Biochim Biophys Acta 1991;1070:1–10.
77 Uehara Y, Nipper V, McCall AL: Chronic insulin hypoglycaemia induces GLUT-3 protein in rat brain neurons. Am J Physiol Endocrinol Metab 1997;272:E716–E719.
78 Boyle PJ, Nagy RJ, O'Connor AM, Kempers SF, Yeo RA, Qualls C: Adaptation in brain glucose uptake following recurrent hypoglycaemia. Proc Natl Acad Sci USA 1994;91:9352–9356.
79 Boyle PJ, Kempers SF, O'Connor AM, Nagy RJ: Brain glucose uptake and unawareness of hypoglycemia in patients with insulin dependent diabetes mellitus. N Engl J Med 1995;333: 1726–1731.
80 Segel SA, Fanelli CG, Dence CS: Blood-to-brain glucose transport, cerebral glucose metabolism, and cerebral blood flow are not increased after hypoglycaemia. Diabetes 2001;50:1911–1917.
81 Borg WP, During MJ, Sherwin RS, Borg MA, Brines ML, Shulman GI: Ventromedial hypothalamic lesions in rats suppress counterregulatory responses to hypoglycaemia. J Clin Invest 1994;93: 1677–1682.
82 Nordfeldt S, Jonsson D: Short-term effects of severe hypoglycaemia in children and adolescents with type 1 diabetes: A cost-of-illness study. Acta Paediatr 2001;90:137–142.
83 Rewers A, Chase HP, Mackenzie T, Walravens P, Roback M, Rewers M, Hamman RF, Klingensmith G: Predictors of acute complications in children with type 1 diabetes. J Pediatr 2002;141:739–740.
84 Nordfeldt S, Samuelsson U: Serum ACE predicts severe hypoglycaemia in children and adolescents with type 1 diabetes. Diabetes Care 2003;26:274–278.
85 Ludvigsson J, Nordfeldt S: Prevention of hypoglycaemia in diabetic children and adolescents. Diab Nutr Metab 2002;15:395–402.
86 Ludvigsson J, Heding L: Beta cell function in children with diabetes. Diabetes 1978;27:230–234.
87 Lalli C, Ciofetta M, Del Sindaco P, Torlone E, Pampanelli S, Compagnucci P, Cartechini MG, Bartocci L, Brunetti P, Bolli GB: Long-term intensive treatment of type 1 diabetes with the short-acting insulin analogue lispro in variable combination with NPH insulin at mealtime. Diabetes Care 1999;2:468–477.
88 Pramming S, Thorsteinsson B, Bendtson I, Ronn B, Binder C: Noctural hypoglycaemia in patients receiving conventional treatment with insulin. BMJ 1985;291:376–379.
89 Nordfeldt S, Ludvigsson J: Adverse events in intensively treated children and adolescents with type 1 diabetes. Acta Pediatr 1999;88:1184–1193.
90 Ludvigsson J, Nordfeldt S: Prevention of hypoglycaemia in children. Symposium on 'hypoglycaemia 2001 from Research to Practice', Assisi, 2001, p 40, abstr.
91 Boland EA, Grey M, Oesterle A, Fredrickson L, Tamborlane WV: Continuous subcutaneous insulin infusion: A new way to lower risk of severe hypoglycaemia, improve metabolic control, and enhance coping in adolescence with type 1 diabetes. Diabetes Care 1999;22:1779–1784.
92 Soltèsz G, Acsàdi G: Association between diabetes, severe hypoglycaemia and electroencephalographic abnormalities. Arch Dis Child 1989;64:992–996.
93 Jones TW, Davis EA: Hypoglycaemia in children with type 1 diabetes: Current issues and controversies. Pediatr Diab 2003;4:143–150.
94 Miniatis AK, Klingensmith GJ, Slover RH: Continuous subcutaneous insulin infusion therapy for children and adolescents: An option for routine care. Pediatrics 2001;107:351–356.
95 Ludvigsson J, Hanas R: Continuous subcutaneous glucose monitoring improved metabolic control in pediatric patients with type 1 diabetes: A controlled crossover study. Pediatrics 2003;11: 933–938.
96 Chase HP, Lockspeiser T, Peery B, Shepherd M, MacKenzie T, Garg SK: The impact of the diabetes control and complications trials an humalog insulin on glycohemoglobin levels and severe hypoglycaemia in type 1 diabetes. Diabetes Care 2001;24:430–434.
97 Ford-Adams ME, Murphy NP, Moore EJ, Edge JA, Ong KL, Acerini CL, Dunger DB: Insulin lispro: A potential role in preventing nocturnal hypoglycaemia in young children with diabetes mellitus. Diab Med 2003;20:656–660.

98 Murphy Np, Keane SM, Ong KK: Randomized cross-over trial of insulin glargine plus lispro or NPH insulin plus regular human insulin in adolescents with type 1 diabetes on intensive insulin regimens. Diabetes Care 2003;26:799–804.
99 Tupola S, Saar P, Rajantie J: Abnormal electroencephalogram at diagnosis of insulin-dependent diabetes mellitus may predict severe symptoms of hypoglycemia in children. J Pediatr 1998;133: 792–794.
100 Pillar G, Schuscheim G, Weiss R, Malhotra A, McCowen KC, Shlitner A, Peled N, Sheadeh N: Interactions between hypoglycaemia and sleep architecture in children with type 1 diabetes mellitus. J Pediatr 2003;142:163–168.
101 Chase P, Kim LM, Owen S, MacKenzie T, Klingensmith G, Murtfeld R, Garg SK: Continuous subcutaneous glucose monitoring in children with type 1 diabetes. Pediatrics 2001;107:222–226.
102 Sulli N, Shashaj B: Continuous subcutaneous insulin infusion in children and adolescent with diabetes mellitus: Decreased HbA1c with low risk of hypoglycemia. J Pediatr Endocrinol Metab 2003;16:393–399.

F. Chiarelli, MD
Department of Pediatrics, Ospedale Policlinico
Via dei Vestini, 5, IT–66100 Chieti (Italy)
Tel. +39 08 71 35 80 15, Fax +39 08 71 57 48 31, E-Mail chiarelli@unich.it

Chiarelli F, Dahl-Jørgensen K, Kiess W (eds): Diabetes in Childhood and Adolescence.
Pediatr Adolesc Med. Basel, Karger, 2005, vol 10, pp 314–328

# Diabetic Retinopathy in Children and Adolescents with Type 1 Diabetes

*C. Bittner*[a], *O. Kordonouri*[b], *T. Danne*[a]

[a]Kinderkrankenhaus auf der Bult, Hannover, und
[b]Klinik für Allgemeine Pädiatrie, Charité, Campus Virchow-Klinikum,
Medizinische Fakultät der Humboldt Universität zu Berlin,
Berlin, Deutschland

In the western hemisphere diabetic retinopathy counts for most cases of loss of vision; the risk to suffer visual impairment is up to 20-fold higher for diabetic subjects compared to healthy controls. The clinical stages of nonproliferative and sight-threatening proliferative retinopathy stages are well classified [1]. Since proliferative changes are rare during adolescence, there has been some controversy in the past whether retinal screening is necessary during pediatric care. Initial investigations on the frequency of retinopathy in patients with juvenile-onset type 1 diabetes gave conflicting results as they were performed by ophthalmoscopy known to have a high inter- and intraobserver variation. Yet, they indicated the severity of the problem as at least more than half of the patients had visible retinal changes after 20 years of diabetes duration [2, 3]. Stereophotographic ophthalmophotography via a dilated pupil improved the reproducibility of the examination and indicated that the frequency of retinal changes was between 67 and 78% after 16 years of diabetes and more than 90% in long-standing diabetes [4, 5]. Only few population-based studies are available [6–8]. The recent population-based Swedish survey of 557 children with an average age of 14 years and diabetes duration of 8 years indicated a prevalence of 14.5% for any retinopathy and 2.3% for proliferative and preproliferative changes [7]. Females are known to be more at risk as males [9]. Since diabetic retinopathy is thus seriously present already in childhood, there is in fact a necessity of a proper follow-up of the retinal status by the pediatric diabetologist [10, 11].

## Pathoanatomy and Pathohistology in Diabetic Retinopathy

The opportunity of direct ophthalmological observation allows the classification of retinal changes not only by structural but also by functional aspects. Retinal blood vessels do not have autonomic nervous system innervation and attempt to maintain constant blood flow through an autoregulative mechanism. Hyperglycemia by itself impairs this autoregulation [12]. Initially, this leads to a phase of increased retinal blood flow [13] and venous dilatation. The two major characteristics of early retinopathy are increased capillary permeability and progressive vascular closure. At the cellular level, there is loss of pericytes and thickening of the basement membrane followed by proliferation and degeneration of endothelial cells. An increase of programmed cell death (apoptosis) could be identified as a central mechanism leading to a loss of not only pericytes but also endothelial cells, indicating that the latter may have a strong proliferative capacity under circumstances of hyperglycemia [14]. The changes of the extracellular matrix together with the impaired interaction between pericytes and endothelial cells eventually lead to a disturbed blood-retinal barrier. It has to be kept in mind that recent results indicate that not only vascular cells but also other cells such as Müller cells, the principal glia of the retina, are altered in diabetes and may contribute to these changes [15]. The resulting predominance of vasoconstricting mechanisms including hemorheological abnormalities finally results in focal thrombosis and vascular closure.

The first morphological lesions are microaneurysms which evolve in areas of capillary hypoperfusion and they first appear in the peripheral temporal region [16]. Those microaneurysms are no longer thought to be areas of local weaknesses of the vessel wall in areas of pericyte loss but rather abortive attempts at intraretinal neovascularization. Local factors of the retina contribute to the localization of these lesions [17]. Using the sensitive fluorescence angiography technique, microaneurysms were detected in all adolescents and young adults after 18 years of diabetes duration in the Berlin Retinopathy Study [18] (fig. 1). Although this rate was slightly lower in two other studies [19, 20], it is generally well accepted that all patients with diabetes will develop minimal retinopathy after more than 20 years of diabetes duration. While microaneurysms are initially hypercellular and perfused they may hyalinize and become occluded and are falsely thought to disappear. In a more advanced

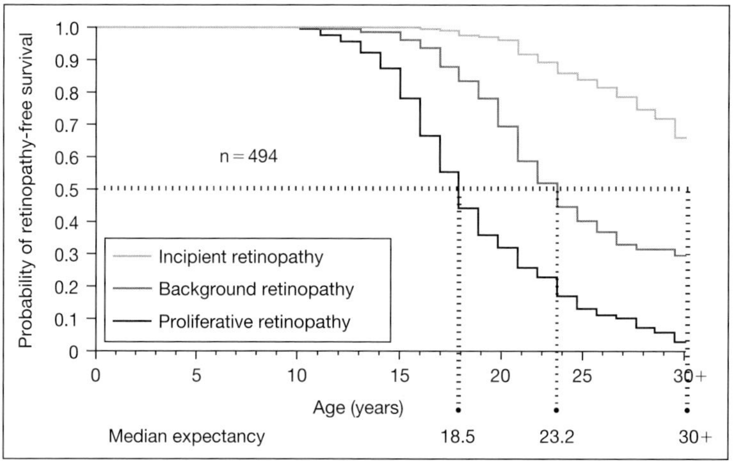


*Fig. 1.* Development of retinopathy in children and adolescents with diabetes detected by fluorescein angiography. Data from the Berlin Retinopathy study [11].

stage of retinopathy, the impairment of the blood-retinal barrier leads to the deposition of hard exudates (extracellular accumulation of lipids) and soft exudates ('cotton-wool spots', nerve fiber layer infarctions caused by obstruction of terminal retinal arterioles) and hemorrhages (fig. 2a, b). This stage is called background retinopathy and can be seen by fluorescein angiography on average after 14.6 (median age: 23.3) years. At this time retinal changes can also be seen by ophthalmoscopy although the diagnosis of background retinopathy by ophthalmoscopy is delayed (median expectancy: 21.1 years of diabetes) [11]. In a report of a cohort of well-controlled adolescents using mydriatic fundus photography, the median expectancy for mild nonproliferative retinopathy was found to be 16.6 years [21]. Thus, in comparing such data the method for retinal detection and the average glycemic control of the study population has to be taken into consideration.

Retinopathy may progress from this stage to vision-threatening proliferative retinopathy when the partial ischemia stimulates neovascularization (fig. 2c). These structurally and functionally deficient new vessels tend to rupture and lead to intraretinal and vitreous hemorrhages that eventually lead to loss of sight and tractional retinal detachment resulting in blindness. Vision-threatening proliferative retinopathy may develop in up to 70% of youth-onset patients after 30 years of diabetes [20]. After a latency period of approximately 5 years, the incidence rate of proliferative retinopathy rises steadily to a plateau of 0.3–0.4% new cases per year after 10–15 years of diabetes

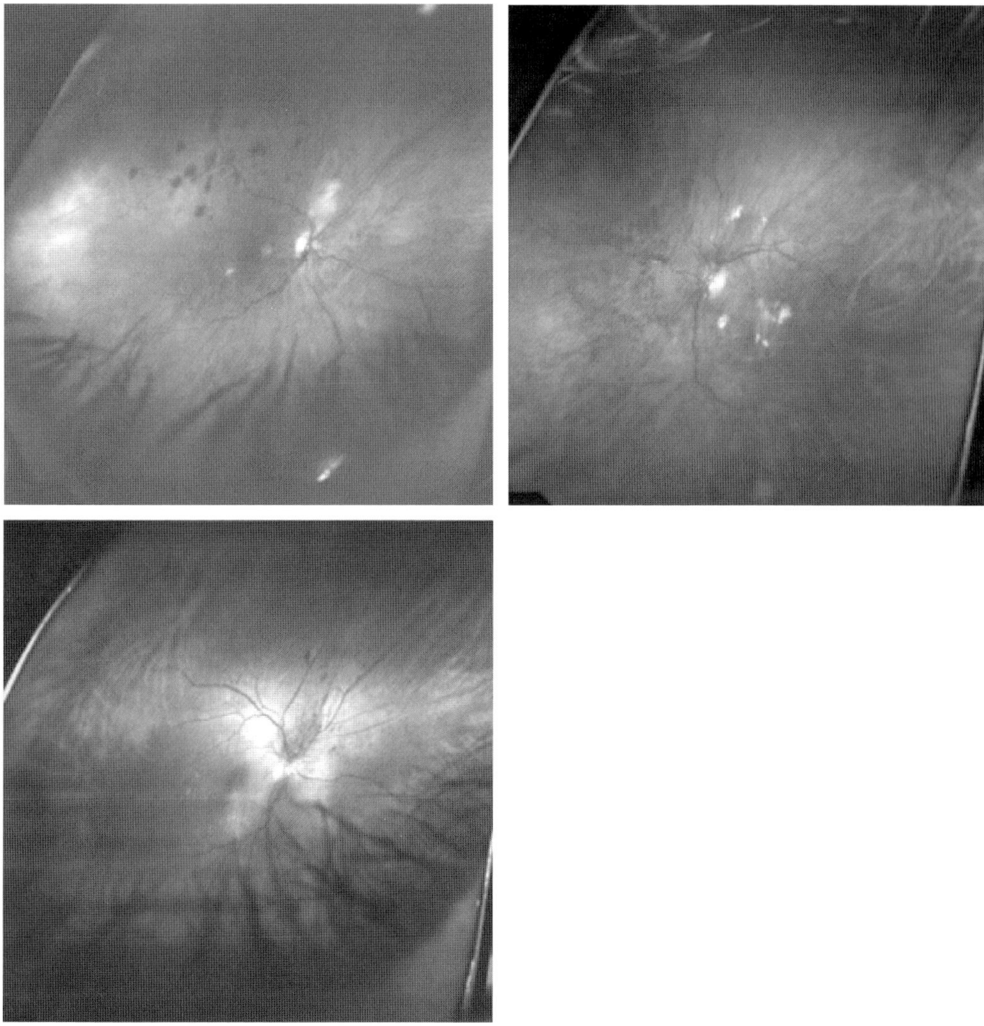

a b c

*Fig. 2.* Examples of diabetic retinopathy detected with non-mydriatic ultra-wide-field, laser-panoramic fundus photography (courtesy of D. Anderson, www.optos.com). *a* Nonproliferative diabetic retinopathy with venous occlusion and retinal bleeding. *b* Nonproliferative diabetic retinopathy with cotton-wool-spots and hard exudates. *c* Proliferative diabetic retinopathy with peripheral neovascularization.

and remains stable thereafter [22]. Although the prognosis has improved considerably in recent years due to the advances in laser therapy and vitroretinal surgery, early detection and treatment appears important to yield best results [23].

## Pathogenesis and Pathophysiology of Diabetic Retinopathy

Hyperglycemia is found to be the superior pathogenetic factor either for microangiopathy in general and consequently also for retinopathy. The pathogenetic concepts by which high glucose leads to retinal changes include genetic conditions like variants of the glycoprotein 1a subunit of the platelet-collagen receptor (C807T, Glu 505 Lys) leading to a more serious risk to reach advanced stages of retinopathy after a long diabetes duration [24] as well as metabolic concepts such as activation of the polyol pathway [25], activation of protein-kinase C through de novo synthesis of diacylglycerol [26], nonenzymatic glycation and formation of advanced glycation end-products (AGEs) [27] as well as increased oxidative stress [28] and induction of interleukin-6 release [29, 30]. The measurement of urinary 8-OhdG is a biomarker that indicates the level of oxidative stress and correlates to the incidence and severity of diabetic retinopathy; nevertheless, it is still an experimental laboratory assessment [31]. As a parameter for the destabilized control over cell growth regulation mechanisms, the so-called somatostatin-like immunoreactivity is reduced [32].

While inhibition of the polyol pathway by means of an aldose reductase inhibitor was successful in preventing basement membrane thickening in galactosemic animals [33], studies in human diabetes have not been successful so far [34]. Treatment with oral inhibitors of the beta-isoform of protein kinase C has been successful to suppress the growth factor-induced increased retinal permeability [35, 36]. Regarding the well-known additional adverse effects of dyslipidemia like alteration of the coagulation-fibrinolytic system, changes in membrane permeability, damage to endothelial cells and increased atherosclerosis [37], the use of pyridoxamine was found to have membrane-stabilizing lipid-lowering effects [38]. Similarly, treatment of diabetic animals with aminoguanidine, an inhibitor of AGE formation, prevented the accumulation of retinal changes of the AGE [39]. Successful human studies with both compounds have not yet been reported and recent approaches aim more at direct inhibition of the receptors for AGEs (RAGE) or reducing increased oxidative stress induced by AGE formation [40, 41]. Lately, the various mechanisms leading to diabetic angiopathy were joined into one unifying hypothesis by Brownlee [42]. All seem to reflect a single hyperglycemia-induced process of overproduction of superoxide by the mitochondrial electron-transport chain. Three of the major biochemical pathways implicated in the pathogenesis of hyperglycemia-induced vascular damage (the hexosamine pathway, the advanced glycation end-product (AGE) formation pathway and the diacylglycerol (DAG)-protein kinase C (PKC) pathway) are activated by increased availability of the glycolytic metabolites glyceraldehyde-3-phosphate and fructose-6-phosphate.

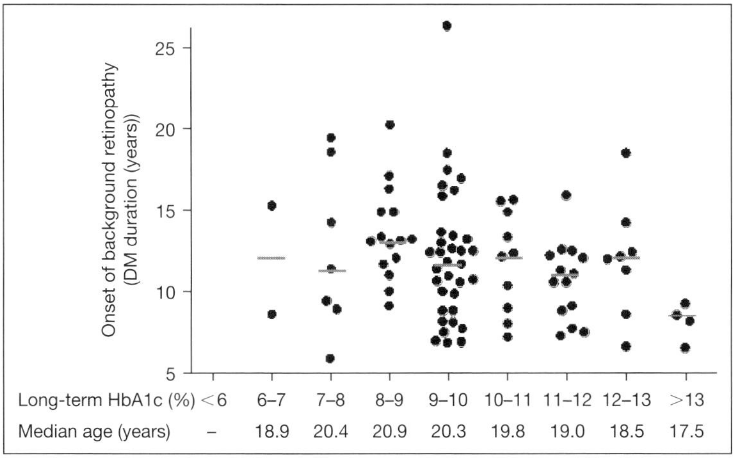


***Fig. 3.*** Presence of background retinopathy despite good long-term glycemic control. Data from the Berlin Retinopathy Study [45].

In experimental diabetic retinopathy, the lipid-soluble thiamine derivative benfotiamine can inhibit these three pathways, as well as hyperglycemia-associated NF-κB activation, by activating the pentose phosphate pathway enzyme transketolase, which converts glyceraldehyde-3-phosphate and fructose-6-phosphate into pentose-5-phosphates and other sugars [43].

Of particular interest is that the retinal removal systems for AGEs appear to be saturable and a threshold of glycemia exists above which a sharp increase in retinal AGE formation is observed [44]. In the Berlin Retinopathy Study (fig. 3) [45], the presence of a threshold HbA1c level (long-term, i.e. from diabetes onset until this analysis) at 9% corresponds approximately to 8.1% of the DCCT [46] for the development of background retinopathy in adolescents. Although the possibility of a threshold model is supported by some other studies [47–49] even the most recent additional analyses from the DCCT group argued against its presence [50]. Nevertheless, the nonlinear relationship between complications and long-term HbA1c indicates that the magnitude of the absolute risk reduction declines exponentially with decreasing HbA1c (fig. 4).

The concomitant findings of increased capillary leakage and focal endothelial cell proliferation as hallmarks of early diabetic retinopathy indicated that these mechanisms could be induced by a growth factor that is able to regulate both [51]. Indeed, the vascular endothelial growth factor (VEGF) is induced by ischemia and has been found in increased concentrations in the ocular fluid probably mediating active intraocular neovascularization [52]. Both AGEs [53] and reactive oxygen intermediates [54] are able to induce

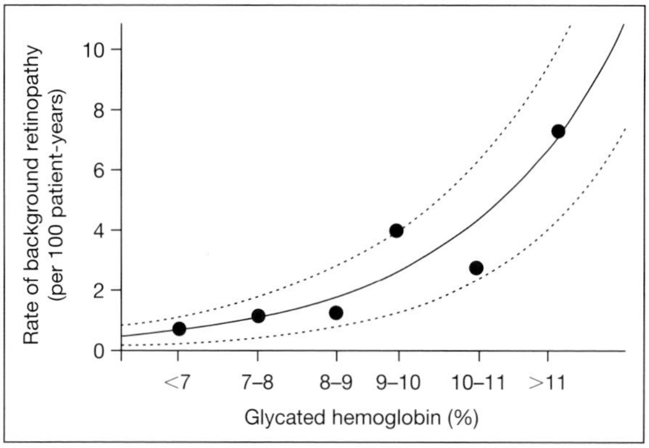


*Fig. 4.* Exponential relationship between level of glycated hemoglobin and incidence of retinopathy [45].

VEGF in endothelial cells and there is evidence that many of the effects of AGEs are actually mediated by increased oxidative stress [55]. Thus, an insufficient antioxidative defence leading to increased growth factor expression may be a common endpoint of the various mechanisms leading to diabetic retinopathy. However, the effect of antioxidants on the development of experimental diabetic retinopathy has been disappointing so far [56, 57].

Regarding the pharmacological treatment of retinopathy supplementing the best possible glycemic control, two studies primarily aimed at the improvement of nephropathy led to novel therapeutic approaches. Danaproid sodium as a mixture of sulfated glycosaminoglycans consisting mainly of heparan sulfate was presumed to have improving effects on nonproliferative retinal findings [58, 59] and the treatment was said to may be worth considering for foveal edema and hard exudates in diabetic maculopathy.

The EUCLID study [60] was designed to investigate the effects of ACE inhibitors on normotensive patients with type 1 diabetes normo- and microalbuminuria. The effect of lisinopril on diabetic retinopathy was studied in a subset of 354 patients (aged 20–59 years) in whom retinal photographs were obtained at baseline and at 24 months [61]. The placebo group had a slightly higher prevalence of retinopathy at baseline (65 vs. 59%, $p = 0.20$) and significantly poorer glycemic control (HbA1c: 7.3 vs. 6.9%, $p = 0.05$). Retinopathy progressed by at least one level in 21 of 159 (13.2%) patients on lisinopril and 39 of 166 (23.4%) on placebo giving an odds ratio after adjustment for center and glycemic control of 0.55 [0.30–1.03] ($p = 0.06$). Lisinopril was associated with a delayed progression to proliferative retinopathy (0.18 [0.04–0.82], $p = 0.03$). The authors suggest that ACE inhibition may decrease retinopathy progression in nonhypertensive patients who have type 1 diabetes with little or no nephropathy, but stated that their assumption needs to be confirmed before using the therapy in clinical practice.

### Practical Advice for the Detection of Retinopathy

The Consensus Guidelines from ISPAD (www.ispad.org) recommend that retinal examinations should always be performed in mydriasis and more elaborate diagnostic procedures with photographic documentation (conventional fundus photography or fluorescein angiography) should be pursued when even minimal retinal changes are apparent by fundoscopy. This photographic documentation may also be important as a measure of quality control. Several methods for classification have been developed for the conventional fundus photography that covers approximately only 30–60° of the peripheral retina [62–64] and controversy also exists on the number of visual fields that are necessary for classification [65]. Nevertheless, one has to be aware of a high intra- and interobserver variability [66]. Non-mydriatic fundus photography has been proposed as a simple and cost-efficient way to screen for diabetes-related eye disease, but interpretation of results are often difficult and reflexes and other artefacts resulting in photographs of unacceptable quality are particular frequent in adolescents [67]. Fluorescein angiography allows not only studying the structural changes with a high reproducibility, but also gives information on functional abnormalities such as fluorescein leakages [1]. Recently, a new technique has been invented to simplify and optimize the retinal screening: non-mydriatic ultra-wide-field, laser-panoramic fundus photography offers a handsome, quick and easily performable method to obtain digital pictures covering 200° of the peripheral retina without the need of mydriasis by scanning two different layers of the retina with two lasers of distinct wavelengths, that even can be sent to an external ophthalmologist (www.optos.com) (fig. 2a–c). The opportunity to perform the retinal screening at the diabetologists office could be an advantage with regard to the still unacceptable low rate of annually performed eye examinations in eligible patients [68] and ameliorates the documentation for follow-up investigations; whether the technique is superior to the conventional screening methods or not has still to be proven in clinical trials. The hitherto existing minimal recommended standard is a stereoscopic slit-lamp biomicroscopic examination by an experienced ophthalmologist, because outstanding experience is needed to correctly identify those early changes. Thus, it is strongly recommended that each pediatric diabetes centre should seek collaboration with an ophthalmologist demonstrating special interest in pediatric diabetes patients. This leads to the following recommendations [69] for the onset of periodic retinal examinations, as no clinically relevant changes were found before: after 5 years of diabetes duration in patients with prepubertal onset, but not before 11 years of age, and above age 15 in all others. Although minimal retinal changes can already be observed in prepubertal children [7], the youngest children to have developed preproliferative retinopathy was an 11-year-old boy in pubertal Tanner stage 2 and a 13-year-old girl (Tanner 3) in the Swedish study. This is in agreement with the results from a Swedish survey [7]. The youngest age at which proliferative changes were observed was age 17 in the Berlin study and age 21 in the Swedish survey. One has to bear in mind that for children who had no permanent access to standard medical care (for example due to insufficient insulin availability), an earlier examination may be advisable. In addition, an initial eye examination at onset may be recommended to rule out concomitant eye disease [70].

### Risk Factors for Retinopathy

Glycated hemoglobin is presently the best parameter to extrapolate the individuals risk for the development of late complications [71]. An analysis of the adolescent subgroup of the DCCT cohort [72] showed a reduction of the risk to develop retinopathy by 53% following intensified treatment and care and achieving better glycemic control compared to subjects on routine care. The risk of progression of pre-existing retinal changes was reduced by 70% [71, 73]. In an ongoing trial that investigates the feasibility of non-mydriatic ultra-wide-field, laser-panoramic fundus photography, the first results seem to indicate a decrease in the incidence of retinopathy in diabetic children and adolescents [unpubl. data]. Possibly these findings could be related to the continuing efforts to achieve the best possible metabolic control showing lower HbA1c during the last years. However, additional factors are likely to modify the individual child's risk to develop microangiopathy [74] (fig. 4).

The first evidence for the importance of pubertal hormones for the development of late complications resulted from the virtual absence of severe fundus changes in growth hormone-deficient patients with type 1 diabetes [75, 76]. An influence of sex steroids on neovascularization could also be demonstrated in animal experiments [77]. Furthermore, as described above, clinically relevant retinal changes or diabetes-related microproteinuria are rarely found before puberty [78, 79] and it was suggested that the prepubertal duration of diabetes might be of little importance for the later development of retinopathy [80]. This observation has not been substantiated in other studies [11, 21, 81, 82, 83], but there was some evidence that children who manifested their diabetes before the age of 5 years possibly do have protective factors [84]. However, in agreement with other studies [85–87] puberty led to an acceleration of retinal changes in the Berlin Retinopathy Study [11].

Other studies have demonstrated that the presence of high-normal diastolic blood pressure results in a higher incidence of retinopathy [88, 89]. Therefore, tracking of blood pressure measurements is important to closely follow patients who exhibit a blood pressure rise above their previous level.

Abnormal lipid profiles have been found to be related to the development of retinopathy also in young patients with type I diabetes [90]. In long-standing childhood-onset diabetes progression of retinopathy was associated with higher triglyceride and LDL-cholesterol levels [91]. Little information is available in pediatric patients. The Berlin Retinopathy Study found some evidence for the contribution of elevated triglycerides [92] and lower HDL-cholesterol levels [90] in adolescents developing retinopathy. The diagnostic relevance of lipoprotein(a) and other lipid markers is controversial at this time [93].

There is some evidence elucidated by the DCCT that severe retinopathy is also determined by familial factors [94], possibly mediated by an association of microangiopathy with one of the genes that are associated with the development of type I diabetes, i.e. for the HLA-DR4 region [95], or being caused by a relationship to genes regulating major factors influencing the development of angiopathy such as arterial hypertension. However, presently none of the genetic markers has proven to be clinically useful in identifying high risk patients sufficiently. Cigarette smoking has been demonstrated as an important independent variable for the development and progression of retinopathy [96] in adults with diabetes. Although there is evidence that addictive behavior may be less frequent in adolescents with diabetes than in their peers [97], tobacco consumption is prevalent in a substantial number of young adults with diabetes [98] and should be addressed and discouraged as early as possible.

In conclusion, it should be stressed that the diabetic retinopathy is still a frequent complication also in pediatric patients despite the current efforts improving glycaemic control from the onset of the disease. As an effective treatment of diabetic retinopathy is not yet available, any effort to prevent the development of retinopathy through improved glycemic control is of utmost importance.

## References

1 Danne T, Kordonouri O, Enders I, Hövener G: Monitoring for retinopathy in children and adolescents with type 1 diabetes. Acta paediatrica 1998;87(suppl 425):35–41.

2 Larsson Y, Lichtenstein A, Ploman KG: Degenerative vascular complications in juvenile diabetes treated with a free diet. Diabetes 1953;1:449–458.

3 Lestradet H, Papoz L, de Menibus CH, Levasseur, Besse J, Billaud L, Battistelli F, Tric P, Lestradet F: Long-term study of mortality and vascular complications in juvenile-onset (type I) diabetes. Diabetes 1981;30:175–179.
4 Palmberg P, Smith M, Waltmann S, Krupin T, Singer P, Burgess D, Wendtlant T, Achtenberg J, Cryer P, Santiago J, White N, Kilo C, Daughaday W. The natural history of retinopathy in juvenile onset diabetes. Ophthalmology 1981;88:613–618.
5 Frank RN, Hoffman WH, Podgor MJ, Joondeph HC, Lewis RA, Margherio M, Nachazel DP, Weiss H, Christopherson KW, Cronin MA: Retinopathy in juvenile onset diabetes mellitus of short duration. Diabetes 1982;31:874–882.
6 Klein R, Klein BE, Moss SE, Davis MD, De Mets DL: Retinopathy in young-onset diabetic patients. Diabetes Care 1984;8:311–315.
7 Joner G, Brinchmannn-Hansen O, Torres CG, Hanssen KF. A nationwide cross-sectional study of retinopathy and microalbuminuria in young Norwegian type 1 (insulin-dependent) diabetic patients. Diabetologia 1992;35:1049–54.
8 Kernell A, Dedorsson I, Johansson B, Wickström CP, Ludvigsson J, Tuvemo T, et al: Prevalence of diabetic retinopathy in children and adolescents with IDDM. Diabetologia 1997;40:307–310.
9 Hayward LM, Burden ML, Burden AC, Blackledge H, Raymond NT, Botha JL, et al.: What is the prevalence of visual impairment in the general and diabetic population: Are there ethnic and gender differences? Diabet Med 2002;19:27–34.
10 Cutfield W: Screening for retinopathy in childhood: Do the ayes have it? J Pediatr 1998;132: 760–761.
11 Danne T, Kordonouri O, Hövener G, Weber B. Diabetic angiopathy in children. Diab Med 1997;14:1012–25.
12 Ernest JT, Goldstick TK, Engermann RL: Hyperglycemia impairs retinal oxygen autoregulation in normal and diabetic dogs. Invest Ophthalmol Visc Sci 1983;24:985–989.
13 Grunwald JE, Bruckner AJ, Schwartz SS, Braunstein SN, Baker L, Petrig BL, Riva CE: Diabetic glycemic control and retinal blood flow. Diabetes 1990;39:602–607.
14 Mizutani M, Kern TS, Lorenzi M: Accelerated death of retinal microavascular cells in human and experimental diabetic retinopathy. J Clin Invest 1996;97:2883–2890.
15 Mizutani M, Gerhardinger C, Lorenzi M: Muller cell changes in human diabetic retinopathy. Diabetes 1988;47:445–449.
16 Tang J, Mohr S, Du Y-P, Kern TS: Non-uniform distribution of lesions and biochemical abnormalities within the retina of diabetic humans. Curr Eye Res 2003;27:7–13.
17 Kern TS, Engermann RL: Vascular lesions distribute non-uniformly within the retina. Exp Eye Res 1990;60:545–549.
18 Burger W, Hövener G, Düsterhus R, Hartmann R, Weber B: Prevalence and development of retinopathy in children and adolescents with diabetes mellitus. A longitudinal study. Diabetologia 1986;29:17–22.
19 Klein R, Klein BEK, Moss SE, Davis MD, DeMets DL: The Wisconsin Epidemiologic Study of diabetic retinopathy. II. Prevalence and risk of diabetic retinopathy when age at diagnosis is less than 30 years. Arch Ophthalmol 1984;102:520–526.
20 Orchard TJ, Dorman JS, Maser RE, Becker DJ, Drash AL, Ellis D, LaPorte RE, Kuller LH: Prevalence of complications in IDDM by sex and duration. Pittsburgh Epidemiology of Diabetes Complications Study II. Diabetes 1990;39:1116–1124.
21 Holl RW, Lang GE, Grabert M, Heinze E, Lang GK, Debatin KM: Diabetic retinopathy in pediatric patients with type 1 diabetes: Effects of diabetes duration, prepubertal and pubertal onset of diabetes, and metabolic control. J Pediatr 1998;132:790–794.
22 Krolewski AS, Warram JH, Christlieb AR, Busick EJ, Kahn CR: Risk of proliferative diabetic retinopathy in juvenile-onset type I diabetes. A 40 year follow up study. Diabetes Care 1986;9: 443–452.
23 Early Treatment Diabetic Retinopathy Study Group: Early photocoagulation for diabetic retinopathy. ETDRS report number 9. Ophthalmology 1991;98:766–785.
24 Reiner AP, Agardh E, Teramura G, Gaur P, Gaur LK, Agardh C-D: Diabetes duration may modify the association between genetic variation in the glycoprotein Ia subunit of the platelet collagen receptor and risk of severe diabetic retinopathy: A working hypothesis. Thromb Haemost 2003;89:142–148.

25 Kinoshita JH, Nishimura C: The involvement of aldose reductase in diabetic complications. Diab Metab Rev 1988;4:323–337.
26 Koya D, King GL: Protein kinase C activation and the development of diabetic complications. Diabetes 1998;47:859–866.
27 Brownlee M: Glycation and diabetic complications. Diabetes 1994;43:836–841.
28 Baynes JW: Role of oxidative stress in development of complications in diabetes. Diabetes 1991;40:405–412.
29 Nakamura N, Hasegawa G, Obayashi H, Yamazaki M, Ogata M, Nakano K, et al: Increased concentration of pentosidine, an advanced glycation end product, and interleukin-6 in the vitreous of patients with proliferative diabetic retinopathy. Diabetes Res Clin Pract 2003;61:93–101.
30 Funatsu H, Yamashita H, Noma H, Mimura T, Yamashita T, Hori S: Increased levels of vascular endothelial growth factor and interleukin-6 in the aqueous humor of diabetics with macular edema. Am J Ophthalmol 2002;133:70–77.
31 Wu LL, Chiou C-C, Chang P-Y, Wu JT: Urinary 8-OhdG: A marker of oxidative stress to DANN and a risk factor for cancer, atherosclerosis and diabetics. Clin Chim Acta 2004;339:1–9.
32 Simo R, Lecube A, Sararols L, Garcia-Arumi J, Segura RM, Casamitsana R, et al: Deficit of somatostatin-like immunoreactivity in the vitreous fluid of diabetic patients possible role in the development of proliferative retinopathy 81. Diabetes Care 2002;25:2282–2286.
33 Robinson WG, Kador PF, Kinoshita JH: Retinal capillaries: Basement membrane thickening by galactosemia prevented with aldose reductase inhibitor. Science 1983;221:1177–1179.
34 Sorbinil Retinopathy Trial Research Group: A randomized trial of Sorbinil, an aldose reductase inhibitor in diabetic retinopathy. Arch Ophthalmol 1990;108:1234–1244.
35 Ishii H, Jirousek MR, Koya D, Takagi C, Xia P, Clermont A, Bursell SE, Kern TS, Ballas LM, Heath WF, Stramm LE, Feener EP, King GL. Amelioration of vascular dysfunctions in diabetic rats by an oral PKC beta inhibitor. Science 1996;272:728–731.
36 Aiello LP, Bursell SE, Clermont A, Duh E, Ishii H, Takagi C, Mori F, Ciulla TA, Ways K, Jrousek M, Smith LE, King GL: Vascular endothelial growth factor-induced retinal permeability is mediated by protein kinase C in vivo and suppressed by an orally effective beta-isoform selective inhibitor. Diabetes 1997;46:1473–1480.
37 Misra A, Kumar S, Vikram NK, Kumar A: The role of lipids in the development of diabetes microvascular complications: Implications for therapy. Am J Cardiovasc Drugs 2003;3:325–338.
38 Metz TO, Alderson NL, Thorpe SR, Baynes JN: Pyridoxamine, an inhibitor of advanced glycation and lipoxidation reactions: A novel therapy for treatment of diabetic complications. Arch Biochem Biophys 2003;419:41–49.
39 Hammes HP, Martin S, Federlin K, Geisen K, Brownlee M: Aminoguanidine treatment inhibits the development of experimental diabetic retinopathy. Proc Natl Acad Sci USA 1991;88: 11555–11558.
40 Bierhaus A, Ziegler R, Nawroth PP: Molecular mechanisms of diabetic angiopathy – clues for innovative therapeutic interventions. Horm Res 1998;50(suppl 1):1–5.
41 Mendez JD: Advanced glycation end product and chronic complication of diabetes mellitus. Gac Med Mex 2003;139:49–55.
42 Brownlee M: Biochemistry and molecular cell biology of diabetic complications. Nature 2001;414:813–820.
43 Hammes HP, Du X, Edelstein D, Taguchi T, Matsumura T, Ju Q, Lin J, Bierhaus A, Nawroth P, Hannak D, Neumaier M, Bergfeld R, Giardino I, Brownlee M: Benfotiamine blocks three major pathways of hyperglycemic damage and prevents experimental diabetic retinopathy. Nat Med 2003;9:294–299.
44 Hammes HP, Wellensiek B, Klöting I, Sickel L, Bretzel RG, Brownlee M: The relationship of glycaemic level to advanced glycation end-product (AGE) accumulation and retinal pathology in the spontaneous diabetic hamster. Diabetologia 1998;41:165–170.
45 Danne T, Weber B, Hartmann R, Enders I, Burger W, Hövener G: Long-term glycaemic control has a nonlinear association to the frequency of background retinopathy in adolescents with type I diabetes. Follow-up of the Berlin Retinopathy Study. Diabetes Care 1994;17:1390–1396.
46 Danne Th, Weber B, Dinesen B, Mortensen HB: Threshold of HbA1c for the effect of hyperglycemia on the risk of diabetic microangiopathy (letter). Diabetes Care 1996;19:183.

47 Krolewski AS, Laffel LMB, Krolewski M, Quinn M, Warram JH: Glycosylated haemoglobin and the risk of microalbuminuria in patients with insulin-dependent diabetes mellitus. N Engl J Med 1995;332:1251–1255.
48 Mathiesen ER, Ronn B, Strom B, Foght V, Deckert T: The natural course of microalbuminuria in insulin-dependent diabetes: A ten year prospective study. Diab Med 1995;12:482–487.
49 Nagaraj RH, Kern TS, Sell DB, Fogarty J, Engerman RL, Monnier VM: Evidence of a glycaemic threshold for the formation of pentosidine in diabetic dog lens but not in collagen. Diabetes 1996;45:587–594.
50 DCCT Research Group: The absence of a glycemic threshold for the development of long-term complications: The perspective of the Diabetes Control and Complications Trial. Diabetes 1996; 45:1289–1298.
51 Leung DW, Cachianes G, Kuang WJ, Goedel DV, Ferrara N: Vascular endothelial growth factor is a secreted angiogenic mitogen. Science 1989;246:1306–1309.
52 Aiello LP, Avery RL, Arrigg PG, Keyt BA, Jampel HD, Shah ST, Pasquale LR, Thieme H, Iwamoto MA, Park JE, et al: Vascular endothelial growth factor in ocular fluid of patients with diabetic retinopathy and other retinal disorders. N Engl J Med 1994;331:1480–1487.
53 Lu M, Kuroki M, Amano S, Tolentino M, Keough K, Kim I, Bucala R, Adamis AP: Advanced glycation end-products increase retinal vascular endothelial growth factor expression. J Clin Invest 1998;101:1219–1224.
54 Kuroki M, Voest EE, Amano S: Reactive oxygen intermediates increase vascular endothelial growth factor expression in vitro and in vivo. J Clin Invest 1996;98:1667–1675.
55 Giardino I, Edelstein D, Brownlee M: BCL-2 expression or antioxidants prevent hyperglycemia-induced formation of intracellular advanced glycation end-products in bovine endothelial cells. J Clin Invest 1996;97:1422–1428.
56 Hammes HP, Bartmann A, Engel L, Wülfroth P: Antioxidant treatment of experimental daibetic retinopathy with nicartine. Diabetologia 1997;40:629–634.
57 Kern TS, Kowrulu RA, Engermann R: Effects of antioxidants on the development of retinopathy in diabetes and galactosemia. Invest Ophthalmol Vis Sci 1996;37:S970.
58 van der Pijl JW, van der Woude FJ, Geelhoed-Duijvestijn PH, Frohlich M, van der Meer FJ, Lemkes HH, van Es LA: Danaparoid sodium lowers proteinuria in diabetic nephropathy. J Am Soc Nephrol 1997;8:456–462.
59 van der Pijl, van der Woude FJ, Swart W, van ES LA, Lemkes HH: Effect of danaparoid sodium on hard exsudates in diabetic retinopathy. Lancet 1997;350:1743–1745.
60 The EUCLID Study Group: Randomized placebo-controlled trial of lisinopril in normotensive patients with insulin dependent diabetes and normoalbuminuria and microalbuminuria. Lancet 1997;349:1787–1792.
61 Chaturvedi N, Sjolie AK, Stephenson JM, Abrahamian H, Keipes M, Castellarin A, Rogulja-Pepeonik Z, Fuller JH: Effects of lisinopril on progression of retinopathy in normotensive people with type 1 diabetes. Lancet 1998;351:28–31.
62 Early Treatment of Diabetic Retinopathy Study Research Group: Grading diabetic retinopathy from stereoscopic colour fundus photographs – an extension of the modified Airlie House classification. ETDRS report number 10. Ophthalmology 1991;98:786–806.
63 Klein R, Klein BE, Magli YL, Brothers RJ, Meuer SM, Moss SE, et al: An alternative method of grading diabetic retinopathy. Ophthalmology 1986;93:1183–1187.
64 Aldington SJ, Kohner EM, Meuer S, Klein R, Sjolie AK. Methodology for retinal photography and assessment of diabetic retinopathy: The EURODIAB IDDM complications study. Diabetologia 1995;38:437–444.
65 Moss SE, Meuer SM, Klein R, Hubbard LD, Brothers RJ, Klein SE: Are seven standard photographic fields necessary for classification of diabetic retinopathy? Invest Ophthalmol Vis Sci 1989;30:823–828.
66 Milton RC, Ganley JP, Lynk RH: Variability in grading diabetic retinopathy from stereo fundus photographs: comparison of physician and lay readers. Br J Ophthalmol 1977;61:192–201.
67 Buxton MJ, Sculpher MJ, Ferguson BA, Humphreys JE, Altman JF, Spiegelhalter DJ, Kirby AJ, Jacob JS, Bacon H, Dubridge SB, et al: Screening for treatable diabetic retinopathy: A comparison of different methods. Diabet Med 1991;8:371–377.

68 Massin P: Screening for diabetic retinopathy. Sang Thrombose Vaisseaux 2003;15:249–255.
69 Laron Z (ed): ISPAD, IDF, WHO (European Region). Consensus Guidelines for the Management of Insulin-Dependent (Type 1) Diabetes mellitus (IDDM) in Childhood and Adolescence. Tel Aviv, Freud Publishing House, 1995.
70 Lang-Muritano M, La Roche GR, Stevens JL, Gloor BR, Schoenle EJ: Acute cataracts in newly diagnosed IDDM in five children and adolescents. Diab Care 1995;18:1395–1396.
71 DCCT Research Group: The effect of intensive treatment of diabetes on the development and progression of long-term complications in insulin-dependent diabetes mellitus. N Engl J Med 1993;329:977–986.
72 DCCT Research Group: Effect of intensive diabetes treatment on the development and progression of long-term complications in adolescents with insulin-dependent diabetes mellitus: Diabetes Control and Complications Trial. J Pediatr 1994;125:177–188.
73 The Diabetes Control and Complications Trial: The effect of intensive diabetes treatment on the progression of diabetic retinopathy in insulin-dependent diabetes mellitus. Arch Ophthalmol 1995;113:36–51.
74 Kovacs M, Mukerji P, Drash A, Iyengar S: Biomedical and psychiatric risk factors for retinopathy among children with IDDM. Diabetes Care 1995;18:1592–1599.
75 Merimee TJ: A follow-up study of vascular disease in growth-hormone-deficient dwarfs with diabetes. N Engl J Med 1978;298:1217–1222.
76 Alzaid AA, Dinneen SF, Melton LJ, Rizza RA: The role of growth hormone in the development of diabetic angiopathy. Diabetes Care 1994;17:531–534.
77 Williamson JR, Rowold E, Chang K, Marvel J, Tomlinson M, Sherman WR, Ackermann KE, Berger RA, Kilo C: Sex steroid dependency of diabetes-induced changes in polyol metabolism, vascular permeability, and collagen cross-linking. Diabetes 1986;35:20–27.
78 Rogers DG, White NH, Shalwitz RA, Palmberg P, Smith ME, Santiago JV: The effect of puberty on the development of early diabetic microvascular disease in insulin-dependent diabetes. Diab Res Clin Pract 1987;3:39–44.
79 Murphy RP, Nanda M, Plotnick L, Enger C, Vitale S, Patz A: The relationship of puberty to diabetic retinopathy. Arch Ophthalmol 1990;108:215–218.
80 Kostraba JN, Dorman JS, Orchard TJ, Becker DJ, Ohki Y, Ellis D, Doft BH, Lobes LA, LaPorte RE, Drash AL: Contribution of diabetes duration before puberty to development of microvascular complications in IDDM subjects. Diabetes Care 1989;12:686–693.
81 McNally PG, Raymond NT, Swift PGF, Hearnshaw JR, Burden AC: Does the prepubertal duration of diabetes influence the onset of microvascular complications? Diab Med 1993;10:905–905.
82 Algvere P: Prepubertal diabetes duration increases the risk of retinopathy. Acta Paediatr 1994;83:341.
83 Burger W, Hartmann R, Hövener G, Danne Th, Weber B: Realistic objectives and rational approaches to the treatment of children and adolescents with diabetes aiming at the prevention of secondary complications; in Weber B, Burger W, Danne Th (eds): Structural and Functional Abnormalities in Subclinical Diabetic Angiopathy. Pediatr Adolesc Endocr. Basel, Karger, 1992, vol 22, pp 210–219.
84 Donaghue KC, Fairchild JM, Craig ME, Chan AK, Hing S, Cutler LR, et al: Do all prepubertal years of diabetes duration contribute equally to diabetes complications? Diabetes Care 2003;26:1224–1229.
85 Bonney M, Hing SJ, Fung AT, Stephens MM, Fairchild JM, Donaghue KC, Howard NJ, Silink M: Development and progression of diabetic retinopathy. Adolescents at risk. Diab Med 1995;12: 967–973.
86 Klein BEK, Moss SE, Klein R: Is menarchy associated with retinopathy? Diab Care 1990;13:1034–1038.
87 Goldstein DE, Blinder KJ, Ide CH, Wilson RJ, Wiedmeyer HM, Little RR, England JD, Eddy M, Hewett JE, Anderson SK: Glycaemic control and development of retinopathy in youth-onset insulin-dependent diabetes mellitus. Ophthalmology 1993;100:1125–1132.
88 Chase HP, Garg SK, Jackson WE, Thomas MA, Harris S, Marshall G, Crews MJ: Blood pressure and retinopathy in type I diabetes. Ophthalmology 1990;97:155–159.
89 Klein BE, Klein R, Moss SE, Palta M. A cohort study of the relationship of diabetic retinopathy to blood pressure. Am J Epidemiol 1983;118:228–238.

90 Kordonouri O, Danne Th, Hopfenmüller W, Enders I, Hövener G, Weber B: Lipid profiles and blood pressure: Are they risk factors for the developemt of early background retinopathy and incipient nephropathy in children with insulin-dependent diabetes mellitus? Acta Paediatr 1996;85:43–48.
91 Lloyd CE, Klein R, Maser RE, Kuller LH, Becker DJ, Orchard TJ: The progression of retinopathy over 2 years: The Pittsburgh Epidemiology of Diabetes Complications (EDC) Study. J Diab Compl 1995;9:140–148.
92 Weber B, Burger W, Hartmann R, Hövener G, Malchus R, Oberdisse U: Risk faktors for the development of retinopathy in children and adolescents with type I (insulin-dependent) diabetes. Diabetologia 1986;29:23–29.
93 Willems D, Dorchy H, Dufrasne D: Serum lipoprotein (a) in type I diabetic children and adolescents: Relationships with HbA1c and subclinical complications. Eur J Pediatr 1996;155:175–178.
94 The Diabetes Control and Complications Study Group: Clustering of long-term complications in families with diabetes in the diabetes control and complications trial. Diabetes 1997;46:1829–1839.
95 Cruickshanks KJ, Vadheim CM, Moss SE, Roth MP, Riley WJ, Mclaren NK, Langfield D, Sparkes RS, Klein R, Rotter JI: Genetic marker associations with proliferative retinopathy in persons diagnosed with diabetes before 30 years of age. Diabetes 1992;41:879–885.
96 Marshall G, Garg SK, Jackson WE, Holmes DL, Chase HP: Factors influencing the onset and progression of diabetic retinopathy in subjects with insulin-dependent diabetes mellitus. Ophthalmology 1993;100:1133–1139.
97 Glasgow AM, Tynan D, Schwartz R, Hicks JM, Turek J, Driscol C, O'Donell RM, Getson PR: Alcohol and drug use in teenagers with diabetes mellitus. J Adolesc Health 1991;12:11–14.
98 Masson EA, MacFarlane IA, Priestley CJ, Wallymahmed ME, Flavell HJ: Failure to prevent nicotine addiction in young people with diabetes. Arch Dis Child 1992;67:100–102.

Thomas Danne, MD
Kinderkrankenhaus auf der Bult
Janusz-Korczak-Allee 12, DE–30173 Hannover (Germany)
Tel. +49 511 8115 340, Fax +49 511 8115 344, E-Mail danne@hka.de

Chiarelli F, Dahl-Jørgensen K, Kiess W (eds): Diabetes in Childhood and Adolescence.
Pediatr Adolesc Med. Basel, Karger, 2005, vol 10, pp 329–346

# Complications and Consequences

*Thomas M. Kapellen, Angela Galler, Klemens Raile, Wieland Kiess*

Universitätsklinik und Poliklinik für Kinder und Jugendliche, Universität Leipzig, Leipzig, Germany

With modern diabetes management growth and development in children and adolescents with diabetes should be undistinguishable from those in healthy subjects. However, comorbidity including autoimmune disorders like autoimmune thyroiditis, adrenal insufficiency, celiac disease or eating disorders could lead to disturbance of growth and pubertal development. Such comorbidity could also have a negative impact on metabolic control. Awareness of these possible complications and monitoring therefore are mandatory for good clinical diabetes management.

## Growth and Development

Over the last decades the prognosis with regard to growth and pubertal development in children and adolescents with type 1 diabetes mellitus has improved considerably with better disease management. The introduction of frequent insulin injections, glucose monitoring and better caloric intake has achieved near-normal glucose levels. The latter is thought to be responsible for good growth perspectives in children with diabetes.

In 1930, Mauriac first described a condition of poorly controlled diabetes with short stature and hepatomegaly. Some of these patients could have been misdiagnosed as having celiac disease. Although Mauriac syndrome is fortunately rare, subtle abnormalities in growth and above normal weight gain are still frequently observed in children and adolescents with type 1 diabetes.

Published data on height at diagnosis and height development in children and adolescents with diabetes are quite controversial. Many data show an increased growth velocity before diabetes onset. Hypponen et al. [34] and the

Eurodiab Study group found increased height and early growth in children with type 1 diabetes before disease manifestation. There is no doubt that metabolic control affects height development. Children with prepubertal onset of diabetes had an even more pronounced loss of final height than patients with poor metabolic control but later onset of diabetes [31]. Other authors report on reduced final height, especially in girls, which is related to advanced bone age before puberty [4]. Puberty seems not to be delayed in some study populations [4] but has been reported to be late-normal in others [54].

Disturbances in the IGF-axis with lower IGF1 levels and IGFBP3 levels in diabetic children are obvious [74]. In contrast, both spontaneous and stimulated growth hormone secretion is elevated in pediatric and adolescent diabetics. This paradox can be explained by a reduced rate of hepatic growth hormone receptors reflected by low IGFBP 3 levels [20].

Major attention should be paid to weight development and body composition in patients with diabetes. Recent studies have reported greater BMI increase in adolescents with diabetes than in nondiabetic adolescents. This was shown especially in girls [14, 77].

### Thyroid Disease

The most frequent autoimmune disease in type 1 diabetes affects the thyroid. The etiology of autoimmunity in pancreas and thyroid is a T-cell-mediated disease and seems to be due to a common genetic susceptibility. Two immune-regulatory genes (HLA = human leukocyte antigen and CTLA-4 = cytotoxic T-lymphocyte-associated protein 4) contribute to the susceptibility for both diseases [47].

Positivity for thyroid autoantibodies in children with type 1 diabetes shows considerable variability in different countries. Incidence and prevalence numbers vary between 3 and 50% [10, 45, 65] compared to a suggested rate of 3–10% in nondiabetic children and adolescents [40, 50, 84]. The largest cohort analysis was published by Kordonouri et al. [45] reporting a rate of 21.6% of thyroid antibodies in a group of 7,097 children and adolescents with type 1 diabetes. In this study, patients with antibody positivity were older, had a longer duration of diabetes and had developed diabetes later in life. 63% of patients with positive thyroid antibodies were girls. Increasing rates of thyroid antibodies with age were also seen in adults [37].

The majority of patients with positive thyroid antibodies have normal thyroid function. Elevated TSH levels as a marker for subclinical hypothyroidism are found in about 15% in the antibody-positive patient group. Overt primary hypothyroidism due to autoimmune thyroiditis is seen in 3–5% of the patients [10, 23, 44]. Clinical findings of hypothyroidism like goiter, weight gain, fatigue, cold intolerance and bradycardia are rare because of screening for TSH and autoantibodies in patients with type 1 diabetes.

Since screening is both efficient and cost effective there is no longer any controversy about thyroid antibody screening in diabetic patients with type 1 diabetes. Screening is performed in our institution once a year. In case of significant antibody levels (especially thyroperoxidase antibodies), a longitudinal survey of diabetic children over 5 years showed a higher risk of later development of TSH elevation and subclinical or clinical hypothyroidism [44]. Therefore, in patients with elevated TPO/TGA antibodies thyroid function (TSH and free T4) should be measured routinely. Ultrasound of the thyroid gland could provide further information on the development of Hashimoto's disease with typical patterns like increased volume of the gland and areas of lower echogenicity within the thyroid. There is no consensus on the time point of introduction of treatment with thyroxin! In our opinion, only in the case of subclinical or clinical hypothyroidism or significant antibody levels plus ultrasound findings should treatment with thyroxin be introduced.

The impact of subclinical hypothyroidism on metabolic control in children and adolescents with type 1 diabetes mellitus was studied by Mohn et al. [55]. In this retrospective case-control study, 13 patients with subclinical hypothyroidism had significantly more symptomatic and severe hypoglycemic events during the 12 months prior to diagnosis. There was no difference in HbA1c, insulin requirement or growth between the two groups as in the cohort of Kordonouri et al. [45]. After introduction of thyroxin substitution, the rate of hypoglycemia decreased rapidly and after 6 months there was no longer any difference between the groups.

Hyperthyroidism is less common than hypothyroidism in association with diabetes but still more common than in the general population. There are less published data available with a frequency of subclinical disease in about 2–3% and overt hyperthyroidism or thyrotoxicosis in only a few patients [49, 67, 79]. Hyperthyroidism may be due to Grave's disease or the hyperthyroid phase of Hashimoto's thyroiditis, and should be considered if there is unexplained weight loss with normal appetite, agitation, sweating, tachycardia, tremor or unexplained problems with metabolic control.

There should be no difference in treatment strategies between patients with diabetes and the nondiabetic population. Therefore, antithyroid drugs still remain the initial treatment of choice. However, in the non-European countries (especially the US) radioactive iodine is used more frequently. There are no long-term safety data available until now and radioactive iodine has not been shown to be superior to antithyroid drug treatment at the moment.

***Table 1.*** Incidence, onset, genetics and clinical characteristics of polyendocrine autoimmune syndromes type I compared to type II (according to Dittmar and Kahaly [18])

| | Type I | Type II |
|---|---|---|
| Incidence | <1:100,000/year | 1–2/100,000/year |
| Male:female ratio | 3:4 | 1:3 |
| Age at onset | childhood, age 3–5 | adults 4th or 5th decade |
| Genetics | monogenic autosomal-recessive AIRE gene on chromosome 21 HLA-association | polygenic dominant inheritance chromosome 6 HLA-association |
| Concomitant disease | mucocutaneous candidiasis | none |
| Autoimmune endocrinopathies | hypoparathyroidism (80–85%)<br>Addison's disease (60–70%)<br>type 1 diabetes (<20%)<br>hypogonadism (12%)<br>thyroid disease (10%)<br>hypopituitarism (0–2%) | thyroid disease (70–75%)<br>type 1 diabetes (50–60%)<br>Addison's disease (40–50%)<br>hypoparathyroidism (0–5%) |
| Nonendocrine autoimmune diseases | vitiligo, alopecia areata, autoimmune gastritis, pernicious anemia, autoimmune hepatitis, Sjögrens syndrome, myasthenia gravis | |

## Other Endocrine Disorders

In addition to thyroid autoimmune diseases, diabetes is occasionally associated with Addison's disease (primary adrenal insufficiency). This rare condition has been described even in children [32]. Often a combination of Addison's disease, autoimmune thyroiditis or Graves' disease and type 1 diabetes is seen as a so-called polyglandular autoimmune syndrome (PAS). There are clinical, epidemiological and genetic differences between PAS type I (also known as autoimmune polyendocrinopathy, candidiasis and ectodermal dystrophy = APDEAC or MEDAC = multiple endocrine deficiency autoimmune candidiasis syndrome) and PAS type II (table 1).

Besides these major three components patients can develop vitiligo, hypogonadism and alopecia to variable degrees. In most patients (48%) type 1 diabetes is the first manifestation of PAS.

Addison's disease must be considered if unsuspected hypoglycemic episodes, especially in the early morning, are combined with decreasing insulin requirement. If a patient then shows clinical signs such as increased skin pigmentation, fatigue, weight loss or hyponatremia and hyperkalemia further diagnostics should be introduced.

High ACTH levels and anti-adrenal antibodies are argumentative for Addison's disease. However, up to 2% of all patients with type 1 diabetes mellitus have detectable anti-adrenal antibodies without being diagnosed as having adrenal insufficiency [61]. Jaeger et al. [37] found anti-adrenal antibodies in about 0.7% of the general population and 1.0–1.1% in diabetes patients and their first-degree relatives. Therefore, screening for anti-adrenal antibodies seems to be neither effective, specific, nor cost effective.

If ACTH is still within normal levels diagnosis is confirmed by a low cortisol response to a Synacthen® test.

Treatment of adrenal insufficiency with glucocorticoids and mineralocorticoids is lifelong. In these patients, insulin requirement, especially in the morning, could exceed the amounts usually required by patients with normal adrenal function. A comprehensive education of dose adjustment in case of stress, infections or sports activities should be performed for patients and their relatives. For emergency cases like accidents, surgery or sick days an emergency passport with information about glucocorticoid dose adjustment should be handed out (table 2).

In patients with more than two confirmed autoimmune diseases (especially including Addison's disease) a screening for further antibodies of PAS is recommended in regular intervals. However, the clinical relevance and benefit for an individual patient has not been shown in systematic studies.

### Celiac Disease

Celiac disease (CD), also known as gluten-sensitive enteropathy, is characterized by chronic small intestinal inflammation as a result of inappropriate T cell-mediated immune response to ingested gluten proteins of wheat. In addition to screening using the measurement of specific antibodies to gliadine, endomysium (EMA) and tissue transglutaminase (tTGA), the diagnosis of CD should be verified by jejunal biopsy. Typical findings in the small bowel mucosa are villous atrophy, lymphocytic infiltration and hypertrophy of the crypts. Sensitivity and specificity for EMA and tTGA reach almost 100% [17]. Clinical symptoms should disappear after introduction of a gluten-free diet as antibody titers also decrease. Subsequent jejunal biopsy would show healing of the mucosa with avoidance of gluten [69].

The typical clinical picture of CD is malabsorption, chronic diarrhea, and failure to thrive presenting in early childhood. Such typical presentations seem

*Table 2.* Emergency plan for surgery and severe infections (Hospital for Children and Adolescents, University of Leipzig)

| | |
|---|---|
| *Surgery day* | |
| Initial bolus injection of hydrocortisone | |
| Infants | 25 mg |
| Toddlers | 50 mg |
| School-age | 100 mg |
| Adolescents | 200 mg |
| Continuous infusion of 200 mg/m$^2$ body surface for 24 h | |
| 1/3 glucose 20% 2/3 isotonic solution | |
| Insulin bypass | |
| Measurement of glucose levels every hour | |
| Measurement of sodium and potassium every 4–6 h | |
| *1st and 2nd postoperative days* | |
| Hydrocortisone 4- to 6-fold dose of prior dosage | |
| Fludrocortisone dosage as prior to surgery | |
| *3rd and 4th postoperative days* | |
| Hydrocortisone 2- to 3-fold dose of prior dosage | |
| Fludrocortisone dosage as prior to surgery | |
| *5th postoperative day* | |
| Hydrocortisone and fludrocortisone as prior to surgery | |

to disappear, and silent or latent CD are becoming more prevalent with subsequent screening of persons at risk (table 3).

In the normal population, the prevalence of celiac disease is estimated as 0.1 to 0.3% with two thirds of diagnoses in adulthood [39, 51]. Antibody screening in children showed silent CD in 0.5–1% in Sweden and the US [11, 30]. In contrast, screening for endomysium antibodies or tissue transglutaminase antibodies in patients with type 1 diabetes mellitus was positive in 6–12% in different countries (table 4). Celiac disease was confirmed by jejunal biopsy in 60–100% of positive screening (i.e. 4.6–10.4% of all children and adolescents).

The frequency of celiac disease in patients with diabetes is 6–10 times higher than in the normal population. Comorbidity of both diseases may be explained by a similar genetic background associated with HLA DQ2 and 8 and similar triggers for autoimmune disease. Dieterich et al. [17] demonstrated that most CD-specific antibodies are directed to the enzyme tissue transglutaminase. The activity of this enzyme creates gliadine peptides that bind to HLA DQ2 molecules expressed on the surface of intestinal antigen-presenting cells. These are recognized by CD-specific intestinal T cells.

*Table 3.* Different clinical manifestations of celiac disease

| Form of manifestation | Symptoms | Estimated prevalence (Book [9]) |
|---|---|---|
| Typical CD | malabsorption, failure to thrive chronic diarrhea | <1% |
| Silent CD | short stature, iron deficiency, possible mild abdominal symptoms | 10–20% |
| Latent CD | no clinical symptoms | 80–90% |

*Table 4.* Prevalence of positive antibody screening and celiac disease proven by biopsy in children and adolescents with type 1 diabetes mellitus in different countries

| Reference | Country | Patients | Prevalence of positive EMA/TGA, % | Biopsy-proven celiac disease, % |
|---|---|---|---|---|
| Aktay et al. [2] | USA | 218 | 7.7 | 4.6 |
| Arato et al. [5] | Hungary | 205 | 11.7 | 8.4 |
| Al-Ashwal et al. [1] | Saudi Arabia | 123 | 8.1 | 4.9 |
| Crone et al. [13] | Austria | 157 | 10.2 | 5.7 |
| Gillet et al. [25] | Canada | 233 | 8.2 | 6.0 |
| Hanokoglu et al. [27] | Israel | 109 | 8.3 | – |
| Hansen et al. [26] | Denmark | 106 | 10.4 | 10.4 |
| Speikerkoetter et al. [72] | Germany | 205 | 6.3 | 3.4 |

Screening for celiac disease – when and how?

There is no consensus on these questions. It seems to be reasonable to treat patients with diabetes and celiac disease as early as possible because the risk of developing further autoimmune disease [59, 80] and lymphomas may then be reduced [48]. The development of those diseases is proportional to the time of exposure to gluten in clinically diagnosed patients with CD [81]. Intestinal lymphomas have been described in up to 4% of patients with adult disease. Undiagnosed and untreated CD could double the mortality due to the development of malignancies [21]. Corrao et al. [12] reported a significant excess of mortality during the first 3 years after the diagnosis of celiac disease in those patients with malabsorption symptoms, but not in those diagnosed by antibody screening alone (latent CD). The mortality rate increased with the delay of diagnosis and with poor compliance to a gluten-free diet. Anyway, it still remains uncertain whether malignancies will develop in subjects with silent or latent CD over a longer period of time.

There is evidence that introduction of a gluten-free diet has an impact on glycemic control and weight gain in patients with diabetes. Amin et al. [4] report on a 12-months' follow-up in 11 children and adolescents with diabetes and celiac disease and case-by-case control subjects. They found a significant improvement in HbA1c in the group of celiac patients after the introduction of a gluten-free diet. BMI SDS improved also and was equal to that of the control subjects after the follow-up period. In this study, only 1 patient demonstrated typical clinical signs of the disease, and 4 subjects had mild abdominal symptoms categorized as silent disease. Other authors did not find an effect of the gluten-free diet on metabolic control [42].

Another aspect is the possible development of osteoporosis in patients with CD. Gluten withdrawal for 1 year in children with CD shows normalization of bone mineralization. In adult patients, bone mineral density values will no longer reach normal values after diet introduction [6, 71]. There is agreement that antibody screening should be done at the onset of diabetes. Some authors report on transient antibody positivity at the time of diabetes manifestation.

## Eating Disorders

In young women in westernized countries disorders of eating behavior are common. Thinness is en vogue and dietary restraint is pursued. With the increasing rate of overweight and obese adolescents borderline eating disorders including binge eating are seen more frequently. The management of type 1 diabetes in children and adolescents is focused on food regimen and insulin treatment in order to achieve good metabolic control. In this context, control of food consumption is critical. On the other hand, food has to be used to treat hypoglycemic events. Extra food has to be taken during sports activities to avoid low blood sugar levels.

The rates of eating disorders in the general population compared to patients with diabetes are given in table 5. In addition to these specified disorders, there is a wide field of borderline disorders (subthreshold disorders) with dieting behaviors, body imaging behaviors or purging and binge-eating behaviors not meeting the full criteria for DMS-IV. These are addressed by the Diagnostic and Statistical Manual for Primary Care (DSM-PC) which provides diagnostic codes for these disorders. Prevalence is quoted to be even higher than that of the specific diseases with rates of 7.1% of boys and 8.9% of girls in a large cohort of schoolchildren from grades 5 to 12 [22].

The frequency of eating disorders or subthreshold disorders seems to be more frequent in females and males with type 1 diabetes than in nondiabetic individuals. In a cross-sectional study, Jones et al. [38] found eating disorders meeting DMS-IV criteria in about 10% of females with diabetes (age 12–19 years) and in only about 4% of controls. None of the females met criteria for anorexia nervosa but 1% had bulimia nervosa and another 9% binge-eating disorder. There seems to be no special association with anorexia nervosa and type 1 diabetes mellitus but with eating disorders including binging [66]. Subthreshold disorders were even more common (diabetes 14%, controls 8%). Even more adolescents with diabetes reported unhealthy weight control practices. Neumark-Szainer et al. [57] found about 38% of females and 16% of males to report about fasting, skipping meals, eating very little, or even using diet pills, vomiting, skipping insulin or using less insulin. In this study there was unfortunately no control group. Correlations with HbA1c showed poor metabolic control in the groups with more unhealthy behaviors. Other authors found a correlation of BMI with greater body dissatisfaction [53]. This greater body dissatisfaction may trigger a cycle of dieting and binge-eating especially in young women for whom body weight and shape are central to their self-image. There is a clear association of eating disturbance and metabolic control and diabetes-related complications. In addition to impaired metabolic control [38, 53, 57, 66], acute complications like diabetic ketoacidosis are more frequent [63]. Microvascular diabetic complications seem to occur even earlier and more frequently in young patients with diabetes. In a 4-year follow-up, Rodin et al. [66] reported on a group of 91 girls (age 12–18 years). In this group of adolescent girls, the authors found dieting in 38%, binge eating in 45%, insulin omission in 14% and self-induced vomiting in 8%. These behaviors were even more frequent at follow-up after 4 years. HbA1c was significantly higher in the group of girls with highly disordered eating (11.1%) compared to girls with moderate disorder (8.9%) and nondisordered behaviors (8.7%). Prevalence of retinopathy was fourfold higher at follow-up in the highly disordered group (86%) compared to the nondisordered group (24%). Disordered eating status in this study was in fact even more predictive for retinopathy than duration of diabetes.

Besides the weight gain problem with consecutive self-image dissatisfaction, patients with diabetes have a unique opportunity to control weight by insulin omission. This induces hyperglycemia and glucosuria. Practice of insulin omission is frequently used in girls of mid-teen age (11–14%) and even more often seen in adolescence and young adulthood (34%) [68]. Other risk factors for the development of eating disorders in adolescents with diabetes can be found in

***Table 5.*** Rates of eating disorders in a stringent manner of diagnostic criteria (Diagnostic and statistical manual of mental disorders IV = DSM-IV) in the general population compared to patients with diabetes (according to Hoek et al. [29] and Jones et al. [38])

| Disorder | Definition (based on DSM-IV) | Epidemiology |
|---|---|---|
| Anorexia nervosa | 1. Refusal to maintain body weight greater than normal weight (less than 85%) for age and height.<br>2. Intense fear of weight gain<br>3. Disturbance in the way in which one's body weight or shape is experienced:<br>– undue influence of body weight or shape on self-evaluation<br>– denial of seriousness of the current low body weight<br>4. In postmenarchal age: amenorrhoea | Prevalence: 0.3–0.5% of young women<br>Female:male ratio 10:1<br>In adolescents up to 14:6<br>Incidence: 8/100,000/year<br>Diabetics: 0–0.2% |
| Bulimia nervosa | 1. Recurrent episodes of binge-eating characterized by both:<br>– eating in a discrete period of time an amount of food that is definitely larger than most people would eat during a similar period of time and under similar circumstances.<br>– a sense of lack of control during the episode<br>2. Recurrent inappropriate compensatory behavior to prevent weight gain: self-induced vomiting, misuse of laxatives or diuretics, fasting, excessive exercise<br>3. Recurrent episodes of binge-eating at least twice a week for 3 months | Prevalence: 0.5–1% of young women, 0.1% of young men<br>Incidence: 12/100,000/year<br>Diabetes: females 1% (vs. 0.5%) |

*Table 5* (continued)

| Disorder | Definition (based on DSM-IV) | Epidemiology |
|---|---|---|
| Binge-eating disorder | 1. Recurrent episodes of binge-eating<br>2. at least 3 of the following:<br>– rapid eating<br>– eating until becoming uncomfortable<br>– eating large amounts when not hungry<br>– eating alone because of embarrassment<br>– disgust, depression or guilt because of eating patterns | Prevalence suggested 1–4% in women<br>Male:female 2:3<br>Up to 30% of individuals in weight-control programs<br>Diabetes: females 9% (vs. 4%) |

the family function. Girls with diabetes report less support, poorer communication and less trust in the relationships with their parents [52].

Pediatric diabetes teams should therefore be aware of eating disorders especially in the group of adolescent girls. Intervention can be made in ambulatory settings with specialized psychologists who have experience with both eating disorders and diabetes. In life-threatening weight loss, patients have to be stabilized with parenteral nutrition. In these cases, collaboration with specialized psychiatrists is essential. Further research is needed in order to develop preventive strategies for eating disorders in the high-risk group of adolescent girls with diabetes.

## Skin and Joints

Patients with diabetes are at higher risk than nondiabetic subjects to develop several skin disorders. In children, only few data exist on the development of skin problems.

Lipodystrophy expressed as lipoatrophy and lipohypertrophy is a typical cutaneous manifestation at the injection sites of patients with diabetes. The reduction of subcutaneous adipose tissue is now seen less frequently with the use of human insulin. The etiopathogenesis and specialness of both conditions seems to be controversial [64]. Local trophic effects could explain tissue growth. Raile et al. [64] showed a strong association of lipoatrophy and lipohypertrophy with insulin antibodies. Not changing the injections site has been reported to be an independent risk factor for lipohypertrophy [28]. Raile et al. [65] found lipohypertrophy in almost half of all children and adolescents with diabetes whereas lipoatrophy was seen in only 5% of the pediatric patients.

Clinical experience and experimental data suggest that insulin absorption from lipodystrophic injection sites is disturbed and therefore those sites should be avoided for the injection of insulin [78]. Rotation of the injection sites should help avoid lipodystrophy.

The development of scleroderma-like changes of the hand and limited joint mobility (LJM) has been described in diabetes [19, 24, 35, 83]. LJM is another common complication in patients with diabetes affecting about up to 35% of children and adolescents. Infante et al. [36] describe a decreasing rate of LJM in the hands and fingers over the last 20 years (from 31 to 7%) that is most likely the result of better glycemic control during these two decades. Also, LJM not only affects the fingers and hands but also the feet, elbows, neck and spine. Typical is a positive praying sign expressing a limited interphalangeal joint extension when putting the palms in opposition. There are reports on the association of LJM with microvascular complications in children and adults [19, 24].

There is an association with scleroderma-like skin syndrome and LJM in patients with diabetes. Scleroderma-like changes of the fingers and hands are seen in up to 39% of diabetes patients [83]. Ichthyosiform skin changes were seen even more frequently in the study of Yosipovitch et al. [83] (48%).

Necrobiosis lipoidica diabeticorum (NLD) is a less common skin change in patients with diabetes. The prevalence in children is reported to be 0.06% in a population-based setting and up to 10% in an older hospital-based survey [16, 82]. Typically, a well-circumscribed reddish lesion can be found with sometimes central ulceration as usually found in the pretibial region. O'Toole et al. [60] reported that only a minority of the patients with NLD attending their dermatology outpatient clinic suffered from diabetes (11%). The etiology of NLD remains unclear but successful treatment with immunomodulating drugs could suggest an underlying immune process. Treatment of this rare condition also remains controversial. There are no well-conducted clinical trials. Most frequently reported are topical, systemic or intralesional corticosteroids. Newer reports recommend immunomodulative or immunosuppressive therapy strategies or PUVA [15, 58, 73, 75]. As limited joint mobility NLD is also associated with a higher frequency of microvascular complications [82].

Our group found a higher frequency of paronychia in adolescents with diabetes and particularly girls than in controls (34.4 vs. 23%; $p < 0.01$). Patients with paronychia were older and had a longer duration of diabetes while there was no difference in long-term HbA1c between the groups. Vibration perception in all measured regions was impaired, compared to healthy adolescents.

Subclinical neuropathy and microalbuminuria was found to be more frequent in patients with paronychia than in those without [41].

### Other Consequences

There are various other consequences regarding psychosocial development, education, partnership, and choice of profession.

Psychosocial development in our experience could be disturbed especially in families with minor psychosocial problems before the manifestation of diabetes. Therefore, in a multidisciplinary pediatric diabetes team a psychologist with experience with the care of pediatric patients and diabetes should be available. Diagnostic tools for the assessment of diabetes treatment satisfaction, lifestyle satisfaction and childhood development should be available and used in these conditions. Interventions should be carried out in an ambulatory setting. An experienced pediatric psychiatrist should also be accessible in cooperation with the diabetes team in the in-patient setting.

The psychopathology of adolescents with diabetes includes, besides eating disorders, especially noncompliance with medical treatment. This condition is a challenge for every pediatric diabetes team and can last for years in some cases. Diagnosable psychiatric disorders can be hidden and have to be searched for.

Normal psychosocial development depends on normal integration in social life. Therefore, toddlers should have access to kindergarten. Nursery school teams should be educated on diabetes management especially regarding hypoglycemia. In our experience, education by our diabetes nurse in the kindergarten is always welcome. Some nursery school teams even inject insulin and adjust doses. If insulin injection is needed while the child is staying in kindergarten another alternative is management by a pediatric community nurse.

In addition, diabetes education should be readily available in all schools. Teachers and classmates should be informed about diabetes in an age-dependent manner. Some children tend to withhold the diagnosis and management of diabetes from their classmates. This should be carefully evaluated and discussed before reintegration of the patient with diabetes into daily routine. If children and adolescents with diabetes take part in sports activities, the coach and team should be aware of possible hypoglycemic events and prevention and treatment of them. Children and adolescents with diabetes should have access to all the activities their classmates might have. With this concept, psychosocial development should be secured.

Another major step in life is choice of career. In several countries, legal regulations restrict a free choice of career. In Germany, for example, military service and use of weapons is prohibited for people suffering from diabetes.

There are several jobs where a diabetes patient could put himself at risk in case of a hypoglycemic attack. This is particularly so in jobs with conveyance of persons. Other possible problems are from metabolic disturbances due to shift working. Therefore, a job-seeking adolescent with diabetes should have access to comprehensive professional counseling.

Transition from pediatric into adult care should be handled in a well-planned and structured manner. The importance of a good transition was studied by several groups in the past few years. Kipps et al. [43] showed that the differences of quality of transition depend on the process. This process could significantly influence the future of metabolic control and diabetes complications in every patient. The cooperation with an adult diabetes clinic could provide a bridge for patients and pediatric diabetologists to manage the transition period successfully.

Peer groups and partnerships play a major role in adolescence. The way of dealing with the chronic disease can be positively and negatively influenced by peers depending also on the self-esteem and self-management of each individual diabetes patient. In discussions with adolescents, one can recognize the wish to not be different from their peers. Self-esteem and self-image could be boosted by group work, for example in diabetes camps. In our group, these camps are also used to bring up discussions on contraception and family planning. This approach is well accepted and welcomed by the adolescents.

## Conclusion

Pediatricians dealing with children and adolescents with diabetes should be aware of concomitant diseases and their complications. The frequency of these conditions is often underestimated. In addition, an accumulation of these complications in adolescence together with psychosocial problems could critically affect metabolic control and diabetes management of the adolescent patient with diabetes. Screening for different conditions should be a matter of fact. Evaluation of the psychosocial situation should be provided at certain intervals. Computed quality management programs or paper data sheets could help deal with this in a comprehensive way.

## References


1 Al-Ashwal AA, Shabib SM, Sakati NA, Attia NA: Prevalence and characteristics of celiac disease in type I diabetes mellitus in Saudi Arabia. Saudi Med J 2003;24:1113–1115.

2 Aktay AN, Lee PC, Kumar V, Parton E, Wyatt DT, Werlin SL: The prevalence and clinical characteristics of celiac disease in juvenile diabetes in Wisconsin. J Pediatr Gastroenterol Nutr 2001;33:462–465.

3 American Academy of Pediatrics: Policy statement identifying and treating eating disorders. Pediatrics 2003;110:204–211.
4 Amin R, Ahmed ML, Murphy N, Acerini CL, Edge J, Dunger DB: A longitudinal study of the effects of a gluten free diet on glycemic control and weight gain in subjects with type 1 diabetes and celiac disease. Diabetes Care 2002;25:1117–1122.
5 Arato A, Korner A, Veres G, Dezsofi A, Ujpal I, Madacsy L: Frequency of coeliac disease in Hungarian children with type 1 diabetes mellitus. Eur J Pediatr 2003;162:1–5.
6 Barera G, Mora S, Brambilla P, Ricotti A, Menni L, Beccio S, Bianchi C: Body composition in children with celiac disease and the effects of a gluten-free diet: A prospective case-control study. Am J Clin Nutr 2000;72:71–75.
7 Barera G, Bonfanti R, Viscardi M, Bazzigaluppi E, Calori G, Meschi F, Bianchi C, Chiumello G: Occurrence of celiac disease after onset of type 1 diabetes: A 6-year prospective longitudinal study. Pediatrics 2002;109:833–838.
8 Bryden KS, Neil A, Mayou RA, Peveler RC, Fairburn CG, Dunger DB: Eating habits, body weight, and insulin misuse. Diabetes Care 1999;22:1956–1960.
9 Book LS: Diagnosing celiac disease in 2002: Who, why, and how? Pediatrics 2002;109:952–954.
10 Burek CL, Rose NR, Guire KE, Hoffman WH: Thyroid autoantibodies in black and in white children and adolescents with type 1 diabetes mellitus and their first degree relatives. Autoimmunity 1990;7:157–167.
11 Carlsson AK, Axelsson IE, Borulf SK, Bredberg AC, Ivarsson SA: Serological screening for celiac disease in healthy 2.5-year-old children in Sweden. Pediatrics 2001;107:42–45.
12 Corrao G, Corazza GR, Bagnardi V, Brusco G, Ciacci C, Cottone M, Guidetti CS, Usai P, Cesari P, Pelli MA, Loperfido S, Volta U, Calabro A, Certo M: Mortality in patients with coeliac disease and their relatives: A cohort study. Lancet 2001;i:356–361.
13 Crone J, Rami B, Huber WD, Granditsch G, Schober E: Prevalence of celiac disease and follow-up of EMA in children and adolescents with type 1 diabetes mellitus. J Pediatr Gastroenterol Nutr 2003;37:67–71.
14 Danne T, Kordonouri O, Enders I, Weber B: Factors influencing height and weight development in children with diabetes. Results of the Berlin Retinopathy Study. Diabetes Care 1997;20:281–285.
15 De Rie MA, Sommer A, Hoekzema R, Neumann HA: Treatment of necrobiosis lipoidica with topical psoralen plus ultraviolet A. Br J Dermatol 2002;147:743–747.
16 De Silva BD, Schofield OM, Walker JD: The prevalence of necrobiosis lipoidica diabeticorum in children with type 1 diabetes. Br J Dermatol 1999;141:593–594.
17 Dieterich W, Ehnis T, Bauer M, Donner P, Volta U, Riecken EO, Schuppan D: Identification of tissue transglutaminase as the autoantigen of celiac disease. Nat Med 1997;3:797–801.
18 Dittmar M, Kahaly GJ: Extensive personal experience. Polyglandular autoimmune syndromes: Immunogenetics and long-term follow-up. J Clin Endocrinol Metab 2003;88:2983–2992.
19 Duffin AC, Donaghue KC, Potter M, McInnes A, Chan AK, King J, Howard NJ, Silink M: Limited joint mobility in the hands and feet of adolescents with type 1 diabetes mellitus. Diabet Med 1999;16:125–130.
20 Dunger D, Ahmed L, Ong K: Growth and body composition in type 1 diabetes mellitus. Horm Res 2002;58:66–71.
21 Ferguson A, Kingstone K: Coeliac disease and malignancies. Acta Paediatr Suppl 1996;412:78–81.
22 Field AE, Camargo CA Jr, Taylor CB, Berkey CS, Frazier AL, Gillman MW, Colditz GA: Overweight, weight concerns, and bulimic behaviors among girls and boys. J Am Acad Child Adolesc Psychiatry 1999;38:754–760.
23 Franzese A, Buono P, Mascolo M, Leo AL, Valerio G: Thyroid autoimmunity starting during the course of type 1 diabetes denotes a subgroup of children with more severe diabetes. Diabetes Care 2000;23:1201–1202.
24 Frost D, Beischer W: Limited joint mobility in type 1 diabetic patients: Associations with microangiopathy and subclinical macroangiopathy are different in men and women. Diabetes Care 2001;24:95–99.
25 Gillett PM, Gillett HR, Israel DM, Metzger DL, Stewart L, Chanoine JP, Freeman HJ: High prevalence of celiac disease in patients with type 1 diabetes detected by antibodies to endomysium and tissue transglutaminase. Can J Gastroenterol 2001;15:297–301.

26 Hansen D, Bennedbaek FN, Hansen LK, Hoier-Madsen M, Hegedu LS, Jacobsen BB, Husby S: High prevalence of coeliac disease in Danish children with type I diabetes mellitus. Acta Paediatr 2001;90:1217–1220.
27 Hanukoglu A, Mizrachi A, Dalal I, Admoni O, Rakover Y, Bistritzer Z, Levine A, Somekh E, Lehmann D, Tuval M, Boaz M, Golander A: Extrapancreatic autoimmune manifestations in type 1 diabetes patients and their first-degree relatives: A multicenter study. Diabetes Care 2003;26: 1235–1240.
28 Hauner H, Stockamp B, Haastert B: Prevalence of lipohypertrophy in insulin-treated diabetic patients and predisposing factors. Exp Clin Endocrinol Diab 1996;104:106–110.
29 Hoek HW, van Hoeken D: Review of the prevalence and incidence of eating disorders. Int J Eat Disord 2003;34:383–396.
30 Hoffenberg EJ, Barriga GS, Eisenbarth F: Prospective study of the frequency of celiac disease in children in Colorado: Initial results. J Pediatr Gastroenterol Nutr 2001;33:494–498.
31 Holl RW, Grabert M, Heinze E, Sorgo W, Debatin KM: Age at onset and long-term metabolic control affect height in type 1 diabetes mellitus. Eur J Pediatr 1998;157:972–977.
32 Hugle B, Dollmann R, Keller E, Kiess W: Addison's crisis in adolescent patients with previously diagnosed diabetes mellitus as manifestation of polyglandular autoimmune syndrome type II-report of two patients. J Pediatr Endocrinol Metab 2004;17:93–97.
33 Hunter I, Greene SA, MacDonald TM, Morris AD: Prevalence and etiology of hypothyroidism in the young. Arch Dis Child 2000;83:207–210.
34 Hypponen E, Virtanen SM, Kenward MG, Knip M, Akerblom HK: Obesity, increased linear growth, and risk of type 1 diabetes in children. Diabetes Care 2000;23:1755–1760.
35 Infante JR, Rosenbloom AL, Silverstein JH, Garzarella L, Pollock BH: Changes in frequency and severity of limited joint mobility in children with type 1 diabetes mellitus between 1976–78 and 1998. J Pediatr 2001;138:33–37.
36 International Society for Pediatric and Adolescent Diabetes: Consensus guidelines 2000. Zeist, Medical Forum International, 2000.
37 Jaeger C, Hatziagelaki E, Petzold R, Bretzel RG: Comparative analysis of organ-specific autoantibodies and celiac disease associated antibodies in type 1 diabetic patients, their first degree relatives and healthy control subjects. Diabetes Care 2001;24:27–32.
38 Jones JM, Lawson ML, Daneman D, Olmsted MP, Rodin G: Eating disorders in adolescent females with and without type 1 diabetes: Cross sectional study. BMJ 2000;320:1563–1566.
39 Johnston SD, Watson RG, McMillan SA, Sloan SA, Love AH: Prevalence of celiac disease in Northern Ireland. Lancet 1997;350:1370.
40 Kabelitz M, Liesenkotter KP, Stach B, Willgerodt H, Stablein W, Singendonk W, Jager-Roman E, Litzenborger H, Ehnert B, Gruters A: The prevalence of anti-thyroid peroxidase antibodies and autoimmune thyroiditis in children and adolescents in an iodine replete area. Eur J Endocrinol 2003;148:301–307.
41 Kapellen TM, Galler A, Kiess W: Higher frequency of paronychia (nail bed infections) in pediatric and adolescent patients with type 1 diabetes than in nondiabetic peers. J Pediatr Endocr Metabol 2003;16:751–758.
42 Kaukinen K, Salmi J, Lahtela J, Siljamaki-Ojansuu U, Koivisto A, Oska H, Collin P: No effect of gluten-free diet on metabolic control of type 1 diabetes in patients with diabetes and celiac disease. Diabetes Care 1999;22:1747–1749.
43 Kipps S, Bahu T, Ong K, Ackland FM, Brown RS, Fox CT, Griffin NK, Knight AH, Mann NP, Neil HA, Simpson H, Edge JA, Dunger DB: Current methods of transfer of young people with type 1 diabetes to adult services. Diab Med 2002;19:649–654.
44 Kordonouri O, Deiss D, Danne T, Dorow A, Bassir C, Gruters-Kieslich A: Predictivity of thyroid autoantibodies for the development of thyroid disorders in children and adolescents with type 1 diabetes. Diab Med 2002;19:518–521.
45 Kordonouri O, Klinghammer A, Lang EB, Grüters-Kieslich A, Grabert M, Holl RW: Thyroid autoimmunity in children and adolescents with type 1 diabetes. Diabetes Care 2002;25:1346–1350.
46 Krassas GE: Treatment of juvenile Graves' disease and its ophthalmic complication: the 'European way'. Eur J Endocrinol 2004;150:407–414.

47 Levin L, Tomer Y: The etiology of autoimmune diabetes and thyroiditis: Evidence for common genetic susceptibility. Autoimmun Rev 2003;2:377–386.
48 Logan R, Rifkind E, Turner I, Ferguson A: Mortality in coeliac disease. Gastroenterology 1989;97:265–271.
49 Lorini R, d'Annunzio G, Vitali L, Scaramuzza A: IDDM and autoimmune thyroid disease in the pediatric age group. J Pediatr Endocrinol Metab 1996;9(suppl 1):89–94.
50 Loviselli A, Velluzzi F, Mossa P, Cambosu MA, Secci G, Atzeni F, Taberlet A, Balestrieri A, Martino E, Grasso L, Songini M, Bottazzo GF, Mariotti S; Sardinian Schoolchildren Study Group: The Sardinian Autoimmunity Study. 3. Studies on circulating antithyroid antibodies in Sardinian schoolchildren: Relationship to goiter prevalence and thyroid function. Thyroid 2001;11: 849–857.
51 Madirano CO, Lorenzo HA, Fernadez CC, Arnalich FF, Vazques RJ: Coeliac disease in the adulthood. An Med Interna 1998;15:327–333.
52 Maharaj S, Rodin G, Connolly J, Olmsted M, Daneman D: Eating problems and the observed quality of mother-daughter interactions among girls with type 1 diabetes. J Consult Clin Psychol 2002;69:950–958.
53 Meltzer LJ, Bennett Johnson S, Prine JM, Banks RA, Desrosiers PM, Silverstein JH: Disordered eating, body mass, and glycemic control in adolescents with type 1 diabetes. Diabetes Care 2001;24:678–682.
54 Meyer K, Deutscher J, Anil M, Berthold A, Bartsch M, Kiess W: Serum androgen levels in adolescents with type 1 diabetes: Relationship to pubertal stage and metabolic control. J Endocrinol Invest 2000;23:362–368.
55 Mohn A, Di Michele S, Di Luzio R, Tumini S, Chiarelli F: The effect of subclinical hypothyroidism on metabolic control in children and adolescents with type 1 diabetes mellitus. Diab Med 2002;19:70–73.
56 Nielsen S, Emborg C, Molbak A-G: Mortality in concurrent type 1 diabetes and anorexia nervosa. Diabetes Care 2002;25:309–312.
57 Neumark-Sztainer D, Patterson J, Mellin A, Ackard DM, Utter J, Story J, Sockalosky J: Weight control practices and disordered eating behaviours among adolescent females and males with type 1 diabetes. Diabetes Care 2002;25:1289–1296.
58 Nguyen K, Washenik K, Shupack J: Necrobiosis lipoidica diabeticorum treated with chloroquine. J Am Acad Dermatol 2002;46(2 suppl)S34–S36.
59 Not T, Tommassini A, Tonini G, Buratti E, Pocecco M, Tortul C, Valussi M, Crichiutti G, Berti I, Trevisiol C, Azioni E, Neri E, Torre G, Martelossi S, Soban M, Lenhardt A, Cattin L, Ventura A: Undiagnosed coeliac disease and risk of autoimmune disorders in subjects with type 1 diabetes. Diabetologia 2001;44:151–155.
60 O'Toole EA, Kennedy U, Nolan JJ, Young MM, Rogers S, Barnes L: Necrobiosis lipoidica: Only a minority of patients have diabetes mellitus. Br J Dermatol 1999;140:283–286.
61 Peterson R, Salmi H, Hyoty H, Miettinen A, Ilonen J, Reijonen H, Knip M, Akerblom HK, Krohn K: Steroid 21-hydroxylase autoantibodies in insulin-dependent diabetes mellitus. Chidhood Diabetes in Finland (DiMe) Study group. Clin Immunol Immunopathol 1997;82:37–42.
62 Pestoni C, Ferreiros MM, de la Torre C, Toribio J: Two girls with necrobiosis lipoidica and type I diabetes mellitus with transfollicular elimination in one girl. Pediatr Dermatol 2003;20:211–214.
63 Polonsky WH, Anderson BJ, Lohrer PA, Aponte JE, Jacobson AM, Cole CF: Insulin omission in women with IDDM. Diabetes Care 1994;17:1178–1185.
64 Raile K, Noelle V, Landgraf R, Schwarz HP: Insulin antibodies are associated with lipoatrophy but also with lipohypertrophy in children and adolescents with type 1 diabetes. Exp Clin Endocrinol Diab 2001;109:393–396.
65 Radetti G, Paganini C, Gentili L, Bernasconi S, Betterle C, Borkenstein M, Cvijovic K, Kadrnka-Lovrencic M, Krzisnik C, Battelino T, et al: Frequency of Hashimoto's thyroiditis in children with type 1 diabetes mellitus. Acta Diabetol 1995;32:121–124.
66 Rodin G, Olmsted MP, Rydall AC, Maharaj SI, Colton PA, Jones JM, Bianucucci LA, Daneman D: Eating disorders in young women with type 1 diabetes mellitus. J Psychosom Res 2002;53: 943–949.
67 Roldan MB, Alonso M, Barrio R: Thyroid autoimmunity in children and adolescents with type 1 diabetes mellitus. Diab Nutr Metab 1999;12:27–31.

68 Rydall AC, Rodin GM, Olmsted MP, Devenyi RG, Daneman D: Disordered eating behavior and microvascular complications in young women with insulin-dependent diabetes mellitus. N Engl J Med 1997;336:1849–1854.
69 Schober E, Rami B, Granditsch G, Crone J: Coeliac disease in children and adolescents with type 1 diabetes mellitus: To screen or not, to treat or not? Horm Res 2002;57(suppl 1):97–100.
70 Schwartz SA, Weissberg-Benchell J, Perlmuter LC: Personal control and disordered eating in female adolescents with type 1 diabetes. Diabetes Care 2002;25:1987–1991.
71 Semrad CE: Bone mass and gastrointestinal disease. Ann NY Acad Sci 2000;904:564–570.
72 Spiekerkoetter U, Seissler J, Wendel U: General screening for celiac disease is advisable in children with type 1 diabetes. Horm Metab Res 2002;34:192–195.
73 Stanway A, Rademaker M, Newman P: Healing of severe ulcerative necrobiosis lipoidica with cyclosporin. Austr J Dermatol 2004;45:119–122.
74 Strasser-Vogel B, Blum WF, Past R, Kessler U, Hoeflich A, Meiler B, Kiess W: Insulin-like growth factor (IGF)-I and –II and IGF-binding proteins-1, -2, and -3 in children and adolescents with diabetes mellitus: Correlation with metabolic control and height attainment. J Clin Endocrinol Metab 1995;80:1207–1213.
75 Tidman M: Management of necrobiosis lipoidica. Clin Exp Dermatol 2002;27:328–337.
76 The EURODIAB Substudy 2 Study Group: Rapid early growth is associated with increased risk of childhood type 1 diabetes in various European populations. Diabetes Care 2002;10: 1755–1760.
77 Thon A, Heinze E, Feilen KD, Holl RW, Schmidt H, Koletzko S, Wendek U, Nothjunge J: Development of height and weight in children with diabetes mellitus: Report on two prospective multicentre studies, one cross-sectional, one longitudinal. Eur J Pediatr 1992;151: 258–262.
78 Thow JC, Johnson AB, Marsden S, Taylor R, Home PD: Morphology of palpably abnormal injection sites and effects on absorption of isophane (NPH) insulin. Diab Med 1990;7:795–799.
79 Umpierrez GE, Latif KA, Murphy MB, Lambeth HC, Stentz F, Bush A, Kitabchi AE: Thyroid dysfunction in patients with type 1 diabetes: A longitudinal study. Diabetes Care 2003;26: 1181–1185.
80 Valerio G, Maiuri L, Troncone R, Buono P, Lombardi F, Palmieri R, Franzese A: Severe clinical onset of diabetes and increased prevalence of other autoimmune diseases in children with celiac disease diagnosed before diabetes mellitus. Diabetologia 2002;45:1719–1722.
81 Ventura A, Magazzu G, Greco L, Sige P: Duration of exposure to gluten and risk for autoimmune disorders in patients with celiac disease. Gastroenterology 1999;97:265–271.
82 Verrotti A, Chiarelli F, Amerio P, Morgese G: Necrobiosis lipidica diabeticorum in children and adolescents: A clue for underlying renal and retinal disease. Pediatr Dermatol 1995;12: 220–223.
83 Yosipovitch G, Hodak E, Vardi P, Shraga I, Karp M, Sprecher E, David M: The prevalence of cutaneous manifestations in IDDM patients and their association with diabetes risk factors and microvascular complications. Diabetes Care 1998;21:506–509.
84 Zois C, Stavrou I, Kalogera C, Svarna E, Dimoliatis I, Seferiadis K, Tsatsoulis A: High prevalence of autoimmune thyroiditis in school children after elimination of iodine deficiency in northwestern Greece. Thyroid 2003;13:485–489.

Dr. Thomas M. Kapellen
Universitätsklinik und Poliklinik für Kinder und Jugendliche
Universität Leipzig, Oststrasse 21–25, DE–04317 Leipzig (Germany)
Tel. +49 341 97 972 60 00, Fax +49 341 97 972 60 09, E-Mail kapt@medizin.uni-leipzig.de

Chiarelli F, Dahl-Jørgensen K, Kiess W (eds): Diabetes in Childhood and Adolescence.
Pediatr Adolesc Med. Basel, Karger, 2005, vol 10, pp 347–361

# Type 2 Diabetes mellitus in Childhood

*Maria Antonietta Piscopo, Andrea Rigamonti, Gaia Biancamaria Chiesa, Sonia Bettini, Angela Azzinari, Riccardo Bonfanti, Matteo Viscardi, Franco Meschi, Giuseppe Chiumello*

Pediatric Department, Endocrine Unit, Scientific Institute H San Raffaele, Vita-Salute University, Milan, Italy

In the past, type 2 diabetes mellitus (T2DM) was considered a disease of adults and older individuals, not a pediatric condition. Over the last decade, however, in the USA and the rest of the world there has been a disturbing trend of increasing cases of T2DM in children and adolescents, mirroring the increasing rates of obesity. This emerging epidemic of T2DM in youth has alerted health care providers to increase awareness in the scientific community [1].

T2DM is a serious condition that can have a detrimental impact on health, quality of life and life expectancy. Due to its chronic nature, which necessitates lifelong maintenance, it is also a tremendous economic burden on the health care system.

## Epidemiology

Although T2DM has historically been characterized as adult-onset diabetes, it has been shown to be on the rise in young people in recent years, comprising some 30% of new cases of diabetes in the second decade of life [2]. The mean age at diagnosis of T2DM in young people is 12–14 years. The recent increase in the incidence of T2DM is thought to be related to the increasing prevalence of obesity in young people, which has reached epidemic proportions in the US and is disproportionately high in young people of a particular ethnic background [3, 4]. In 1988–1994, The Third National Health and Nutrition Examination Survey (NHANES III) recruited a representative sample of US adolescents aged 12–19 years, and showed that the prevalence of T2DM and type 1 diabetes in the US pediatric population is 0.41% (4/1,000) [5].

The incidence of T2DM in young people is particularly high in minority populations. Pima Indians have the highest documented prevalence of T2DM in the world. Pima youth in the age range 5–14 years have an incidence rate of T2DM of 1 in 1,000 person-years. T2DM has also been documented in first Nation Youth in Manitoba, with a prevalence of at last 0.53 per 1,000 in the age range 7–14 years [6–8]. Among Japanese's youth T2DM is seven times more frequent than type 1 diabetes, showing a 30-fold increase in incidence over the past 20 years concomitant with changing food patterns and increasing obesity [9, 10]. Similar alarming statistics have also been obtained recently in other parts of the world [11]. Recent studies have demonstrated that 21% of diabetic patients of Mexican-American descent had T2DM, compared with only 3% of their white counterparts [3]. In another study, 69% of pediatric diabetics with T2DM in the Greater Cincinnati area were African-American, although this ethnicity constituted only 14.5% of the general population. The odds ratio for the development of T2DM in African-American compared with white youths was 3.5 in boys and 6.1 in girls; African-American girls have been shown to be at particularly high risk for obesity, compared with boys and white girls [4]. In San Antonio, Tex., USA, 123 youths with T2DM were diagnosed between 1990 and 1998, accounting for 18% of all new diabetes cases [12].

New papers are reporting cases of T2DM also in Europe: in the year 2000, a retrospective epidemiological study has investigated the prevalence of T2DM in children in Birmingham (UK); in 12 months 67 children presented with diabetes, of whom 4 were new presentations of T2DM. The prevalence of T2DM in those aged under 18 is 0.038 per 1,000, with an annual incidence of 1.52 per 100,000 [13].

In a recent Italian study, the prevalence of glucose intolerance and its determinants with levels of glycemia were studied in 710 grossly obese Italian children of European origin aged 6–18 years. In these grossly obese children, the prevalence of impaired glucose tolerance was 4.5%, and both insulin resistance and impaired insulin secretion contribute to the elevation of glycemia [14].

## Pathophysiology

Ethnic and geographic differences in the incidence of T2DM indicate that the disease is a complex metabolic disorder of heterogeneous etiology, with social, behavioral and environmental risk factors unmasking the underlying genetic susceptibility of individuals.

There is clearly a strong hereditary component to the disease, which is likely to be multigenic in nature. In adults, the concordance rate of T2DM in monozygotic twins is approximately 90%, and the lifetime risk of developing T2DM in a first-degree relative is approximately 40%. The important role of genetic determinants is well illustrated when differences in the prevalence of T2DM in various racial groups are considered. However, even though genetic susceptibility to T2DM is important, the rapid increase observed in the prevalence of this disorder has occurred too quickly to be the result of increased gene frequency and altered genetic pool.

Although the pathogenesis of T2DM is controversial, it is generally agreed that: (1) the disease has strong genetic and environmental components; (2) its inheritance is polygenic; (3) impaired insulin sensitivity and secretion, each of which is under genetic control, are both important elements in its pathogenesis; (4) most patients are obese; (5) obesity, especially intra-abdominal obesity, causes insulin resistance and is under genetic control [15].

As we know, glucose homeostasis depends on the balance between insulin secretion by pancreatic β-cells and insulin action. Insulin resistance alone is not sufficient for hyperglycemia to develop, and inadequate β-cell insulin secretion is necessary. There has been considerable debate about whether insulin resistance or insulin hyposecretion is the primary defect in T2DM in adults. The constellation of clinical characteristics in children with T2DM suggests that the initial abnormality is impaired insulin action, later compounded with β-cell failure.

Familiar trends in diabetes risk might be transmitted across generations by environmental as well as genetic factors. Marked increases in body mass index (BMI) in pubertal and young adult woman predispose to glucose intolerance and overt diabetes during pregnancy [16]. Gestational diabetes promotes fetal overgrowth, and children born large for gestational age in diabetic pregnancies are themselves at higher risk of childhood obesity and T2DM. Though this vicious cycle of glucose intolerance has been demonstrated most convincingly in PIMA Indians, we are likely to witness in the not too distant future a surge in the incidence of gestational diabetes in other high-risk groups [17].

It is well recognized that resistance to insulin-stimulated glucose uptake is a characteristic finding in patients with T2DM and impaired glucose tolerance. Cross-sectional and longitudinal studies in populations at high risk for developing T2DM demonstrate that hyperinsulinemia and insulin resistance are present in the prediabetic normoglycemic state. The evolution from normal to impaired glucose tolerance is associated with worsening of insulin resistance. In patients with T2DM, impaired insulin action and insulin secretory failure are both present. The failure of the β-cell to continue to hypersecrete insulin underlines the transition from insulin resistance, with compensatory hyperinsulinemia and normoglycemia, to clinical diabetes, with overt fasting hyperglycemia and increased hepatic glucose production.

It has been proposed that hyperglycemia may worsen both insulin resistance and insulin secretory abnormalities, thus enhancing the transition from impaired glucose tolerance to diabetes or aggravating diabetes. In this way, hyperglycemia may beget more hyperglycemia, a concept called glucose toxicity. Glucose toxicity-induced abnormalities of insulin secretion and action can be ameliorated by correction of hyperglycemia [18].

## Risk Factors

*Obesity and Lifestyle*

Obesity seems to precede T2DM and may cause diabetes in genetically predisposed individuals.

Cross-sectional and longitudinal studies have shown that excessive body weight and increased abdominal fat distribution are major risk factors for adult-onset T2DM in virtually all populations.

In healthy young people, increased adiposity is directly correlated with insulinemia and negatively with insulin sensitivity, suggesting that body fat may be related to risk of T2DM. The negative impact of obesity in the pathogenesis of glucose metabolism disturbances is evident early in childhood in both white and black children.

In addition to the degree of obesity, the duration of obesity and location of body fat are also important risk factors for T2DM. Maximum lifetime BMI is associated cross-sectionally with T2DM, independent of current BMI. The risk of T2DM is positively related to the number of years of being obese. Furthermore, the site of body fat, particularly central fat, is a predictor of T2DM, independent of the presence of obesity. In children, the relative roles of different compartments of adiposity are less clear, and their relation to T2DM still needs to be investigated further [19–21].

*Family History*

One of the most consistent findings in youth with T2DM is the presence of a first- or second-degree relative with T2DM [22]. Of Mexican-American children with T2DM, 80% have an affected first-degree relative. Among black children with T2DM, 95% have a family history of T2DM, often with multiple affected family members in more than one generation. In healthy black children, a family history of T2DM is a risk factor for insulin resistance. These children manifest around a 25% decrease in insulin sensitivity compared with black children who have no family history of T2DM [23].

*Ethnic Factors*

The emerging epidemic of T2DM in youth appears to be mostly affecting children from minority ethnic groups. Among Pima Indian children, who have the highest reported rates of T2DM, genetic predisposition to insulin resistance appears to play a major role. This genetic predisposition to insulin resistance is manifested early in life by the presence of hyperinsulinemia in nondiabetic Pima Indian children compared with Caucasian children [24]. T2DM is more common in African-American children than in Caucasian children. African-American children are more hyperinsulinemic and insulin resistant than Caucasian children. It is possible that children of certain ethnic groups have a genetic predisposition to insulin resistance, which in the presence of environmental modifiers could increase their risk of T2DM and result in disease expression during physiological states of insulin resistance [25]. The 'thrifty' genotype hypothesis represents one attempt to explain the high prevalence of obesity and T2DM in these ethnic populations. This hypothesis postulates that, in a hunter-gatherer society, the thrifty genotype promoted fat deposition and conferred a survival advantage when food supplies were unpredictable and scarce. However, with the adoption of the more sedentary lifestyle typical of today's society and increased energy intake from abundant food supplies, such a metabolic phenotype has become a disadvantage predisposing to obesity and T2DM [26].

## Fetal Origins of T2DM and Maternal Influences

Growth retardation in the intrauterine environment may predispose individuals to be at increase risk for obesity, hypertension, metabolic syndrome, T2DM, and cardiovascular disease later on in life. Fetal malnutrition is thought to relate to metabolic syndrome via negative effects on functioning of kidney, pancreas, hypothalamic-pituitary-adrenal axis, sympathetic system, and muscle, liver and adipose tissue.

The relation of the prevalence of T2DM to birth weight is U-shaped. Multiple epidemiological studies developed in North America and Europe appear to broadly confirm the association of low birth weight in babies born at term, with the glucose metabolism impairment in the adult life. The prevalence of T2DM has been reported at 13–25% for low birth weight (<2,500 g). Exposure to maternal gestational diabetes has also been noted as a predictor for childhood obesity and T2DM. Gestational diabetes, in fact, creates a hyperglycemic intrauterine environment and may alter glucose and insulin metabolism in the offspring. In over nutrition conditions (birth weight >4,000 g), the prevalence of T2DM has been reported to be 8–18% [27].

Growth of tissues has critical periods at different times and the intrauterine environment can be one mechanism which may cause permanent changes in pancreas structure and hormone secretion pattern [28].

Recently, emerging evidence suggests that several maternal factors may be associated with childhood obesity, including maternal smoking during pregnancy, breastfeeding behavior, and parental dietary behavior and control feeding.

Maternal smoking may be related to poor diet during pregnancy, and a suboptimal nutritional environment in utero could result in fetal growth retardation [29].

Recent studies have shown that low birth weight is associated with a high prevalence of T2DM in British adults. Similar results have been discussed in a population-based study of 3.061 Pima Indians aged 5–29 years; in Pima Indian children and young adults, lower birth weight is associated with higher serum insulin concentration (and presumably lower insulin sensitivity), especially when related to their smaller body size. In conclusion, low-birth-weight Pima Indians are more insulin resistant than those with normal birth weight and this may explain their increased risk for T2DM [24].

## Puberty

Puberty appears to play a major role in the development of T2DM in children. The majority of youth with T2DM are diagnosed at puberty. During puberty, there is increased resistance to the action of insulin, resulting in hyperinsulinemia [16]. Insulin responses during an oral glucose tolerance test (OGTT) increase significantly from toddler age to adolescence. After puberty, basal and stimulated insulin responses decline. Hyperinsulinemic-euglycemic clamp studies demonstrate that insulin-mediated glucose disposal is on average 30% lower in adolescents between Tanner stages II and IV compared with prepubertal children in Tanner stage I and compared with young adults [30–32]. In the presence of normal pancreatic β-cell function, puberty-related insulin resistance is compensated by increased insulin secretion [33].

The causes of insulin resistance during puberty have been under investigation. Both growth hormone (GH) and sex steroids are likely candidates; however, the transient nature of pubertal insulin resistance is out of tempo with the increasing levels of sex steroids, which remain elevated in young adults while insulin resistance subsides. On the other hand, GH secretion increases during puberty simultaneously with the decrease in insulin action [34]. Studies have demonstrated that insulin-stimulated glucose metabolism correlates inversely with GH and/or insulin-like growth factor I level [31]. Administering GH to adolescents who are not GH deficient is associated with a deterioration in insulin action, whereas testosterone or dihydrotestosterone administration has no such effect. Thus, increased GH secretion during normal puberty is most probably responsible for the insulin resistance that evolves during puberty, and both these changes subside with the completion of puberty [35].

Given this information, it is not surprising that the peak age for T2DM is in mid-puberty. In an individual who has a genetic predisposition for insulin resistance, compounded with environmental risk exposure, the additional burden of insulin resistance during puberty may tip the balance from a state of compensated hyperinsulinemia with normal glucose tolerance to inadequate insulin secretion and glucose intolerance that continues beyond puberty.

### Polycystic Ovary Syndrome

Polycystic ovarian syndrome (PCOS) is another condition associated with insulin resistance. Women with PCOS are at increased risk of T2DM because they have profound insulin resistance, independent of obesity, and they have abnormalities in β-cell function. In women with PCOS, 31% have impaired glucose tolerance and 7.5–16% have T2DM [37]. Adolescents with PCOS have evidence of skeletal muscle insulin resistance with 40% reduction in insulin-stimulated glucose disposal, compared with body composition-matched non-hyperandrogenic control subjects. Those adolescents with PCOS who have impaired glucose tolerance have a 50% decrement in first-phase insulin secretion [38].

### Acanthosis nigricans

Acanthosis nigricans, a marker of insulin resistance, is a frequently associated finding in up to 90% of youth with T2DM. This skin lesion is characterized by velvety hyperpigmented patches in intertriginous areas. The medical importance of acanthosis nigricans is its association with insulin resistance/hyperinsulinism and features of syndrome X. The prevalence of this skin lesion is reported to be highest in black children (13.3%), followed by

Hispanics (5.5%) and Caucasian (0.5%). The presence of acanthosis nigricans during routine physical examination should alert health care providers to the presence of insulin resistance/hyperinsulinemia and may prove a useful guide for screening individuals at risk for T2DM [39].

### Diagnosis

The differential diagnosis of children and adolescents with excessive weight gain and obesity includes insulin resistance with or without diabetes mellitus, hypercortisolemia, hypothyroidism, excessive caloric consumption, and chromosomal disorders (e.g. Prader-Labhart-Willi syndrome). T2DM is diagnosed when fasting plasma glucose exceeds 126 mg/dl or if checked randomly glucose is >20 mg/dl or at 2 h after eating a meal or during a glucose tolerance test confirmed on different days. When obesity is present along with evidence of insulin resistance (acanthosis nigricans and/or insulin-to-glucose ratio >0.20) with no islet autoantibodies, then the child has T2DM. The presence of autoantibodies, with or without obesity, indicates type 1A (autoimmune) diabetes. It should be remembered that there is evidence of the presence of β-cell autoimmunity in adults with T2DM (4–15%); this situation is called latent autoimmune diabetes of the adult (LADA) and has also been described in children with clinical features of T2DM [36].

If the patient is African-American and has a family history of diabetes, the presentation is more acute, insulin sensitivity is normal, acanthosis and autoantibodies are absent, and the obesity is not marked, then the patient most likely has atypical diabetes [16, 40].

Normal insulin sensitivity and absence of obesity, acanthosis nigricans, and autoantibodies in a Caucasian patient with a family history of diabetes (autosomal-dominant in three or more generations) is consistent with maturity-onset diabetes of youth (MODY). The absence of autoantibodies in a patient who is not markedly obese and who does not have a family history is typical of type 1B (idiopathic) diabetes.

In newly diagnosed children and adolescents, T2DM accounts for about 10–20%, atypical diabetes 5–10%, type 1B 5–7%, and MODY is rare.

Because T2DM may remain asymptomatic for a prolonged period, the American Diabetes Association now recommends the screening of overweight children (BMI >85th percentile for age and sex) who have 2 or more of the following risk factors: family history of diabetes in a first- or second-degree relative; American Indian, black, Hispanic, or Asian/Pacific Islander ethnicity; signs of insulin resistance (acanthosis nigricans, hypertension, dyslipidemia, polycystic ovary syndrome).

Screening should be initiated at age 10 years (or at puberty) and performed every 2 years. Acceptable screening methods include fasting blood glucose or a 2-hour OGTT, but not glycosylated hemoglobin because of its low clinical sensitivity [41, 16].

## Prevention

As noted previously, the recent surge in T2DM in adolescents is related at least in part to increased prevalence of obesity among populations at risk for the disease. Therefore, preventive measures among pediatric patients should focus on obese subjects with a family history of T2DM.

No established guidelines are available to differentiate safe and low-risk obesity from dangerous and high-risk obesity in pediatric patients. A recent report documents high rates of glucose intolerance and unsuspected T2DM among obese subjects with BMI above the 95th percentile for age and gender. Consequently, subjects with BMI exceeding the 95th percentile for age and gender must be considered at risk. Nevertheless, some (particular pubertal) obese patients may have no apparent defects in insulin production or action and display no evidence of fasting hyperglycemia or glucose intolerance [41].

Glucose tolerance in obese patients is best assessed using a standard OGTT, which is reproducible and reliable in obese adolescents. Those with IGT (2 h glucose, 140–199 mg/100 ml) or IFG (fasting glucose, 111–125 mg/100 ml) are at the greatest risk of developing T2DM.

Such patients require immediate intervention to prevent further deterioration in blood glucose control. In adults with IGT, intensive lifestyle intervention has been shown in long-term studies to significantly reduce (by 31–58%) the rate of development of T2DM. In theory, intensive lifestyle intervention should also benefit pediatric patients who are at risk for developing T2DM [42].

However, lifestyle intervention is difficult, time-consuming, and, in many cases of childhood obesity, ineffective. Treatment failure may exacerbate insulin resistance, dyslipidemia, and glucose intolerance, leading to irreversible β-cell dysfunction and overt T2DM. Insulin resistance, dyslipidemia, and glucose intolerance in adolescents may also predispose to steatohepatitis and the development of arterial fatty plaques [40].

Recent investigations suggest that pharmacological agents may complement the effects of lifestyle intervention and reduce the risk of diabetes in selected patients. Metformin, trioglitazone, and acarbose reduce the risk of T2DM development in adults with IGT (Diabetes Prevention Program, TRIPOD, STOP-NIDDM). This is probably also true in adolescents with IGT.

## Therapy

The ideal goal of treatment is normalization of blood glucose values and HbA1c. Successful control of the associated comorbidities, such as hypertension and hyperlipidemia, is also important.

The ultimate goal of treatment is to decrease the risk of the acute and chronic complications associated with diabetes. There is strong evidence from a UK Prospective Diabetes Study that normalization of blood glucose decreases the frequency of microvascular complications of T2DM in adults. Macrovascular outcomes were not significantly decreased [43].

The early age of onset of T2DM in children may particularly increase the risk of microvascular complications, which are known to be directly related to duration of hyperglycemia and diabetes.

The initial treatment of T2DM will vary depending on the clinical presentation. The spectrum of the disease at diagnosis ranges from asymptomatic hyperglycemia to diabetic ketoacidosis and hyperglycemic hyperosmolar nonketotic states.

Clinical features suggesting initial treatment with insulin include dehydration, presence of ketosis, and acidosis. Patients who are not ill at diagnosis can be managed initially with medical nutrition therapy and exercise, but most will require drug therapy [44].

There are five types of glucose-lowering oral agents available for the treatment of type 2 diabetes:

1. Biguanides: decrease hepatic glucose output and enhance primarily hepatic and also muscle insulin sensitivity without a direct effect on β-cell function (metformin)
2. Sulfonylureas: promote insulin secretion (acetohexamide, chlorpropramide, gliclazide, glimepiride, glipizide, glyburide, tolazamide, and tolbutamide)
3. Meglitinide: short-term promotion of glucose-stimulated insulin secretion (repaglinide)
4. Glucosidase inhibitors: slow hydrolysis of complex carbohydrase and slow carbohydrate absorption (acarbose and miglitol)
5. Thiazolidenediones: improve peripheral insulin sensitivity (troglitazone, rosiglitazone, and pioglitazone) [45].

All children with T2DM should receive comprehensive self-management education.

Referral to a dietician with knowledge and experience in the nutritional management of children with diabetes is necessary. Dietary recommendation should be culturally appropriate, sensitive to family resources, and provided to all caregivers. Encouraging healthy eating habits by the entire family is very important.

Daily physical activity increasing caloric expenditure, is an important component of therapy. Exercise can decrease insulin resistance and is an important component of weight management. Decreasing sedentary activity, such as television watching and computer use, has been shown to be an effective way to increase daily physical activity in children. Involvement of family members can provide positive reinforcement and make overall family health a higher priority [41, 42].

Successful treatment with diet and exercise is defined as cessation of excessive weight gain with normal linear growth, near-normal fasting blood glucose values (<126 mg/dl), and near-normal HbA1c (less than 7%). Successful diabetes management without oral medication or insulin occurs in fewer than 10% of adult patients with diabetes over time [42].

If treatment goals with nutrition education and exercise are not met, pharmacological therapy is initiated. The first oral agent used should be metformin. Metformin has the advantage over sulfonylureas of having a similar reduction in HbA1c and overall glucose levels without the risk of hypoglycemia. In addition, weight is either decreased or remains stable, and LDL cholesterol and triglyceride levels decrease.

Treatment with metformin also may normalize ovulatory abnormalities in girls with PCOS and increase the risk of unplanned pregnancy. Therefore, preconception and pregnancy counseling should be part of the treatment regimen for all girls and women of childbearing age with T2DM. No oral agent should be used during pregnancy, highlighting the importance of counseling adolescents with T2DM about sexuality and pregnancy.

Due to the concern about lactic acidosis, metformin is contraindicated in patients with impaired renal function and should be discontinued with the administration of radiocontrast material. Metformin should not be used in patients with known hepatic disease, hypoxemic conditions, severe infections or alcohol abuse [45].

A recent study evaluated the safety and efficacy of metformin at doses to 1,000 mg twice daily in 82 subjects aged 10–16 years for up to 16 weeks in a randomized double-blinded placebo-controlled trial. Metformin significantly improved glycemic control (42 mg/dl) and reduced HbA1c (7.5 vs. 8.6 mg/dl). Improvement was seen in both sexes and in all race subgroups. The drug did not have a negative impact on body weight or lipid profile, adverse events were similar to those reported in adults treated with metformin (abdominal pain, diarrhea, nausea and headache). No cases of clinical hypoglycemia or lactic acidosis [46] have been reported.

If monotherapy with metformin is not successful over a reasonable period of time (3–6 months), several alternatives can be considered. Some clinicians would add sulfonylurea, whereas others might add insulin. Other insulin secretogogues are acceptable as well as glucosidase inhibitors, but these are used less frequently in children. With greatly elevated blood glucose levels or in very symptomatic patients, starting treatment with insulin (bedtime insulin alone, twice-a-day insulin or multidose insulin regimens) may most effectively bring hyperglycemia and symptoms under control. When glucose control is established, adding metformin while decreasing insulin is a therapeutic option [47].

### Monitoring for Complications

All types of diabetes increase the risk for microvascular and macrovascular complications, including myocardial infarction, stroke, renal failure, blindness, and neuropathy. However, risk for developing these complications may be substantially greater in T2DM than in type 1 [41].

The cumulative incidence of nephropathy after 30 years of postpubertal diabetes is significantly higher in T2DM (44.4%) than in type 1 diabetic patients (20.2%). Moreover, the incidence of nephropathy among type 1 diabetic patients has declined in the past two decades, whereas it is has not among T2DM patients.

Elevated blood glucose, common to both types of diabetes, affects the blood vessels through several mechanisms. Acutely, hyperglycemia increases blood pressure, promotes blood clot formation, and reduces endothelium-dependent blood flow, effects that appear to be mediated by oxidative stress. In the long-term, hyperglycemia induces formation of advanced glycosylation end products that damage the vascular endothelium. For these reasons, good glycemic control reduces diabetes complication rates. However, unlike type 1, T2DM is strongly associated with two additional cardiovascular disease risk factors: obesity and hyperinsulinemia [48].

Dilated eye examination should be performed in adolescents with T2DM according to the ADA's standards of medical care. Screening for microalbuminuria should also be performed yearly. It is unclear whether foot examinations are important in this age group; however, these examinations are painless, inexpensive, and provide an opportunity for education about foot care. We suggest tests for elevated blood pressure and lipid abnormalities. However, studies to detect macrovascular disease are probably not indicated. It is important to carefully control hypertension and in this case ACE inhibitors are the agents of choice in children with microalbuminuria. Children with T2DM may be hyperlipidemic. In this case weight loss, increased activity, and improvement in glycemic control often results in improvement of lipid levels [49, 50].

## Conclusion

The progression of disease from childhood to adulthood is often silent; by the time of diagnosis, many adults with T2DM already have microvascular and macrovascular complications. Intergenerational cycles and social/cultural factors perpetuate the familial and ethnic patterns of chronic illness. These facts underscore the central importance of reproductive and pediatric medicine in the prevention of adult disease.

The prevalence of T2DM in the US may increase by as much as 65% during the next 50 years, and if societal trends in obesity are not controlled, we can expect further increases in the prevalence of childhood disease and gestational diabetes. Such changes will place enormous burdens on the medical, financial, and social communities [16].

As pediatric endocrinologists caring for individual patients, we must aggressively manage hyperglycemia, dyslipidemia, and hypertension to prevent long-term complications. However, we must also define the metabolic, genetic, and lifestyle factors that increase the risk of chronic metabolic and cardiovascular disease more precisely and identify, at an early age, those families and children at highest risk. We will then, in collaboration with representatives of the lay community, be able to implement individual and societal measures that will prevent diabetes.

## References


1 Arslanian S: Type 2 diabetes in children: Clinical aspects and risk factors. Horm Res 2002; 57:19–28.

2 Rosenbloom AL, Joe JR, Young RS, Winter ME: Emerging epidemic of type 2 diabetes in youth. Diabetes Care 1999;22:345–354.

3 Glaser NS: Non-insulin-dependent diabetes mellitus in childhood and adolescence. Pediatr Clin N Am 1997;44:307–337.

4 Pinhas-Hamiel O, Dolan LM, Daniels SR: Increased incidence of non-insulin-dependent diabetes mellitus among adolescents. J Pediatr 1996;128:608–615.

5 Campagna Anne-Fagot, Saaddine Jinan B, Flegal Katherine M, Beckles Gloria LA: Diabetes, impaired fasting glucose, and elevated HbA1c in US adolescents: The Third National Health and Nutrition Examination Survey. Diabetes Care 2001;24:834–837.

6 Dabelea D, Pettit DJ, Jones KL, Arslanian SA: Type 2 diabetes mellitus in minority children and adolescents: An emerging problem. Endocrinol Metab Clin N Am 1999;28:709–729.

7 Blanchard JF, Dean H, Anderson K, Wajda A, Ludwig S, Depew N: Incidence and prevalence of diabetes in children aged 0–14 in Manitoba, Canada, 1985–1993. Diabetes Care 1997;20: 512–515.

8 Dean HJ, Mundy RL, Moffatt M: Non-insulin-dependent diabetes mellitus in Indian children in Manitoba. Can Med Assoc J 1992;147:52–57.

9 Kitagawa T, Owada M, Urakami T, Tajima N: Epidemiology of type 1 (insulin dependent) and type 2 (non-insulin-dependent) diabetes mellitus in Japanese children. Diab Res Clin Pract 1994:24 (suppl):S7–S13.

10 Kitagawa T, Owada M, Urakami T, Yamauchi K: Increased incidence of non-insulin-dependent diabetes mellitus among Japanese schoolchildren correlates with an increased intake of animal protein and fat. Clin Pediatr 1998;37:111–115.
11 Kadiki OA, Reddy MR, Marzouc AA: Incidence of insulin-dependent diabetes (IDDM) and non-insulin-dependent diabetes (NIDDM) in Benghazi, Libya. Diab Res Clin Pract 1996;32:165–173.
12 Hale DE, Danney MM: Non-insulin dependent diabetes in Hispanic youth. Diabetes 1998; 47:A28.
13 Fagot-Campagna: Prevalence of type 2 diabetes in children in Birmingham. BMJ 2001;322:1428.
14 Invitti C, Guzzaloni G, Gilardini L, Morabito F, Viberti G: Prevalence and concomitants of glucose intolerance in European obese children and adolescents. Diabetes Care 2003;26:118–124.
15 Gerich JE: The genetic basis of type 2 diabetes mellitus: Impaired insulin secretion versus impaired insulin sensitivity. Endocr Rev 1998;19:491–503.
16 American Diabetes Association: Type 2 diabetes in children and adolescents. Pediatrics 2000;105: 671–680.
17 Freemark M: Pharmacologic approaches to the prevention of type 2 diabetes in high risk pediatric patients. J Clin Endocrinol Metab 2003;88:3–13.
18 Kahn SE: The relative contributions of insulin resistance and beta-cell dysfunction to the pathophysiology of type 2 diabetes. Diabetologia 2003;46:3–19.
19 Sinha R, Fish G, Teague B: Prevalence of impaired glucose tolerance among children and adolescents with marked obesity. N Engl J Med 2002;346:802–810.
20 Boyko EJ, Fujimoto WY, Leonetti DL, Newell-Morris L: Visceral adiposity and risk of type 2 diabetes. Diabetes Care 2000;23:456.
21 Pietrobelli A, Faith MS, Allison DB, Gallagher D, Chiumello G, Heymsfield SB: Body mass index as a measure of adiposity among children and adolescents: A validation study. J Pediatr 1997;132:204–210.
22 Arslanian S: Type 2 diabetes mellitus in children: Pathophysiology and risk factors. J Pediatr Endocrinol Metab 2000;13:1385–1394.
23 Danadian K, Balasekaran G, Lewy V, Meza M, Robertson R, Arslanian SA: Insulin sensitivity in African-American children with and without family history of type 2 diabetes. Diabetes Care 1999;22:1325–1329.
24 Dabelea D, Pettit D, Hanson R, Imperatore G, Bennett PH, Knowler WC: Birth weight, type 2 diabetes, and insulin resistance in Pima Indian children and young adults. Diabetes Care 1999;22:944–950.
25 Campagna AF, Pettit DJ, Engelgau MM, Burrows NR, Geiss LS, Valdez R, Beckles GLA, Saaddine J, Gregg EW, Williamson DF, Narayan KMV: Type 2 diabetes among North American children and adolescents: An epidemiologic review and a public health perspective. J Pediatr 1999;5:664–672.
26 Hales CN, Barker DJ: Type 2 diabetes mellitus: The thrifty phenotype hypothesis. Br Med Bull 2001;60:5–20.
27 Hernandez V, Zarate A: Fetal weight at weight as predisposing risk factor for type 2 diabetes in adulthood. Ginecol Obstet Mex 2001;69:390–398.
28 Wei JN, Sung FC, Li CY, Chang CH: Low birth weight and high birth weight infants are both at increased risk to have type 2 diabetes among schoolchildren. Diabetes care 2003;26:343–348.
29 Hales CN: The role of poor fetal and infant growth in non-insulin-dependent diabetes. Bull Mem Acad R Med Belg 1993;148:281–285.
30 Kobayashi K, Amemija S, Higashida K, Ishihara T, Sawanobori E, Mochizuki M, Kikuchi N, Tokuyama K, Nakazawa S: Pathogenic factors of glucose intolerance in obese Japanese adolescents with type 2 diabetes. Metabolism 2000;49:186–191.
31 Amiel SA, Sherwin RS, Simenson DC, Lauritano AA, Tamborlane WV: Impaired insulin action in puberty. N Engl J Med 1986;315:215–219.
32 Moran A, Jacobs DR, Steinberger J, Hong CP, Prineas R, Luepk R, Sinaiko AR: Insulin resistance during puberty. Diabetes 1999;48:2039–2044
33 Caprio S, Plewe G, Diamond MP, Simonson DC, Boulware SD, Sherwin RS, Tamborlane WV: Increased insulin secretion in puberty: A compensatory response to reduction in insulin sensitivity. J Pediatr 1989;114:963–967.

34 Metzger DL, Kerrigan JR, Rogol AD: Gonadal steroid hormone regulation of the somatotropic axis during puberty in humans: Mechanism of androgen and estrogen action. Trends Endocrinol Metab 1994;5:290–296.
35 Arslanian SA, Danadian K, Suprasongin C: GH treatment in adolescents with non-GH deficient short stature (NGHD-SS): Physical, biochemical and metabolic changes. Pediatr Res 1999; 45.84A.
36 Hathout E, Thomas W, El-Shahawy M, Nahab F, Mace J: Diabetic autoimmune markers in children and adolescents with type 2 diabetes. Pediatrics 2001;107:102–106.
37 Ehrmann DA, Barnes RB, Rosenfield RL, Cavaghan MK, Imperial J: Prevalence of impaired glucose tolerance and diabetes in woman with polycystic ovary syndrome. Diabetes Care 1999;22:141–146.
38 Lewy VD, Danadian K, Witchel SF, Arslanian S: Early metabolic abnormalities in adolescent girls with polycystic ovarian syndrome. J Pediatr 2001;138:38–44.
39 Stuart CA, Gilkinson CR, Smith MM, Bosma AM, Keenan BS, Nagamani M: Acanthosis nigricans as a risk factor for non-insulin-dependent diabetes mellitus. Clin Pediatr 1998;37:73–79.
40 Hansen JR, Fulop MJ, Hunter MK: Type 2 diabetes mellitus in youth: A growing challenge. Clin Diab 2000;18:320–325.
41 Ludwig DS, Ebbeling CB: Type 2 diabetes mellitus in children. JAMA 2001;286:112–123.
42 Huang TK, Goran MI: Prevention of type 2 diabetes in young people: A theoretical perspective. Pediatr Diab 2003;4:38–56.
43 Owada M, Nitadori Y, Kitagawa T: Treatment of NIDDM in youth. Clin Pediatr 1998;37:117–122.
44 Lee Jones K: Non-insulin dependent diabetes in children and adolescents: The therapeutic challenge. Clin Pediatr 1998;37:103–110.
45 Lee Jones K, Arslanian S, Peterokova V, Park JS, Tomlimson M: Effect of metformin in pediatric patients with type 2 diabetes. Diabetes Care 2002;25:89–94.
46 Cuse K, DeFronzo RA: Metformin. A review of its metabolic effect. Diab Rev 1998;6:89–131.
47 Hamiel OP, Zeitler P: Barriers to the treatment of adolescent type 2 diabetes, a survey of provider perceptions. Pediatric Diabetes 2003;4:24–28.
48 Yokoyama H, Okudaira M, Otani T, Sato A, Miura J, Takaike H, Yamada H, Muto K, Uchigata Y, Ohashi Y, Iwamoto Y: Higher incidence of diabetic nephropathy in type 2 than in type 1 diabetes in early-onset diabetes in Japan. Kid Int 2000;58:302–311.
49 Yokohama H, Okudaira M, Otani T, Watanabe C, Takaine H, Miuira J, Yamada H, Mutou H, Satou A, Uchigata Y, Iwamoto Y: High incidence of diabetic nephropathy in early-onset Japanese NIDDM patients. Diabetes Care 1998;7:1080–1085.
50 Goran MI, Ball GDC, Cruz ML: Obesity and risk of type 2 diabetes and cardiovascular disease in children and adolescents. J Endocrinol Metab 2002;88:1417–1427.

Prof. Giuseppe Chiumello
Centro di Endocrinologia dell'Infanzia e dell'Adolescenza
Istituto Scientifico H San Raffaele, Università Vita-Salute
via Olgettina 60, IT–20190 Milano (Italy)
Tel. +39 02 26432623, Fax +39 02 26432626, E-Mail chiumello.giuseppe@hsr.it

Chiarelli F, Dahl-Jørgensen K, Kiess W (eds): Diabetes in Childhood and Adolescence.
Pediatr Adolesc Med. Basel, Karger, 2005, vol 10, pp 362–372

# Beta-Cell Function Replacement by Islet Transplantation and Gene Therapy

*Luca Falqui*

Department of Medicine, Diabetes and Endocrinology,
San Raffaele Scientific Institute and University, Milan, Italy

## Replacing the Lost β-Cell Function: An Unsolved Issue

The concept of replacing exogenous insulin therapy with an endogenous, novel cellular source of insulin emerged over 30 years ago, when chemical diabetes in rodents was reverted by syngeneic islet transplantation [1]. It was only in 1986, however, that the development of a method for human islet isolation [2] led to the first attempts at islet transplants in man [3, 4]. In the following years, several international centers started clinical programs of islet transplantation, with variable results [5, 6]. Only since 2000 has the introduction of a new immunosuppressive regimen, now known as the 'Edmonton protocol' [7], and of several refinements of the entire procedure led to consistent success. Despite this improvement, chronic immunosuppression and scarcity of transplantable islets make islet transplantation a treatment for a niche of diabetic patients. Therefore, alternative cellular replacement therapies, including gene therapy and β-cell development from stem cells, have been intensively sought.

## The Procedure for Islet Isolation and Transplant

The islets are obtained from pancreas retrieved from brain-dead multiorgan donors. A careful surgical procedure and correct preservation of the pancreatic gland before the isolation are crucial for islet yield and viability. In 1986, Ricordi et al. [2] devised a method that enables a controlled mechanical and enzymatic dissociation of the pancreatic gland. Through a series of improvements and modifications to meet the cGMP requirements, this method has evolved over these years to become the 'standard procedure' currently used by the majority of centers involved in clinical islet transplants. The process is based on the injection of a blend of proteolytic enzymes (mostly collagenase) into the pancreatic duct, the gland is then loaded into a chamber where the enzymatic digestion is accelerated by a controlled mechanical shaking. Depending on the activity of that specific collagenase lot, and on some characteristic of the pancreas itself (i.e. donor age, amount of fibrotic tissue and fat), the process may approximately require 10–30 min. A key feature of the method is that as soon as islets are liberated from the pancreatic tissue, they are eluted into a separated section of the circuit where rapid cooling stops enzyme action; thus, islets are preserved from further digestion and possible damage. At the end of the digestion phase, islets are separated from exocrine fragments on density gradients of human albumin, performed on and automated system (COBE centrifuge), rinsed and finally collected in specifically designed plastic bags.

The clinical procedure of islet transplantation consists of an infusion of the suspension of islets into a distal branch of the portal vein. By a percutaneous transhepatic puncture, in local anesthesia and under ultrasonography visualization, the vessel is cannulated, and islets are slowly infused by gravity. Islets lodge in pre-terminal or terminal branches of the portal tree, depending on size. The portal vein pressure is monitored, and the infusion rate is reduced or temporarily interrupted if an increase is detected. At the end of the procedure, the catheter is retracted and a fibrin plug is left in the vein wall to prevent bleeding.

## Clinical Results

The overall clinical outcome of islet transplantation in type 1 diabetic patients is documented in the International Registry [8]. In a series of more than 450 transplants performed from 1990 to 2000 in many centers, only 8% of patients achieved or maintained insulin independence. A careful look at these data reveals, however, that they are influenced by the 'center effect'. Indeed, the Milan and Giessen groups were able to report a success rate of 50% of insulin independence at 1 year. Careful surgical harvest of pancreas pre-isolation, an experienced team performing the isolation procedure and a dedicated post-transplant management of patients and of immune suppressive therapy are key elements to success. Several immunosuppressive regimens have been developed to prevent islet rejection with acceptable adverse effects. These regimens are based on the combination of drugs with different effects on the immune system. A short course of anti-thymocyte globulin, or OKT3, followed by an

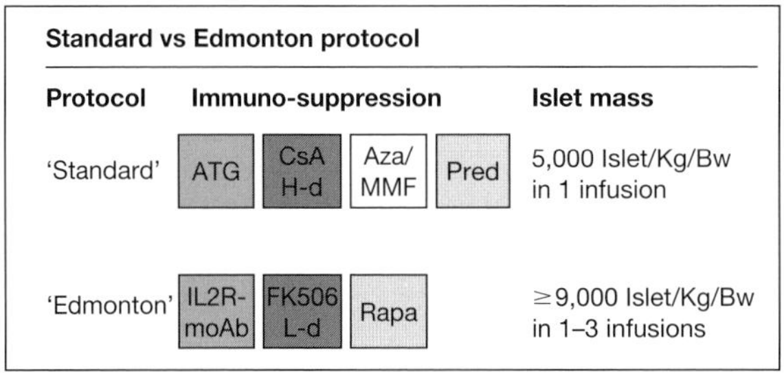


***Fig. 1.*** A comparison of the most important differences between the Standard Islet Transplantation Procedure and the Edmonton Protocol is reported. ATG = Antitymocyte globulin; CSA = cyclosporine; H-d = high dosage; AZA = azathioprine; MMF = mycophenolate mofetil; Pred = prednisone; Il-2R Ab = monoclonal antibody against IL-2 receptor; FK506 = tacrolimus; L-d = low dosage; Rapa = rapamycin.

anticalcineurin drug, cyclosporin or tacrolimus, plus azatioprine and predisone (at high dose, tapered over time) had been employed in a large majority of islet transplants performed at different centers up to 2000.

In 2000, the Edmonton group reported of a series of seven islets transplants in which a dramatic 100% success rate at 1 year was obtained [7]. Subsequent reports from the same group in a larger series of patients confirmed a 80% insulin independence at 1 year, and 2 of the initial 3 patients remaining insulin-free beyond 4 years [9]. These results have been achieved introducing a series of refinements in several aspects of islet isolation and transplant procedures. Among many, two factors may represent the key to success: the first, the use of a new immunosuppressive regimen, where a monoclonal antibody against IL-2 receptor was used as induction therapy, and rapamycin (sirolimus) plus low-dose FK-506 (tacrolimus) for maintenance therapy. Steroid was excluded from the scheme. A second factor, likely of similar relevance, has been the larger number of islets implanted into each patient (fig. 1). This islet mass has been obtained from 2 or 3 pancreases, and was implanted into patients in two or three procedures, approximately at monthly intervals. The complete procedure consolidated in the so-called 'Edmonton Protocol' has been progressively adopted by many centers with comparable result [10].

## Complications and Adverse Effects of the Procedure

The complications may occur during the implantation phase or develop as adverse effects of the immunosuppressive treatment. A transient increase (×3–5) of liver enzymes has been reported in most cases in the peri-transplant period. Infrequent complications include peritoneal bleeding, development of arteriovenous fistula and thrombosis of a peripheral portal branch. All these events appeared to be of mild or moderate entity, and resolved spontaneously without specific treatment. Frequent adverse effects of the immunosuppressive therapy were mouth ulcer, amenorrhea, hyperlipidemia, and arthritis. More important, in a very few cases an impairment of renal function occurred which required a modification of the immunosuppressive regimen [11].

## Impact of Islet Transplantation of Diabetes Complications

Recent studies have shown that islet transplantation can provide excellent glycemic control over many years with normal HbA1c levels. These results raise the possibility that islet transplantation may affect the outcome of diabetic complications provided that rejection and recurrence of autoimmunity can be prevented by non-toxic immunosuppressive drugs. Long-term studies in non-uremic diabetic recipients of whole pancreas transplantation have shown that many years (up to 10) of near-normal glycemic control were needed to arrest the progression or to reverse diabetic lesions in the native kidney [12]. The current survival time of islet transplants in non-uremic diabetic patients is insufficient to provide the information. However, Fiorina et al. [13] have recently reported a significant improved survival of renal transplants in uremic diabetic patients after islet-kidney transplants, compared to intensified insulin treatment (83 vs. 51% at 7 years). Remarkably, HbA1c levels were similar in both groups, pointing to an additional advantage provided by the transplant, beyond metabolic control. Among the possible factors, the authors pointed to a positive association between persistent C-peptide secretion (>0.5 ng/ml) and renal survival and reduced albumin excretion, even in the patients who had returned to insulin therapy. This suggestion is supported by a study that demonstrated improved renal function after administration of C-peptide in type 1 diabetes [14] making the association more convincing. However, additional studies in larger groups are needed to confirm this finding.

## Gene Therapy

A potentially unlimited source for cellular replacement therapy of type I diabetes may be obtained by conferring the property to synthesize insulin to non-endocrine cells. Several non-endocrine cells – skin, muscle and liver cells – can be engineered to synthesize proinsulin by a relatively simple gene transfer procedure [15–17]. These cells, however, release the intact pro-hormone since they lack the β-cell specific convertases for proinsulin conversion to mature insulin. To circumvent this obstacle, the proinsulin DNA sequence has been genetically modified at the A-chain/C-peptide and C-peptide/B-chain junctions to generate cleavage motifs recognized by the ubiquitous protease furin [18]. This enables non-endocrine cells to convert and release the '*fur*in-sensitive *h*uman *pro**I*nsulin' (FurHPI) mostly (60–80%) in a mature insulin form, which retains all the biological activity of wild-type insulin [19]. The implantation of insulin-producing human fibroblasts into the peritoneum of diabetic rodents frankly reduced blood glucose levels. However, since these cells released insulin in a non-regulated manner, cell overgrowth and lack of regulation led to uncontrolled, irreversible hypoglycemia [20].

## Gene Therapy for Glucose-Regulated Insulin Release

To be proposed for clinical application, any 'surrogate β-cell' should be capable of releasing insulin in response to blood glucose variations in a properly regulated manner [21]. Ideally, a 'surrogate β-cell' should reproduce the dynamics of insulin secretion of the endocrine pancreas, which responds to acute elevations in blood glucose with a burst of insulin release within 15–30 s. This response relies on the endocrine cell machinery of granule formation, storage and regulated exocytotic secretion that is absent in non-endocrine cells, which therefore release insulin through the constitutive, non-regulated pathway.

To maintain circulating insulin levels in the narrow therapeutic range, several authors have attempted to develop a glucose-responsive regulation of the synthesis of transgeneic insulin in cells that are naturally responsive to glucose. Liver cells have been extensively studied because, similarly to β-cells, they possess the property of 'sensing' extracellular glucose variations, due to the expression of the glucose transporter 2 (Glut-2) and glucokinase [22] and because the expression of several genes is modulated in response to carbohydrates levels [23]. This property is mediated by the binding of a liver-specific transcription factor, named carbohydrate responsive element binding protein (ChREBP), to short DNA elements named *c*arbo*h*y*d*rate-*r*esponsive *e*lements (ChoREs) or *g*lucose *r*esponsive *e*lements (GlREs). ChoREs/GlREs were first identified in the liver-type pyruvate kinase (L-PK) gene promoter and, subsequently, in the regulatory regions of several other genes, including spot 14, fatty acid synthase, acetyl-CoA carboxylase and glucose-6-phosphatase [reviewed in 24]. This property has prompted several authors to use

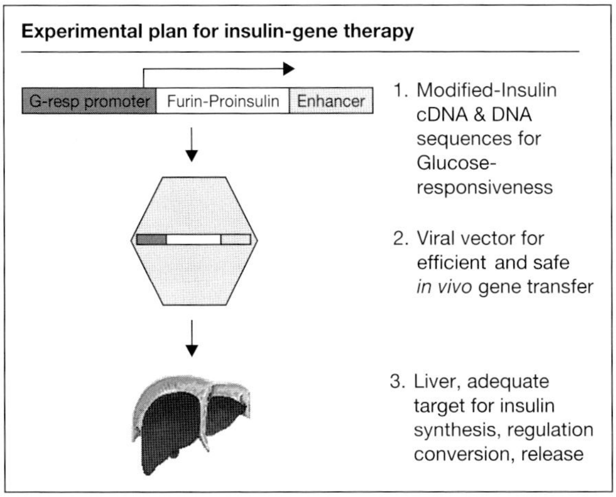


***Fig. 2.*** Experimental plan for insulin gene therapy. The general scheme of insulin-gene therapy is outlined. An 'expression cassette', coding for a modified insulin protein (FurHPI) under the transcriptional control of a glucose-responsive promoter is inserted into a vector (a genetically modified virus). Once injected intravenously, the vector delivers the therapeutic DNA to liver cells.

glucose-responsive promoters or selected sequences to control the expression of the insulin transgene in liver cells (fig. 2). An expression cassette was generated in which the glucose-responsive DNA sequence from the abovementioned genes was functionally linked to the FurHPI cDNA. In some cases, regulatory elements from other mammalian or viral genes have been added to modulate insulin expression. The 'cassette' was inserted into an adenoviral vector, which was amplified in packaging cells to obtain high titer preparations. Finally, the vector suspension was injected into diabetic rodents, in the general circulation or directly into the portal vein. This insulin-gene therapy approach resulted in the synthesis, processing and release of human insulin from rodent livers and in the consequent reduction of blood glucose levels. Insulin levels depended on the amount of vector particles injected; with appropriate dosage, within 1 week after gene therapy, normal or near-normal fasting glycemia was achieved and non-fasting hyperglycemia was largely reduced. After glucose load, treated animals normalized blood glucose within 2–4 h, and very importantly, tolerated a 16–24 hour fast without hypoglycemia. Since liver cells progressively eliminate the Adenoviral vectors, insulin expression persisted for up to 3 months after a single injection [25–26]. The most conclusive results have been obtained by Lee et al. [27] who used a parvovirus-derived vector (adeno-associated virus) as a gene delivery vehicle. They used the full-length (3.1 kb) L-PK promoter to regulate the synthesis of a short-chain insulin analogue which does not require processing. This approach resulted in the long-term correction of diabetes in NOD mice and diabetic rats, both in the fasting and in the fed state. No spontaneous hypoglycemia was reported. However, during a glucose tolerance test, the kinetics of insulin levels displayed a time to peak of 4 h and a return to basal level after 6 h, which is delayed when compared to insulin kinetics in normal animals. Consequently, late mild hypoglycemia occurred. Overall, these results demonstrate that a simple procedure of insulin gene therapy to the liver is capable to replace basal insulinization in rodents, and that a certain degree of glucose responsiveness is achieved. No side effects were observed and only minimal hypoglycemia was induced under a provocative test. This represents a strong proof of principle of the potential of insulin gene therapy, but in the view of a future clinical translation, it raises the question of a possible need for a faster activation and repression of insulin synthesis.

### Drug-Induced Insulin Release in Engineered Cells

Ideally, glucose should control insulin release from a 'surrogate β-cell'. In alternative, the insulin release could respond to a drug, so as to mimic the condition of type 2 diabetes. Such a pharmacological control of insulin release was developed by Rivera et al. [28], who engineered insulin protein so that it accumulated as aggregates in the endoplasmic reticulum of a candidate 'surrogate β-cell'. Insulin release was then stimulated by a synthetic small-molecule drug that induces protein disaggregation. Experiments in vitro and in vivo demonstrated rapid and transient secretion insulin. However, a major limitation to this approach was that that small molecule has to be administrated by injection. More recently, the same group [29] proposed a different pharmacological control system, based on the oral administration of the immunosuppressive drug rapamycin. To obtain regulated expression, they placed expression of the FurHPI under the control of a transcription system inducible by rapamycin and performed experiments of hepatic gene transfer in rodents by adenoviral vectors. Insulin release from mouse liver was negligible in the absence of rapamycin, was inducible in a dose-dependent manner upon its administration, and reversible following drug withdrawal. The response of the inducible system was rather slow, requiring hours to be activated; moreover, rapamycin is a powerful immunosuppressant. These results indicate however that a pharmacological regulation may constitute a possible alternative to self-regulated, glucose-responsive insulin release from a 'surrogate β-cell', provided a non-toxic, oral compound with fast activity is found.

## Islet Neogenesis in the Liver by Gene Transfer

In search of a 'surrogate β-cell' capable of timely regulated insulin secretion, an intriguing new possibility has emerged from embryogenesis studies that have identified in the gut endoderm the common origin for the pancreas and the liver. This common origin has suggested the possibility to redirect liver cells into β-cells by inducing the expression of key transcription factor(s) of β-cells development with a gene transfer approach. In the first study [30], insulin promoter factor 1 (Ipf1, also known as Pdx-1) was expressed in the liver by an early generation Adenoviral vector. Ipf1 is required for the development of the pancreas, and in mature β-cells, for fully competent insulin secretion [31]. The hepatic expression of Ipf1 produced reduction of glucose levels in diabetic mice for approximately 10 days. Later on, Kojima et al. [32] demonstrated that since Ipf1 also regulates exocrine cell gene expression, Ipf1 gene transfer induced the co-expression of insulin and trypsin. Trypsin production was associated with fatal liver inflammation. Therefore, these Authors turned to a transcription factor, Neurod1, that is expressed only in developing and adult β-cells, and to betacellulin, a β-cell growth factor. Using an adenoviral constructs of recent generation as gene transfer vehicle, which led to prolonged expression of both genes, they detected in the liver clusters of cells that contained the hormones, insulin, glucagon, pancreatic polypeptide and somatostatin, normally expressed in pancreatic endocrine cells. More strikingly, this gene-transfer procedure led to normalization of glucose levels in diabetic mice, and to normal insulin secretion under glucose challenge. Clearly, many issues remain unsolved, i.e. which is the origin and the long term fate of these cells; in addition these findings need to be confirmed by other studies in different animal models. There is no doubt, however, that this study opens new exciting perspectives towards the development of fully competent 'surrogate β-cells' for the treatment of diabetes.

## The Autoimmunity Issue

A critical aspect for any cell or gene replacement therapy of type 1 diabetes is the possibility of autoimmune recurrence against new insulin-producing cells. It is well known that a pancreas transplant from an HLA identical twin or sibling is susceptible to immune recognition that leads to selective β-cell destruction [33]. The key autoantigen(s) that triggers immune response is still unknown. Insulin, or its precursor proinsulin, has been proposed as one of the candidates because of the presence of anti-insulin antibodies and insulin-reactive T cell clones, both in human and in the non-obese diabetic (NOD) mouse [reviewed in 34]. It is, however, possible that insulin-producing cells, different from β cells, may escape autoimmune recognition or attack. This subject has been initially addressed by Lipes et al. [35], who demonstrated that transgenic insulin-producing pituitary cells were not destroyed by the autoimmune system when transplanted into syngeneic NOD mice, which were perfectly capable to eliminate a simultaneous islet graft. More recently, Olson et al. [26] and Lee et al. [27] did not observe autoimmune reactivity against insulin-producing liver cells in the BB rat or in the NOD mouse. However, whether 'substitutive insulin-producing cells' could be susceptible to autoimmune recurrence in man remains to be established.

## Conclusions and Perspectives

The results recently obtained in the islet transplantation clinical trials demonstrate that this β-cell replacement strategy is capable of normalizing blood glucose levels and to free IDDM patients from insulin injection for a long time. A positive impact on diabetic complications is also observed. Despite its efficacy, the treatment is conditioned by the small number of organ donors, the high-cost procedure, and by the strict requirement for a chronic immunosuppression. For these reasons, the procedure is currently indicated to limited number of adult type 1 diabetic subjects, with severe autonomic neuropathy and hypoglycemia unawareness.

Among the potential alternative sources of transplantable insulin-secreting cells there are islets from xenogeneic donors, genetically engineered rodent β-cell lines and human allogeneic stem cells cultured or engineered to become β-cells. All these approaches, however, rely on immunosuppressive treatments or on the development of safe and biocompatible devices for containment and immune isolation of immortalized cells of non-human sources [36]. Currently, unsolved issues in the delivery vehicle efficiency and safety preclude a clinical application of gene therapy. However, if the safety issue is solved, a liver-directed gene therapy approach may provide diabetic subjects with the level of functional correction sufficient to restore blood glucose values in the near-normal range needed to prevent complications, in the absence of demanding insulin treatment, surgical risks and immunosuppression.

## Acknowledgments

I thank Sabina Martinenghi and Antonio Secchi for careful revision of the manuscript.

## References


1 Ballinger W, Lacy P: Transplantation of intact pancreatic islets in rats. Surgery 1972;72:175–186.

2 Ricordi C, Lacy PE, Finke EH, Olack BJ, Sharp DW: Automated method for isolation of human pancreatic islets. Diabetes 1988;37:413–420.

3 Scharp DW, Lacy PE, Santiago JV, McCullough CS, Weide LG, Falqui L, Marchetti P, Gingerich RL, Jaffe AS, Cryer PE, et al: Insulin independence after islet transplantation into type I diabetic patient. Diabetes 1990;39:515–518.

4 Scharp DW, Lacy PE, Santiago JV, McCullough CS, Weide LG, Boyle PJ, Falqui L, Marchetti P, Ricordi C, Gingerich RL, et al: Results of our first nine intraportal islet allografts in type 1, insulin-dependent diabetic patients. Transplantation 1991;51:76–85.

5 Ricordi C, Tzakis AG, Carroll PB, Zeng YJ, Rilo HL, Alejandro R, Shapiro A, Fung JJ, Demetris AJ, Mintz DH, et al: Transplantation 1992;53:407–414.

6 Secchi A, Socci C, Maffi P, Taglietti MV, Falqui L, Bertuzzi F, De Nittis P, Piemonti L, Scopsi L, Di Carlo V, Pozza G: Islet transplantation in IDDM patients. Diabetologia 1997;40:225–231.

7 Shapiro AM, Lakey JR, Ryan EA, Korbutt GS, Toth E, Warnock GL, Kneteman NM, Rajotte RV: Islet transplantation in seven patients with type 1 diabetes mellitus using a glucocorticoid-free immunosuppressive regimen. N Engl J Med 2000;343:230–238.

8 Brendel M, Hering B, Schultz A, Bretzel R: International Islet Registry Report. Giessen, University of Giessen, 1999, pp 1–20.

9 Ryan EA, Lakey JR, Paty BW, Imes S, Korbutt GS, Kneteman NM, Bigam D, Rajotte RV, Shapiro AM: Successful islet transplantation: Continued insulin reserve provides long-term glycemic control. Diabetes 2002;51:2148–2157.

10 Shapiro AM, Ricordi C, Hering B: Edmonton's islet success has indeed been replicated elsewhere. Lancet 2003;362:1242.

11 Maffi P: 3nd International Islet Isolation Workshop/Network of Islet Centers in Europe (NICE), Milan, 2004.

12 Fioretto N, Steffes MW, Sutherland DE, Goetz FC, Mauer M: Reversal of lesions of diabetic nephropathy after pancreas transplantation. N Engl J Med 1998;339:69–75.

13 Fiorina P, Folli F, Zerbini G, Maffi P, Gremizzi C, Di Carlo V, Socci C, Bertuzzi F, Kashgarian M, Secchi A: Islet transplantation is associated with improvement of renal function among uremic patients with type 1 diabetes mellitus and kidney transplantation. J Am Soc Nephrol 2003;14: 2150–2158.

14 Johansson BL, Borg K, Fernquist-Forbes E, Kernell A, Odgren T, Wahren J: Beneficial effects of C-Peptide on incipient nephropathy and neuropathy in patients with type 1 diabetes mellitus. Diabet Med 2000;17:181–189.

15 Vollenveider F, Irminger J-C, Gross DJ, Villa-Komaroff L, Halban PA: Processing of proinsulin by the transfected hepatoma (FAO) cells. J Biol Chem 1992;267:14629–14636.

16 Kolodka TM, Finegold M, Moss L, Woo SLC: Gene therapy for diabetes mellitus in rats by hepatic expression of insulin. Proc Natl Acad Sci USA 1995;92:3293–3297.

17 Yoshimoto K, Murakami R, Moritani M, Ohta M, Iwawana H, Nakauchi H, Itakura M: Loss of ganciclovir sensitivity by exclusion of thymidine kinase gene from transplanted proinsulin-producing fibroblasts as a gene therapy model for diabetes. Gene Ther 1996;3:230–234.

18 Groskreutz DJ, Sliwkowski MX, Gorman CM: Genetically engineered proinsulin constitutively processed and secreted as mature, active insulin. J Biol Chem 1994;269:6241–6245.

19 Simonson GD, Groskreutz DJ, Gorman CM MacDonald MJ: Synthesis and processing of genetically modified human proinsulin by rat myoblast primary cultures. Hum Gene Ther 1996;7: 71–78.

20 Falqui L, Martinenghi S, Severini GM, Corbella P, Taglietti MV, Arcelloni C, Sarugeri E, Monti LD, Paroni R, Dozio N, Pozza G, Bordignon C: Reversal of diabetes in mice by implantation of human fibroblasts genetically engineered to release mature human insulin. Hum Gene Ther 1999;10: 1753–1762.

21 Halban PA, Kahn SE, Lernmark A, Rhodes CJ: Gene and cell-replacement therapy in the treatment of type 1 diabetes: How high must the standards be set? Diabetes 2001;50:2181–2191.

22 German MS: Glucose sensing in pancreatic islet beta cells: The key role of glucokinase and the glycolytic intermediates. Proc Natl Acad Sci USA 1993;90:1781–1785.
23 Vaulont S, Kahn A: Transcriptional control of metabolic regulation genes by carbohydrates. FASEB J 1994;8:28–35.
24 Towle H: Metabolic regulation of gene transcription in mammals. J Biol Chem 1995;270: 23235–23238.
25 Barry SC, Ramesh N, Lejnieks D, Simonson WT, Kemper L, Lernmark A, Osborne WR: Glucose-regulated insulin expression in diabetic rats. Hum Gene Ther 2001;12:131–139.
26 Olson DE, Paveglio SA, Huey PU, Porter MH, Thule PM: Glucose-responsive hepatic insulin gene therapy of spontaneously diabetic BB/Wor rats. Hum Gene Ther 2003;14:1401–1413.
27 Lee HC, Kim SJ, Kim KS, Shin HC, Yoon JW: Remission in models of type I diabetes by gene therapy using a single-chain insulin analogue. Nature 2000;408:483–488.
28 Rivera VM, Wang X, Wardwell S, Courage NL, Volchuk A, Keenan T, Holt DA, Gilman M, Orci L, Cerasoli F Jr, Rothman JE, Clackson T: Regulation of protein secretion through controlled aggregation in the endoplasmic reticulum. Science 2000;287:826–830.
29 Auricchio A, Gao GP, Yu QC, Raper S, Rivera VM, Clackson T, Wilson JM: Constitutive and regulated expression of processed insulin following in vivo hepatic gene transfer. Gene Ther 2002;914:963–971.
30 Ferber S, Halkin A, Cohen H, Ber I, Einav Y, Goldberg I, Barshack I, Seijffers R, Kopolovic J, Kaiser N, Karasik A: Pancreatic and duodenal homeobox gene 1 induces expression of insulin genes in liver and ameliorates streptozotocin-induced hyperglycemia. Nat Med 2000;6:568–572.
31 Edlund H: Pancreatic organogenesis: Developmental mechanisms and implications for therapy. Nat Rev Genet 2002;3:524–532.
32 Kojima H, Fujimiya M, Matsumura K, Younan P, Imaeda H, Maeda M, Chan L: NeuroD-betacellulin gene therapy induces islet neogenesis in the liver and reverses diabetes in mice. Nat Med 2003;9:596–603.
33 Gruessner AC, Sutherland DE: Analyses of pancreas transplant outcomes for United States cases reported to the United Network for Organ Sharing (UNOS) and non-US cases reported to the International Pancreas Transplant Registry (IPTR). Clin Transplant 1999:51–69.
34 Roep BO: The role of T-cells in the pathogenesis of type 1 diabetes: From cause to cure. Diabetologia 2003;46:305–321.
35 Lipes MA, Cooper EM, Skelly R, Rhodes CJ, Boschetti E, Weir GC, Davalli AM: Insulin-secreting non-islet cells are resistant to autoimmune destruction. Proc Natl Acad Sci USA 1996;93: 8595–8600.
36 De Vos P, Hamel AF, Tatarkiewicz K: Considerations for successful transplantation of encapsulated pancreatic islets. Diabetologia 2002;45:159–173.

Dr. L. Falqui
Dipartimento di Medicina Generale, Endocrinologia e Diabetologia
DIMER, Istituto Scientifico Universitario H San Raffaele
Via Olgettina 60, IT–20132 Milan (Italy)
Tel. +39 02 2643 7656, Fax +39 02 2643 4155, E-Mail falqui.luca@hsr.it

# Author Index

# Subject Index